PROMOTING HEALTH

The Primary Health Care Approach
7E

PROMOTING HEALTH

The Primary Health Care Approach
7E

JANE TAYLOR
PhD (Pub Hlth), M Hlth Prom, Grad Cert Int Hlth, BEd
Associate Professor and Discipline Lead Health Promotion & Public Health
School of Health and Sports Sciences, University of Sunshine Coast, QLD

LILY O'HARA
PhD (Pub Hlth), MPH, Postgrad Dip Hlth Prom, BSc
Associate Professor of Public Health (Health Promotion)
Department of Public Health, College of Health Sciences, QU Health,
Qatar University, Doha

LYN TALBOT
Dr Pub Hlth, M Hlth Sc, Grad Dip Hlth Sc, Grad Cert Higher Ed, RN
Corporate and Community Planner—Strategy, City of Greater Bendigo, VIC

GLENDA VERRINDER
PhD, M Hlth Sc, Grad Dip Hlth Sc, Grad Cert Higher Ed, Cert CHN, RN, RM
Senior Lecturer, La Trobe Rural Health School, School of Science, Health and Engineering,
La Trobe University, VIC

ELSEVIER

ELSEVIER

Elsevier Australia. ACN 001 002 357
(a division of Reed International Books Australia Pty Ltd)
Tower 1, 475 Victoria Avenue, Chatswood, NSW 2067

ISBN: 978-0-7295-4353-8

Notice
Practitioners and researchers must always rely on their own experience and knowledge in evaluating and using any information, methods, compounds or experiments described herein. Because of rapid advances in the medical sciences, in particular, independent verification of diagnoses and drug dosages should be made. To the fullest extent of the law, no responsibility is assumed by Elsevier, authors, editors or contributors for any injury and/or damage to persons or property as a matter of products liability, negligence or otherwise, or from any use or operation of any methods, products, instructions, or ideas contained in the material herein.

National Library of Australia Cataloguing-in-Publication Data

 A catalogue record for this book is available from the National Library of Australia

---

Senior Content Strategist: Melinda McEvoy
Content Project Manager: Shubham Dixit
Edited by Jo Crichton
Proofread by Annabel Adair
Design by Georgette Hall
Index by Innodata Indexing
Typeset by New Best-set Typesetters Ltd
Printed in Singapore by Markono Print Media Pte Ltd

CONTENTS

PREFACE

Health and wellbeing are resources that enable people to live, learn, play, work, flourish and thrive. Unfortunately, there are major disparities in people's health status around the world. There is strong evidence that physical, mental, social and spiritual health and wellbeing are experienced unequally, and that most of those differences are unfair or inequitable. Addressing the factors that contribute to such inequities is the central challenge for health practitioners wanting to engage in critical health promotion in a comprehensive primary health care context.

This is a time of significant change internationally. Political instability and social uncertainty are the result of an erosion of 'public goods', persistent poverty, energy and food insecurity and, most recently, the global COVID-19 pandemic. It is a time of increasing awareness of the impact of globalised economic activities on the health and wellbeing of people and the social, cultural, economic, political and physical environments in which we live. There is deep concern about global climate change, ecological sustainability and the implications for human health and survival. The Sustainable Development Goals have set goals and targets in 17 areas, all of which impact on the health and wellbeing of people around the world, and while there has been good progress towards these, many are not on track to be achieved by 2030. As such, there has never been a greater need for critical health promotion.

Taking action on the socio-ecological determinants of health to enhance health and reduce health inequities is the basis for critical health promotion practice in a comprehensive primary health care context. The concepts and skills presented in this updated edition of *Promoting Health: The Primary Health Care Approach* provide an essential resource for such practice.

This edition builds on the sound philosophical approach of the previous six editions. The key principles of critical health promotion and comprehensive primary health care – equity, social justice and community empowerment – underpin both parts of the book. Part 1 addresses health promotion development and key concepts and introduces the *Framework of health promotion practice in a comprehensive primary health care context.* Each chapter in Part 2 of the book focuses on one part of the framework. Throughout the book, current policy and practice initiatives have been updated. The use of health promotion theories and models has been strengthened, and new examples from practice have been introduced in the book and on the Evolve website.

The Ottawa Charter for Health Promotion continues to provide a relevant and useful framework for improving health. At the start of Chapters 3 to 9, there are questions for the health practitioner to consider in relation to each action area of the Ottawa Charter. At the end of each chapter, the relevant International Union for Health Promotion and Education (IUHPE) Core Competencies for Health Promotion are identified. Each chapter also presents reflective questions that may be used to prompt personal reflection or to guide group exploration.

We hope that *Promoting Health: The Primary Health Care Approach* (7th ed.) engages health practitioners from a broad range of disciplines and supports them in their critical health promotion practice in a comprehensive primary health care context to achieve better health and wellbeing outcomes for all.

Jane Taylor
Lily O'Hara
Lyn Talbot
Glenda Verrinder

INTRODUCTION

This seventh edition of *Promoting Health* affirms the use of critical health promotion within a comprehensive primary health care context, to address health and wellbeing priorities in all settings from the local through to the global. The philosophy underpinning comprehensive primary health care (CPHC) remains as relevant now as it was when first endorsed by the World Health Organization in 1978 and expressed within the Declaration of Alma-Ata.

The term 'comprehensive primary health care' is used throughout this book to reflect a comprehensive approach to primary health care. It does not refer to primary-level services. Central to CPHC are principles to guide all action to create health and wellbeing. These principles tell us what is important and *how* we should do what we do. They include social justice, equity, community empowerment and ecological sustainability, and the need to work with people to enable them to make decisions about health and wellbeing priorities most important to them.

The socio-ecological determinants of health and wellbeing are well established and need to be the focus of effort both within and outside of the healthcare sector. Addressing the socio-ecological determinants of health and wellbeing requires sound health promotion knowledge and skills to plan, implement and evaluate health promotion policies and programs.

The Ottawa Charter for Health Promotion (WHO, 1986) operationalises CPHC principles set out in the Declaration of Alma-Ata (WHO, 1978) in a framework for health promotion practice. The Charter has been reaffirmed repeatedly by people working in health promotion worldwide, and continues to provide a relevant guide for professional practice in health promotion. Health promotion action to improve health and wellbeing must primarily work to change the environments that structure health and wellbeing opportunities, as well as to support individuals to address the determinants of health and wellbeing over which they have control. To undertake these actions, health practitioners need an extensive set of skills. This book focuses on assisting health practitioners from a broad range of disciplines to develop the competencies essential for critical health promotion practice within a CPHC context.

While health promotion is a discipline of its own that can lead to professional accreditation, health promotion is also everyone's responsibility. Health promotion is a broad-ranging activity, which must be embraced by as many people as possible within and outside the health sector. Teachers, therapists road safety workers, engineers, mediators, human rights investigators, community workers, local government workers and many more play a role in health promotion action. Active participation by members of the community in all aspects of health promotion action is also essential. Community members have a role to play in forming partnerships with practitioners and agencies to develop environments that are conducive to the health and wellbeing of the community.

Everyone has opportunities to promote health and wellbeing, whether it be to lobby for changes to improve the socio-ecological determinants of health and wellbeing, to work to make community settings more health promoting, to assist individuals to learn about health-enhancing behaviour, or to engage people meaningfully in the decision-making processes that affect their health. There is a full range of health promotion practice roles, from policy advocacy and building health-enhancing settings, through to providing communities with support in making changes in their communities to improve health, conducting health education, providing health information, and conducting screening and surveillance activities on behalf of particular groups. Health practitioners in particular, have roles as advocates for communities and for consideration of the health perspective on priorities outside the health sector, which have an impact on health and wellbeing.

By virtue of these roles, health practitioners can take a leadership role in the creation of health and wellbeing. Professional associations such as the International Union for Health Promotion and Education (IUHPE), health promotion and public health associations, and the associations of other health-specific disciplines, play an important role in advocating for the health and wellbeing of the community and in modelling the effectiveness of a true multidisciplinary approach.

This book provides detailed practical guidance for students and practitioners new to health promotion, whether their role is specifically in health promotion or involves incorporating health promotion into their work in another health discipline or in wider fields of practice. In this book we encourage health practitioners to take up the challenge to work as health activists, and promote health and wellbeing in ways which enable communities and individuals to flourish and thrive.

If countries continue to support a burgeoning illness-management system, the costs to the health of the community will continue to rise. Inequalities in health status and lack of access to appropriate health services will become even worse. However, if a comprehensive primary health care challenge is taken up by all whose work impacts on health, as well as by community members who find their health jeopardised by the circumstances in which they live, then the positive effect could be quite profound.

Different terms are used to describe the workforce involved in promoting health and wellbeing. The term 'health workers' is used extensively in the women's health movement, because it implies a more equal relationship between professionals and their patients or clients. The term 'health promotion practitioner' is used to describe the workforce role where the primary purpose is to enhance health and wellbeing. These specialist practitioners need to possess or develop a full range of health promotion competencies. The term 'health practitioner' is used throughout this book in recognition that many health promotion activities are undertaken by workers whose primary qualification may be from a different discipline, and who is undertaking health promotion activities within a wider field of practice.

In this book, the terms 'low-income', 'middle-income' and 'high-income countries' are used. Low-income countries are home to 9% of the world's population. Alternative terms for low-income countries include 'third world' or 'developing nations' but these terms are not used in this book as they are perjorative. They suggest that the low-income nations are deficient, and reflect the parochialism of high-income countries. The majority of the world's population now live in middle-income countries (76%). High-income countries are home to 16% of the world's population but consume around 80% of its collective resources. High-income countries are often referred to as the 'developed' or 'first' world. For the same reason as described above, these terms are not used because they imply a hierarchy of countries based on levels of economic development.

Health promotion draws on many areas of expertise. In deciding which skills and topics to include in this book, we gave strong consideration to the International Union for Health Promotion and Education Health Promotion Competencies, and to topics commonly examined in university health science programs. In this book, we have used real-life examples from our own professional practice fields and often in our local geographic areas. This was a deliberate decision in order to illustrate the diversity and wisdom in health promotion. We encourage health practitioners to examine the health promotion practice around them and to draw on the wisdom and expertise of what is working locally. We hope that these examples will encourage health practitioners to become involved in showcasing their health promotion work, thus demonstrating that health promotion is a meaningful part of many health workers' practice.

HOW TO USE THIS BOOK

The book is structured into two distinct but interrelated parts covering nine chapters.

- Part 1 comprises three chapters and addresses health promotion development and concepts. The chapters present an overview of the development of health promotion within a comprehensive primary health care (CPHC) context. Concepts fundamental to health promotion practice are discussed in some detail. The *Framework for health promotion practice within a CPHC context* is introduced and used throughout the remainder of the book.

- Part 2 provides guidance to health practitioners undertaking health promotion in a comprehensive primary health care context. Chapters in Part 2 are underpinned by principles and concepts fundamental to the health and wellbeing of people. They are based on and presented in reference to the *Framework of health promotion practice in a comprehensive primary health care context* introduced in Chapter 1.

Chapters are interrelated but also designed to stand alone. Readers can dip in and out of chapters and each chapter will direct them to the relevant theoretical concepts and content presented elsewhere in the book.

Part 1: Health promotion development and concepts
Chapter 1

Chapter 1 establishes the foundations for health promotion practice within a comprehensive primary health care (CPHC) context. The current state of health and wellbeing and health inequalities within and between countries are examined along with the socio-ecological determinants of the health and wellbeing of people. The World Health Organization's (WHO) global responses to addressing health inequalities and creating health and wellbeing through a CPHC approach and health promotion are presented. We describe CPHC as a developmental process where the principles of equity, social justice and empowerment underpin the work for the socio-ecological changes necessary to improve health and wellbeing. The role that CPHC and health promotion have played in improving the health and wellbeing of populations is also discussed. The *Framework for health promotion practice within a CPHC context* is presented as a foundation for subsequent chapters. The purpose of this framework is to guide and support health practitioners undertaking health promotion work fulltime or as a component of their role.

Chapter 2

Chapter 2 presents a closer examination of the core concepts informing health promotion practice within a CPHC context. It commences with a discussion of the terms 'health', 'wellbeing', 'quality of life' and 'salutogenesis'. Concepts related to the individual-level socio-ecological determinants of health and wellbeing, such as personal values, attitudes and beliefs, opportunities for education and individual responsibility for health and wellbeing are discussed. This is followed by a discussion of concepts related to the population-level socio-ecological determinants of health and wellbeing, including human capital and those particular to the social, cultural, economic, political and physical environments. The chapter concludes with important considerations relevant to health promotion practice in community settings.

Chapter 3

Chapter 3 builds on the ideas presented about the socio-ecological determinants of health and wellbeing and core health promotion concepts presented in previous chapters. It especially explores ecological sustainability and human health and wellbeing, focusing on the relationship between people and their social and natural environments. Links between the health and wellbeing of people, the health of the physical environment and the implications for health promotion within a CPHC context are made.

Part 2: Health promotion practice

Chapter 4

Chapter 4 describes the health promotion practice cycle that consists of community assessment, program planning, implementation and evaluation, and the underlying values and principles of critical health promotion. This content underpins the five broad strategy areas of health promotion action of the *Framework of health promotion practice in a comprehensive primary health care context* presented in Chapter 1. The health promotion practice cycle facilitates the development of a research base for health promotion action in a way that both strengthens the relevance of health promotion work and enables health practitioners to be accountable for their health promotion practice.

Chapter 5

Chapter 5 examines health promotion action that develops healthy public policy to create environments and settings that support health and wellbeing. The chapter unpacks the first broad strategy area of health promotion action in the *Framework of health promotion practice in a comprehensive primary health care context*. The meaning of healthy public policy, the policymaking process and the role of health practitioners in advocating for and creating healthy public policy are explored. Examples of healthy public policy at local, regional, national and international levels are provided. Frameworks for promoting health in various settings where people live, learn, work and play, such as cities, schools, health services and workplaces, are also explored.

Chapter 6

Chapter 6 discusses community development action to support social and environmental change, which is the second broad strategy area of health promotion action in the *Framework of health promotion practice in a comprehensive primary health care context*. Community development is an essential component of the socio-ecological approach to health promotion, because it relates to making changes in the settings of people's lives that improve their health and wellbeing. We examine community development as a way of working with communities on the health and wellbeing priorities they identify to achieve changes to the environment and to enable community empowerment. The chapter also examines the role of social enterprise and social entrepreneurship in community development, challenges for community development, and the evaluation of community development.

Chapter 7

Chapter 7 explores health education and health literacy to develop knowledge and skills for health and wellbeing, which is the third broad strategy area of health promotion action in the *Framework of health promotion practice in a comprehensive primary health care context*. The role of health literacy as a social determinant of health and wellbeing and an outcome of effective health education and empowerment of people is explored. Behaviour change theories and models, and learning and teaching theory as a basis for planning health education strategies are presented. Skills required for health practitioners to undertake effective education at group and community levels, including using adult learning principles and a range of teaching–learning activities, and theory, tips and skills for working with groups, are provided.

Chapter 8

Chapter 8 discusses health information and social marketing to address health and wellbeing priorities, which is the fourth broad strategy area of health promotion action in the *Framework of health promotion practice in a comprehensive primary health care context*. We explore how social marketing can be used to contribute to raising levels of knowledge in the community about particular health and wellbeing priorities, to support the implementation of a change to policy, or as a means of advocacy for a desired social change. Social marketing knowledge and skills required by health practitioners, as well as those required to prepare health communication materials are also presented. If the strategies in Chapters 7 and 8 are used alone, the approach is regarded as a behavioural approach, and is not consistent with CPHC. These strategies must be used in conjunction with all of the others in the *Framework of health promotion practice in a comprehensive primary health care context*, if the socio-ecological approach is to be used in a CPHC context.

Chapter 9

Chapter 9 focuses on vaccination, screening, risk assessment and surveillance for population health and wellbeing to monitor and reduce risk of disease conditions, which is the fifth and final broad strategy area of health promotion action in the *Framework of health promotion practice in a comprehensive primary health care context*. These four health enhancing strategies are mostly carried out in primary health care services and can make a significant contribution to the health status of the population. If the strategies in Chapter 9 are used alone, the approach is regarded as a biomedical approach which is not consistent with CPHC. If they are used in conjunction with those strategies in Chapters 7 and 8, but not the other chapters, then this approach is regarded as selective primary health care, and likewise, is not consistent with CPHC. These strategies must be used in conjunction with all of the others in the *Framework of health promotion practice in a comprehensive primary health care context*, if the socio-ecological approach is to be used in a CPHC context.

Critical reflection on health promotion study and professional practice

Questions for reflection are included in each chapter to encourage users to explore some of the important practice issues raised in the chapter.

These have been designed to encourage active and self-directed learning, and to assist educators with in-class discussions. An answer guide to all reflective questions is available to educators on the Evolve website accompanying the text. Short quizzes for each chapter are also available to educators on the Evolve website. In the practice-based Chapters 4 to 9, reflective questions framed in reference to the action areas of the Ottawa Charter appear at the commencement of the chapter. The use of the Ottawa Charter illustrates its direct applicability to health promotion practice, and assists the health practitioner to think broadly and strategically about practice challenges and to reflect on and critique their professional role and the health promotion philosophy of their organisation.

The purpose of *Promoting Health* is to set out the core principles that guide practitioners to engage in critical health promotion. In doing this, an 'ideal' set of circumstances and ways of working are described, which may be more difficult to put into practice than they seem. A more global perspective is taken in the early chapters, and content of specific relevance to health promotion in New Zealand and Australia is included. You are encouraged to read widely and examine the many other examples currently available, and to work with your colleagues to develop your own health promotion competence and ways of practising.

Health promotion competencies

Considerable work has been done since the 1990s to establish the core professional competencies for health promotion practice, which are described in detail in Chapter 1. This text enables health practitioners to develop an introductory-level understanding of core knowledge, values, attitudes and skills essential for health promotion professional accreditation. The IUHPE health promotion competency statements highlighted at the end of each chapter relate to the content of that chapter.

REFERENCES

World Health Organization (WHO). (1978). Declaration of Alma-Ata. Retrieved from http://www.who.int/publications/almaata_declaration_en.pdf.

World Health Organization (WHO). (1986). The Ottawa charter for health promotion. Retrieved from https://www.who.int/healthpromotion/conferences/previous/ottawa/en/.

ACKNOWLEDGEMENTS

In completing this seventh edition of *Promoting Health: The Primary Health Care Approach*, there are a number of people whose contributions must be acknowledged. Andrea Wass wrote the first and second editions and we pay tribute to her work and acknowledge the contribution of others to those two editions. Lyn Talbot and Glenda Verrinder assumed authorship for editions three through to six, and Jane Taylor and Lily O'Hara have joined the authorship team for this seventh edition.

We (Jane and Lily) thank and acknowledge the sustained contribution of Lyn and Glenda for editions three to six along with their colleagues and family that supported them along the way. We thank Lyn and Glenda also for inviting us to join them in co-writing this seventh edition.

Thanks are extended to the students and practitioners who have contributed to the discussion and refinement of many ideas presented in this work, and who have participated in 'field testing' some of the material. Thanks are also extended to colleagues and practitioners who have provided case examples drawn from their practice.

For this edition we particularly thank Susanne Fincham for her assistance with the electronic referencing of the book.

Finally, we would like to thank Melinda McEvoy from Elsevier for inviting us to write the seventh edition, and Shubham Dixit and Shruti Raj Srivastava for their support throughout the process.

Lily O'Hara is Associate Professor of Public Health at Qatar University in Doha, Qatar. She has a PhD from the University of the Sunshine Coast, Master of Public Health from Queensland University of Technology, Postgraduate Diploma in Health Promotion (Distinction) from Curtin University, and a Bachelor of Science from the University of Queensland. Most recently, she completed a Certificate 3 in Vocational Assessment from the Council for Awards in Care, Health and Education, UK. Lily is a public health and health promotion educator and practitioner with experience in Australia, United Arab Emirates (UAE) and Qatar. She has worked in health promotion practice roles with Queensland Health, Cancer Council Queensland, a multi-national pharmaceutical company, a small private health promotion company, and the Department of Health in Abu Dhabi, UAE. Lily is a former national president and a Life Member of the Australian Health Promotion Association. Lily has worked in academic roles at the University of the Sunshine Coast, Queensland University of Technology, Emirates College for Advanced Education, Abu Dhabi University and Qatar University. Lily has worked on community, workplace, school and health service-based programs addressing a broad range of health and wellbeing issues. Her research focuses on analysing public health approaches to body weight and their inequitable impact on people with larger bodies. She is also developing and evaluating ethical, evidence-based, salutogenic health promotion initiatives for body liberation using the social justice-based Health at Every Size approach. Lily's research also focuses on developing the ethical and technical competencies of the health promotion workforce, and she is the co-author of the Red Lotus Critical Health Promotion Model.

Jane Taylor is Associate Professor of Public Health at the University of the Sunshine Coast (USC). She has a PhD from USC, Master of Health Promotion and Graduate Certificate in International Health from Curtin University, and a Bachelor of Education from the University of Tasmania. Jane is the Discipline Leader for Public Health at USC with 25 years of professional health promotion experience. She worked as a health promotion practitioner in community and government sectors on a range of community-based health promotion programs including women's health, Aboriginal and Torres Strait Islander health, school health promotion and public health service delivery in rural and remote Queensland prior to joining USC in 2004. Jane was involved in establishing public health and health promotion programs at USC and teaches philosophical and technical health promotion courses at undergraduate and postgraduate levels. In 2018, USC health promotion programs received accreditation with the International Union for Health Promotion and Health Education which Jane provided leadership for. Jane's health promotion research focuses on strengthening the theoretical foundations of health promotion to support a critical (social justice and equity focused) practice approach. This involves using modern health promotion values and principles to design, implement, evaluate and critique health promotion policies and programs, and undertake research. She is also interested in the role of health promotion in reorienting health services to deliver comprehensive primary health care and health promotion workforce development.

Lyn Talbot has a Doctor of Public Health, Master of Health Sciences, Graduate Diploma of Public and Community Health, and a Graduate Certificate in University Teaching and

Learning, all from La Trobe University. Lyn commenced her professional life as a registered nurse at the Alfred Hospital, Melbourne, and spent a number of years in hospital-based clinical nurse education before moving to a university teaching role at La Trobe University, Bendigo, where she was Course Coordinator and Head of the then Department of Public Health. She was a member of the Royal College of Nursing, Australia, and the Australian Health Promotion Association, and was a Rotary Ambassadorial Scholar. Following on from her university role, Lyn was the Corporate and Community Planner for the City of Greater Bendigo until her recent retirement.

Glenda Verrinder is an Honorary Associate in the La Trobe Rural Health School, College of Science, Health and Engineering, La Trobe University. Glenda has a PhD, Master of Health Sciences, Graduate Diploma of Public and Community Health, and a Graduate Certificate in University Teaching and Learning, all from La Trobe University and a Certificate in Community Nursing from Royal District Nursing Service. Glenda commenced her professional life as a registered nurse and midwife primarily working in community nursing. Her roles at La Trobe University and the Public Health Association of Australia reflect her interests in human ecology and health, ecological sustainability and promoting health.

GLOSSARY

This glossary is modified from the following sources.

Australian Health Promotion Association. (2009). Core competencies for health promotion practitioners. Retrieved from https://www.healthpromotion.org.au/images/docs/core _competencies_for_hp_practitioners.pdf.

Bajayo, R. (2012). Building community resilience to climate change through public health planning. Health Promotion Journal of Australia, 23(1), 30–36. doi:10.1071/HE12030.

Baum, F. (2008). The new public health (3rd ed.). South Melbourne: Oxford University Press.

Baum, F., & Sanders, D. (1995). Can health promotion and primary health care achieve health for all without a return to their more radical agenda. Health Promotion International, 10(2), 154.

Green, L. W. (2005). New features and updated citations. In L. W. Green & M. W. Kreuter, Health program planning: an educational and ecological approach. New York: McGraw-Hill.

Gregg, J., & O'Hara, L. (2007). The Red Lotus Health Promotion Model: a new model for holistic, ecological, salutogenic health promotion practice. Health Promotion Journal of Australia, 18(1), 12-19. doi:10.1071/HE07012.

Hawe, P., Degeling, D. E., & Hall, J. (1995). Evaluating health promotion. Sydney: McLennon & Petty.

Intergovernmental Panel on Climate Change (IPCC). (2007). Fourth assessment report. Retrieved from https://www.ipcc.ch/assessment-report/ar4/.

International Union for Health Promotion and Education. (n.d.). Health promotion practitioners. Retrieved from http://www.iuhpe.org/index.php/en/practitioner.

Ivestopedia. (n.d.). Neoliberalism. Retrieved from http://www.investopedia.com/terms/n/neoliberalism.asp

Keen, M., Brown, V., & Dyball, R. (2005). Social learning: a new approach to environmental management. In M. Keen, V. A. Brown, & R. Dyball (Eds.), Social learning in environmental management: towards a sustainable future. London: Earthscan Publications Ltd.

McKnight, J., & Kretzmann, J. P. (2005). Mapping community capacity. In M. Minkler (Ed.), Community organizing and community building for health (2nd ed.). New Brunswick: Rutgers University Press.

Moberg, F., & Simonsen, S. H. (n.d.). What is resilience? An introduction to socio-ecological research. Stockholm Resilience Centre. Retrieved from http://www.stockholmresilience.org/download/18.10119fc11455d3c557d6d21/1459560242299/SU_SRC_whatisresilience_sidaApril2014.pdf.

Navarro, V. (1976). The underdevelopment of health of working America: causes, consequences and possible solutions. American Journal of Public Health, 66(6), 538–547. doi:10.2105/AJPH.66.6.538.

Nutbeam, D. (1998). Health promotion glossary. Health Promotion International, 1(4), 349–364.

Rockstroem, J., Steffen, W., Noone, K., et al. (2009). Planetary boundaries: exploring the safe operating space for humanity. Ecology and Society, 14(2), 32. doi:10.5751/ES-03180-140232.

Smith, B. J., Tang, K. C., & Nutbeam, D. (2006). WHO health promotion glossary: new terms. Health Promotion International, 21(4), 340–345. doi:10.1093/heapro/dal033.

Talbot, L., & Verrinder, G. (2018). Promoting health: the primary health care approach (6th ed.). Sydney: Elsevier Australia.

United Nations. (1987). Report of the World Commission on Environment and Development: our common future. Retrieved from http://www.un-documents.net/wced-ocf.htm

Walsh, J., & Warren, K. (1979). Selective primary health care: an interim strategy for disease control in developing countries. In F. Baum (Ed.), The new public health (2008) (3rd ed.). Melbourne: Oxford University Press.

World Health Organization (WHO). (1986). The Ottawa Charter for Health Promotion. Retrieved from https://www.who.int/healthpromotion/conferences/previous/ottawa/en/.

World Health Organization (WHO). (n.d.-a). Introduction to healthy settings. Retrieved from http://www.who.int/healthy_settings/about/en/.

World Health Organization (WHO). (n.d.-b). Social determinants of health. Retrieved from https://www.who.int/social_determinants/en/.

advocacy for health a combination of individual and social actions designed to gain political commitment, policy support, social acceptance and systems support for a particular health goal or program (Nutbeam, 1998).

'bottom-up' decision making community involvement in planning, implementing and evaluating local strategies to address health and wellbeing priorities that the community has identified.

burden of disease a measurement of the gap between a population's current health and the optimal state where all people attain full life expectancy without suffering major ill-health (Smith et al., 2006).

capacity building the development of knowledge, skills, commitment, structures, systems and leadership to enable effective health promotion. It involves actions to improve health at three levels: the advancement of knowledge and skills among practitioners; the expansion of support and infrastructure for health promotion in organisations; and the development of cohesiveness and partnerships for health and wellbeing in communities (Smith et al., 2006).

climate change a change in the state of the climate that can be identified by changes in the mean and/or variability of its properties and that persists for an extended period, typically decades or longer (Intergovernmental Panel on Climate Change (IPCC), 2007).

community the group of people that one feels connected to, beyond the family. In modern, highly urban societies, individuals rarely belong to a single distinct community but maintain membership of various communities based on factors such as geography, occupation, social contact, values, leisure interests and other important features of their lives (e.g. gay community, hearing and non-hearing communities, religious community, academic community) (Hawe et al., 1995).

community assessment the first stage in the health promotion practice cycle and involves gathering existing and new evidence to determine the health and wellbeing assets, needs and priorities of a community as a foundation for planning health promotion action.

community assets the combination of unique capabilities that exist within communities; for example, knowledge, skills, physical and service resources and infrastructure, social capital, etc. upon which to build health and wellbeing at the community level (Bajayo, 2012; McKnight & Kretzmann, 2005).

community building an orientation to community development practice that accentuates building the capacities of complex and multidimensional communities, rather than overcoming an identified problem.

community development the process of facilitating the development of a community's skills and abilities to improve the conditions that affect their health and wellbeing. It often involves helping the community identify priority issues and facilitating their efforts to bring about change in these areas (Hawe et al., 1995).

community participation/involvement involving people in processes related to their health and wellbeing. Some people use this term to refer to involving people in health promotion activities. Others use it to refer to involvement in decision-making structures that affect health, including intersectoral approaches to health promotion. Most effective participation occurs when a community's skills have been developed (community development); that is, when a community is skilled in the processes of participation and decision making (Hawe et al., 1995).

comprehensive primary health care (CPHC) a developmental process where the principles of equity, social justice and empowerment underpin the work for socio-ecological changes necessary to improve health and wellbeing.

contributing factor any aspect of behaviour, society or the environment, or anything that contributes to a risk or protective factor for a health issue (e.g. lack of access to condoms is a contributing factor for unsafe sex, which is a risk factor for contracting HIV). Contributing factors *predispose, enable* or *reinforce* risk or protective factors (Green, 2005).

critical health promotion a social justice approach to health promotion that is underpinned by a system of values and related principles that supports the reflective process of explicitly identifying and challenging dominant social structures and discourses that privilege the interests of the powerful and contribute to health and wellbeing inequities.

Critical health promotion values and principles a system of values and related principles that characterise critical health promotion practice. Critical health promotion values include: holistic health paradigm; salutogenic approach; ecological science; focus determined by equity; working with people as an ally; assuming people are doing the best for their wellbeing; comprehensive use of evidence; portfolio of multiple strategies; empowering engagement strategies; respecting personal autonomy; maximum beneficence; and non-maleficence as a priority consideration.

disease prevention includes actions to reduce the risk of disease (primary prevention), detect the presence of disease very early, often before it is symptomatic (secondary prevention) and reduce the consequences of disease once it is already established (tertiary prevention) (Nutbeam, 1998).

ecological science as applied in critical health promotion is the application of systems theory and, therefore, recognition that: people exist in multiple ecosystems which are comprised of social, cultural, political, economic, built and natural environments; these ecosystems operate at all levels from the individual to the family, group, community, population and planetary levels; all parts within these ecosystems impact on each other; and the whole of any ecosystem is greater than the sum of the parts (Gregg & O'Hara, 2007).

ecological sustainability both a process and an outcome. It is a process of change that improves the long-term health of humans and ecological systems (Talbot & Verrinder, 2018).

empowerment a social-action process that promotes participation of people, organisations and communities towards the goal of increased individual and community control, political efficacy, improved quality of community life and social justice.

empowerment for health a process through which people gain greater control over decisions and actions affecting their health (Nutbeam, 1998).

enabling taking action in partnership with individuals or groups to empower them through the mobilisation of human and material sources, to promote and protect their health (Nutbeam, 1998).

enabling factor any characteristic of an individual, group or environment that facilitates health behaviour or other conditions affecting health, including any skill or resource required to attain that condition. Enabling factors can facilitate conditions that lead to ill-health or conditions that lead to good health (e.g. lack of easy access to contraception, availability of nutritious take-away food) (Green, 2005).

epidemiology the study of the distribution and determinants of health-states or events in specified populations and the application of this study to improving health outcomes (Nutbeam, 1998).

equality all individuals are equal and entitled to their human rights without discrimination of any kind. To protect human rights, law must enshrine these values, but there must also be processes to ensure that the results of their implementation do not produce disadvantage or discrimination.

equity in health means fairness. Equity in health means that people's *needs* guide the distribution of opportunities for wellbeing (Nutbeam, 1998).

evaluation the process by which we decide the worth or value of something. For health promotion, this process involves measurement and observation (*evaluation research*) and comparison with some criterion or standard (Hawe et al., 1995).

evidence-based health promotion the use of information derived from formal research and systematic investigation to identify causes and contributing determinants of health priorities and the most effective health promotion actions to address these in given contexts and populations (Smith et al., 2006).

global health the transnational impacts of globalisation on health determinants and health issues which are beyond the control of individual nations (Smith et al., 2006).

goal (program goal, health goal) the desired long-term outcome of a health promotion program, such as a reduction of a health problem or improvement in health status. It is *measurable* (Hawe et al., 1995).

health a state of physical, mental, social and spiritual wellbeing and not merely the absence of disease or infirmity. Health is a *resource* for everyday life, not the object of living. It is a positive concept emphasising social and personal resources as well as physical capabilities. Health is determined by the *relationship* between individuals and the environments in which they live, work and play (Nutbeam, 1998).

health communication interpersonal or mass communication activities which are directed towards improving the health status of individuals and populations. It may involve the integration of mass and multimedia communication with more local and/or personal traditional forms of communication (Nutbeam, 1998).

health education consciously constructed opportunities for learning which are designed to facilitate voluntary changes in behaviour towards a predetermined goal. It can be applied to individuals, groups, organisations and communities (Hawe et al., 1995).

health impact assessment a combination of procedures, methods and tools by which a policy, program, product or service may be judged concerning its effects on the health of the population (Smith et al., 2006).

health literacy the cognitive and social skills that determine the motivation and ability of individuals to gain access to, understand and use information in ways that promote and maintain good health (Nutbeam, 1998).

health outcome a change in the health status of an individual, group or population which is attributable to a planned health promotion program (Nutbeam, 1998).

health policy a formal statement or procedure within institutions that defines priorities and the parameters for action in response to health assets and needs, available resources and other political pressures (Nutbeam, 1998).

health promotion competencies a combination of the essential knowledge, abilities, skills and values necessary for the practice of health promotion (adapted from Shilton et al., 2001, in IUHPE, n.d.). Core competencies are defined as the minimum set of competencies that constitute a common baseline for all health promotion roles; that is, they are what all health promotion practitioners are expected to be capable of doing to work efficiently, effectively and appropriately in the field (Australian Health Promotion Association, 2009).

health promotion practice work which reflects health promotion as defined in the Ottawa Charter and successive charters and declarations to promote health and wellbeing, and reduce health inequities (Nutbeam, 1998).

health promotion practitioner a person who works to promote health and wellbeing, and reduce health inequities using the actions described by the Ottawa Charter and successive charters and declarations to promote health and reduce health inequities.

health promotion setting the place or social context in which people engage in daily activities in which environmental, organisational and personal factors interact to affect health and wellbeing (WHO, n.d.-a).

healthy public policy any form of legislation, standard of practice, code, bylaw or policy that contributes to the health and wellbeing of people. It is characterised by an explicit concern for health and equity and by accountability for health impact. The main aim of building healthy public policy is to create supportive social, cultural, economic, political, natural and built environments that enable people to live well and thrive (Nutbeam, 1998).

holistic health the co-existing social, spiritual, mental and physical aspects of wellbeing; also referred to as health of the mind, body and spirit.

impact evaluation follows *evaluability assessment* in the steps of *program evaluation* and is the first step in testing a completed health promotion program's performance. Impact evaluation is concerned with evaluating the immediate effects of the program; that is, its effect on those factors which contribute to or cause the health priority. Corresponds to the measurement of program *objectives*. It should include an assessment of both intended and unintended effects (Hawe et al., 1995).

intersectoral collaboration a recognised relationship between part or parts of different sectors of society which has been formed to take action on an issue to achieve health outcomes or intermediate health outcomes in a way which is more effective, efficient or sustainable than might be achieved by the health sector acting alone (Nutbeam, 1998).

mediation a process through which the different interests (personal, social, economic) of individuals and communities and different sectors (public and private) are reconciled in ways that promote and protect health (Nutbeam, 1998).

medico-industrial complex the health industry, which is composed of multibillion-dollar enterprises including medical practices, hospitals, nursing homes, insurance companies, drug manufacturers, hospital supply and equipment companies, real estate and construction businesses, health systems consulting and accounting firms, and banks. The concept conveys the idea that an important (if not the primary) function of the healthcare system is business (i.e. to make profits) with two other secondary functions, research and education (Navarro, 1976).

need health needs are those states, conditions or factors in the community that, if absent, prevent people achieving optimum physical, mental, social and spiritual health and wellbeing, such as basic health services, information, a safe physical environment, good food, housing, productive work, and a network of emotionally supportive and stimulating relationships (Hawe et al., 1995).

needs assessment a systematic procedure for determining the nature and extent of health needs in a population, the causes and contributing factors to those needs and the human, organisational and community resources which are available to respond to these (Smith et al., 2006).

neoliberalism a policy model of social studies and economics that transfers control of economic factors from the public sector to the private sector. It draws on the basic principles of neoclassical economics, suggesting that governments must limit subsidies, make reforms to tax law in order to expand the tax base, reduce deficit spending, limit protectionism and open markets up to trade (Ivestopedia, n.d.; or see Baum & Sanders, 1995).

network a grouping of individuals, organisations and agencies organised on a non-hierarchical basis around common issues or concerns, which are pursued proactively and systematically based on commitment and trust (Nutbeam, 1998).

objective the desired impact of a health promotion program; an improvement of factors that contribute to the health priority. It is measurable (how much improvement, by when, by whom) (Hawe et al., 1995).

outcome evaluation the final phase of health promotion program evaluation and the second of a two-step process that tests the performance of a program. Outcome evaluation answers the question of to what extent the program has achieved its goal, and at what cost (Hawe et al., 1995).

planetary boundaries quantified boundaries determined by scientists within which humanity can continue to develop and thrive for generations to come. Boundaries have been developed for climate change, biosphere integrity, land system change, freshwater use, biogeochemical flows (nitrogen and phosphorus cycles), atmospheric aerosol loading, stratospheric ozone depletion, and novel entities (Rockstroem et al., 2009).

predisposing factor any characteristic of an individual, a community or an environment that predisposes behaviour or other conditions related to a health priority. Includes knowledge, belief, attitude and socio-economic status (Green, 2005).

primary health care essential health care made accessible at a cost a country and a community can afford with methods that are practical, scientifically sound and socially acceptable (Nutbeam, 1998).

process evaluation measures the activity of the health promotion program, specifically program reach, participant satisfaction, implementation of program activities, performance of materials or other components and ongoing quality assurance (Hawe et al., 1995).

program (health promotion program) a coherent series of goals, objectives, strategies and activities which are carried out with a group of participants for the purpose of improving the health and wellbeing status of the group. A health promotion program is planned in response to an identified health priority and is based on scientific theory and evidence of effectiveness (Hawe et al., 1995).

program evaluation assessment of health promotion program effectiveness; the process of determining the value or the degree of success of a program in achieving predetermined goals and objectives; includes unintended effects (Hawe et al., 1995).

program planning the second step in the health promotion practice cycle, following community assessment. The process of articulating what you are trying to achieve with your program, why you are doing it and how you will go about it. Includes setting goals and objectives, selecting strategies, designing activities for the program and developing the evaluation plan (Hawe et al., 1995).

public health the science and art of promoting health, preventing disease, and prolonging life through the organised efforts of society (Nutbeam, 1998).

quality of life the perception of individuals that their needs are being met and that they are not being denied opportunities to achieve happiness and fulfilment, regardless of health status or social and economic conditions (Nutbeam, 1998).

reinforcing factor any reward or punishment or any feedback following or anticipated as a consequence of health behaviour (Green, 2005).

re-orienting health services characterised by a more explicit concern for the achievement of population health outcomes in ways in which the health system is organised and funded. This must lead to a change in attitude and organisation of health services which focuses on the needs of the individual as a whole person balanced against the needs of population groups (WHO, 1986).

resilience the long-term capacity of a system to deal with change and continue to develop (Moberg & Simonsen, n.d.).

resilience thinking recognition that systems are dynamic interactions between people and their environments (Moberg & Simonsen, n.d.).

salutogenic approach in health promotion practice emphasises a focus on those factors that create and support holistic health and wellbeing, happiness and meaning in life (Gregg & O'Hara, 2007).

selective primary health care (SPHC) based on the illness system and a biomedical model of health care (Walsh & Warren, 1979, cited in Baum, 2008).

settings for health the place or social context in which people engage in daily activities in which environmental, organisational and personal factors interact to affect health and wellbeing (Nutbeam, 1998).

social capital the degree of social cohesion which exits in communities; the processes between people which establish networks, norms and social trust, and facilitate coordination and cooperation for mutual benefit (Nutbeam, 1998).

social marketing the application of commercial marketing techniques to the analysis, planning, implementation and evaluation of programs designed to influence the behaviour of specific audiences in order to improve individuals and society (Smith et al., 2006).

socio-ecological determinants of health the individual and environmental factors which determine the health and wellbeing status of individuals or populations and the dynamic interactions between them.. Environmental factors include factors in the social, cultural, political, economic, built and natural environments (WHO, n.d.-b).

strategy in health promotion, the type of approach used to bring about desired changes in the determinants and contributing determinants of health and wellbeing. The health promotion strategies included in the Ottawa Charter for Health Promotion are enable, mediate and advocate. The action areas included in the Ottawa Charter which are used to develop a strategy portfolio include: building healthy public policy, creating supportive environments, strengthening community action, developing personal skills and reorienting health services (WHO, 1986).

supportive environments for health social, economic, cultural, political, natural and built environments where people live, learn, work and play that provide protection from threats to health and support people to live well (Nutbeam, 1998).

sustainable development development that meets the needs of the present without compromising the ability of future generations to meet their own needs (United Nations, 1987).

sustainable health promotion actions those actions that can maintain their benefits for communities and populations beyond their initial stage of implementation. Sustainable actions can continue to be delivered within the limits of finances, expertise, infrastructure, natural resources and participation by stakeholders (Smith et al., 2006).

systems thinking the understanding of a phenomenon within the context of a larger whole (Keen et al., 2005).

wellbeing the optimal state of health: the realisation of the fullest potential of an individual physically, psychologically, socially, spiritually and economically; and the fulfilment of one's role expectations in the family, community, place of worship, workplace and other settings (Smith et al., 2006).

PART 1
HEALTH PROMOTION DEVELOPMENT AND CONCEPTS

The first part of this book, Chapters 1 to 3, presents an overview of the origins of health promotion as a discipline of practice within a comprehensive primary health care (CPHC) context. Key underlying principles and concepts fundamental to the health and wellbeing of people, which inform health promotion practice, are explored. The particular principles and concepts presented apply to health promotion practice anywhere in the world, although there is a focus on Australia and Aotearoa New Zealand. Part 1 frames health promotion practice from a sustainability perspective. The professional competencies required for effective health promotion action are described. This section of the book includes the *Framework for health promotion practice within a CPHC context* to guide and support health practitioners undertaking health promotion work full time or as a component of their role in any setting. This framework provides the foundation for Chapters 4 to 9 in Part 2 of this book.

1 Health promotion in context

INTRODUCTION

This chapter establishes the foundations for health promotion practice within a comprehensive primary health care (CPHC) context. The current state of health and wellbeing and health inequalities within and between countries are examined. This is followed by an exploration of the broad range of determinants that contribute to health status and health inequities or unfair health inequalities. These are characterised as the socio-ecological determinants of health and wellbeing. The World Health Organization's (WHO) global responses to addressing health inequalities and creating health and wellbeing through a CPHC approach and health promotion are then identified. There are three main premises underpinning these foundations which apply everywhere in the world. The first premise is that health can be conceptualised as 'a state of physical, mental and social wellbeing, and not merely the absence of disease or infirmity' (World Health Organization [WHO], 1948) and is determined by the complex interactions of a broad range of socio-ecological determinants of health. The second premise is that how long people live, and how healthy they are, varies greatly within and between countries, and although they are not the major determinants of health, health services can make a significant and important contribution to reducing health inequalities (ABC Radio National, 2016; CSDH, 2008; Duckett, 2016). The third premise is that even though addressing the socio-ecological determinants of health through health promotion action could significantly improve health and wellbeing, health services are still predominantly focused on managing illness and treating conditions after they have arisen.

In this chapter we discuss the role that CPHC and health promotion have played in improving the health and wellbeing of populations. We describe CPHC as a developmental process where the principles of equity, social justice and empowerment underpin the work for the socio-ecological changes necessary to improve health and wellbeing. The aim of CPHC is to address the conditions that generate both good health and wellbeing and poor health. We present a framework for health promotion practice (revised from Talbot & Verrinder, 2005, 2018) that health practitioners can use to guide their health promotion practice within a CPHC context. First, we need to understand what the current health status is around the world and how it varies within and between countries.

HEALTH STATUS AND HEALTH INEQUALITIES

As described above, health is a complex, holistic concept that includes physical, mental, social and spiritual wellbeing, and not just the absence of disease or injury. There are many ways of measuring health and wellbeing, with the most common being life expectancy, mortality and morbidity rates. In this section we explore the current situation with respect to inequalities in life expectancy, maternal and child mortality, and self-rated health.

Life expectancy at birth reflects the overall mortality rates of a population and is one of the core indicators of health status. The World Health Statistics 2019 report states that global life expectancy in 2016 was 72 years of age (WHO, 2019b). However, there are major inequalities in life expectancy within and between countries. Infant mortality is much higher in babies born to women with no education compared with those who have been to school, life expectancy at birth varies enormously based on postcode, and maternal mortality rates for Indigenous Australians are substantially higher than those of non-Indigenous Australians (AIHW, 2019a).

Health inequalities between countries are strongly related to economic development. The World Bank classifies countries as low-income, lower middle-income, upper middle-income, and high-income countries, based on the gross national income (GNI) per person in each country in US dollars. In 2019, countries with a 2018 per capita GNI of US$1025 or less were classified as low-income, between US$1026 and US$3995 as lower middle-income, between US$3996 and US$12,375 as upper middle-income, and US$12,376 or more were classified as high-income countries (World Bank, 2019).

In low-income countries, life expectancy at birth in 2016 was 62.7 years, and there was a steady gradient upwards, with people in lower middle-income countries expected to live to 67.9 years, people in upper middle-income countries to 75.2 years, and people in high-income countries expected to live to 80.8 years, 18.1 years longer than people in low-income countries (WHO, 2019b). The age that people die is the major reason for this gap. In low-income countries, almost a third of all deaths occur in children aged under 5 years, with many of these deaths from preventable or treatable conditions related to poverty, such as infectious and parasitic diseases, maternal and perinatal conditions, and nutritional diseases. In high-income countries, the majority of people who die are old with most deaths from chronic conditions such as cardiovascular disease and cancer (WHO, 2019b). Targets for improvements in mortality and other health indicators are included in the United Nations Sustainable Development Goals (United Nations [UN], 2015) in recognition that ensuring healthy lives and promoting the wellbeing of people at all ages is essential to sustainable development.

In 2015, 193 member states of the United Nations (UN) agreed to a global sustainable development agenda to address challenges related to poverty and inequality as well as peace and justice, climate change and environmental degradation (UN, 2015). This agenda resulted in the 2016 Sustainable Development Goals (SDGs), replacing the Millennium Development Goals (MDGs) which concluded in 2015. The 2030 Agenda for Sustainable Development strongly reinforced health as a political, development and humanitarian priority for all countries. There are 17 interconnected SDGs (Fig. 1.1) and 169 targets for member states to achieve by 2030 in order to end poverty and promote prosperity and people's wellbeing while protecting the environment.

Sustainable Development Goal 3 is to ensure healthy lives and promote wellbeing for all at all ages. Known in short as Good Health and Well-being, SDG 3 includes 13 targets for maternal and child health, communicable and non-communicable diseases (NCDs), mental health, sexual and reproductive health care services, exposure to pollution and contamination, injuries and road traffic accidents and tobacco control. SDG 3 also focuses on universal health coverage, equitable and affordable access to high-quality vaccines and medicines, sustainable financing, a strong health workforce and capacity to address health emergencies.

Achieving the targets in SDG 3 will also depend on the achievement of other SDGs including ending poverty (SDG 1), food security (SDG 2), education (SDG 4), gender equality (SDG 5), clean water and sanitation (SDG 6), affordable and clean energy (SDG 7), decent work and economic growth (SDG 8), reducing other inequalities (SDG 10), cities (SDG 11), consumption and production (SDG 12), climate change (SDG 13), peace, justice and strong institutions (SDG 16), and partnerships for the goals (SDG 17). To attain the goal of healthy lives for all at all ages, around 50 SDG targets across 14 SDGs must be achieved (WHO, 2019b).

With a decade remaining, there has been progress in many areas (UN, 2019). The 2019 Sustainable Development Goals Report (UN, 2019), which provided progress against targets for each of the 17 SDGs, noted reduced rates of maternal and child mortality and improvements in some infectious diseases, resulting in increased life expectancy globally. However, major inequalities still exist within and between countries. For example, women

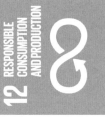
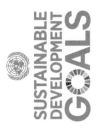

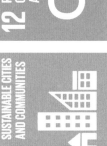

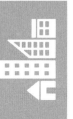
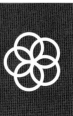
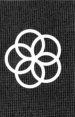
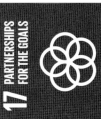

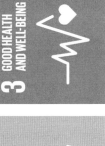
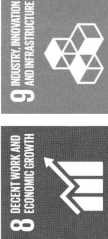

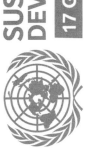
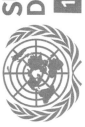
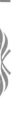

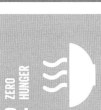

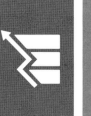
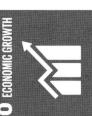
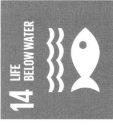

FIGURE 1.1 Sustainable Development Goals
Source: *United Nations, 2015.*

in the poorest countries face 15 times the risk of dying during pregnancy or from complications of childbirth, compared with women in middle- or high-income countries. Between 1990 and 2013, life expectancy stagnated in Europe and decreased in Africa (WHO, 2015b). In Europe, this is due mainly to adverse mortality trends in the former Soviet Union countries due to political and economic change and instability. The decrease in Africa is due mainly to mortality from HIV/AIDS, where 10% of maternal deaths are due to the aggravating effect of HIV infections (WHO, 2012, 2015c).

Health inequalities in Australia and New Zealand
Australia

Over the past two decades, Australia has consistently ranked in the top 10 of member countries of the Organisation for Economic Co-operation and Development (OECD) for life expectancy at birth (AIHW, 2014), with an overall life expectancy of 82.9 years in 2016 (WHO, 2019b). In 2019, Australia had the eighth-highest life expectancy among OECD member countries (OECD, 2019).

Although Australians as a whole have high levels of health by world standards, significant health inequalities exist. Population groups with worse than average health include Australia's Aboriginal and Torres Strait Islander peoples ('Indigenous Australians'), those with low socio-economic resources, people living in rural or remote areas, sole parents, and people living with disability or mental illness. In 2015–2017, life expectancy at birth for Indigenous males was 71.6 years and for Indigenous females was 75.6 years (Australian Government, 2020). Life expectancy for Indigenous males was 8.6 years lower than that for non-Indigenous males and 7.8 years lower for Indigenous females than for non-Indigenous females (Australian Government, 2020). From 2006 to 2018, age-standardised mortality rates for both Indigenous and non-Indigenous people improved by almost 10%, meaning that the gap has not narrowed. If these trends continue, Australia will not meet the *Closing the Gap* target of eliminating the difference in life expectancy between Indigenous and non-Indigenous Australians by 2030 (Australian Government, 2020).

Life expectancy for Indigenous Australians varies considerably dependent on location. For Indigenous Australians living in remote and very remote areas, life expectancy in 2015–2017 was 65.9 years for men and 69.6 years for women, while for Indigenous Australians living in major cities it was 72.1 years for men and 76.5 years for women, a gap of 6.2 and 6.9 years respectively (AIHW, 2019a). Indigenous Australians living in remote parts of the country have a life expectancy below the global average of 69.8 years for men and 74.2 years for women, and similar to males in Pakistan and Mongolia (65.7 years) and females in Guyana (69.0 years) and Rwanda (69.9 years) (WHO, 2019b).

Together with life expectancy, maternal mortality and child mortality rates are widely used as indicators of the overall development of a country or population. SDG target 3.1 is to reduce the global maternal mortality rate to less than 70 deaths per 100,000 live births by 2030. In 2017, the maternal mortality rate in Australia was 6 deaths per 100,000 (AIHW, 2019a). However, between 2012 and 2017, the age-standardised maternal mortality rate for Indigenous Australian women was 26.5 deaths per 100,000 (AIHW, 2019a), which is less than the overall SDG target of 70 but more than four times the overall rate for Australia.

SDG target 3.2 is to end preventable deaths of newborns and children under 5 years of age, with all countries aiming to reduce under-5 mortality to at least as low as 25 per 1000 live births by 2030. Child mortality rates in Australia are very low at 3.7 deaths per 1000 live births (UN Interagency Group for Child Mortality Estimation, 2019), but there are considerable inequalities within the population. Indigenous Australian children are still more than twice as likely to die before the age of 5 years than non-Indigenous children (AIHW, 2018).

Self-rated health is another valid and reliable health indicator used to assess overall health status and health inequalities (AIHW, 2018). It is usually assessed with the question 'In general, how would you rate your health?' with the possible responses being 'excellent', 'very good', 'good', 'fair' or 'poor'. Australia's Health 2018 reports that in 2014–15, 57% of Australians aged 15 and over described their health as 'excellent' or 'very good' (AIHW, 2018), with no significant change over the period from 2011 to 2012. Self-rated health scores also provide evidence of inequalities between Indigenous and non-Indigenous Australians. In 2014–15, an estimated 40% of Indigenous Australians aged 15 and over rated their health as 'excellent' or 'very good', compared with 56% of Australians in general (AIHW, 2018). Self-rated health status also varies geographically; however, the relationship is reversed, with Indigenous Australians living in remote and very remote areas more likely to rate their health positively than those in regional areas or major cities (AIHW, 2018). These differences demonstrate that when rating one's own health status, people may be thinking about health more holistically, and considering mental, emotional, social and spiritual aspects of wellbeing in their self-assessment. Therefore, it is vital when assessing health status to include both subjective and objective measures as complementary indicators of health (AIHW, 2018).

Geographical 'hotspots' of health inequality have been identified in Victoria and Queensland (Duckett, 2016), and a disproportionately high level of disadvantage is experienced in a small number of communities within Victoria (Vinson et al., 2015). *Dropping off the Edge 2015* shows that 11 postcodes in Victoria accounted for a nine-fold overrepresentation in disadvantage for life opportunities in areas such as social wellbeing, health and community safety, and access to housing, education and employment (Vinson et al., 2015). These postcodes had high unemployment, greater interaction with the criminal justice system, low levels of education, and significant levels of disability. Likewise, the social disadvantages Indigenous Australians experience in relation to housing, education, income and employment have contributed to the differences in health outcomes between Indigenous and non-Indigenous Australians (AIHW, 2018).

New Zealand

The New Zealand Health Survey (Ministry of Health, 2019a) shows similar health status to Australia. In 2019, New Zealand ranked 15th among OECD member countries (OECD, 2019) with an overall life expectancy of 82.2 years in 2016 (WHO, 2019b). However, significant inequalities exist within the population. In 2012–14, life expectancy at birth for Māori males was 73.0 years compared to 80.3 years for non-Māori males, and 77.1 years for Māori females compared with 83.9 years for non-Māori females (Statistics New Zealand, 2018). There was a rapid increase in Māori life expectancy until the early 1980s, after which it stabilised, while non-Māori life expectancy continued to increase, resulting in a widening gap between Māori and non-Māori people. However, since the 1990s, life expectancy for Māori has increased at a slightly faster rate than for non-Māori, resulting in a progressive narrowing of the gap. By 2012–14, the gap between Māori and non-Māori life expectancy at birth had decreased to 7.1 years (Statistics New Zealand, 2018).

The maternal mortality rate in New Zealand in 2017 was 9 deaths per 100,000 live births (WHO, 2019b). In combined data from 2006 to 2015, there was a significantly higher maternal mortality rate among Māori (26.3 per 100,000) and Pacific women (23.8 per 100,000) compared with New Zealand European women (13.5 per 100,000) (Perinatal

Maternal Mortality Review Committee, 2017). In 2018, the child mortality rate in New Zealand was 5.7 deaths per 1000 live births (UN Interagency Group for Child Mortality Estimation, 2019). However, in 2012–14 the child mortality rate for Māori was almost 50% higher than the rate for non-Māori (Ministry of Health, 2019b).

The proportion of people in New Zealand reporting their health as 'excellent', 'very good' or 'good' in 2018/19 was 86.2%, a significant decrease from 87.5% in 2017/18 and 89.3% in 2011/12. However, for those aged 75 years and older, the opposite is true, with a significant increase in the proportion of older people rating their health positively over the same time period.

Māori and Pacific adults are slightly less likely to report that their health was 'good', 'very good' or 'excellent' than non-Māori and non-Pacific adults. People living in the most socio-economically deprived areas are also less likely to report 'good', 'very good' or 'excellent' health compared with those living in the least deprived areas (Ministry of Health, 2019a).

Human Development Index

Life expectancy and mortality rates are not the only measures of the robustness of the health of a population. Created by the United Nations Development Program, the Human Development Index (HDI) is a single number for each country (United Nations Development Program [UNDP], 2019). Average achievements in health (life expectancy at birth: SDG 3), education (expected years of schooling: SDG 4.3, and mean years of schooling: SDG 4.6) and income (gross national income per capita: SDG 8.5) are calculated, and then those achievements are 'discounted' according to how they are distributed among the country's population. The HDI is therefore a measure of achievements adjusted for inequality. Australia (ranked 6th in 2019) and New Zealand (ranked 14th) are both considered very high index countries. A 20-year-old young adult born in the year 2000 in a very high index country is more than likely to be enrolled in higher education (55% of 20-year-olds) and on the path to being a highly skilled worker in a globalised and competitive world. Only 1% of children born in such countries will have died before the age of 20. In stark contrast, 17% of children born in countries with a low human development index will have died before age 20. If they survive, only 3% will be in higher education at age 20, and they can expect their lives to be 13 years shorter than those in high index countries (UNDP, 2019). At the age of 20, their massively unequal opportunities for health, education and employment have set them on vastly different life trajectories.

People and planetary happiness

The happiness of people and the planet are further indicators of health and wellbeing status. Happiness indicators are being used increasingly by governments to guide policy and assess overall wellbeing (Helliwell et al., 2019). Produced by the United Nations Sustainable Development Solutions Network, the first World Happiness Report in 2012 was released in support of a UN meeting on 'Wellbeing and Happiness: Defining a New Economic Paradigm', and subsequent reports have been produced in most years since. The reports demonstrate that subjective wellbeing measures, collectively referred to as 'happiness', are valid and reliable indicators of the quality of people's lives. Three happiness indicators are included in the reports: life evaluation, positive affect and negative affect. For life evaluation, people are asked to select a number between 0 and 10, where 0 represents the worst possible life and 10 the best possible life. Positive affect (emotion) is assessed by asking people to recall the frequency of happiness, laughter and enjoyment on the previous day. Negative affect is assessed by asking people to recall the frequency of worry, sadness and anger on the previous day. The World Happiness Reports present the findings on each of these measures and analyse the relationship between the happiness measures and six other factors: gross domestic product (GDP) per capita, social support, healthy life expectancy, freedom to make life choices, generosity, and absence of corruption. These factors are used to explain the variation in happiness between countries.

The World Happiness Report 2019 (Helliwell et al., 2019) showed the Scandinavian and north-west European countries dominated the life evaluation rankings, with Finland in first place, followed by Denmark, Norway, Iceland, the Netherlands, Switzerland and Sweden. New Zealand was ranked in 8th place and Australia in 11th. Countries with the lowest rankings were Syria, Malawi, Yemen, Rwanda, Tanzania, Afghanistan, Central African Republic, and South Sudan (lowest). Significant inequalities exist between the top and bottom countries, with average life evaluations in the top 10 countries more than double those in the bottom countries. Income inequalities between the countries contributed the most to these differences, followed by inequalities in social support, and healthy life expectancy.

The Happy Planet Index (HPI) incorporates the life evaluation data used in the World Happiness Report and extends it to include life expectancy and ecological footprint, which is a per capita measure of the amount of land that a nation requires to sustain its consumption (Jeffrey et al., 2016). The Happy Planet Index was developed by the New Economics Foundation, a British think tank that promotes social, economic and environmental justice. The 2016 Happy Planet Index ranked Costa Rica as the highest-ranking country, followed by Mexico, Colombia, Vanuatu and Vietnam; a very different list of countries to those at the top of the Human Development Index or any other usual measure of development. New Zealand was ranked in 38th position and Australia in 105th position, due predominantly to a significantly larger ecological footprint than higher-ranking countries.

SOCIO-ECOLOGICAL DETERMINANTS OF HEALTH AND WELLBEING

These various indicators of health and wellbeing clearly show that the conditions in which people are born, live, work and play influence the distribution of health and wellbeing among people. While there are many actions that a person can take to protect their own or their family's health, very often the context of their lives makes it impossible to take those actions. Perhaps they have been disempowered in some way, are alienated from society, or living in poverty. Or perhaps their health and wellbeing are not related to behaviours at all, but are directly impacted by exposure to discrimination or stigma, or poor-quality housing, or other environmental factors that have a direct effect on physical, mental, spiritual or social wellbeing.

The WHO's *Civil Society Report on Commission of Social Determinants of Health* (2007) explored the following determinants of health to provide guidance on actions to tackle inequalities created by these factors.

1. Social gradient: The lower a person's socio-economic position, the worse their health, even after accounting for possible differences in behaviours. Personal and social empowerment and freedom are significant for health outcomes at every level in society.

2. Health system factors: The degree to which the health system promotes equitable access to services, whether it actively perpetuates injustices, and the amount of out-of-pocket expenses all affect health outcomes.

3. Urban settings: Across the world a high proportion of urban dwellers live in slums, deprived of the basic public health services of housing, water, sanitation and food security.

4. Early development: Great variation in child mortality within and between nations is not explained by biological or other individual factors but by differences in environmental determinants.

5. Employment conditions: Availability of work, the work environment and employment contract conditions reflect the social gradient; those at lower levels often have unsafe work conditions and lower levels of control.

6. Education and life course: The benefits of education accumulate across the life course for individuals and families, and across generations in society.

7. Priority public health conditions related to behaviour within the social context: Tobacco, alcohol and drug use, and nutrition are international issues of concern and are socially patterned, demanding social solutions.

8. Women and gender equity: Gender inequality gives an indication of wider inequalities across society. Gender bias particularly marginalises women in the workforce, in their property rights and in economic and social life.

9. The shape of society: Health inequities reflect the unequal distribution of power in a society and the opportunities for decision making and accessing resources this brings. The degree to which household, workplace and national economic and social policies are underpinned by equity principles is a key indicator.

10. Globalisation of trade, communications and transport influence conditions within nations and relations between them: There are potential benefits and risks, with clear evidence that the globalisation of trade has increased inequalities between nations.

These factors all operate beyond the individual level, and have been termed the social determinants of health, to reflect the fact that they are functioning on the level of society, rather than the individual level. However, they extend well beyond the social environment and also include cultural, economic, political, natural and built environments. These environments interact with individual factors (human biology, socio-economic position, knowledge, values, attitudes, beliefs, behaviours and skills) to determine health and wellbeing outcomes. Collectively these environmental and individual factors are referred to as the socio-ecological determinants of health and wellbeing (e.g. AIHW, 2018; Craig et al., 2015; PHM et al., 2014; Wilkinson & Pickett, 2009). The links between the individual and environmental determinants of health and wellbeing for individuals, communities and populations are now well understood.

In the 20th century, improvements in health and wellbeing in affluent nations resulted primarily from improved living conditions, particularly sanitation, water supply and access to nutritious food, and investments in public infrastructure such as education and health services. In parallel, economic security was achieved by industrial growth, technological advancement, trade and the development of a skilled workforce to support it. Furthermore, advances in scientific knowledge and access to health care have been factors in prolonging life expectancy and quality of life for those who can afford to pay. As a result, life expectancy for the populations of high-income nations increased by around 20 years during the 20th century (WHO, 2015c).

During the latter part of the 20th century, a number of low- to middle-income countries (LMICs) were encouraged to embrace globalised trade. Many people within these nations emerged from poverty and the changes are reflected in improvements in their population health status and life expectancy. Like the health gains in affluent nations, population health improvements in these nations reflect the changing shape of their societies, their economic, public health and social policies, and the quality of their healthcare systems; however, there are still significant inequities within all societies. While economic growth has contributed to many improvements, it should also be noted that a focus on economic growth alone can be detrimental to the health of some within a population due to a country's choices around taxation, wealth distribution and neoliberal-inspired policies including austerity measures that reduce spending overall on public services such as education and health. Neoliberalism is a policy model that transfers control of economic factors to the private sector from the public sector. This model has had a profound effect on health.

The philosophy of a democratically elected government will determine to what extent equity is a principle underpinning public policy. For example, wealth redistribution through taxation is highly influential on health status. Nations such as those in Scandinavia that tend to have a graded taxation system with higher taxation rates for the wealthy are able to fund more and better social services, such as universal health care, dental care, transport, child care and housing assistance for their poor. When democratically elected governments adopt a neoliberal or user-pays approach to health policy, health risks for vulnerable members of society increase (PHM et al., 2014).

Depending on their contribution to good health and wellbeing, or poor health and wellbeing, any of the socio-ecological determinants may be referred to as protective or risk factors. Labonté (1997) differentiates between the determinants of health and illness in two separate models (Figs 1.2 and 1.3). In the determinants of illness, he includes physiological risk factors, behavioural risk factors, psychosocial risk factors, and risk conditions that

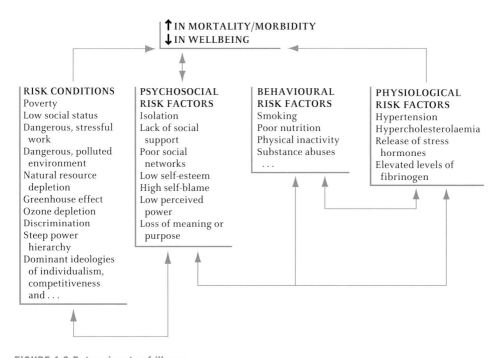

FIGURE 1.2 Determinants of illness
Source: Labonté, 1997.

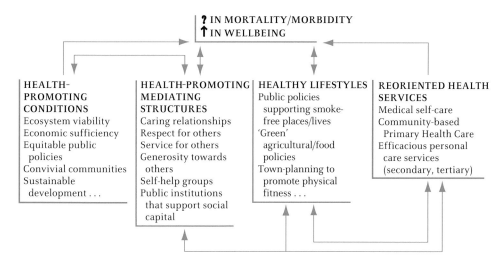

FIGURE 1.3 Determinants of health
Source: *Labonté, 1997.*

contribute to increased morbidity and mortality, and reduced wellbeing. In the determinants of health, he includes reoriented health services, policies and environments that support healthy lifestyles, health promoting mediating structures and health promoting conditions. Inequalities in the risk or protective factors for health and illness lead to unequal health outcomes. When the socio-ecological determinants are unfairly distributed, the inequalities are regarded as inequitable. Particular subpopulations or groups suffer the cumulative effects of a number of socio-ecological determinants of health. These groups are notably people living in poverty, those from cultural, ethnic and social minority groups, and people from isolated rural communities, who tend to have worse health. Additionally, they have less access to medical practitioners and specialist health professionals, and suffer more accidents and chronic illnesses. Poverty results in poorer health status, not necessarily because of lower differential access to funds, but because the poor are more exposed to discrimination, violence and dangerous workplaces, and often take more risks with their health.

The iceberg model

The iceberg model provides a useful way to understand the role of individual and environmental-level determinants of health and wellbeing, and the relationships between these determinants and health and wellbeing outcomes (Fig. 1.4). The iceberg is divided into three sections. The top section visible above the waterline refers to what is apparent: the measurable states of physical, mental, social and spiritual health and wellbeing. These observable states of health and wellbeing include life expectancy, mortality rates, morbidity rates, self-rated health, healthy life years (HeaLYs), disability-adjusted life years (DALYs) and quality-adjusted life years (QALYs) (Hyder et al., 2012), and other indicators of health and wellbeing status. The section immediately below the iceberg waterline is connected to the observable states of health and wellbeing and can be identified and measured without too much difficulty. Here we see the individual physiological and behavioural factors that are commonly the focus of much public health and medical

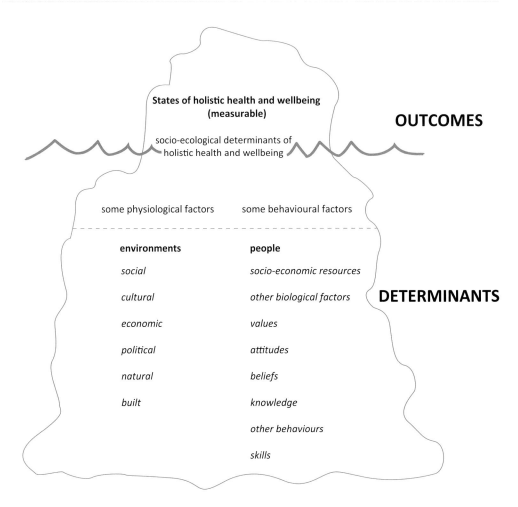

FIGURE 1.4 The iceberg model
Source: *Revised from Talbot & Verrinder, 2005. Originally adapted from Travis & Ryan, 2004.*

attention, including hypertension, high cholesterol levels, smoking, poor nutrition, physical inactivity and substance use. Tools are readily available to identify these risk or protective factors for poor health and wellbeing. Beneath these more obvious factors though, well below the waterline and therefore much more difficult to detect, are the majority of socio-ecological determinants, covering a broad range of risk and protective factors at both individual and environmental levels. These are often referred to as the causes of the causes.

Given the outcome of the *Titanic*'s encounter with an iceberg, it is tempting to think about the submerged section of the iceberg as a hidden but significant threat to health and wellbeing, and indeed many of the socio-ecological determinants contribute to poor health outcomes and greater health inequity. But remember, health is not just the absence of disease, and as such the submerged section of the iceberg can also be interpreted as a significant contributor to good health and wellbeing, and greater health equity. The base of the iceberg is essential for its stability, and therefore also represents the vast range of factors that contribute to protecting and promoting the health and wellbeing of people. Including a focus on strengths and assets for good health and wellbeing is referred to as a salutogenic approach, which is further discussed in Chapter 2. The iceberg model can be used to examine the immediate and contributing determinants of any health priority. To demonstrate this, we use it to examine heart disease and breastfeeding.

Heart disease

We know about the physiological and behavioural risk factors for heart disease (*immediately below the iceberg waterline*). But what are the risk factors that are not so easily observable? What are the structural issues? What are the socio-ecological factors that contribute to the physiological and behavioural risk factors? What are the causes of the causes (*way below the iceberg waterline*)? For example, a polluted environment contributing to poor living conditions, or the overarching economic imperative to make money and consume goods leading to overtime or a poor workplace environment, or exposure to race or weight-based discrimination all cause stress and contribute directly to the physiological risk factors for heart disease. Other socio-ecological factors contribute to the behavioural risk factors. Perhaps fresh food is not available, which is very likely in remote areas. A person may have grown up in a family where physical activity was not valued. Perhaps there was a lack of physical education at school. They may have poor body image and been fat shamed by their health provider. Perhaps there is no convenient, safe or affordable facility for physical activity. Smoking may be the normal behaviour valued among friends and family. Having a low income may mean not being able to afford a range of nutrient-rich foods. Working two jobs may mean lack of time or energy for food preparation. These factors will worsen for successive generations and for groups with the least power in society. We need to ask who are these people? Where do they live? Do they receive adequate social support?

Breastfeeding

The health and wellbeing benefits (*above the iceberg waterline*) of exclusively breastfeeding infants to six months and continuing to breastfeed while introducing appropriate foods up to two years is well established for both infants and their mothers. For example, breastfeeding ensures an infant's nutritional requirements are met, protects against common childhood illnesses and some long-term chronic conditions, and contributes to physical growth and cognitive development. For mothers, breastfeeding protects against breast and ovarian cancers later in life, aids spacing of children due to delay of the menstrual period, contributes to a quicker recovery from childbirth and facilitates maternal emotional fulfilment.

In Australia, the majority of babies are being breastfed when discharged from hospital. However, by six months breastfeeding rates drop substantially with only 15%–18% of infants exclusively breastfed to six months. A similar story of high initiation followed by high early cessation is reported globally in the developed world. Individual physiological and behavioural factors (*immediately below the iceberg waterline*) that influence whether a mother exclusively breastfeeds up to six months include the age of the mother, whereby those under 25 years of age (especially teenage mothers), those who have had multiparous and/or a caesarean birth, and Indigenous women are less likely to continue to breastfeed. Mothers that have smoked during pregnancy are more likely to cease breastfeeding before six months.

At the individual level (*way below the iceberg waterline*) factors that influence continuation of breastfeeding include a mother's intention to bottle-feed during the antenatal period, whether or not she perceives her breastmilk supply to be sufficient, pain and discomfort experienced during breastfeeding, the need to return to work early, not having enough time, and emotional reasons such as depression, stress and coping with other children. Infant-related issues such as an unsettled baby, inadequate weight gain, attachment problems, reflux, troublesome sleeping patterns and poor interest from the baby in breastfeeding also influence the continuation of breastfeeding. Women that attend antenatal classes are also more likely to continue to breastfeed than those who do not. The range of environmental determinants (*also way below the iceberg waterline*) such as the introduction of infant formula during the postnatal hospital stay, ineffective support from healthcare professionals and informal networks for mothers to continue to breastfeed, living in rural areas where there is limited access to ongoing support once leaving hospital, exposure to intimate partner violence, and poor partner support, all influence whether or not a mother continues to breastfeed her infant.

Lead by the WHO Commission for the Social Determinants of Health, and supported by national, regional and local research (e.g. see AIHW, 2018; Craig et al., 2015; and *Fair Society Healthy Lives [The Marmot Review]*, 2010), the socio-ecological determinants of health are gradually being incorporated into the language of health service provision, especially in the community sector. However, this is occurring much more slowly in the medical sector where the biomedical and behavioural health paradigm is still dominant. The planning frameworks, funding application proformas and reporting documents used by agencies, such as state government health departments and associations (e.g. health promotion foundations such as VicHealth in Victoria and Healthway in South Australia and District Health Boards in New Zealand Whakapā ki Aotearoa) provide useful examples of how the socio-ecological determinants can be integrated into practice. A comprehensive whole-of-government approach is needed if we are to fully protect and maximise the health of the community. Such an approach would need to consider the health consequences of public policy in all areas, including policy within the health sector and extending beyond to other sectors such as taxation, transport, urban planning, environment, education, etc. This idea will be taken up further in the following chapters.

WHO GLOBAL RESPONSES TO HEALTH AND WELLBEING

The World Health Organization (WHO) is a global health agency established in 1948 under the auspices of the United Nations to improve the health of the world's people. It currently comprises 194 member states, with headquarters in Geneva and offices in 150 countries across six regions. Each region has a regional office: regional office for the Americas/Pan American Health Organization (AMRO/PAHO) in Washington DC, USA; regional office for Europe (EURO) in Copenhagen, Denmark; regional office for Africa (AFRO) in Brazzaville, Congo; regional office for South-East Asia (SEARO) in New Delhi, India; regional office for the Eastern Mediterranean (EMRO) in Cairo, Egypt; and regional office for the Western Pacific (WPRO) in Manila, Philippines. Australia and New Zealand are part of the Western Pacific Region.

The WHO defined health as 'a state of complete physical, mental and social wellbeing and not merely the absence of disease or infirmity' in the constitution of the WHO in 1948 (WHO, 1948). The tenets of the constitution are:

- *the enjoyment of the highest attainable standard of health is one of the fundamental rights of every human being without distinction of race, religion, political belief, economic or social condition*

- *the health of all peoples is fundamental to the attainment of peace and security and is dependent upon the fullest cooperation of individuals and states*
- *the achievement of any state in the promotion and protection of health is of value to all*
- *unequal development in different countries in the promotion of health and control of disease, especially communicable disease, is a common danger*
- *healthy development of the child is of basic importance*
- *the ability to live harmoniously in a changing total environment is essential to such development*
- *the extension to all peoples of the benefits of medical, psychological and related knowledge is essential to the fullest attainment of health*
- *informed opinion and active cooperation on the part of the public are of the utmost importance in the improvement of the health of the people, and, finally,*
- *governments have a responsibility for the health of their peoples, which can be fulfilled only by the provision of adequate health and social measures.*

(World Health Organization, 1948)

The WHO has produced landmark documents such as the Declaration of Alma-Ata (WHO, 1978) (Appendix 1), the Ottawa Charter for Health Promotion (WHO, 1986) (Appendix 2) and affirming declarations such as the Rio Political Declaration on Social Determinants of Health (SDH) (WHO, 2011), Shanghai Declaration on Promoting Health in the 2030 Agenda for Sustainable Development (WHO, 2016a) (Appendix 3) and the Declaration of Astana on Primary Health Care (WHO, 2018) (Appendix 4). As a body of work, these documents demonstrate the evolution of the organisation's response to emergent health and wellbeing priorities through primary health care and health promotion.

Primary health care
The Declaration of Alma-Ata

In 1978, the WHO and United Nations Children's Fund (UNICEF) held a major international conference on primary health care in Alma-Ata in the USSR (now known as Almaty, Kazakhstan) which was attended by representatives from 134 nations. The outcome of the conference was the Declaration of Alma-Ata (WHO, 1978). Through this declaration, the member states of the WHO defined and outlined a way forward for health systems based on primary health care.

> *Primary health care is essential health care based on practical, scientifically sound and socially acceptable methods. PHC is made universally accessible to the community through their full participation and at a cost that the community and country can afford to maintain at every stage of their development in the spirit of self-reliance and self-determination.*
>
> *(WHO, 1978)*

This followed growing concern in the 1960s and 1970s that the health status of some populations had not improved as predicted, despite investment in and rapid growth of healthcare systems. Globally, there had been the belief that medical knowledge and technology would solve health problems, but there was a growing scepticism of the role and power of medicine itself and the value of medical treatment (e.g. Illich, 1975). It became increasingly apparent that medical services alone had a limited effect on the health of populations and that it was public health actions that were responsible for most population health improvement (McKeown, 1979). Despite wide-ranging evidence that social conditions such as poverty, living conditions and education have a great impact on health and wellbeing, few countries had acted specifically to improve these conditions.

There were differences between high-income and low-income countries. High-income countries had invested heavily in acute medical care systems; however, low-income countries could not afford this investment and people in these countries often lacked access to even basic healthcare services. Some countries, including high-income countries, began to review their health systems and the approach to health and illness care. In Australia, for example, the Labor Government began to invest in community-controlled and community-based multidisciplinary health services in 1973. The Lalonde Report (Lalonde, 1974) had a significant impact in Canada and other high-income countries. In that report, health was represented as being dependent on biological, environmental and lifestyle factors and access to health systems. This was a dramatic shift away from the focus on the biological determinants of health and medical interventions that had dominated health sector thinking in high-income countries in the first part of the 20th century.

Inspiration for the Declaration of Alma-Ata was drawn from the Chinese model of barefoot doctors and the participation of Australia's National Aboriginal and Islander Health Organisation representatives in drafting the declaration. Ever since, 'Aboriginal community-controlled health services have been the torch bearers for comprehensive primary health care in Australia' (PHM et al., 2014, p. 395).

This conference and declaration continue to be regarded as a critically important milestone in the enhancement of health equalities. Since then, this philosophy has been reiterated internationally in numerous documents, including those in the appendices of this book. The prerequisites for health outlined in the declaration included peace, shelter, education, social security, social relations, food, income, empowerment of women, a stable ecosystem, sustainable resource use, social justice, respect for human rights and equity (WHO, 1978). The declaration set out a philosophy designed to ensure these prerequisites for health are met; an approach for the comprehensive delivery of primary health care; and a level of care for health improvement through the entire health system (Vuori, 1986).

Primary health care philosophy

The PHC philosophy enables societies to act on the prerequisites for health specified in the Declaration of Alma-Ata (WHO, 1978) and address the socio-ecological determinants of health and wellbeing. The philosophy provides a foundation for improving daily living conditions, tackling the inequitable distribution of power, money and resources, and measuring and understanding health priorities and assessing the impact of action (WHO, 2011, 2015d). The Declaration of Alma-Ata (WHO, 1978) provided the foundation for PHC to be seen as the key to achieving a level of health and wellbeing that permitted people of the world to lead a socially and economically productive life. Three major principles are embedded in the Declaration of Alma-Ata:

1. Equity
2. Social justice, and
3. Empowerment.

Equity means fairness, and social justice requires a commitment to fairness. Empowerment is a process which enables people to participate in a way that improves their lives

> ## INSIGHT 1.1 CPHC as a philosophy for health services: New Zealand Ministry of Health
>
> In New Zealand, 20 district health boards (DHBs) plan, manage, provide and purchase healthcare services for the population of their district (local geographic area) to ensure services are arranged effectively according to the specific demography and needs of their population. DHBs manage funding for primary care, hospital services, public health services, aged care services and services provided by other non-government health providers, including Māori and Pacific providers. DHB objectives reflect the notion of CPHC; for example, 'promoting the inclusion and participation in society and the independence of people with disabilities; reducing health disparities by improving health outcomes for Māori and other population groups; reducing—with a view toward elimination—health outcome disparities between various population groups' (Ministry of Health, n.d.; 2018). Furthermore, DHBs are expected to 'show a sense of social responsibility [and] to foster community participation in health improvement' (Ministry of Health, n.d.; 2018).
>
> The *New Zealand Health Strategy: Future direction* (Ministry of Health, 2016) also addresses the underlying tenets of CPHC philosophy, as evidenced via the following:
>
> - Acknowledging the special relationship between Māori and the Crown under the Treaty of Waitangi
> - The best health and wellbeing possible for all New Zealanders throughout their lives
> - An improvement in health status of those currently disadvantaged
> - Collaborative health promotion, rehabilitation and disease and injury prevention by all sectors
> - Timely and equitable access for all New Zealanders to a comprehensive range of health and disability services, regardless of ability to pay
> - A high-performing system in which people have confidence
> - Active partnership with people and communities at all levels, and
> - Thinking beyond narrow definitions of health and collaborating with others to achieve wellbeing.
>
> *Sources: Ministry of Health, 2016, 2018, n.d.*

and achieves social justice. These three key principles underpin all PHC activities and are discussed in more detail in Chapter 2. The New Zealand Ministry of Health Matatu Hauora provides an example of CPHC as a philosophy for health services (Insight 1.1).

Primary health care approaches

Since the Declaration of Alma-Ata (WHO, 1978) two different approaches to PHC have emerged. The terms 'selective' and 'comprehensive' are good descriptors of the different approaches to, or ways of doing, primary health care. In short, selective primary health care (SPHC) (Walsh & Warren, 1979, cited in Baum, 2008) uses a biomedical model of health, while comprehensive primary health care (CPHC) focuses on socio-ecological changes necessary to improve health and wellbeing. CPHC includes treatment, rehabilitation, palliation, prevention and health promotion. In the CPHC approach, provision of medical care is only one aspect, whereas SPHC concentrates primarily on treating poor health. Thus, while CPHC focuses on the process of empowerment and increasing people's control over the influences on their health, SPHC operates in a way that assumes that the health system alone creates health, and ensures that control over health is maintained by health practitioners. The different approaches can be characterised as an individual approach in

SPHC versus a system approach in CPHC (Green & Raeburn, 1988, cited in Baum, 2008, p. 35). Strong health systems based on CPHC are more efficient and yield better health outcomes and improved equity.

Rifkin and Walt (1986) suggested differences in the definitions, and the policy and practice implications of confusing the two approaches. In line with the Alma-Ata Declaration (WHO, 1978), CPHC practice defines health as a state of complete physical, mental and social wellbeing; addresses inequalities through equity and social justice measures; considers the impact of education, housing, food and income; acknowledges the value of community development; and recognises the expertise of individuals in their own health. It is an intersectoral enterprise in which the socio-ecological determinants of health, and the concept of generational and intergenerational equity, are embedded in all policies. It involves the redistribution of wealth through taxation to enable investment in 'public goods' and policy decisions are based on evidence or the precautionary principle. Community participation in decision making is also conducted in a way that empowers individuals and communities. Rifkin and Walt argue that SPHC practice assumes that health is the absence of disease rather than the broader WHO definition; focuses on the eradication and prevention of diseases; and locates action for health almost solely within the realms of specialists trained to treat disease. Limitations of the SPHC approach are reflected in the following points.

- Through the emphasis on disease, the need to address issues of equity, social justice and empowerment, which are at the root of many health problems, is ignored.

- Non-medical actions, such as the provision of education, housing and food, which have a greater bearing on health and wellbeing than health services, are discounted.

- The value of community development as a strategy for improving health is unrecognised or used as a technique for increasing community compliance with medically defined solutions, rather than as a mechanism for community empowerment, thus intensifying the power of health practitioners.

- The great expertise that people have with regard to their own lives and the issues that affect them is disregarded.

Arguing for a comprehensive over a selective approach is not to argue against the important role of the primary health care system in addressing specific illness and disease conditions. Clearly, we must address diseases that cause human suffering and premature death. However, by *only* addressing those diseases, we risk perpetually attempting to address the end result of the problem instead of the root causes of poor health and wellbeing. CPHC addresses health and wellbeing priorities within their socio-ecological context, using a process where the expertise that ordinary people have and their right to exert control over their own lives are recognised.

CPHC has been the linchpin for Aboriginal community-controlled health services (ACCHSs) in Australia. It is essential in tackling the broad socio-ecological determinants of health and improving greater access to culturally acceptable, affordable health care. ACCHSs have played a critical role in developing 'better-informed Aboriginal health policy development' (PHM et al., 2014, p. 396) and have provided a CPHC strategy for organising health care. As noted by Ah Chee (2015), 'Aboriginal community-controlled health services are key to *Closing the Gap by 2030* (Hoy, 2009) and they are needed now, more than ever'. The National Aboriginal Community Controlled Health Organisation (NACCHO) is a good example of a CPHC approach or 'way of doing' primary health care (Insight 1.2).

INSIGHT 1.2 CPHC as an approach for the delivery of health care: National Aboriginal Community Controlled Health Organisation (NACCHO)

NACCHO is 'a living embodiment of the aspirations of Aboriginal communities and their struggle for self-determination' (NACCHO, n.d.). It represents over 143 Aboriginal community-controlled health services (ACCHSs) in urban, regional and remote Australia. The organisation aims to increase the capacity of ACCHSs in health policy development and in controlling and delivering effective health care. These services are initiated and operated by the local Aboriginal communities to deliver 'holistic, comprehensive and culturally appropriate health care to the community which controls it, through a locally elected Board of Management'. NACCHO's work includes the following:

- *Promoting, developing and expanding the provision of health and wellbeing services through local ACCHSs.*
- *Liaison with organisations and governments within both the Aboriginal and non-Aboriginal community on health and wellbeing policy and planning issues.*
- *Representation and advocacy relating to health service delivery, health information, research, public health, health financing and health programs.*
- *Fostering cooperative partnerships and working relationships with agencies that respect Aboriginal community control and holistic concepts of health and wellbeing.*

Source: NACCHO, n.d.

Médecins Sans Frontières (MSF) provides another example of CPHC as an approach to the delivery of health care. MSF dispenses essential drugs such as vaccines, and assists local communities with water and sanitation programs. MSF also provides training of local personnel to work with disadvantaged groups in remote healthcare centres and slums. MSF works at both reducing the risk of illness and treating disease by providing essential medical care, and also assists with essential infrastructure support in a socially acceptable and empowering way to improve living conditions and health care. Other potential priorities set by local communities are also acknowledged (MSF, n.d.).

Primary health as a level of CPHC delivery

The term 'primary care' is often used to refer to primary-level health services or a level of care; that is, the first point of contact with the health system for people with health issues. The primary health networks (PHNs) in Australia are a good example of primary health as a level of service delivery (Australian Government, 2018) (Insight 1.3). In a CPHC system, this level of care needs to be the most comprehensive. In this way, issues can be dealt with where they begin. Primary-level health services include ACCHSs, community health centres, pharmacies and local governments. Non-government organisations (NGOs) and community groups are also an important part of CPHC services. However, these services can only be regarded as CPHC services if the CPHC philosophy underpins the way in which those first-level services are provided; that is, if the work is guided by the principles of equity, social justice and empowerment. Community participation in decision making, collaboration with other sectors within the community to deal effectively with health issues, and incorporation of health promotion, is essential to the work. There are examples worldwide of successful CPHC organisations that have improved the health of populations (PHM et al., 2014), including ACCHSs. Programs in India, South America and Asia have 'shown consistent commitment to equitable, broad-based and multi-sectoral

> ## INSIGHT 1.3 Primary health as a level of care: Primary Health Networks in Australia
>
> Since 2015, 31 Primary Health Networks (PHNs) have been established with the aim of improving 'primary health care' in Australia (Australian Government, 2018). They are Commonwealth government-funded not-for-profit companies that are legally independent of government. The PHNs' objectives are to 'improve the efficiency and effectiveness of medical services for patients, particularly those at risk of poor health outcomes, and to improve coordination of care … PHNs will achieve these objectives by working directly with general practitioners, other primary health care providers, secondary care providers and hospitals to facilitate improved outcomes for patients'. These objectives are achieved through three key roles. First, PHNs commission (not provide) a range of primary health care services, such as, general practice, prevention and screening, early intervention, treatment and management regionally to address local needs. Commissioned services are 'clinically focused, with general practice at the heart of improving the delivery of primary health care'. Second, they provide practice support to other providers to develop the capacity of the health workforce and delivery of high-quality care. Third, they work collaboratively with local health service providers to integrate health services to improve the patient experience and use of resources. The seven priorities for PHNs are mental health, Aboriginal and Torres Strait Islander health, population health, health workforce, digital health, aged care and alcohol and other drugs. You can access the PHN in your local area via the interactive map locator and explore the work the organisation is undertaking.
>
> *Source: Australian Government, 2018.*

development', with each reflecting their own histories (PHM et al., 2011, p. 51). For example, Reeve and colleagues (2015) evaluated primary care partnerships between ACCHSs, a hospital and a community health service in Western Australia between 2006 and 2012. The strategy involved the integration of health promotion, health assessments and chronic disease management with an acute primary care service. They found that occasions of service increased to very remote outlying communities in particular. Health assessment uptake increased which in turn led to people being placed on a care plan and quality-of-care indicators showed improvements. There was a downward trend in mortality.

The Declaration of Astana

The WHO continues to affirm the philosophy of CPHC (WHO, 2011, 2015d, 2018) and calls for a global commitment to the enhancement of health equity by acting on the socio-ecological determinants of health and wellbeing. Most recently, 40 years after the Alma-Ata Declaration, the Astana Declaration on Primary Health Care was ratified at the 2018 Global Conference on Primary Health Care in Astana, Kazakhstan. The Astana Declaration reinforces the vision of the 1978 Alma-Ata Declaration and the 2030 SDGs, and outlines a new vision for PHC into the 21st century (WHO, 2018). The Declaration envisions:

> ***governments and societies*** *that prioritize, promote and protect people's health and wellbeing, at both population and individual levels, through strong health systems;*
>
> ***primary health care and health services*** *that are high quality, safe, comprehensive, integrated, accessible, available and affordable for everyone*

*and everywhere, provided with compassion, respect and dignity by health
professionals who are well-trained, skilled, motivated and committed;*

enabling and health-conducive environments *in which individuals and
communities are empowered and engaged in maintaining and enhancing
their health and well-being;*

partners and stakeholders *aligned in providing effective support to national
health policies, strategies and plans* (WHO, 2018).

The Declaration acknowledges and reiterates the important role of health promotion
in the pursuit of this vision and meeting the health and wellbeing needs of all peoples
across the life span through CPHC.

HEALTH PROMOTION

Ottawa Charter for Health Promotion

The 1986 Ottawa Charter for Health Promotion (Appendix 2) was built on the progress
made through the Declaration of Alma-Ata and defines health promotion as 'the process of
enabling people to increase control over, and to improve, their health' (WHO, 1986). The
Charter was the outcome of the first WHO International Conference on Health Promotion
held in Ottawa, Canada, in 1986. The aim was to increase the relevance of the CPHC
approach to high-income countries that had largely ignored the Declaration of Alma-Ata.
Like the Declaration of Alma-Ata, the Ottawa Charter for Health Promotion was a landmark
document, laying out a clear statement of action that continues to provide guidance for
health practitioners around the world to improve the health and wellbeing of populations.

The Ottawa Charter for Health Promotion highlights the collective role of organisations,
systems, communities and individuals in achieving positive wellbeing. The five action areas
of the Charter (Fig. 1.5) are designed to promote health and wellbeing in the following ways.

1. Building healthy public policy. It is not health policy alone that influences
    health—all public policy should be examined for its impact on health and,
    where policies have a negative impact on health, work to change them needs to
    be done. For example, if a local government has a policy of allowing industrial
    complexes near residential areas, this would need to change if it was having a
    negative impact on residents' health.

2. Creating environments which support healthy living. The protection of both
    the natural and built environment is important for health. In the built
    environment, living, work and leisure environments need to be organised in
    ways that do not create or contribute to poor health. For example, affordable
    child care for working parents needs to be provided. The natural environment
    needs to be conserved for health. These will come through the establishment of
    healthy public policy.

3. Strengthening community action. Communities themselves are the experts in
    their own community and can determine what their needs are, and how they
    can best be met. Thus, greater power and control remain with the people
    themselves, rather than totally with the 'experts'. Community development is
    one means by which this can be achieved.

4. Developing personal skills. If people are to feel more in control of their lives
    and have more power in decisions that affect them, they may need to develop

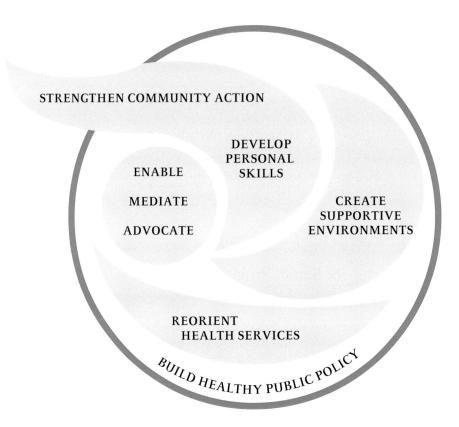

FIGURE 1.5 The Ottawa Charter for Health Promotion
Health promotion emblem (English version) from The Ottawa Charter for Health Promotion
Source: *World Health Organization, 1986.*

more skills. This could include being provided with necessary information, training or other resources that would enable people to take action to promote or protect their health. Those who work in the health system must work towards enabling people to acquire the necessary knowledge and skills to make informed decisions.

5. Reorienting health care. Health promotion is everybody's business and intersectoral collaboration is the key. Within the health system there needs to be a balance between health promotion and curative services. One prerequisite for this reorientation is a major change in the way in which health practitioners are educated.

The five action areas of the Charter, used collectively within any population and setting, are designed to be used as a portfolio of strategies addressing the full range of health and wellbeing determinants, not as a menu from which to pick and choose. Comprehensive initiatives utilising *all* action areas therefore yield far greater health and wellbeing outcomes than when they are used singularly (Kickbusch, 1989). A strength of the Ottawa Charter (WHO, 1986) is that it draws on and incorporates the philosophy of CPHC, and in addition to the five action areas described above:

1. is done with and by the people, not for them—it encourages participation in decision making at all levels;

2. usually involves a range of different approaches that include structural and policy changes for people in the context of their everyday lives, not just a focus on individual behaviour-change approaches; and

3. is directed at improving people's control over the determinants of their health.

The Ottawa Charter continues to provide a vehicle to understand the socio-ecological determinants of health and guide practice. As Ludovika Singh (cited in de Leeuw, 2011, p. ii159) said:

> *Time flows like a river*
>
> *The Charter is a boulder in the stream*
>
> *Its erosion forms a wide and fertile estuary*

Subsequent global health promotion charters and declarations

Each international health promotion conference, since the first in Ottawa, has reaffirmed the philosophy that underpins CPHC as outlined in the Declaration of Alma-Ata, and the action areas of the Ottawa Charter for Health Promotion have been celebrated and built upon each time. These benchmark conferences have been followed by international health promotion conferences in Adelaide (WHO, 1988), Sundsvall (WHO, 1991), Jakarta (WHO, 1997), Mexico City (WHO, 2000), Bangkok (WHO, 2005), Nairobi (WHO, 2009), Helsinki (WHO, 2013a) and most recently Shanghai (WHO, 2016a), all of which provide global direction for health promotion action through a series of charters, declarations and statements. The nine global conferences, the resulting declaration or charter, and the focus of each are presented in Table 1.1. Weblinks to these documents are available in the *More to Explore* section at the end of this chapter. Of particular importance, the most recent declaration, *The Shanghai Declaration on promoting health in the 2030 Agenda for Sustainable Development* (WHO, 2016a) (Appendix 3), acknowledges the role of health promotion in progressing all the SDGs (UN, 2015) and reinforces the need for increased investment in health promotion to address increasing inequities through good governance and collaborative effort. The Shanghai Declaration call to action states:

> *We recognize that health is a political choice and we will counteract interests detrimental to health and remove barriers to empowerment—especially for women and girls. We urge political leaders from different sectors and from different levels of governance, from the private sector and from civil society to join us in our determination to promote health and wellbeing in all the SDGs. Promoting health demands coordinated action by all concerned, it is a shared responsibility. With this Shanghai Declaration, we, the participants, pledge to accelerate the implementation of the SDGs through increased political commitment and financial investment in health promotion.*
>
> *(WHO, 2016a)*

The Shanghai Declaration also emphasises the ongoing need for national and global-level policies that support the development of health and social justice. This reinforces the importance of a Health in All Policies (HiAP) approach first introduced via the *Adelaide Statement on Health in All Policies* in Adelaide, in 2010 (WHO, 2010a) and revisited at the 8th Global Conference in Helsinki in 2013 (WHO, 2013a). The HiAP approach recognises that responsibility for many of the socio-ecological determinants of health falls outside of the health sector; for example, housing, transport, education, and that many population health gains are dependent on other sectors and all levels of government considering how

TABLE 1.1 WHO global health promotion charters, declarations and statements

Conference year & location	WHO health promotion charter, declaration or statement	Focus of charter, declaration or statement
1986 Ottawa, Canada	The Ottawa Charter for Health Promotion	First global health promotion charter to guide countries to set up health promotion strategies and programs. The Charter reaffirmed social justice and equity identified in the Alma-Ata Declaration (WHO, 1978) as prerequisites for health to be achieved through the strategies of advocacy and mediation.
1988 Adelaide, Australia	Adelaide Recommendations on Healthy Public Policy	Called for all countries to develop healthy public policies to address health gaps between countries. It also emphasised the responsibility of developed countries in ensuring that their policies positively impact the health of developing countries.
1991 Sundsvall, Sweden	Sundsvall Statement on Supportive Environments for Health	Called for policy and decision makers across all sectors and levels to engage in creating environments in which people live to be supportive of health.
1997 Jakarta, Indonesia	Jakarta Declaration on Leading Health Promotion into the 21st Century	Proposed a way forward for health promotion action into the 21st century. It acknowledged changes in the determinants of health and set out priorities for health promotion which included: promoting social responsibility for health, increasing investment for health development, consolidating and expanding partnerships for health, increasing community capacity and empowering individuals, and securing an infrastructure for health promotion.
2000 Mexico City, Mexico	Mexico Ministerial Statement for the Promotion of Health: From Ideas to Action	Acknowledged health promotion as a key component of public policies and programs in all countries. This culminated in a *Framework for Countrywide Plans of Action for Health Promotion* for use by governments of all member countries.
2005 Bangkok, Thailand	Bangkok Charter for Health Promotion in a Globalized World	Identified challenges, actions and commitments in addressing the determinants of health and wellbeing within a globalised world through health promotion.
2009 Nairobi, Kenya	Nairobi Call to Action	Identified commitments and strategies needed to close the gap in health through health promotion.

TABLE 1.1 WHO global health promotion charters, declarations and statements—cont'd

Conference year & location	WHO health promotion charter, declaration or statement	Focus of charter, declaration or statement
2013 Helsinki, Finland	The Helsinki Statement on Health in All Policies	Affirmed commitment to health equity and reiterated the importance of the uptake of a *Health in all Policies* approach by all countries across all sectors to achieve improved public health outcomes.
2016 Shanghai, China	Shanghai Declaration on promoting health in the 2030 Agenda for Sustainable Development	Pledged a commitment to the accelerated implementation of the United Nations Sustainable Development Goals through investment in health promotion.

they contribute to health and wellbeing through their policy agendas. More details about the HiAP approach and examples of the adoption of this initiative in Australia and New Zealand are provided in Chapter 5.

Implementing the Ottawa Charter action areas

As presented earlier in this chapter, the Ottawa Charter action areas provide a solid foundation along with a socio-ecological determinants approach for CPHC. There are, however, some challenges for organisations and practitioners implementing the five action areas to truly fulfil the promise of the Charter locally and globally. At the core of the work is a commitment to empowerment, community engagement and political action, and there is a need to strengthen and validate the role of advocacy, mediation and enabling (de Leeuw, 2011). Health promotion experts have reflected on the Charter and highlight areas for vigilance. Many raise concerns about the impact of neoliberalism. (See the entire issue of *Health Promotion International*, 26 [S2]. Analysis of progress made in achieving the five action areas of the Ottawa Charter for Health Promotion and the continuing challenges facing practitioners, including the impact of neoliberalism, is made by international experts in health promotion.) The PHM and others (2014, p. 1) argue that neoliberal globalisation has produced a global health crisis. Baum and Sanders (2011) argue that transnational corporations (TNCs) pose a major threat to improving health inequalities. They reason that to counteract this, a Health in All Policies approach should be used to monitor and enforce TNCs' accountability for health (WHO, 2013a). They suggest that part of this process should include undertaking health impact assessments (see Chapters 3 and 9) and health equity impact assessments on their activities. Similarly, Wallerstein and colleagues (2011) are concerned about TNCs, and the accompanying social and environmental devastation, which, in their view, has challenged the effectiveness of community action to create health. However, they propose that there are new mechanisms for community engagement (see Chapter 6) that continue to emerge and provide examples of a reorientation of health promotion through the growth of healthy city and healthy community initiatives and other current community-organising strategies where 'the principle of community is given greater value, and with it the ideas of agency, equality, autonomy and solidarity' (Wallerstein et al., 2011, p. ii234). Poor health promotion literacy (see Chapter 7) within the health sector is raised by Whitehead and Irvine (2011). They argue that developing the literacy of health practitioners who remain unaware of, or unengaged with, health promotion practice is the main reform required for the future of developing personal skills, which is the fourth action area of the Ottawa Charter for Health Promotion.

Health promotion professional competencies

Health promotion professional competencies refer to the foundation knowledge, skills, values and attributes required for professional health promotion practice. Over the past 15 years several countries, including Australia (Australian Health Promotion Association, 2009; Shilton et al., 2001) and Aotearoa New Zealand (Health Promotion Forum of New Zealand, 2012), and at the global level the International Union for Health Promotion and Education (IUHPE) (Barry et al., 2012) have developed health promotion competency frameworks. These competency frameworks include a range of knowledge, and ethical and technical competencies required for best-practice health promotion action, and align with the philosophy of CPHC. They are designed for those in designated full-time health promotion roles and those in non-designated health promotion roles who undertake health promotion work as part of their role. In addition, they are used to design tertiary health promotion curricula, workforce development training, health promotion position descriptions, and inform credentialling or accreditation of the health promotion profession. Competencies for each nation vary according to the local practice context and the challenge in developing competencies for the international workforce is to develop robust and meaningful competencies for use in a broad context.

In Australia, the Australian Health Promotion Association, which is the peak professional body for health promotion in Australia, introduced the *Core Competencies for Health Promotion Practitioners* for Australia in 2009 (AHPA, 2009). These competencies have been used extensively within Australia and informed the development of competency frameworks by other countries and at the international level. Similarly, in 2012 the Health Promotion Forum of New Zealand, the peak professional health promotion body in New Zealand, published the *Health Promotion Competencies for Aotearoa New Zealand* (HPFNZ, 2012). Weblinks to these competency frameworks are included in the More to Explore section at the end of this chapter.

IUHPE core competencies and professional standards for health promotion

The IUHPE core competencies and professional standards for health promotion comprise nine domains of action which are underpinned by explicit ethical values and a knowledge domain (IUHPE, n.d.). Ethical values inform the context within which all the other competencies are practised (Fig. 1.6).

> *The IUHPE Core Competencies and Professional Standards for Health Promotion are underpinned by an understanding that Health Promotion has been shown to be an ethical, principled, effective and evidence-based discipline and that there are well-developed theories, strategies, evidence and values that determine good practice in Health Promotion. The term 'Health Promotion action' is used in the context of these competencies and standards to describe programmes, policies and other organised Health Promotion interventions that are empowering, participatory, holistic, inter-sectoral, equitable, sustainable and multi-strategy in nature, which aim to improve health and reduce health inequities.*
>
> *(Barry et al., 2012, p. 4)*

The knowledge domain describes the core concepts and principles that make health promotion practice distinctive. The remaining nine domains—enable change, advocate

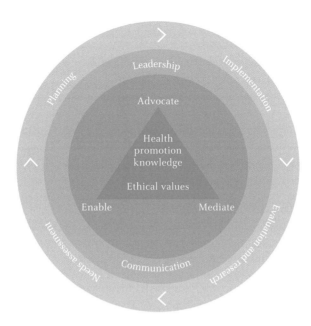

FIGURE 1.6 International Union for Health Promotion and Education's Core Competencies for Health Promotion
Source: IUHPE, n.d.

for health, mediate through partnership, communication, leadership, assessment, planning, implementation, and evaluation and research—each deal with a specific area of health promotion practice with their associated competency statements articulating the necessary skills needed for competent practice. It is the combined application of all the domains, the knowledge base and the ethical values which constitute the IUHPE Core Competencies Framework for Health Promotion (Barry et al., 2012, p. 7).

Health promotion competencies are also included in public health and other health professional frameworks. For example, the Council of Academic Public Health Institutions Australasia (CAPHIA), the peak organisation for public health departments in universities in Australia, New Zealand and Papua New Guinea, includes health promotion as one of eight public health competency areas of practice in its Foundation Competencies for Public Health Graduates in Australia, 2nd ed. (CAPHIA, 2016). Other frameworks that explicitly specify competencies and/or acknowledge health promotion as a component of professional work include:

- Code of conduct for registered health practitioners (Aboriginal and Torres Strait Islander Health Practice Board of Australia, 2014)
- Practice standards for mental health social workers (Australian Association of Social Workers, 2013)
- Professional competencies of the newly qualified dentist/dental hygienist, dental therapist and oral health therapist/dental prosthetist (Australian Dental Council, 2016)
- Australasian competency standards for paramedics (Paramedics Australia, 2011)
- Physiotherapy practice thresholds in Australia and Aotearoa New Zealand (Physiotherapy Board of Australia & Physiotherapy Board of New Zealand, 2015)

- Registered nurse accreditation standards (Australian Nursing & Midwifery Accreditation Council, 2012)
- Podiatry competency standards for Australia and New Zealand (Australian and New Zealand Podiatry Accreditation Council, 2015)
- Accreditation standards for pharmacy programs in Australia and New Zealand (Australian Pharmacy Council, 2020)
- National competency standards for dietitians in Australia (Dietitians Association of Australia, 2015)
- Environmental health course accreditation policy (Environmental Health Australia, 2014).

IUHPE health promotion accreditation system

The articulation of health promotion competencies has contributed significantly to the profession through the establishment of an international health promotion accreditation system by the IUHPE (Battel-Kirk and the IUHPE Global Accreditation Organisation Board of Directors, 2016; IUHPE, n.d.). The first global IUHPE Health Promotion Accreditation System was launched in 2016 at the 22nd IUHPE World Conference on Health Promotion in Brazil. This voluntary accreditation system is overseen by the IUHPE Global Accreditation Organisation and accreditation criteria are based on the Core Competencies and Professional Standards for Health Promotion. The purpose of the system is to '... promote quality assurance, competence and mobility in Health Promotion practice, education and training globally' and is available to individual practitioners and tertiary health promotion courses. Tertiary institutions that offer health promotion courses can apply for accreditation through the IUHPE Global Accreditation Organisation to become an 'IUHPE Accredited Health Promotion Course'. Accreditation is for a period of three years, after which re-accreditation needs to be sought. Students graduating from an 'IUHPE Accredited Health Promotion Course' are eligible to apply to become an 'IUHPE Registered Health Promotion Practitioner'. Practitioners that have a health promotion qualification from a health promotion course not accredited with the IUHPE Accreditation System, a course from a relevant discipline and two years' health promotion experience, or three years' experience in health promotion in the past five years, are eligible to apply either directly through the IUHPE online application system or via their regional- or country-level National Accreditation Organisation (NAO). An NAO is a health promotion body approved by the IUHPE Global Accreditation Organisation to undertake registration of individual health promotion practitioners. The Australian Health Promotion Association is the NAO for Australian health promotion professionals wanting to apply for registration. Individual practitioner registration is also for a period of three years after which re-registration needs to be sought and is dependent on continuing professional development in the field. Weblinks to the IUHPE Health Promotion Accreditation System and the Australian Health Promotion Association Health Promotion Practitioner Registration System are included in the More to Explore section at the end of this chapter.

A FRAMEWORK FOR HEALTH PROMOTION PRACTICE WITHIN A CPHC CONTEXT

We now present a framework of health promotion practice within a CPHC context (Fig. 1.7). The framework is underpinned by the socio-ecological determinants of health and wellbeing,

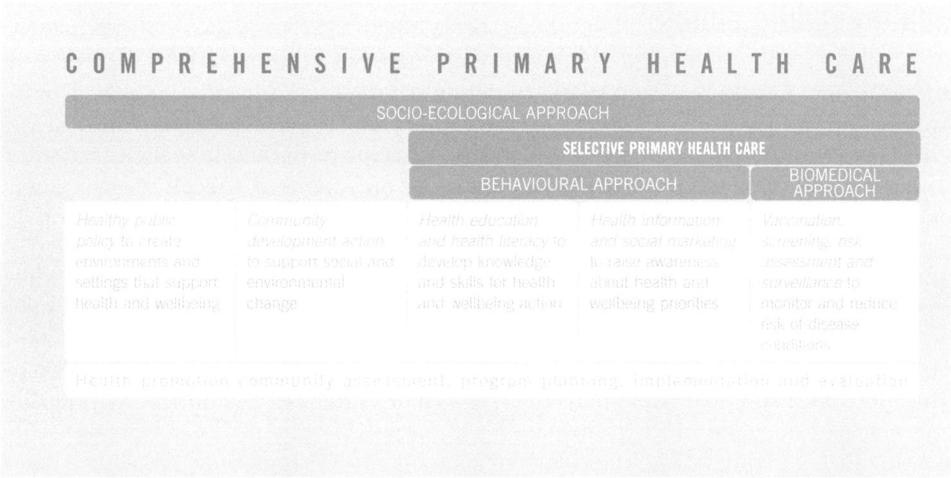

FIGURE 1.7 Framework for health promotion practice
Source: *Revised from Talbot & Verrinder, 2018. Originally adapted from Labonté, 1992.*

the Ottawa Charter for Health Promotion five action areas and three strategies (WHO, 1986) and a best practice community assessment, planning, implementation and evaluation process. The framework includes a portfolio of five broad strategy areas of health promotion action.

The purpose of the framework is to guide and support health practitioners undertaking health promotion work. The components of the framework and the five broad strategy areas of health promotion action are outlined briefly below. Each is then discussed more fully in Chapters 4 to 9, which aim to describe health promotion practice and draw on current health promotion case examples.

Health promotion community assessment, planning, implementation and evaluation

Health promotion community assessment, planning, implementation and evaluation are founded on best practice research knowledge and professional skills. These stages of a health promotion program , which are addressed in detail in Chapter 4 are underpinned by a set of ethical and technical values and principles (see Fig. 4.1 in Chapter 4). Throughout the cycle, health practitioners first identify health and wellbeing priorities of communities and examine the range of interrelated socio-ecological determinants of health and wellbeing that contribute to identified priorities. They then work out what health promotion strategies are needed to address the determinants of the identified priorities, and then implement these strategies. They need to evaluate the short-term impact of the strategies on the determinants of the health and wellbeing priority being addressed, and the long-term outcome(s) on the health and wellbeing priority. Finally, practitioners communicate the processes, short-term impacts and long-term outcomes of health promotion action to relevant community and professional audiences. The range of professional health promotion competencies required to undertake this scope of health promotion work were described earlier in this chapter (Barry et al., 2012). Competencies particular to the different health promotion strategy portfolio components are presented in Chapters 5 to 9.

Healthy public policy

Developing healthy public policy to create environments and settings that support health and wellbeing has been central to effective health promotion practice since the Ottawa Charter for Health Promotion (WHO, 1986). This action area is addressed in detail in Chapter 5. Healthy public policy describes the decisions enshrined in legislation, policy, strategic plans, rules, standards, codes of practice, or operations of a sector of government or an organisation, made on behalf of the relevant population or group to protect their health and wellbeing. Healthy public policy can be very broad and include policy at international, national, state and local government levels, regulatory activities including executive orders, local laws, ordinances, and organisational position statements, and formal and informal rules. Policies in particular settings, for example schools and workplaces, provide structural and regulatory support that cannot be implemented so readily elsewhere. The aim is to ensure that regulations relating to that setting, service directions, priorities and practices integrate CPHC principles. For example, the City of Greater Bendigo uses the One Planet Living policy framework to guide its process to become the world's most liveable community (City of Greater Bendigo, n.d.). Other examples of healthy public policy include SunSmart schools, antidiscrimination laws, and organisational health and wellbeing policies.

Community action

Community action to support social and environmental change aims to empower and build the capacity of communities (both geographic localities and communities of common purpose or interest) to develop and sustain improvements in their social and physical environments. This action area is addressed in detail in Chapter 6. Health promotion in this component of the portfolio typically comprises community organisation and development activities across whole communities or populations, such as local community capacity-building plans and activities. Examples include the many creative and innovative projects presented in *Fairer Health: Case Studies on Improving Health for All* (VicHealth, 2009), the *Transitioning Towns Toolbox* (McKinna & Wall, 2013) and the *All Ages All Ability Action Plan* (City of Greater Bendigo, 2019).

Advocacy is an important aspect of community action and involves a combination of individual, peer and social actions designed to gain political commitment, policy support, structural change, social acceptance and systems support for a particular goal. It includes direct political lobbying and may be carried out by health practitioners on behalf of a vulnerable community, or by the community itself. This involves change being made by people in their own locality or change at policy or planning level by a budget-holder, on behalf of another group of constituents, workers or population groups. Changes are likely to be sustained over time if community members are directly involved in identifying priorities and planning and implementing a response. Once in place, policies and economic regulatory activities can be a powerful lever for those seeking to make that setting more health promoting.

Health education and health literacy

Health education and health literacy focus on developing the knowledge and skills required for health and wellbeing action. These concepts are addressed in detail in Chapter 7. Health education is the provision of education to individuals or groups, and working with individuals as they develop self-awareness and personal skills with the aim of improving their knowledge, attitudes, self-efficacy and individual capacity for change. Activities may be organised around population groups with a common learning need, such as adolescents, culturally and linguistically diverse groups, same-sex attracted youth, Indigenous people or groups affected by a specific condition. Such groups are prioritised because of greater health and wellbeing needs, and they become the focus for specific health promotion and capacity-building strategies. The health literacy of individuals, commonly known as functional health literacy, refers to the knowledge, skills and capacity of people to access, understand and use health-related information to make decisions supportive of their health and wellbeing. For example, how to navigate the healthcare system, health-related information provided by a healthcare provider, or via printed or electronic media sources. The development of strategies to enhance the health literacy of people and the health literacy capability of health-related organisations and systems is an important component of health promotion work.

Health information and social marketing

Health information and social marketing are used to raise awareness about health and wellbeing priorities. These concepts are addressed in detail in Chapter 8. Social marketing programs are designed to advocate for change and influence the voluntary behaviour of priority audiences to benefit this audience and society as a whole. The aim is to shift attitudes, influence people's view of themselves and their relationships with others, change lifelong habits, values or behaviours, and make a sustained change in their personal health and wellbeing behaviour(s). Social marketing and health information typically use persuasive and cultural change processes (not just information). Health promotion activities are usually organised around behaviours, such as smoking, physical activity and ways to improve mental health, but are also now widely used to promote behaviours for enhancing environmental sustainability (French et al., 2009; McKenzie-Mohr, 2011).

The aim of health information programs is to create awareness of the determinants of health and illness, the services and support available to help maintain or improve health and wellbeing, and personal responsibility for actions affecting health and wellbeing. Examples include any of the various health awareness weeks. Programs can involve raising public awareness about a health priority through use of mass or limited-reach media; for example, advertising in newspapers, magazines, pamphlets and fliers or on radio, television and so forth at local, state and national levels. It may also involve a mix of promotional strategies including public relations and face-to-face communications (French et al., 2009; McKenzie-Mohr, 2011). Health information and social marketing health promotion actions are considered a behavioural approach because they seek to engage individuals in making informed choices to change to more health-enhancing behaviours, such as quitting smoking or eating a more nutritious diet. Naturally, some people will find this more difficult than others due to other determinants impacting a person's life.

Screening, individual risk assessment and surveillance

Screening, risk assessment and surveillance are used to monitor and reduce risk of disease conditions. These strategies are addressed in detail in Chapter 9. They are based on medical and epidemiological evidence that identifies opportunities to reduce the risk or enhance the early detection of diseases. For example, immunisation programs are based on scientific knowledge about immunology and improve public health for minimal costs. Equity is enhanced by government strategies, such as providing free immunisation, and by improving access for vulnerable population groups. Screening involves the systematic use of a test or investigatory tool to detect individuals at risk of developing a specific disease that is amenable to prevention or treatment at an early stage of detection. Activities include medical approaches designed to improve physiological risk factors for disease and early detection of some cancers.

Screening and individual risk-assessment activities are aimed at early detection of disease rather than the maintenance or improvement of good health. With early detection of a disease, complications that may further compromise the health of an individual may be avoided. Health promotion strategies in this area usually require individuals to initiate an activity to enhance their current or future health, such as attending screening, or to change an existing behaviour. The approaches do not alter the underlying life conditions for the individual. Individual risk factor assessment involves a more comprehensive process of detecting overall risk of a single disease or multiple diseases. These can include genetic, biological, psychological and behavioural risks. Surveillance activities are designed to inform potential whole-of-population responses to health risks that could have the capacity to affect large numbers of people. Potential risks posed by rapidly spread infectious diseases, such as influenza, involve global strategies to minimise spread.

COMPREHENSIVE PRIMARY HEALTH CARE INTO THE FUTURE

The CPHC approach has provided better knowledge and understanding of the socio-ecological determinants of health and wellbeing, and equity has been a core concern in CPHC, public health and health promotion organisations. There is ongoing acknowledgement that inequalities in social, economic and environmental circumstances continue to increase and erode conditions for health and wellbeing. Evidence also suggests that the CPHC approach delivers better health outcomes at lower costs in a socially acceptable way (Macinko et al., 2003; PHM et al., 2014; WHO, 2008b). CPHC is the only approach to health care that is capable of reducing the burden of disease among the poorest of the poor, and in doing so raise the health status of the population overall. To work within a CPHC approach is to work on the root causes of health and wellbeing, and illness. Greater impacts will be achieved when health promotion practice within a CPHC context becomes an integral, appropriately funded stream in national policy, in parallel with policies towards ensuring ecological sustainability (Ife & Tesoriero, 2006; Pettigrew et al., 2015).

In the decades following the Declaration of Alma-Ata, lessons for implementing a CPHC approach have emerged. First, while the WHO continues to promote a CPHC approach, its effect in practice has been described as limited (PHM et al., 2014). Adoption of an SPHC approach has resulted in disproportionate spending on medical care, which remains largely unchanged in most nations. Second, the rise of neoliberalism has brought about economic changes (including increased disparities between rich and poor), caused social and ecological degradation, and reduced spending on health care in some countries (Gillam, 2008; Labonté & Schrecker, 2006; PHM et al., 2014). Third, the implementation of UHC is not truly 'universal' in many countries (PHM et al., 2014) and the interpretation of UHC varies from country to country (WHO, 2016b). Inequities have been aggravated by health sector reform where local health services have been left unsupported and co-payments for services introduced or increased (PHM et al., 2014). Fourth, while SPHC has provided much-needed relief to address some behavioural and biomedical challenges, such as antiviral treatment for HIV transmission, action tackling the socio-ecological determinants of health and wellbeing has often been neglected. The reorientation of health systems to include health promotion has been patchy (Ziglio et al., 2011). Finally, intersectoral collaboration and community participation in health-related decisions have not necessarily been supported in this work (PHM et al., 2011).

Consequently, although life expectancy has risen overall globally, there are widening health inequalities within and between countries and some gains have been lost (WHO, 2015a). For these reasons, CPHC is more important than ever. There are, however, some challenges for the WHO, national governments and health practitioners to implement these strategies to improve population health. WHO reports provide expert information to guide government policy and funding decisions on specific subjects; for example, health research (WHO, 2012), health systems financing and universal coverage (WHO, 2010c, 2013c), primary health care (WHO, 2008b), and the health workforce (WHO, 2006, 2010b).

Health systems financing

There is great inequity in global healthcare spending, whereby richer countries spend more on health resources than do poorer countries (UNDP, 2011; WHO, 2019a). Globally, healthcare spending has grown substantially due to growth of the medico-industrial complex, referring to the health system which has an important (if not primary) function of making profits and two secondary functions, research and education (Navarro, 1976). Non-demographic factors such as technology and administrative costs have been important drivers of healthcare costs (Bryant & Sonerson, 2006; Mooney, 2012). This growth has occurred primarily in affluent countries such as those that are members of the OECD. However, higher spending on health care does not necessarily reflect that the system is based on equity, nor does it mean that universal access to basic public health services, such as sanitation, water supply and immunisation, is available. Over the past decade some LMICs are moving closer to various forms of universal health coverage (UHC); for example, China, Mexico, Rwanda, Turkey, South Africa, Brazil, Mexico and Tunisia (PHM et al., 2014) and the Western Pacific Region of the WHO (WHO, 2016b). UHC is one of the targets for the SDGs. However, these developments are not without challenges and it will be important to see how this coverage affects human development and life expectancy indices within each country. It is important to reiterate that 'universal healthcare, while critical, does not guarantee equal opportunity to be healthy. Universal solutions (aimed at the entire population) can be very effective in improving average health, but do not necessarily alter underlying health disparities' (Turrell et al., 2006 in Duckett, 2016, p. 4). Insight 1.4 provides an overview of the overall healthcare system spending in Australia.

INSIGHT 1.4 Overall healthcare system spending, Australia

The focus of the Australian healthcare system's spending overall has been largely on the provision of acute illness care services to individuals. This means that attention and resources are focused on treating health problems, rather than the determinants of health issues. This is reflected in the Australian health budget. In 2017–18, Australia spent 10% of its GDP on health services (AIHW, 2019b). The majority of health spending went on hospitals (40%) and primary health care (34%). Over the decade from 2007–08 to 2017–18, Australian Government expenditure on public hospitals increased by an average of 3.9% per year, and 3.3% per year for primary health care; these were the highest rates of increased funding of any component of the Australian health budget. From 2016–17 to 2017–18, spending declined on private hospitals, research, medical expenses tax rebates, patient transport services, and public health (AIHW, 2019b). There is scope for Australia to focus more of its health expenditure on the promotion and protection of health and wellbeing using a socio-ecological framework.

Source: AIHW, 2019b.

Development of equitable health systems

Evidence shows that more-equal societies are healthier and so it is reasonable to suggest that reducing socio-ecological inequalities should be the primary aim of health systems. Health systems are defined as 'the ensemble of all public and private organisations, institutions and resources mandated to improve, maintain or restore health' (The Tallinn Charter: health systems for health and wealth, cited in Kutzin & Sparkes, 2016). They encompass both personal and population services, as well as activities to influence the policies and actions of other sectors to address the socio-ecological determinants of health and wellbeing. If the system is to be 'universally accessible to the community through their full participation and at a cost that the community and country can afford' (WHO, 1978) then UHC is essential and health promotion must be part of the suite of strategies to improve health and wellbeing. Commitment to health equity is an essential part of effective stewardship. Health ministries are responsible for protecting citizens' health and ensuring quality care is provided. Pro-equity healthcare strategies differ from country to country. Access to health care is one measure of equity. Globally, this usually takes three forms. In the poorest countries, most of the population have equal but deficient access to health care. The people with the highest income in these countries find ways to obtain care. In richer countries, general access is better but people in the middle and upper income groups benefit most, and the people with lower incomes usually have to queue for care. In some countries, most of the population has adequate access to health care but a small minority, often the poorest, are deprived (WHO, 2003, p. 123).

The World Bank, however, favours 'a health system model of mixed public/private service delivery and stratified multi-payer health insurance markets with minimal safety net for the poor' (PHM et al., 2014, p. 255). These preferences reflect the power of neoliberalism and although there are sufficient resources worldwide to meet the challenges in health inequalities, 'many national health systems are weak, unresponsive, inequitable—even unsafe' (WHO, 2006). In Australia, Baum and colleagues concluded that 'a focus on clinical service provision, while highly compatible with neoliberal reforms, will not on its own produce the shifts in population disease patterns that would be required to reduce demand for health services and promote health' (2016, p. 43). They argue that CPHC is much better suited to that task. It is worth noting that only 10 to 15% of gains in life expectancy are estimated to be attributable to health care (Leys, 2009, p. 6 in PHM et al., 2014) but CPHC has made an important contribution to gains in quality of life for many.

Despite this recognition, it is concerning that the WHO is under continuing pressure to implement SPHC and to 'retreat to a purely technical role and withdraw from any effective engagement with the political and economic dynamics that characterise the global health crisis' (PHM et al., 2014, p. 5). As an organisation, it is funded by member states and contributions from donors. Members from the rich and powerful countries dominate policy directions in their role as donors and non-government agencies are beholden to donor funding and agendas (PHM et al., 2014). TNCs such as those in the pharmaceutical industry exert political influence through donations (Oxfam, 2015). Yet international organisations such as the WHO, UNICEF and the International Labour Organization have expressed concerns about the impacts of the neoliberal agenda.

Health practitioners working in CPHC need to join the discussion about 'public goods' and the negative health and wellbeing impacts of structural adjustments, global financing and austerity measures. Thinking globally means supporting the need to re-regulate global finance, rejecting austerity measures and tax havens, and supporting global tax systems, and everyone needs to confront the question of limits to growth if we are to have a habitable planet (PHM et al., 2014). Acting locally means working towards and within a fair (universally accessible) health system.

Global health workforce

The security of an adequate global health workforce is a priority for healthcare systems. There is not only a shortage of the number of people who make the systems work, but of the right mix of skills from acute care through to health promotion and rehabilitation, particularly in the poorest countries. Rural and isolated areas are most disadvantaged in countries such as Australia (Humphreys, 2012) and across the world. Migration of health practitioners compounds the problem. Affluent nations have actively recruited new health graduates, such as doctors and nurses, from universities in poorer nations overseas in order to meet their workforce shortages (Mooney, 2012). The promise of high wages is hard to resist for new graduates, but the 'brain drain' has a significant effect on the already poor healthcare systems of these nations. Affluent nations have effectively transferred the cost of tertiary education for more professionals to the economies of countries that can least afford it (WHO, 2006). There is an unequal distribution of health practitioners within and between countries. Sheikh (2012, p. 233) reports that 'there is an undeniable correlation between countries facing the greatest burden of maternal and child deaths and those with health workforce shortages'. Cost containment measures, changed priorities, weak education and health management systems, and discrimination contribute to the problem (Sheikh, 2012; WHO, 2006).

To address the challenge of migration, the WHO Global Code of Practice on the International Recruitment of Health Personnel was adopted in 2010. The aim of the Code is to establish and promote voluntary principles and practices for the ethical international recruitment of health personnel and to facilitate the strengthening of health systems. Active recruitment of health personnel from developing countries facing critical shortages of health practitioners is discouraged between member states (WHO, 2010b).

Evidence suggests that offering workers good working conditions, adequate remuneration, the chance to work in a supportive team, the opportunity for further education and being shown respect, develops a healthy workforce. To achieve the goals associated with healthcare systems driven by CPHC philosophy, renewed commitment and new options for education and employment of health practitioners are required (WHO, 2010b). Sheikh (2012) argues that ministries within governments of education, health, public services, labour, foreign affairs, finance and international trade all have a role to play.

Health information systems

A health information system (HIS) based on CPHC principles can be defined as 'an integrated effort to collect, process, report and use health information and knowledge to influence policy-making, program action and research' (WHO, 2003, p. 116). The information can be used for strategic decision making and for program planning, implementation, monitoring and evaluation. Robust health information systems are needed in healthcare systems oriented to CPHC principles so that the needs of the population, particularly those most in need, can be understood and addressed efficiently and effectively. The WHO's *Components of a Strong Health Information System* (WHO, 2008a) provides a framework for countries based on inputs, processes and outputs. The inputs include all health information system resources, the physical and structural prerequisites of an HIS including: the ability of those responsible to lead and coordinate the process; the existence of policies; financial resources; and people with the necessary skills to do the work. The processes used by an

HIS include health indicators from a variety of data sources that produce an accessible, relevant management system that protects the privacy of an individual. The outputs need to be useful evidence for decision making. Information should then be synthesised into usable statistics and widely disseminated.

The lack of appropriate timely evidence threatens healthcare systems. Health research was the focus of the *World Health Report 2013—Research for Universal Health Coverage* (WHO, 2013c). At the international level, research initiatives and knowledge to action practices in public health have been encouraged by the WHO. The 2013 report highlighted the significance of conducting and translating health research to improve the health of populations.

CONCLUSION

The purpose of this chapter was to establish the foundations for health promotion practice within a CPHC context. Despite significant gains in various health indicators around much of the world, there remain troubling health inequalities within and between countries. In the last 40 years, particularly through the work of the WHO, we have seen the development of numerous international, national and local policies and programs to support health promotion practice within a CPHC context. These developments occurred as a result of recognition of the socio-ecological determinants of health and wellbeing and their role in exacerbating or ameliorating health inequalities. It is acknowledged that health promotion practice within a CPHC context can contribute to the success of the SDGs (UN, 2015) by addressing the socio-ecological determinants of health and wellbeing and health inequalities.

Practitioners can, in their daily role, promote social and environmental justice and foster healthy, sustainable and peaceful environments by engaging in evidence-based health promotion practice within a CPHC context. To do this, any practitioner engaged in health promotion, either in a designated role or with health promotion as part of their broader role, needs to have the required health promotion competencies to perform the role ethically and effectively. They will also benefit from using frameworks that facilitate best health promotion practice. Many of the key strategies and skills required to do this effectively are discussed in the remainder of this book. Health practitioners are encouraged to develop their knowledge and skills in health promotion so that they may contribute to making life better and fairer for the people in their communities.

MORE TO EXPLORE

THE SOCIO-ECOLOGICAL DETERMINANTS OF HEALTH

- ABC Radio National. (2016, September 3). Health inequalities and the causes of the causes. The 56th Boyer Lecture Series (Sir Michael Marmot): http://www.abc.net.au/radionational/programs/boyerlectures/boyer-lecture-health-inequality-and-the-causes-of-the-causes/7763106
- The School of Life. (2014). Why some countries are poor and others rich. [video] https://www.youtube.com/watch?sns=fb&v=9-4V3HR696k&app=desktop
- WHO. (n.d.). Social determinants of health. Key concepts. http://www.who.int/social_determinants/thecommission/finalreport/key_concepts/en/
- WHO. (2013b). The many paths towards universal health coverage [video] https://www.youtube.com/watch?v=VQ3sHfYzcv8&feature=youtu.be

HEALTH PROMOTION CONFERENCE CHARTERS AND DECLARATIONS

- The Ottawa Charter for Health Promotion: https://www.who.int/healthpromotion/conferences/previous/ottawa/en/
- Adelaide Recommendations on Healthy Public Policy: https://www.who.int/healthpromotion/conferences/previous/adelaide/en/
- Sundsvall Statement on Supportive Environments for Health: https://www.who.int/healthpromotion/conferences/previous/sundsvall/en/
- Jakarta Declaration on Leading Health Promotion into the 21st Century: https://www.who.int/healthpromotion/conferences/previous/jakarta/declaration/en/
- Mexico Ministerial Statement for the Promotion of Health: https://www.who.int/healthpromotion/conferences/previous/mexico/statement/en/
- Bangkok Charter for Health Promotion in a Globalized World: https://www.who.int/healthpromotion/conferences/6gchp/bangkok_charter/en/
- Nairobi Call to Action: https://www.who.int/healthpromotion/conferences/7gchp/en/
- The Helsinki Statement on Health in All Policies: https://www.who.int/healthpromotion/conferences/8gchp/statement_2013/en/
- Shanghai Declaration on promoting health in the 2030 Agenda for Sustainable Development: https://www.who.int/healthpromotion/conferences/9gchp/shanghai-declaration/en/

HEALTH PROMOTION COMPETENCIES

- Core Competencies for Australian Health Promotion Practitioners: https://www.healthpromotion.org.au/images/docs/core_competencies_for_hp_practitioners.pdf
- Health Promotion Competencies for Aotearoa New Zealand: http://hauora.co.nz/assets/files/Health%20Promotion%20Competencies%20%20Final.pdf
- International Union for Health Promotion and Education Core Competencies and Professional Standards for Health Promotion: https://www.iuhpe.org/images/JC-Accreditation/Core_Competencies_Standards_linkE.pdf

HEALTH PROMOTION ACCREDITATION SYSTEMS

- Australian Health Promotion Association Health Promotion Registration System: https://registration.healthpromotion.org.au/
- International Union for Health Promotion and Education Health Promotion Accreditation System: www.iuhpe.org/index.php/en/the-accreditation-system; https://www.iuhpe.org/images/JC-Accreditation/System_handbook_Full_LinkA.pdf

IUHPE Core Competencies for Health Promotion

The IUHPE Core Competencies for Health Promotion comprises nine domains of action. Each domain has a set of core competency statements and a detailed outline of the knowledge and skills that contribute to competency in that domain.

The content of this chapter relates especially to the achievement of competency in the health promotion domains outlined below.

1. Enable change	*1.1 Work collaboratively across sectors to influence the development of public policies which impact positively on health and reduce health inequities.* Determinants of health and health inequities
	1.2 Use health promotion approaches which support empowerment, participation, partnership and equity to create environments and settings which promote health. Health promotion models
	1.5 Work in collaboration with key stakeholders to reorient health and other services to promote health and reduce health inequities. Theory and practice of collaborative working
2. Advocate for health	*2.3 Raise awareness of and influence public opinion on health issues.* Ability to work with diverse individuals and groups
	2.4 Advocate for the development of policies, guidelines and procedures across all sectors which impact positively on health and reduce health inequities. Health and wellbeing issues relating to a specified population or group
3. Mediate through partnership	*3.2 Facilitate effective partnership working which reflects health promotion values and principles.* Theory and practice of collaborative working
5. Leadership	*5.2 Use leadership skills which facilitate empowerment and participation (including teamwork, negotiation, motivation, conflict resolution, decision making, facilitation and problem solving).* Emerging challenges in health and health promotion
6. Assessment	*6.4 Identify the determinants of health which impact on health promotion action.* Available data and information sources Social determinants of health
	6.7 Identify priorities for health promotion action in partnership with stakeholders based on best available evidence and ethical values. Health inequalities Evidence base for health promotion action and priority setting

7. Planning	*7.2 Use current models and systematic approaches for planning health promotion action*
	Use and effectiveness of current health promotion planning models and theories
9. Evaluation and research	*9.5 Contribute to the development and dissemination of health promotion evaluation and research processes.*
	Use appropriate evaluation and research methods, in partnership with stakeholders, to determine the reach, impact and effectiveness of health promotion action

In addition, IUHPE specifies knowledge, skills and performance criteria essential for health promotion practitioners to act professionally and ethically, including having knowledge of ethical and legal issues, behaving in an ethical and respectful manner and working in ways that review and improve practice. Full details are available at: http://www.iuhpe.org/index.php/en/the-accreditation-system

Reflective Questions

1. Review the discussion about the WHO definition of health in this chapter. What are the implications for health promotion practice of using this definition, rather than the narrower 'absence of illness' definition?

2. Using the Iceberg Model (Figure 1.4), identify as many individual and environmental determinants as possible that impact on your physical, mental, spiritual and social health and wellbeing.

3. Review the philosophy and scope of activity undertaken by your local District Health Board in New Zealand (see Insight 1.1), Aboriginal Community Controlled Health Organisation (see Insight 1.2) or Primary Health Network in Australia (see Insight 1.3). Discuss whether this philosophy and scope of work is more aligned with a comprehensive or selective primary health care approach.

4. Refer to Table 1.1 which provides an overview of the nine WHO global health promotion charters, declarations and statements. The 2016 Shanghai Declaration on promoting health in the 2030 Agenda for Sustainable Development outlines key actions for health promotion. Identify and discuss the role you might play as a practitioner in contributing to this agenda at global, national and local levels.

5. Health promotion professional competencies refer to the foundation knowledge, skills, values and attributes required for professional health promotion practice. At the global level, the International Union for Health Promotion and Education (IUHPE) has developed a health promotion competency framework which you can access in the More to Explore section of this chapter. Reflect on your current level of competence (emerging, developing, proficient) in each of the nine domains. To do so, consider the competency statements within each domain. What strategies might you use to further develop your health promotion competencies?

REFERENCES

ABC Radio National. (2016). Health inequality and the causes of the causes. The 56th Boyer Lecture Series (Sir Michael Marmot). [Audio podcast]. Retrieved from http://www.abc.net.au/radionational/programs/boyerlectures/2016-boyer-lectures/7802472.

Aboriginal and Torres Strait Islander Health Practice Board of Australia. (2014). Code of conduct for registered health practitioners. Retrieved from https://www.atsihealthpracticeboard.gov.au/Codes-Guidelines/Code-of-conduct.aspx

Ah Chee, D. (2015, Aug. 02). Learn from 'one of the best examples in the world of a comprehensive primary healthcare service' [Blog post]. In M. Sweet (Ed.), The crikey health blog. Retrieved from http://blogs.crikey.com.au/croakey/2015/08/02/learn-from-one-of-the-best-examples-in-the-world-of-a-comprehensive-primary-healthcare-service/.

Australian and New Zealand Podiatry Accreditation Council. (2015). Podiatry competency standards for Australia and New Zealand. Retrieved from http://www.anzpac.org.au/files/Podiatry%20Competency%20Standards%20for%20Australia%20and%20New%20Zealand%20V1.1%20201212%20(Final).pdf.

Australian Association of Social Workers. (2013). Practice standards. Retrieved from http://www.aasw.asn.au/document/item/4551.

Australian Dental Council. (2016). Professional competencies of the newly qualified dentist/dental hygienist, dental therapist and oral health therapist/dental prosthetist. Retrieved from https://www.adc.org.au/Program-Accreditation/Program-Accreditation-Standards.

Australian Government. (2018). PHN – an Australian Government Initiative. Retrieved from https://www1.health.gov.au/internet/main/publishing.nsf/Content/PHN-Home

Australian Government. (2020). Closing the gap report 2020. Retrieved from https://ctgreport.niaa.gov.au.

Australian Health Promotion Association (AHPA). (2009). Core competencies for health promotion practitioners. Retrieved from https://www.healthpromotion.org.au/images/docs/core_competencies_for_hp_practitioners.pdf.

Australian Institute of Health and Welfare (AIHW). (2014). Australia's health 2014. Retrieved from http://www.aihw.gov.au/australias-health/2014/how-healthy/.

Australian Institute of Health and Welfare (AIHW). (2018). Australia's health 2018. Retrieved from https://www.aihw.gov.au/reports-data/health-welfare-overview/australias-health/reports

Australian Institute of Health and Welfare (AIHW). (2019a). Deaths in Australia. Retrieved from https://www.aihw.gov.au/reports/life-expectancy-death/deaths-in-australia

Australian Institute of Health and Welfare (AIHW). (2019b). Health expenditure Australia 2017–18. Health and welfare expenditure series no. 65. Cat. no. HWE 77. Canberra: AIHW. Retrieved from https://www.aihw.gov.au/getmedia/80dcaae7-e50f-4895-be1f-b475e578eb1b/aihw-hwe-77.pdf.aspx?inline=true.

Australian Nursing & Midwifery Accreditation Council. (2012). Registered nurse accreditation standards. Retrieved from https://www.anmac.org.au/sites/default/files/documents/ANMAC_RN_Accreditation_Standards_2012.pdf.

Australian Pharmacy Council. (2020). The accreditation standards for pharmacy programs in Australia and New Zealand. Retrieved from https://www.ccea.com.au/files/1015/0450/1916/CCEA_Accreditation_and_Competency_Standards_2017.pdf.

Barry, M. M., Battel-Kirk, B., Davison, H., et al. (2012). The CompHP project handbooks. International Union for Health Promotion and Education (IUHPE), Paris. Retrieved from: http://www.iuhpe.org/images/PROJECTS/ACCREDITATION/CompHP_Project_Handbooks.pdf.

Battel-Kirk, B. and the IUHPE Global Accreditation Organisation Board of Directors. (2016). The IUHPE health promotion accreditation system handbook. IUHPE, Paris. Retrieved from https://www.iuhpe.org/images/JC-Accreditation/System_handbook_Full_LinkA.pdf

Baum, F. (2008). The new public health, 3rd ed. South Melbourne: Oxford University Press.

Baum, F., Freeman, T., Sanders, D., et al. (2016). Comprehensive primary health care under neoliberalism in Australia. Social Science & Medicine, 68, 43–52. https://doi.org/10.1016/j.socscimed.2016.09.005.

Baum, F., & Sanders, D. (2011). Ottawa 25 years on: a more radical agenda for health equity is still required. Health Promotion International, 26(S2). https://doi.org/10.1093/heapro/dar078.

Bryant, J., & Sonerson, A. (2006). Gauging the cost of aging. Finance and Development International Monetary Fund, 43(3). Retrieved from http://www.imf.org/external/pubs/ft/fandd/2006/09/bryant.htm.

City of Greater Bendigo. (2019). All ages all abilities action plan October 2019. Retrieved from https://www.bendigo.vic.gov.au/sites/default/files/2019-10/All%20Ages%20All%20Abilities%20Action%20Plan%202019.pdf.

City of Greater Bendigo. (n.d.) One planet living. Retrieved from https://www.bendigo.vic.gov.au/About/One-Planet-Living.

Council of Academic Public Health Institutions Australasia. (2016). Foundation competencies for public health graduates in Australia, 2nd ed. Retrieved from http://caphia.com.au/testsite/wp-content/uploads/2016/07/CAPHIA_document_DIGITAL_nov_22.pdf.

Craig, E., Dell, R., Reddington, A., et al. (2015). Te Ohonga Ake: the determinants of health for Māori children and young people in New Zealand. Ministry of Health (New Zealand). Retrieved from http://www.health.govt.nz/publication/te-ohonga-ake-health-maori-children-and-young-people-chronic-conditions-and-disabilities-new-zealand.

CSDH. (2008). Closing the gap in a generation: health equity through action on the social determinants of health. Final Report of the Commission on Social Determinants of Health. World Health Organization. Retrieved from https://www.who.int/social_determinants/thecommission/finalreport/en/

de Leeuw, E. (2011). Editorial: The boulder in the stream. Health Promotion International, 26(S2). https://doi.org/10.1093/heapro/dar083.

Dietitians Association of Australia. (2015). National competency standards for dietitians in Australia. Retrieved from https://daa.asn.au/wp-content/uploads/2017/01/NCS-Dietitians-Australia-with-guide-1.0.pdf.

Duckett, S. (2016). Perils of place: identifying hotspots of health inequality. Grattan Institute. Retrieved from http://grattan.edu.au/report/perils-of-place-identifying-hotspots-of-health-inequality/.

Environmental Health Australia. (2014). Environmental health course accreditation policy. Retrieved from https://www.eh.org.au/documents/item/331.

Fair Society, Healthy Lives (The Marmot Review). (2010). Strategic review of health inequalities in England post 2010. Retrieved from http://www.instituteofhealthequity.org/resources-reports/fair-society-healthy-lives-the-marmot-review/fair-society-healthy-lives-full-report-pdf.pdf

French, J., Blair-Stevens, C., McVey, D., & Merritt, R. (2009). Social marketing and public health: theory and practice. Oxford: Oxford Scholarship.

Gillam, S. (2008). Is the Declaration of Alma-Ata still relevant to primary health care? British Medical Journal, 336, 536–538. https://doi.org/10.1136/bmj.39469.432118.AD.

Green, L., & Raeburn, J. (1988). Health promotion: what is it? What will it become? Health Promotion International, 3(2), 151–159. https://doi.org/10.1093/heapro/3.2.151.

Health Promotion Forum of New Zealand. (2012). Health promotion competencies for Aotearoa New Zealand. Retrieved from http://hauora.co.nz/assets/files/Health%20Promotion%20Competencies%20%20Final.pdf.

Helliwell, J., Layard, R., & Sachs, J. (2019). World happiness report 2019. Retrieved from https://worldhappiness.report/ed/2019/

Hoy, W. (2009). Closing the gap by 2030: aspiration versus reality in Indigenous health. Medical Journal of Australia, 190(10), 542–544.

Humphreys, J. (2012). 'Rural and remote health' in understanding the Australian health care system. Sydney: Elsevier.

Hyder, A. A., Puvanachandra, P., & Morrow, R. H. (2012). Measuring the health of populations: explaining composite indicators. Journal of Public Health Research, 1(3), 222–228. https://doi.org/10.4081/jphr.2012.e35

Ife, J. W., & Tesoriero, F. (2006). Community development: community-based alternatives in an age of globalisation (3rd ed.). Sydney: Pearson Education.

Illich, I. (1975). Limits to medicine: medical nemesis: the expropriation of health. Harmondsworth: Penguin.

International Union for Health Promotion and Education (IUHPE). (n.d.). The IUHPE health promotion accreditation system. Retrieved from www.iuhpe.org/index.php/en/the-accreditation-system.

Jeffrey, K., Wheatley, H., Abdallah, S. (2016) The happy planet index: 2016. A global index of sustainable well-being. London: New Economics Foundation. Retrieved from http://www.happy-planet-index.com/

Kickbusch, I. S. (1989). Good planets are hard to find. WHO Healthy Cities Papers #5. Copenhagen: World Health Organization.

Kutzin, J., & Sparkes, S. (2016). Health systems strengthening, universal health coverage, health security and resilience. Bulletin of the World Health Organization, 94, 2. http://dx.doi.org/10.2471/BLT.15.165050.

Labonté, R. (1992). Heart health inequities in Canada: models, theory and planning. Health Promotion International, 7(2), 119–121.

Labonté, R. (1997). Power, participation and partnerships for health promotion. VicHealth, Melbourne, Ch 2: 13, 21 (c) Victorian Health Promotion Foundation (VicHealth). Retrieved from https://www.vichealth.vic.gov.au/media-and-resources/publications/power-participation-and-partnerships-for-health-promotion

Labonté, R., & Schrecker, T. (2006). Globalization and social determinants of health: analytic and strategic review paper. On behalf of the Globalization Knowledge Network. Institute of Population Health. University of Ottawa. Retrieved from http://www.who.int/social_determinants/resources/globalization.pdf.

Lalonde, M. (1974). A new perspective on the health of Canadians: a working document. Retrieved from http://www.phac-aspc.gc.ca/ph-sp/pdf/perspect-eng.pdf.

Leys, C. (2009). Health, health care and capitalism. In L. Pannitch & C. Leys (Eds.), Morbid symptoms: health under capitalism. Pontypool: Merlin Press.

Macinko, J., Starfield, B., & Shi, L. (2003). The contribution of primary care systems to health outcomes within Organization for Economic Cooperation and Development (OECD) countries, 1970–1998. Health Services Research, 38, 831–865. https://doi.org/10.1111/1475-6773.00149.

McKenzie-Mohr, D. (2011). Fostering sustainable behavior: an introduction to community-based social marketing (3rd ed.). British Columbia, Canada: New Society Publishers.

McKeown, T. (1979). The role of medicine: dream, mirage or nemesis? Oxford: Basil Blackwell.

McKinna, D., & Wall, C. (2013). Transitioning towns toolbox. Loddon Mallee Regional Development Australia. Retrieved from http://www.rdv.vic.gov.au/?a=1159239.

Médecins Sans Frontières (MSF). (n.d.). Retrieved from http://www.msf.org.

Ministry of Health. (2016). New Zealand health strategy: future direction. Retrieved from http://www.health.govt.nz/new-zealand-health-system/new-zealand-health-strategy-future-direction.

Ministry of Health. (2018). New Zealand health system. Retrieved from https://www.health.govt.nz/new-zealand-health-system

Ministry of Health. (2019a). Annual update of key results 2018/19: New Zealand health survey. Retrieved from https://www.health.govt.nz/publication/annual-update-key-results-2018-19-new-zealand-health-survey

Ministry of Health. (2019b). Wai 2575 Māori health trends report. Wellington: Ministry of Health. Retrieved from https://www.health.govt.nz/publication/wai-2575-maori-health-trends-report

Ministry of Health. (n.d.). District health boards. Retrieved from http://www.health.govt.nz/new-zealand-health-system/key-health-sector-organisations-and-people/district-health-boards.

Mooney, G. (2012). Health of nations: towards a new political economy. London: Zed Books.

National Aboriginal Community Controlled Health Organization (NACCHO). (n.d.) Retrieved from https://www.naccho.org.au/about/.

Navarro, V. (1976). The underdevelopment of health of working America: causes, consequences and possible solutions. American Journal Public Health, 66(6), 538–547. https://doi.org/10.2105/AJPH.66.6.538.

Organisation for Economic Co-operation and Development (OECD). (2019). Life expectancy at birth. https://doi.org/10.1787/27e0fc9d-en. Retrieved from https://data.oecd.org/healthstat/life-expectancy-at-birth.htm.

Oxfam. (2015). Oxfam issue briefing—Wealth: having it all and wanting more. Retrieved from https://www.oxfam.org/en/research/wealth-having-it-all-and-wanting-more.

Paramedics Australia. (2011). Australasian competency standards for paramedics. Retrieved from https://nasemso.org/wp-content/uploads/PA_Australasian-Competency-Standards-for-paramedics-2011.pdf.

People's Health Movement (PHM), Medact, Medico International, et al. (2011). Global health watch 3: an alternative world health report. London: Zed Books.

People's Health Movement (PHM), Medact, Medico International, et al. (2014). Global health watch 4: an alternative world health report. London: Zed Books.

Perinatal Maternal Mortality Review Committee. (2017). Eleventh annual report of the perinatal and maternal mortality review committee: reporting mortality and morbidity 2015. Wellington: Health Quality Safety Commission. Retrieved from https://www.hqsc.govt.nz/assets/PMMRC/Publications/2017_PMMRC_Eleventh_Annual_Report.pdf

Pettigrew, L. M., De Maeseneer, J., Padula Anderson, M.-I., et al. (2015). Primary health care and the Sustainable Development Goals. The Lancet, 386(10009), 2119–2121. http://dx.doi.org/10.1016/S0140-6736(15)00949-6.

Physiotherapy Board of Australia & Physiotherapy Board of New Zealand. (2015). Physiotherapy practice thresholds in Australia and Aotearoa New Zealand. Retrieved from https://physiocouncil.com.au/wp-content/uploads/2017/10/Physiotherapy-Board-Physiotherapy-practice-thresholds-in-Australia-and-Aotearoa-New-Zealand.pdf.

Reeve, C., Humphreys, J. S., Wakerman, J., et al. (2015). Strengthening primary health care: achieving health gains in a remote region of Australia. Medical Journal Australia, 202(9), 483–487. https://doi.org/10.5694/mja14.00894.

Rifkin, S., & Walt, G. (1986). Why health improves: defining the issues concerning 'comprehensive primary health care' and 'selective primary health care. Social Science and Medicine, 23(6), 559–566. https://doi.org/10.1016/0277-9536(86)90149-8.

Sheikh, M. (2012). Health workers and the MDGs: inextricably linked. Geneva: Global Health Workforce Alliance, World Health Organization. Health and Welfare, Commonwealth Ministers' Reference Book 2012.

Shilton, T., Howat, P., James, R., & Lower, T. (2001). Health promotion development and health promotion workforce competency in Australia. Health Promotion Journal of Australia, 12(2), 117–123.

Statistics New Zealand. (2018). Life expectancy. Retrieved from https://www.health.govt.nz/our-work/populations/maori-health/tatau-kahukura-maori-health-statistics/nga-mana-hauora-tutohu-health-status-indicators/life-expectancy

Talbot, L., & Verrinder, G. (2005). Promoting health: the primary health care approach, 3rd ed. Sydney: Elsevier.

Talbot, L., & Verrinder, G. (2018). Promoting health: the primary health care approach, 6th ed. Sydney: Elsevier.

Travis, J. W., & Ryan, R. S. (2004). Wellness workbook (3rd ed.). Berkeley, CA: Ten Speed Press.

Turrell, G., Stanley, L., Looper, M. D., & Oldenburg, B. (2006). Health inequalities in Australia: morbidity, health behaviours, risk factors and health service use No. 2. Queensland: Queensland University of Technology and the Australian Institute of Health and Welfare.

United Nations. (2015). Sustainable development knowledge platform. Transforming our world: the 2030 agenda for sustainable development. Retrieved from https://sustainabledevelopment.un.org/post2015/transformingourworld.

United Nations. (2019). The sustainable development goals report 2019. Retrieved from https://unstats.un.org/sdgs/report/2019/The-Sustainable-Development-Goals-Report-2019.pdf

United Nations Development Program (UNDP). (2011). Human Development Report 2011. Retrieved from http://hdr.undp.org/en/content/human-development-report-2011.

United Nations Development Program (UNDP). (2019). Human development report 2019. Beyond income, beyond averages, beyond today: inequalities in human development in the 21st century. Retrieved from http://hdr.undp.org/sites/default/files/hdr2019.pdf

United Nations Interagency Group for Child Mortality Estimation. (2019). Child mortality estimates. Retrieved from https://childmortality.org/

VicHealth. (2009). Fairer health: case studies on improving health for all. Retrieved from https://www.vichealth.vic.gov.au/media-and-resources/publications/fairer-health—case-studies-on-improving-health-for-all.

Vinson, T., Rawsthorne, M., Beavis, A., & Ericson, M. (2015). Dropping off the edge: persistent communal disadvantage in Australia. Curtin, ACT: Jesuit Social Services, Richmond, Victoria, Catholic Social Services.

Vuori, H. (1986). Health for all, primary health care and the general practitioners. Retrieved from https://www.ncbi.nlm.nih.gov/pmc/articles/PMC1960528/pdf/jroyalcgprac00153-0008.pdf

Wallerstein, N., Mendes, R., Minkler, M., & Akerman, M. (2011). Reclaiming the social in community movements: perspectives from the USA and Brazil/South America: 25 years after Ottawa. Health Promotion International, 26(S2), ii226–ii236. https://doi.org/10.1093/heapro/dar077.

Whitehead, D., & Irvine, F. (2011). Ottawa 251—'All aboard the dazzling bandwagon'—developing personal skills: what remains for the future? Health Promotion International, 26(S2). https://doi.org/10.1093/heapro/dar072.

Wilkinson, R., & Pickett, K. (2009). The spirit level: why more equal societies almost always do better. London: Allen Lane.

World Bank. (2019). The classification of countries by income. Retrieved from https://datatopics.worldbank.org/world-development-indicators/stories/the-classification-of-countries-by-income.html

World Health Organization. (1948). World Health Organization constitution. Online. Available: https://www.who.int/about/who-we-are/constitution.

World Health Organization. (1978). Declaration of Alma-Ata. Retrieved from http://www.who.int/publications/almaata_declaration_en.pdf.

World Health Organization. (1986). The Ottawa Charter for Health Promotion. Retrieved from http://www.who.int/healthpromotion/conferences/previous/ottawa/en.

World Health Organization. (1988). Adelaide recommendations on healthy public policy. Retrieved from https://www.who.int/healthpromotion/conferences/previous/adelaide/en/.

World Health Organization. (1991). Sundsvall statement on supportive environments for health. Retrieved from https://www.who.int/healthpromotion/conferences/previous/sundsvall/en/.

World Health Organization. (1997). Jakarta declaration on leading health promotion into the 21st century. Retrieved from https://www.who.int/healthpromotion/conferences/previous/jakarta/declaration/en/.

World Health Organization. (2000). The fifth global conference on health promotion: Health promotion: bridging the equity gap. Retrieved from https://www.who.int/healthpromotion/conferences/previous/mexico/en/hpr_mexico_report_en.pdf.

World Health Organization. (2003). The world health report 2003—shaping the future. WHO, Geneva. Retrieved from http://www.who.int/whr/2003/en/.

World Health Organization. (2005). Bangkok charter for health promotion. Retrieved from https://www.who.int/healthpromotion/conferences/6gchp/en/.

World Health Organization. (2006). The world health report 2006—working together for health. Retrieved from http://www.who.int/whr/2006/en/.

World Health Organization. (2007). Civil society report on Commission of Social Determinants of Health. Retrieved from http://www.who.int/social_determinants/publications/civilsociety/en/index.html.

World Health Organization. (2008a) Components of a strong health information system: frameworks and standards for country Health Information Systems (2nd ed.). The Health Metrics Network. Geneva: WHO.

World Health Organization. (2008b). The world health report 2008—primary health care: now more than ever. Retrieved from http://www.who.int/whr/2008/en/.

World Health Organization. (2009). 7th global conference on health promotion. Retrieved from https://www.who.int/healthpromotion/conferences/7gchp/en/.

World Health Organization. (2010a) Adelaide statement on Health in All Policies. Retrieved from https://www.who.int/social_determinants/hiap_statement_who_sa_final.pdf.

World Health Organization. (2010b). Health workforce: managing health workforce migration—the global code of practice. Retrieved from http://www.who.int/hrh/migration/code/practice/en/.

World Health Organization. (2010c). World health report—health systems financing: the path to universal coverage. Retrieved from http://www.who.int/whr/2010/en/.

World Health Organization. (2011). Rio political declaration on social determinants of health, world conference on social determinants of health, Rio De Janeiro, Brazil, 19–21 October, 2011. Retrieved from http://www.who.int/sdhconference/declaration/Rio_political_declaration.pdf.

World Health Organization. (2012). World health statistics 2012. Retrieved from http://www.who.int/gho/publications/world_health_statistics/EN_WHS2012_Full.pdf.

World Health Organization. (2013a). The Helsinki statement on health in all policies. Retrieved from http://www.who.int/healthpromotion/conferences/8gchp/8gchp_helsinki_statement.pdf?ua=.

World Health Organization. (2013b). The many paths towards universal health coverage [video]. Retrieved from https://www.youtube.com/watch?v=VQ3sHfYzcv8&feature=youtu.be.

World Health Organization. (2013c). World health report 2013—research for universal health coverage. Retrieved from http://www.who.int/whr/en/.

World Health Organization. (2015a) GHO Health in 2015: from MDGs to SDGs. Retrieved from http://www.who.int/gho/publications/mdgs-sdgs/en/.

World Health Organization. (2015b) GHO life expectancy. Retrieved from http://www.who.int/gho/mortality_burden_disease/life_tables/situation_trends_text/en/.

World Health Organization. (2015c) GHO world health statistics 2015. Retrieved from http://www.who.int/gho/publications/world_health_statistics/2015/en/.

World Health Organization. (2015d) Social determinants of health—activities 2015. Retrieved from http://www.who.int/social_determinants/social-determinants-health-activities-2015.pdf.

World Health Organization. (2016a). Shanghai declaration on promoting health in the 2030 Agenda for Sustainable Development. Retrieved from https://www.who.int/healthpromotion/conferences/9gchp/shanghai-declaration.pdf?ua=1

World Health Organization. (2016b). Universal health coverage: moving towards better health. Action framework for the Western Pacific Region. Retrieved from http://iris.wpro.who.int/handle/10665.1/13371.

World Health Organization. (2018). Declaration of Astana, global conference on primary health care. Retrieved from https://www.who.int/docs/default-source/primary-health/declaration/gcphc-declaration.pdf.

World Health Organization. (2019a). Global health expenditure database. Retrieved from http://apps.who.int/nha/database.

World Health Organization. (2019b). World health statistics 2019: monitoring health for the SDGs, sustainable development goals. Retrieved from https://www.who.int/gho/publications/world_health_statistics/2019/en/.

Ziglio, E., Simpson, S., & Tsouros, A. (2011). Health promotion and health systems: some unfinished business. Health Promotion International, 26(S2), ii216–ii225. https://doi.org/10.1093/heapro/dar079.

2

Core concepts informing health promotion practice

INTRODUCTION

Chapter 1 established the foundations for health promotion practice within a comprehensive primary health care (CPHC) context. Some of the underlying concepts relevant to health promotion and CPHC were introduced. The purpose of this chapter is to explore further the range of core concepts informing health promotion practice within a CPHC context. In particular, the chapter presents the links between the socio-ecological determinants of health and wellbeing, and population health outcomes, in light of numerous core concepts that shape people's experience of health and wellbeing.

When discussing the socio-ecological determinants of health and wellbeing, it is somewhat easy to assume an understanding of many of the conceptual terms that are commonly used. We provide detailed definitions and explanations of the terms and their relevance to health promotion practice. Having a good understanding of the terms can assist practitioners to explain the reasons for inequalities, enabling them to provide a clear rationale for their health promotion action and to communicate effectively with the partners and communities that they work with. The iceberg model presented in Chapter 1 illustrates diagrammatically the link between the conditions of people's lives and the health and wellbeing outcomes they experience. Several of the core concepts presented in this chapter that shape people's experiences appear below the waterline of the iceberg. Given the importance of these concepts, using them as a guide in professional practice will raise some challenges and complexities. These concepts are always important considerations, irrespective of the professional practice setting.

The chapter commences with a discussion of the terms 'health', 'wellbeing', 'quality of life' and 'salutogenesis'. In the next section, the chapter outlines concepts related to the individual-level socio-ecological determinants of health and wellbeing, such as personal values, attitudes and beliefs, opportunities for education and individual responsibility for health and wellbeing. The third section of the chapter presents an explanation of core concepts related to population-level socio-ecological determinants of health and wellbeing commencing with a discussion about human capital. Concepts related to the social environment, such as the impact of poverty, human rights, equity, equality and social justice, power and empowerment, social capital and resilience are then explored. The cultural environment concepts of culture, cultural safety and cultural competence are followed by those related to the economic and political environment, including health services, economic capital and economic globalisation and neoliberalism. This section concludes with concepts related to the physical environment, including natural capital, environmental justice and liveability. These intersect with the social, cultural, economic and political environments, and provide the context for people's lives.

There can never be a clear separation between the individual and the environments in which they live. Clearly, there is constant interaction and the significance of each concept in producing health and wellbeing outcomes is a wider debate outside the scope of this book. Here they are discussed principally as they relate to professional health promotion practice within a CPHC context. The final section of the chapter introduces important considerations relevant to health promotion practice in community settings.

HEALTH, WELLBEING, QUALITY OF LIFE AND SALUTOGENESIS

Health

As established in Chapter 1, the health of people from individual through to the population level is influenced by the interrelated socio-ecological determinants of health and wellbeing, and needs to be considered within the context of the everyday lives of people.

In 1948, the World Health Organization (WHO, 1948) defined health as 'a complete state of physical, mental and social wellbeing, and not merely the absence of disease or infirmity'. This is probably the most often cited definition of health. It has been important in highlighting that health is about much more than merely the absence of disease, and much more than a physical state.

Health at the individual level is defined in different ways. The main distinction between definitions of individual health is between defining health as the absence of disease and defining it more broadly as a sense of wellness. The health status of a population is an epidemiological term that draws on births and deaths data and on morbidity and mortality causes and statistics. Health status measures enable comparisons of life expectancy and risk of certain illnesses between populations and groups within populations.

In defining health, it is not sufficient to consider only the health of the person in isolation. If health is defined only in individual terms, then issues of power and control, and the unequal access to opportunities in life because of socio-economic status, ethnicity and gender or environment, for example, are easily ignored. The lower a person's social and economic position, the worse their health tends to be; thus, socio-economic inequality is bad for health. Social gradients in health across an entire population are common globally including in Australia and New Zealand. In many nations, the gap between the wealthiest and poorest of the population is very large—and increasing even further (Mooney, 2012). The greater the disparity between the wealthiest and poorest of a population, the greater the health inequality; poorer people in the same country die younger and suffer more illnesses and injuries than their richer counterparts (Marmot, 2012). These disparities in health can arise from the underlying political philosophy, and they will persist while government inaction to address the socio-ecological determinants of health and wellbeing continues. For example, countries ruled by dictatorship or those with a political philosophy strongly based on individualism offer limited social services, making it harder for vulnerable community members to remain well. Countries with a strong social democratic philosophy provide a safety net for all people that reduces risks to health and wellbeing.

A prevailing challenge for health promotion is that many health practitioners are still educated within the biomedical model of disease. As such, in health policy, health promotion initiatives, and in hospital and illness-care settings there remains a tendency to focus on a narrow definition of health (or ill-health) as the basis for risk reduction and treatment. Consider, for example, the different focus of care that would arise if a holistic definition of health was used as a philosophy for care within the health service sector.

The extent to which people value their health depends on a wide range of factors in addition to the state of their physical bodies. However, the WHO definition of health has been criticised on a number of grounds (e.g. Green & Tones, 2010; Labonté & Laverack, 2008; Naidoo & Wills, 2011). On the one hand, first, it has been argued that the definition is unrealistic and unachievable, because it describes a state of such total wellbeing that it is unlikely that anyone could achieve it for more than a very brief period in their lives. With its focus on perfection, too, it excludes those living with disabilities or long-term medical conditions. Second, it has been criticised for being unmeasurable, describing a general state of wellbeing. It has been pointed out that, despite health having been defined this way since 1948, health statistics still only enable us to measure death and disease, and we remain without effective measures of health when it is defined more broadly. Efforts to define and measure other concepts including wellbeing and quality of life remain contested (Green & Tones, 2010; Scott, 2012). On the other hand, some have criticised the WHO definition for not being broad enough. For example, a number of authors have noted its lack of inclusion of spiritual wellbeing (Raeburn & Rootman, 1998; Teshuva et al., 1997). Indigenous peoples and those in the environmental movements have criticised the WHO definition of individual health from a cultural and ecological worldview. Despite the criticisms that have been made of the WHO definition of health—that it is too broad and unmeasurable, or too narrow and lacking spiritual and ecological dimensions—it remains a pertinent concept, and is an important starting point because it has pointed the way to consideration of the broader determinants of health (Green & Tones, 2010; Naidoo & Wills, 2011).

Notable efforts to define health within a broader socio-ecological context have come from Australia's Aboriginal people, New Zealand's Māori people, and the environmental movement, where concern for spiritual and cultural connectedness and ecological sustainability, respectively, have moved health definitions beyond the individual. For example, Aboriginal health has been defined as:

> ... not just the physical well-being of an individual but refers to the social, emotional and cultural well-being of the whole Community in which each individual is able to achieve their full potential as a human being, thereby bringing about the total well-being of their Community. It is a whole-of-life view and includes the cyclical concept of life-death-life.
>
> *(NACCHO, 2011)*

Māori health and wellbeing models are grounded in wellness philosophy with emphasis on spiritual wellbeing and the importance of whānau (family) as a dimension of wellbeing (Ministry of Health, 2017). Two Māori health and wellbeing models and one model of health promotion are presented in Insight 2.1. Honari and Boleyn (1999, pp. 19–20) provide an environmental context by defining health as 'a sustainable state of wellbeing, within sustainable ecosystems, within a sustainable biosphere'. Svalastog and colleagues (2017) identify that in line with modern constructions of health, many historical definitions also acknowledged a relationship between the holistic health and wellbeing experience of people and the environments in which they lived, particularly the social environment.

How health is defined is very important because definitions determine what are regarded as health priorities and therefore what becomes the focus of health promotion action. If health is defined as merely the absence of disease, health promotion will likely be limited to the reduction of risk of physical and medical ailments rather than taking a holistic view that encompasses mental, social and spiritual health and environmental sustainability. Health promotion action would ignore the significance of positive wellbeing or the social determinants of health that may make people's lives uncomfortable, but which are not medically classified as diseases. Ignoring priorities such as poverty, social connection, discrimination, fear for safety, environmental degradation, or chronic back pain, for example, may leave people suffering from conditions that limit their abilities or reduce their quality of life or the future of humanity. It is quite possible that if we address only medically defined problems, we could be ignoring issues that play an important role in disease causation, including mental illnesses. Furthermore, many environmental health issues are ignored on the grounds that there is no 'evidence' of a problem, when evidence may take 20 years

INSIGHT 2.1 Māori health and wellbeing and health promotion models

Two Māori health and wellbeing models and one health promotion model are described below. These models all appear on the New Zealand (Aotearoa) Ministry of Health (2017) website and have been used extensively to guide health- and wellbeing-related policy and health promotion practice over some years.

The Te Whare Tapa Whā Māori Health Model was developed by Sir Mason Durie (1985). The model presents a Māori perspective of ora (health) which is based on a balance between four dimensions or cornerstones of Māori wellbeing for individuals and collectives of people—taha tinana (physical health), taha wairua (spiritual health), taha whānau (family health) and taha hinengaro (mental health). The premise of this model is that if one of the cornerstones becomes unbalanced in any way, so too does people's wellbeing.

The second model is the Te Wheke model which was developed by Pere and Nicholson (1991). The Te Wheke (octopus) is used symbolically to present the health of the family whereby the whānau (head) of the octopus represents the family and waiora (eyes) the wellbeing of individuals and families. The eight tentacles then represent the following interwoven dimensions of health:

- wairuatanga—spirituality
- hinengaro—the mind
- taha tinana—physical wellbeing
- whanaungatanga—extended family
- mauri—life force in people and objects
- mana ake—unique identity of individuals and family
- hā a koro ma, a kui ma—breath of life from forebears
- whatumanawa—the open and healthy expression of emotion.

The third model is the Te Pae Mahutonga (Fig. 2.1), an Indigenous health promotion model that aligns with Māori worldviews about ora (health) and can be used to guide health promotion action (Durie, 2004). In the Te Pae Mahutonga (Southern Cross Star Constellation) model, four central Southern Cross stars represent areas of ora (health): mauriora (cultural identity), waiora (physical environment), toiora (healthy lifestyles), and te oranga (participation in society). The two pointer stars represent capacities required to effect changes in the ora areas: ngā manukura (community leadership) and te mana whakahaere (autonomy).

Sources: Durie, 1985; 2004; Ministry of Health, 2017; Pere & Nicholson, 1991.

to surface and people's health, and the health of the environment, may have already suffered greatly during this time.

Wellbeing

With the inclusion of social wellbeing, the WHO definition of health does touch on the interrelationship between humans and their physical and social environments. Wellbeing has also been difficult to define (Green & Tones, 2010; Miller & Foster, 2010; Scott, 2012). Many people identify wellbeing in the sense of 'being healthy' or 'happy' within the context of their whole lives rather than by the presence or absence of disease. Wellbeing is the state of being comfortable, well, happy in life and healthy. Wellbeing encompasses both moral or physical welfare and can relate to an individual or to a community situation. Honari and Boleyn (1999) describe wellbeing as 'being physically sound, mentally intact, spiritually happy, socially active, politically aware, economically productive and culturally responsible' (p. 20). They claim that this definition implies a degree of balance in human

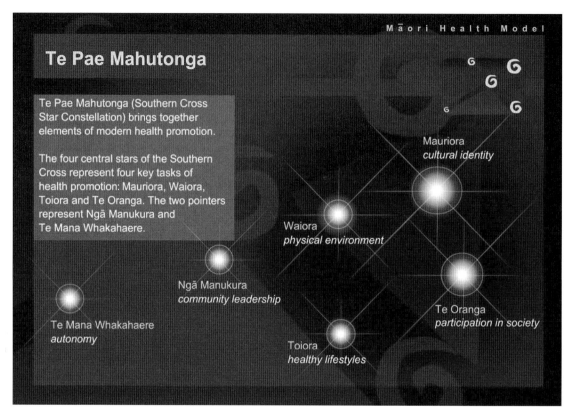

FIGURE 2.1 Southern Cross Model
Source: Durie, 2004; Ministry of Health, 2017.

life factors, which goes far beyond biological life. The Whitehall Wellbeing Working Group (cited in Scott, 2012, p. 5) made the link between personal and wider factors in wellbeing clear by defining wellbeing 'as a positive mental state enhanced and supported by various social, environmental and psychological factors'. Thus, personal capacity, power and social participation are essential elements of wellbeing.

This discussion of wellbeing emphasises the multiple layers of influence on our overall health status, including personal factors (biological, cognitive, emotional, spiritual, social and behavioural); interpersonal factors; and factors from the social, cultural, economic, political, built and natural environments that provide the context of people's lives. There is great potential for improvements in health and wellbeing if greater action is taken on the socio-ecological determinants of health (Brown et al., 2012; Labonté, 2014). The positive and negative influence of the physical environment on health status is detailed further in Chapter 3. The discussion also draws attention to the diverse opportunities for influencing wellbeing through government policy, social programs, health promotion and environmental approaches.

Various nations, including Australia and New Zealand, develop their own priorities and actions, informed by local population and health data, aimed at addressing the socio-ecological determinants affecting the health and wellbeing of their most vulnerable population groups, and enhancing the health and wellbeing of their entire populations. There is now sufficient evidence of the impacts of the socio-ecological determinants of health and wellbeing. This evidence is increasingly being directed at understanding the mechanisms for addressing those determinants most amenable to change, depending on the healthcare system, history and culture, and the prevailing political ideology (Mooney, 2012). There is growing acknowledgement that the narrow focus on economic growth and gross domestic product (GDP) that has characterised measures of national success has failed to address growing social inequalities within or between nations. Other measures, including measures of social wellbeing, provide better insight and a stronger basis for action, including action on environmental sustainability (Cummins et al., 2003; Labonté, 2014; Scott, 2012).

Identifying the determinants of wellbeing provides an important step towards health enhancement. The knowledge also moves the focus away from physical health and the medical health sector, and provides distinct guidance about what aspects of policy, service provision or financial mechanisms to change (Cummins et al., 2003). Specific population data also provide evidence for measurement of progress in improved population wellbeing. This potential for evaluation and tracking the effectiveness of specific strategies is very useful given the complexity of addressing the socio-ecological determinants of health and wellbeing across entire population groups. For example, strategies designed to bring longer-term improvements in mortality and morbidity in some Indigenous communities may be evaluated by incremental improvements in rates of immunisation completion, school completion, or women's participation in health screening for cervical cancer.

Quality of life

Quality of life plays an important part in people's experience of health and wellbeing, including their mental wellbeing, because quality of life encompasses psychosocial dimensions. De Vries reminds us that a sense of wellbeing equates with a sense of wholeness, which is what the term 'health' originally meant. As de Vries points out, 'wholeness is not the same as being happy or living without pain, frustration or handicaps; wholeness may be achieved in the presence of disease or infirmity' (1993, p. 129). This sense of wholeness, or integrity, indicates a positive quality of life. It is interesting to note that this perspective takes the WHO definition of health further, as it suggests that a sense of wholeness may be present even if disease or disability are also present (Naidoo & Wills, 2011). The Australian Institute of Health and Welfare previously used the SF-36™ test in their assessments of wellbeing, but more recently the Organisation for Economic Co-operation and Development (OECD) 'How's Life?' indicator framework is being used which allows international comparisons. This framework groups indicators into three broad dimensions: material living conditions; quality of life; and sustaining wellbeing (OECD, 2015). The SF-36™ is a questionnaire that produces an eight-item sub-scale with a health profile as well as quality of life related to an individual's health status.

It is out of recognition of these dimensions of human wholeness that the notion of quality of life has gained attention in health research. Cross-cultural studies indicate that positive quality of life can be achieved in the following conditions:

- *feeling vital, full of energy*
- *having good social relationships*
- *experiencing a sense of control over one's life and one's living conditions*
- *being able to do things one enjoys*
- *having a sense of purpose in life*
- *experiencing a connectedness to 'community'.*

(Labonté, 1997, p. 15)

Judgements about the items listed above can only be made by the individual, and thus they are often devalued as being 'subjective' assessments, lacking scientific rigour and of limited value in the clinical (medical) setting. These conditions also alert us to the importance of enabling people to make decisions about their own health and quality of life. There is evidence that wellbeing and quality of life have a direct bearing on physical health (Marmot, 2012; OECD, 2015). Wellbeing is sometimes seen as a more useful indicator than quality of life in terms of whole-of-community approaches to health enhancement, especially because wellbeing makes the link between personal factors and social and ecological ones.

Salutogenesis

The salutogenic approach to health and illness was proposed by Aaron Antonovsky, a professor of the sociology of health, in 1979 (Antonovsky, 1996). The rationale behind salutogenesis is that people are, at any time, on a continuum between health and illness, and positive or negative life experiences move them in one direction or the other along the continuum. Antonovsky argued that usual health promotion theory has a primary focus on illness prevention, with identification of risk factors and specific programs to address these and change personal behaviour. Salutogenesis is a focus on the origins of health, rather than on pathological changes; health promotion strategies actively promote health, rather than prevent ill health (Antonovsky, 1996). The focus of health promotion effort needs to be on people, rather than on reducing the risk of acquiring an illness or managing a specific disease—promoting the health of older adults in their community rather than programs to prevent type 2 diabetes, for example. He argued it is morally deficient to regard complex humans by their pathological state—the diabetic patient, smokers, the mentally ill and so on. Antonovsky proposed a theory of salutogenesis that has a focus on building people's sense of coherence, where they develop and maintain a general orientation to the world that is characterised by high coping ability, optimism, self-efficacy and hardiness (Antonovsky, 1996). Salutogenesis is primarily a psychological construct and the sense of coherence is a resource to buffer the person against life's stressors. According to Jonas and colleagues, 'in today's terms it may be defined as a resilience factor' (2014). Even when a person's health is challenged, they are able to move towards wellbeing.

Allen and colleagues (2018) studied a group of people who reported high levels of health, wellbeing and happiness, to determine what they regarded as high-level wellness, and how they attain and maintain this way of being. They found that 'high level wellness is the sense of peace (wellbeing) that comes from knowing, liking and being one's best self' (Allen et al., 2018). Through a series of self-initiated experiential learning cycles, their happy, healthy participants managed to attain and maintain this way of being over time. The authors claim that their 'experiential learning theory of high level wellness links and extends literature on salutogenesis, eudaimonic wellbeing, self-actualization and experiential learning; positioning everyday people as the leaders of their own life-long wellness journeys' (Allen et al., 2018).

Considerable work has been undertaken to develop Antonovsky's salutogenesis theory into a conceptual model and to test it in health promotion research and practice. In the decades since the theory was first proposed, the focus for health promotion has become appropriately broader, in line with the theory of salutogenesis (Gregg & O'Hara, 2007a), with a stronger focus on positive health enhancement and health protection measures (supported by healthy public policy) and on building personal resilience factors (Mittelmark & Bull, 2013). The Red Lotus Health Promotion Model, a new model for holistic, ecological, salutogenic health promotion practice (Gregg & O'Hara, 2007a) (now known as the Red Lotus Critical Health Promotion Model), purposefully incorporates the concept of salutogenesis to ensure those using the model in professional practice focus on those factors that create and support health and wellbeing. To our knowledge, this model is the only health promotion model that is explicit about including the concept of salutogenesis as a core underlying value and principle.

CONCEPTS RELATED TO INDIVIDUAL-LEVEL SOCIO-ECOLOGICAL DETERMINANTS OF HEALTH AND WELLBEING

There are many factors that influence the range of socio-ecological determinants of health and wellbeing at the individual level. This first section presents a number of underpinning concepts, including values, attitudes, beliefs and education, that influence personal or individual-level health-related behaviours. These factors are not always under personal control, but they commonly influence the levels of risk a person takes with their health behaviours. Knowledge of risk behaviours forms the basis of many health promotion behaviour-change strategies.

Values, attitudes and beliefs

Values, attitudes and beliefs are 'constructs'—terms that are used to explain things that cannot be directly observed way below the waterline in the iceberg model (see Fig. 1.4 on page 12). People act in response to their personal and professional values, attitudes and beliefs and we observe these actions or outcomes as particular actions or behaviours.

Values

Values refer to principles or standards that are held by a person or group about what is important, desirable or valuable in life. Values are considered subjective because they cannot be directly observed, and they vary across people and cultures; hence we may describe a cultural 'value system' where people from the same cultural group respond in similar ways. Values are acquired as a part of a person's cultural 'training'—the teachings within families and other groups about what is 'right' and 'wrong' and so on. People sometimes make judgements about others based on differing cultural values. While an individual holds personal values, they become evident in the ways people conduct their public or social lives (Kirschenbaum, 2013). Types of values include ethical and moral values such as honesty and trustworthiness, political values such as commitment to democracy or reconciliation, religious values such as sacrifice and repentance, social values such as equity and justice, and aesthetic values such as gentleness. It is debated whether some values are innate or not.

A person's individual values arise from their life experiences, and although relatively stable, they can change over time. They have a large emotional component; strongly held personal or professional values can be a major influence on the person's behaviour or reaction to a situation. Values provide a 'moral compass' guiding behaviour and most people have strong feelings about defending their personal values, provided they are freely chosen.

Ethical values of health promotion practice

By its nature, health promotion practice involves working with a range of different individuals and communities in a diverse range of possible settings, from acute hospital wards to isolated rural schools. Wherever practice occurs there is potential for the personal values and attitudes of the health promotion practitioners to be markedly different from those of the community members they are working with. Health promotion practice implies a set of values underpinning the service, such as equity, empowerment and social justice.

Values informing health promotion practice may be implicit in the common values and standards expected in society, such as respect for others, or they may be made explicit in the guiding principles of the health agency, perhaps set out in a professional code of practice, mission statement or other strategic planning documents (Forgas et al., 2011). Expected professional values may also be made explicit in a formal contract that a practitioner enters into when they are employed, or in the 'oath' that professionals take when they are formally accepted into a professional role, such as the nurses' codes of professional practice. Professional practice in health promotion implies that a health practitioner's actions will be guided by the values set out in the philosophical frameworks that underpin their practice; primarily, the Declaration of Alma-Ata (see Appendix 1), but also, other complementary documents such as the Universal Declaration of Human Rights (see Appendix 3) and the Earth Charter (see Appendix 4). Equity, social justice and sustainability are key values that are common across these and other philosophical frameworks.

While it is unusual for health practitioners to act deliberately dishonestly or unethically, they frequently find themselves in positions of considerable power, particularly when they are working with a disempowered group or community. In these situations, it is relatively easy for health promotion practitioners to impose their personal values on the community, because they believe it is 'right' or 'best' for the community. They may have the 'wisdom' of experience of having worked with other, similar communities, or 'wisdom' derived from formal education. In acute care and community settings this power can be exercised in simple ways such as the use of the particular jargon of the discipline, which can exclude other practitioners and clients from the discussion or decision making.

There is also the wider debate about the ethics of health promotion itself to consider. Some people argue that health promotion approaches, such as behaviour-change 'requirements' like wearing a helmet when cycling, are an infringement on personal freedoms. Specific health promotion strategies can also be viewed as unethical, especially those dealing with topics that are highly linked to social values and social judgements, such as body weight (Carter et al., 2011). Gregg and O'Hara (2007b, Table 1) outlined the continuum of values and principles evident in health promotion practice. At one end is a practice mode that may be unethical, is professional expert-driven, does not involve participants or community members in decision making, is based on limited evidence, and uses selected individual strategies with a behaviour-change agenda. The other end of the continuum has a salutogenic, holistic focus on wellbeing that will bring sustained improvements to the socio-ecological determinants of health and wellbeing using a broad range of strategies developed in partnership with the community (Gregg & O'Hara, 2007b). As we have outlined throughout this book, the Ottawa Charter provides a framework that will guide the health promotion practitioner towards ethical practice.

Health practitioners need to constantly remind themselves that their work cannot be value-free; values and attitudes are socially constructed (Eckermann et al., 2010). Even though practitioners' actions may be legal, it does not necessarily mean they are moral or ethical. Communities of interest need to be provided with opportunities to express their values through community consultation and partnerships of practice, and health practitioners need to take the time to examine their own values.

Health practitioners can experience a conflict of values as they are required to make choices and adopt priorities as part of their normal working lives. Different aspects of health promotion may compete for priority, and choices made to support one aspect of health promotion may result in a practitioner feeling uncomfortable about the implications of this choice. Similarly, as practice changes through evidence-informed development and experience, it is quite possible that values that seemed acceptable in the past no longer seem appropriate. However, the past cannot be changed, and health practitioners have to come to terms with their previous decisions. Similarly, health practitioners sometimes find themselves in an 'ethical dilemma', a situation where values conflict in a practice setting. They may be forced to make a moral decision about what is the correct way to deal with a situation (Tesoriero, 2010).

The International Union for Health Promotion and Education (IUHPE, 2016) *Core Competencies and Professional Standards for Health Promotion 2016* sets out as a guiding principle the ways in which 'a health promotion practitioner acts professionally and ethically'. These standards should be used as a basis for practice. The IUHPE Health Promotion Competencies are discussed in Chapter 1 and the section presented at the end of every chapter provides principles, knowledge and skills to guide ethical professional health promotion practice.

Attitudes and beliefs

Attitudes are positive or negative personal evaluations about certain socially significant persons, places, objects, activities, events or ideas (Forgas et al., 2011; Gerrig & Zimbardo, 2010). Attitudes are something internal to a person but influence the way the person thinks about (believes), feels about, or behaves in response to, an issue or stimulus. Attitudes consist of cognitive, affective and motor aspects (Kirschenbaum, 2013). The cognitive aspect means that we think about and develop a personal understanding about that thing, such as social media, smoking, violence or service to the community. These are a person's beliefs, their conviction of the truth or reality of a thing, which is not the same as having positive irrefutable knowledge of a fact. Depending on their culture and life experience, people may hold various beliefs about the things that contribute to health and wellbeing and cause illness. These may be based on information that may be verifiable, such as demographic and epidemiological data, or on unreliable sources or hearsay. For example, a person may understand the statistical risks associated with cigarette smoking, or another may argue the risk is low because their grandfather smoked 'all his life until he was 90 and didn't get lung cancer'. Beliefs may vary over time as a result of situational changes. In this context, beliefs about the influence of lifestyle conditions or health-risk behaviours or about personal risk of certain diseases, are likely to affect personal actions.

The affective aspect of attitudes means we are influenced in forming attitudes by our emotions or feelings, such as if we have had a personal experience of someone close to us suffering lung disease, or if we have regularly suffered violence, or have had a family tradition of volunteering for community organisations. We can be persuaded to change our attitude to something in a large variety of ways, including by peer influence, observation, advertising, political messages, increased knowledge or misinformation.

The motor component of attitudes relates to our tendency or likelihood to take action, or behave in a certain way; for example, not smoking, taking assertiveness classes or volunteering to work for a cause or something we believe in. An attitude provides a motive for taking action. Attitudes can change, usually as a result of experience, or vicariously through awareness of the experience of others. The primary focus for a range of advertising strategies or behaviour-change therapies is to change a person's or subgroup of a population's attitude to that element. It is clear that our attitudes affect what we see and how we see it. Studies have shown there is a low correlation between attitudes and behaviour (Ledgerwood & Trope in Forgas et al., 2011). Attitudes can also be powerfully influenced by external forces, such as media cues and images. Attitudes are sometimes irrational, perhaps being based on unbalanced or inaccurate information (Johnson & Boynton in Forgas et al., 2011).

There can be a low correlation between a person's attitudes to a particular matter or risk and their behaviour in relation to the same thing, meaning what they express in their views on a topic and their actions around the same issue are antithetical. A common example occurs with people's attitudes and actions about racism. They commence by stating 'I'm not racist, but ...' and go on to make a negative generalisation about an entire racial group. A similar pattern emerges with incongruence between attitudes and actions towards a number of other '-isms'; for example, sexism, ageism and so forth. For example, an employer may express positive values about female or older staff members but be unwilling to employ suitably qualified female or older applicants. When what someone says is not in line with their observed actions it is termed 'cognitive dissonance'.

Education

The Declaration of Alma-Ata (WHO, 1978) (see Appendix 1) gives recognition to the fundamental role of education in health development. Likewise, the Sustainable Development Goals recognise the central role that education plays in sustainable development (UN, 2015). SDG 4 is quality education with targets related to equitable access to quality child care, and primary and secondary education for all. There has been significant progress made in enrolment in primary education in developing countries, where the level has reached 91%. However, over 50 million children are still not accessing primary education and more than half of these live in sub-Saharan Africa and/or areas affected by conflict (UN, n.d.).

There are both direct and indirect links between education and health and wellbeing outcomes (Anderson et al., 2007). Indirectly, high levels of literacy contribute to reducing social inequalities and improving health and wellbeing. Even in relatively poor areas such as Cuba and Kerala, mass literacy initiatives have contributed to informed political action to improve living standards, population health and life expectancy (Mooney, 2012). Further, access to education leads to safer, better-paid employment and greater resilience in times of social uncertainty. Educated women in poor settings have fewer children with a higher survival rate. In Australia, the *Closing the Gap Report 2020* shows that only two of the four targets related to education of Indigenous Australians were on track: the target to have 95% of Indigenous four-year-olds enrolled in early childhood education, and the target to halve the gap in Year 12 attainment or equivalent. The targets to close the gap in school attendance and halve the gap in reading and numeracy by 2018 were not achieved (Australian Government, 2020).

Directly, education enhances health by providing access to nutritional information and other means of prevention from danger or infection. The children of educated parents have better health for the same reasons; health literacy is 'absorbed' within the household. As the preceding discussion about values and attitudes suggests, those with higher educational attainment are more likely to form positive attitudes to health-enhancing behaviours, based on reliable, accurate information. They are better able to undertake personal research on matters affecting their wellbeing and to make informed decisions to avoid risks to health. In contrast, when educational opportunity is not available, or is disrupted or incomplete, the health of the individual tends to be poorer, especially because of the lifelong barriers to safe, well-paid employment and health literacy.

Individual responsibility

Encouraging people to take responsibility for their own health, both individually and at the levels of the community and the country, is part of the CPHC approach. The re-emergence of these ideas began with the Declaration of Alma-Ata's call for action 'in the spirit of self-reliance' (see Appendix 1), and with the introduction of health education/health literacy approaches designed to encourage voluntary behaviour change, and social marketing messages designed to persuade people to adopt positive values about personal or organisational behaviour change for health maintenance. As the relationships between individual behaviours and illness were identified, calls for changes to individual risk behaviours became more and more common, because an increasing number of diseases were labelled as 'lifestyle' diseases. The inference was that people 'chose' risky behaviours as a part of their lifestyle, and thus it was a matter of individual choice for them to change personal attitudes to health protection and adopt healthier behaviours.

The likelihood that attitudes, beliefs and behaviour can be changed as a result of a person receiving new or accurate information, developing an emotional commitment to making a change, or having a significant health experience or outcome, has been the basis of formulation of a number of behaviour-change models of health education, such as the Health Belief Model (Becker, 1974), the Transtheoretical Model (Stages of Change) (Prochaska & Di Clementi, 1984), the Theory of Planned Behaviour (Ajzen & Fishbein, 1991) and Social Cognitive Theory (Bandura, 1986). These models are presented in more detail in Chapter 7.

Victim blaming

Individuals live their lives in a social context, and there are many factors that influence an individual's lifestyle. As the discussion in the first chapter illustrates, a great many of the determinants of health are the result of the social, economic and political structures in which people live their lives. There are some real dangers, therefore, in focusing only on the role of individual behaviours in disease causation and management. People may be blamed for ill health, and for some of the determinants of ill health, when they do not have control over the factors affecting their health or the freedom to make healthy choices. They may be unable to make changes in their personal health behaviours because of the social, environmental or cultural circumstances of their lives. Making judgements about those who are unable to change has become known as 'blaming the victim'.

Victim blaming occurs when the structural causes of ill health are ignored and attention is focused on the individual or individuals affected by the problem, with the aim of changing their behaviour (Baum, 2016; Laverack, 2012; Mooney, 2012). Victim blaming is a subtle process. Ryan (1976, p. 8) describes it as 'cloaked in kindness and concern'. It occurs when people fail to see the structural causes of deprivation and ill health, and still seek to solve the problem by working to change the individual (Baum, 2016; Laverack, 2012; Mooney, 2012; Ryan, 1976). Victim blaming is therefore another of the negative outcomes of neoliberal political philosophy. Individualism is one of the pillars of neoliberalism—individual credit for success and individual responsibility for personal health. This is a structural cause of inequality and disempowerment, which makes it even harder for vulnerable members of society, those who have chronic illnesses, poor education, who live in poor-quality housing and have insecure employment, to maintain their health. When people are unwell and make increased use of the healthcare system, they pay a high proportion of their income for health care (Mooney, 2012).

One of the real strengths of CPHC and the Ottawa Charter for Health Promotion's five-pronged approach to health promotion action is that the chance of victim blaming occurring is minimised. If health promotion action occurs through working for healthier public policy and creating supportive community environments as well as through further developing the skills of the individual, the structural barriers to ill health are likely to be addressed. It is vital, therefore, that the broad approach to health promotion action described in the Ottawa Charter for Health Promotion is not watered down to the point where structural action disappears and is replaced by more action directed towards the individual (Laverack, 2012).

Victim blaming not only happens to individuals. With a focus on community development and community-based action, when many problems stem from national or international issues, there is a danger that disadvantaged countries or communities may be blamed if they are unable to recover from a disaster or disadvantage (Laverack, 2012; Mooney, 2012).

The issues surrounding individual responsibility for health versus social responsibility for health are complex and interrelated. It is not a case of choosing one over the other, but of what balance there is between the two. Unfortunately, because they have come to represent opposing philosophical and political viewpoints, many discussions present them as opposite to each other, which does not help practitioners clarify how they will address health issues and assist individuals in making changes in their lives (Mooney, 2012). Health promotion practitioners may need to clarify for themselves how to work with the tension between these two aspects of health promotion, to be aware of their own biases, and to keep clear in their minds how both aspects of a problem need to be addressed in whatever balance is appropriate for the issue in question.

Influence of labelling

The concept of labelling is very much related to the notion of victim blaming. The stereotyping or labelling of people, because of their ethnicity, gender, sexuality, age, body size or socio-economic status, can have a powerful impact on the ways they are treated (Moncrieffe & Eyben, 2013; Mooney, 2012). Health practitioners' response to issues and problems that arise may be influenced by beliefs and expectations about particular groups, stages of life or illness experiences. Tesoriero (2010) identifies that the discourse of disadvantage, the way language is used to portray and maintain a negative image of a vulnerable group, can have a strong and lasting effect, and can perpetuate their disadvantage. Disempowerment itself can become a major health issue in communities or for individuals if their strengths are not acknowledged along with disadvantage or unmet needs (Labonté & Laverack, 2008; Laverack, 2012). In the same way, labelling can be a means of social exclusion. The self-identity of people is influenced by the terms used to describe them. Social groups create labels that identify others as 'insiders' or 'outsiders' according to certain criteria. Outsiders lose hope and self-esteem about their sense of belonging in society.

The use of 'strengths perspectives' (Norman, 2012) is increasing in many disciplines, including mental health (e.g. constructivist therapies), nursing (e.g. wellness versus illness), asset-based community assessments (which will be referred to in Chapter 4), and education research (e.g. resilience). Terminology such as 'asset' and 'protective factors' are used instead of 'needs' and 'risk factors'. The identification and building of strengths within individuals, families and communities describes positive relationships, building competencies and opportunities, rather than a 'deficits' focus (Norman, 2012).

Dealing with opposing values and conflicts of interest

Perspectives, or viewpoints, about ways to overcome some health promotion challenges have the potential to create conflict between people or groups with opposing philosophical views or values. This is particularly so where health promotion action has the potential to challenge profit or power, and the role of a health practitioner is to advocate for more equitable power relations. People's view of health and health promotion reflects their broader views about the way the world works. An example of this could be seen by contrasting government policy approaches; a neoliberal approach would argue that those who use the most services should pay the most, whereas a social welfare approach would argue that those with best health should subsidise the health costs of those who need to use more healthcare services. As a result, many of the issues underpinning discussions of health promotion reflect the worldviews of the parties in power, and these have the potential to change.

At a more direct level, conflicting viewpoints can occur when the risks in an unsafe or unhealthy industry or working environment are subsumed in favour of market power or profit having a higher priority. Most high-income nations such as Australia and New Zealand have the protection of workplace health and safety legislation, but their unwillingness to address workers' health considerations has been the basis of some companies moving their industry to countries where there is no legislative protection for workers' health.

Health promotion requires effective communication and joint action with individuals, health practitioners from a variety of backgrounds, professionals from a range of other sectors (e.g. local government, teachers, police, environmental practitioners and road safety workers) and community groups. Key health promotion frameworks and international covenants can be powerful tools for leverage for change in advocacy work.

CONCEPTS RELATED TO POPULATION-LEVEL SOCIO-ECOLOGICAL DETERMINANTS OF HEALTH AND WELLBEING

This section explores and builds on key concepts that relate to the socio-ecological determinants of health referred to in Chapter 1 and outlined in the iceberg model (Fig. 1.4). They are the social and environmental factors which set the context for a person's lifetime health experiences. As outlined in the introduction to the chapter, there can never be a clear separation, or distinction, between the individual and the social; these aspects of life and health are interwoven. Concepts explored in this section include human capital and social, cultural, economic, political and physical environments.

Human capital

The collective sum of human aptitudes and skills impacts on individual and community wellbeing. Communities with a higher proportion of university graduates have indirect health benefits through higher average income, better health literacy and more secure employment. For this reason, these indicators are often cited in discussion on the socio-ecological determinants of health and in liveability indicators (Lowe et al., 2014). Learning, knowledge and skills that build on inherent aptitudes bring economic and non-economic returns to the individual and the wider community. The increased emphasis on the capabilities and impacts of human endeavour has given rise to the concept of human capital.

Human capital relates to the innate and learned capabilities of the individual. It has been defined as 'the knowledge, skills, competencies and attributes embodied in individuals that facilitate the creation of personal, social and economic wellbeing' (Healy & Coté, 2001, p. 18). In a similar vein, Woolcock (1998, p. 154) takes a society-wide perspective and defines human capital as 'a society's endowment of educated, trained and healthy practitioners'—the capabilities that are in their head and hands.

Human capital is multi-faceted in its nature. Skills and competencies may be general (like the capacity to read, write and speak), or highly specific and more or less appropriate in different contexts ... Much knowledge and skill is tacit rather than codified and documented ... Human capital grows through use and experience, both inside and outside employment, as well as through informal and formal learning, but human capital also tends to depreciate through lack of use.

(Healy & Coté, 2001, pp. 18–19)

This quote indicates that human capital is dynamic. It includes capabilities that may be immediately obvious, such as speaking, writing, numeracy and leadership, and also less obvious personal attributes, such as perseverance, capacity for learning, making judgements and ethical decisions, problem-solving capacity and team leadership attributes (Healy & Coté, 2001). Inherent and genetic capabilities or attributes, and health status constitute aspects of human capital because they strongly influence the outcome capabilities of an individual. Key drivers for the development and maintenance of human capital are formal education opportunities and maintaining wellbeing through equitable access to the socio-ecological determinants of health and wellbeing, as set out in the iceberg model presented in Chapter 1 (Fig. 1.4).

Assessing the quality of human capital is a product of the cultural setting the person lives in—valued skills in one cultural setting may seem useless in another setting. This reinforces the importance of policy that supports access to formal education in addition to social and family supports for wellbeing. The habits of learning commenced in the family and school tend to stay with the person into adulthood in their employment opportunities, and hence the impact carries on to their health and wellbeing through secure, fulfilling employment. According to Healy and Coté, 'societies that tend to be less equal in terms of access to education and learning outcomes also tend to be less equal in terms of income distribution' (2001, p. 26).

Additional educational achievements bring returns to the person in terms of their likelihood to remain employed as well as the increased income. Higher educational attainment also enhances creativity, technological advancement, research and innovation in workplaces, with obvious benefits for the economy and for personal health maintenance. Higher levels of human capital, whether measured directly by skills or indirectly by educational attainment, have been found to be strongly associated with higher levels of productivity and workforce participation (Productivity Commission, 2012). Knowledge and human capital act as catalysts to increase productivity relatively evenly across the economy.

In addition to the economic benefits of enhanced human capital, there are also social benefits, and these benefits may be 'possibly larger than the direct labour market and macroeconomic effects' (Healy & Coté, 2001, p. 33). Benefits are evident in lower risk taking, such as the use and abuse of drugs like cigarettes and alcohol, or lower rates of physical inactivity among people with higher levels of education. There are also family-to-child educational benefits and social benefits, such as being less likely to rely on social welfare and unemployment benefits. Enhanced human capital reduces the risk of crime and is associated with higher levels of volunteering, which is an important community asset or strength. In addition, there is growing evidence of the link between human capital and subjective wellbeing (Healy & Coté, 2001). There are clear benefits in addressing the socio-ecological determinants of health and wellbeing to enhance human capital, particularly for the most vulnerable groups in society. The Closing the Gap strategy (Australian Government, 2020) is a very good example of this.

Social environment

Poverty

Sustainable Development Goal 1 is to end poverty in all its forms everywhere (UN, 2015). Poverty is usually defined as a lack of sufficient income, but people's wellbeing does not only depend on their level of income. Poverty is also defined by inequity or disparity. The United Nations (UN) Committee on Economic, Social and Cultural Rights is a committee of independent experts who monitor implementation of these rights internationally. The committee uses the following definition of poverty:

> *a human condition characterized by sustained or chronic deprivation of the resources, capabilities, choices, security and power necessary for the enjoyment of an adequate standard of living and other civil, cultural, economic, political and social rights.*
> **(Office of the United Nations High Commissioner for Human Rights [OHCHR], 2008, p. 6)**

Relative poverty

A distinction is often made between absolute poverty and relative poverty. Absolute poverty is the state described in the definition above where people do not have sufficient resources to meet even basic subsistence needs from day to day. Relative poverty usually relates to life in high-income countries and describes the disadvantaged position of some groups in society, compared with other members of the society. The parameter for this form of poverty is what is regarded as being adequate income to live in that society. Relative poverty within a nation is calculated as the proportion of the population with an income below a certain fraction of the median income (Fritzell et al., 2015). Thus, people are described as 'living below the poverty line'. There is generally disagreement within each country about how the poverty line is defined and measured because social justice advocates will argue for a higher-level measure being necessary to maintain the lifestyle that is common in that society (Fritzell et al., 2015; Harris & White, 2013). Relative poverty is becoming more common as income inequalities between people in high-income countries increase. Relative poverty has similar impacts on mortality rates to absolute poverty, with some of the increased risk possibly being associated with the psychological distress caused by more limited access to, or exclusion from, health and social services that relative poverty causes (Fritzell et al., 2015). In either definition, whether absolute or relative, poverty places people at risk of poorer health and wellbeing.

The first two targets in SDG 1 are to eradicate extreme poverty for all people everywhere, currently measured as people living on less than $1.25 a day, and to reduce the proportion of men, women and children of all ages living in poverty in all its dimensions according to national definitions by at least half (UN, 2015). More than 10% of the world's population live in extreme poverty and are unable to meet their basic needs such as food, education and access to water and sanitation. Poverty is more prevalent in vulnerable communities, and geographically isolated or environmentally vulnerable areas. Worldwide, the poverty rate is more than three times higher in rural areas than in urban areas (UN, 2015). The majority of people living in extreme poverty live in sub-Saharan Africa, and small, fragile and conflict-affected countries often have high poverty rates (UN, n.d.). Women and children are disproportionately affected by poverty. One out of five children live in extreme poverty. Being employed reduces, but does not eliminate poverty, with 8% of employed workers and their families worldwide living in extreme poverty in 2018 (UN, n.d.).

The UN's High Commission for Human Rights argues that normalisation of human rights philosophy into national policy provides a strategic and integrated approach to poverty reduction across the world. Indigenous and minority cultural groups tend to be over-represented among the poor, especially because they have been denied basic human rights (Anderson et al., 2007).

Health is central to poor people's lives and globally there is a clear relationship between poverty and poor health; poverty creates ill health and premature death (Marmot, 2012; Mooney, 2012). There are direct and indirect pathways to this outcome. Families living in poverty experience unhealthy living conditions including substandard housing, unreliable water supply and sanitation, and exposure to chemical and infective agents. Indirectly, poverty results in poor nutrition, which arrests normal development and increases risk of illness (Anderson et al., 2007). Poverty prevents children completing their immunisations and denies people access to the health care and medicines they need when they are ill. Poverty selectively disadvantages females more than males, especially regarding maternal nutrition and educational participation. Thus, illiteracy is a product of poverty and in turn forces them into low-paid and more risky employment.

In nations without well-funded health and social services, illness within a family often creates a spiral of economic decline, whether it is because the primary income-earner is unable to work or because the cost of medical treatment creates a debt that the family is unable to pay. Even within nations such as Australia, New Zealand and Canada with comparatively well-funded public health systems and a range of social benefits, chronic illness forces many to live below the poverty line. Poor people define health holistically, in reference to physical, psychological, social and community wellbeing. They express a range of non-physical reactions to their poverty including shame, humiliation, powerlessness and uncertainty. But they also understand better than many others that physical health is their most valuable asset; good health is crucial to economic survival (Mooney, 2012; WHO & World Bank, 2005, p. 20).

> *Poor people most frequently describe ill-health and 'ill-being' in multidimensional terms, not only as disease but also as hunger, pain, exhaustion, exclusion, isolation, bad relations within the family and with other people, insecurity, fear, powerlessness and anger.*
>
> *(WHO & World Bank, 2005, p. 14)*

Strategies to protect and enhance the health of the poorest people are central to broader goals of poverty reduction and economic growth (International Monetary Fund, 2016) and achievement of the Sustainable Development Goals (UN, 2015).

Human rights

Human rights are internationally agreed standards that apply to all human beings. The international human rights treaties bring legally binding obligations for the governments that sign them to respect them, protect them from infringement and fulfil them. The Universal Declaration of Human Rights (Appendix 3) states that:

> *everyone has the right to a standard of living adequate for the health and wellbeing of himself and his family, including food, clothing, housing and medical care and necessary social services.*
>
> *(UN, 1948)*

Despite this proclamation in 1948, inequalities between countries and within countries are widening. Human rights legislation should form the backbone of social policy.

Human rights are often cited with reference to civil and political rights. There has been less emphasis on economic, social and cultural rights, and governments have been somewhat reluctant to use these as the basis for policy development. This is because of the inherent power they carry and government reluctance to acknowledge the link between human rights and human health and the high costs of implementation (OHCHR, 2008). Human rights are:

- *universal; the birthright of every human being;*
- *aimed at safeguarding the inherent dignity and equal worth of everyone;*
- *inalienable (they cannot be waived or taken away);*
- *interdependent and interrelated (every human right is closely related to and often dependent upon the realisation of other human rights);*
- *articulated as entitlements of individuals (and groups) generating obligations of action and omission, particularly on states;*
- *internationally guaranteed and legally protected.*

(UN, 1948)

Human rights provide a strong framework for ensuring equity and accountability in health system policy and services planning, resource allocation and program evaluation. Human rights treaties provide a framework of protection for a population, but possibly the most powerful is 'the right to health' (the right of everyone to the enjoyment of the highest attainable standard of physical and mental health). This is because the right to health is interdependent with other human rights, such as the rights to food, an adequate standard of living, privacy and access to information. The right to health contains a number of freedoms and entitlements. Freedoms include freedom from torture and from cruel, inhumane or degrading treatment, or treatments against a person's will. Entitlements include the protections provided by a properly functioning health system and the right to healthy natural and work environments. A number of human rights principles are enshrined in the treaties, including the following:

- *Indivisibility. Indivisibility means that civil, cultural, economic, political and social rights are all necessary for the dignity of the human person and are interlinked. Integrated approaches, across government sectors, are essential to ensure human rights are protected.*
- *Equality and non-discrimination. All individuals are equal and entitled to their human rights without discrimination of any kind. To protect human rights, law must enshrine these values, but there must also be processes to ensure that the results of their implementation do not produce disadvantage or discrimination.*
- *Participation and inclusion. Every person is entitled to be an active participant in civil, economic, social, cultural and political life including having their say on any developments that may have an effect on them.*
- *Accountability, transparency and the rule of law. The first component of this, answerability, requires governments and their agencies to be transparent in the decision making and actions. This is designed to provide protection from discrimination against disempowered groups. The second component is redress, which requires institutions*

*to overcome the disadvantage that has occurred if they have not
adhered to the principles.*

(adapted from OHCHR, 2008, pp. 7–8)

When an entire community or population group is deprived of their human rights, they will also experience poverty and poor health. Access to basic human rights is fundamental to opportunities to attain good health. The links between health and human rights fall into three main categories:

1. human rights violations resulting in ill-health
2. reducing vulnerability to ill health through human rights
3. promotion or violation of human rights through health policy, programs or actions of health workers.

Violations of human rights may include things as diverse as torture, slavery or harmful traditional practices. These violations exist today and they have serious health consequences.

Health policies and programs can either promote or violate human rights in the way they are designed or implemented. Equitable access to appropriate and acceptable health services, information, and participation in decision making all enhance health and wellbeing. On the contrary, exposure to discrimination, bias, stereotyping and stigma from health service providers negatively affects health and wellbeing. For example, due to the current government-led 'war on obesity', people with larger bodies receive poorer standard of care and are subjected to higher levels of anti-fat bias and stigmatisation from health professionals, compared with those with smaller bodies (O'Hara & Taylor, 2018). People with larger bodies also face higher levels of discrimination in education, employment and housing, all of which constitute a contravention of human rights (O'Hara & Gregg, 2012).

Human rights principles place clear responsibilities on national governments to enshrine human rights conditions in legislation. They provide clear guidance and mandate for health policymakers and program planners to use equity and social justice as their guiding principles. Human rights principles are clearly congruent with the principles of CPHC.

The United Nations Declaration on the Rights of Indigenous Peoples was adopted in 2007 (UN, 2007). This Declaration provides a mechanism that Indigenous people can use in their advocacy with all levels of government. There has been some controversy over this Declaration with regards to use of the term 'self-determination'. In spite of this opposition, while the text provides no new rights under international law, it does signal the goodwill of nations to acknowledge historical injustices levelled at Indigenous peoples. Australia, Canada, New Zealand and the USA initially voted against the resolution, due in part to disagreement about the definition of the term 'self-determination', but all four countries have since reversed their position and now support the Declaration. There have been efforts made in Australia to set the framework for constitutional reform to recognise Aboriginal and Torres Strait Islander peoples in the nation's constitution (Aboriginal and Torres Strait Islander Social Justice Commissioner, 2015).

*For Indigenous peoples to participate in Australian society as equals requires
that we be able to live our lives free from assumptions by others about
what is best for us. It requires recognition of our values, culture and traditions
so that they can co-exist with those of mainstream society. It requires
respecting our difference and celebrating it within the diversity of the
nation.*

**(Jonas, quoted in Human Rights and Equal Opportunity
Commission, 2003)**

Equity, equality and social justice

The notion of human rights in health is closely related to the concept of equity of opportunity (fairness), rather than 'sameness' of resources or service provision (equality). To engage in activities that are underpinned by principles of equity and social justice requires political and social consciousness on the part of health practitioners. They must be advocates on behalf of communities that they work with. In some ways, the health system itself systematically excludes some groups from equitable access, especially when a universal system fails to meet the needs of people experiencing physical, cultural or geographic barriers to access (AHRC, 2015; Public Health Agency of Canada & WHO, 2008; Tesoriero, 2010). Health practitioners, such as nurses and community health promotion professionals, may feel they are powerless to change these situations, but they have important roles in addressing the inequities through their professional practice (Tesoriero, 2010).

Equity is not the same as equality although the terms are often used interchangeably. Equality is about 'sameness' whereas equity is about 'fairness'. Achieving equality does not necessarily translate into equity of access or equitable opportunities for health and wellbeing gain. Social justice is the collective expression of the principle of equity.

Equity

Equity relates to the quality of being fair or impartial. The principle of equity is strongly related to the protection of human rights. Equity is an ethical value that has been defined by the WHO as:

> the absence of avoidable or remediable differences among groups of people, whether those groups are defined socially, economically, demographically or geographically. Health inequities therefore involve more than inequality with respect to health determinants, access to the resources needed to improve and maintain health or health outcomes. They also entail a failure to avoid or overcome inequalities that infringe on fairness and human rights norms.
>
> (WHO, n.d.)

The Globalization Knowledge Network to the Commission on Social Determinants of Health described three major aspects of health inequities: health disadvantages, due to differences between segments of populations or between societies; health gaps, arising from the differences between the worse-off in a community or society and everyone else; and health gradients, relating to differences across the whole of the population (Labonté et al., 2007). Strategies to reduce inequities within and between nations need to be systematic and have a primary focus on the factors that are creating increased health risks for the most vulnerable people (WHO, 2010).

Equity is about the way resources are shared in order to provide fair access. Reflect back to the socio-ecological determinants of health and wellbeing presented in Chapter 1. Access to the resources needed to maintain health and wellbeing, such as education, employment, housing, supportive relationships and medical care services when needed, is not the same for all people. Unequal access to these resources reflects the underlying social characteristics and the hierarchies of wealth, power, opportunity and influence. Equity relates to the processes needed to ensure fair access to the socio-ecological determinants of health and wellbeing. This implies that some people, because of their life situation, will require additional support just to be able to access resources that other people take for granted. It relates to having values and policies based on enabling access relevant to people's social situation. For instance, some isolated community members need transport assistance or child care in order for them to access education, or culturally sensitive programs may be required for pregnant women from cultural minority groups. Various 'affirmative action' and 'equal opportunity' programs have been established to ensure better access or representation of groups who have not been fairly represented. Gender issues have been a key basis on which equity of access has been argued.

Ethical values are closely related to human rights principles. Human rights provide a basis for setting philosophy, developing strategies and measuring progress towards health equity (Braveman, 2014). As discussed above, human rights refer to the rights of humans everywhere to attain the highest possible standard of health. Inequities in access to resources and services put people who are already disadvantaged, perhaps because they are poor, female, or from a minority racial group, at further disadvantage in terms of human rights to health. Equity principles are needed to address these systematic disadvantages (Braveman, 2014).

Social health policies designed to ensure equity of access become a means of achieving equality of health outcomes. Most strategies to enhance equitable access to the socio-ecological determinants of health and wellbeing are outside the domain of the health sector. They include strategies to redistribute wealth through the taxation system, government pensions or services, which allow selective advantage to those experiencing barriers. Strategies also include health promoting public policy in transport, housing, sanitation, water supply, and education. Equity also means consideration of the needs of future inhabitants of our communities and planet. Although it contributes less to overall population health and wellbeing status, for the people that need it, equity of access to health services is also an important determinant of health and wellbeing. The social and public health policy priorities a government chooses can create the context for the quality of access for their population that is not dependent on the total funds expended (Mooney, 2012).

Equality

The Human Rights Charter considers all people are equal and this is a desirable aspiration. In policy, equality implies a similarity of status or sameness in service provision, and in this context, equality may not be fair to all people. Equality policies in health provide a framework that allows people to have the same means of achieving health. A universal access health insurance system is an example of an equality-based healthcare system.

There is a clear distinction here between policies that provide for equality of service, where people are offered the same support or services irrespective of the circumstances in their lives, and policies that ensure equality of capability or access, where some people are selectively advantaged in order to enable them to access services to the same level that other people in more advantaged circumstances are able to access them.

Equality in health care is an outcome measure; it is about the sameness of a service for all. The aim of equality in health service provision is to create a democratic system in which all people have access to the same services. When equality is achieved, all citizens are entitled to the goods they need to function as free and equal citizens and to avoid oppression by others. When some people are granted easier access or better service, perhaps because they have private health insurance, access is not equal or equitable. Democratic equality also obliges citizens, and people working in the health sector in particular, to promote access equality and to be advocates for change when inequities exist. It is evident that the outcomes are equality of opportunities; equality of access is achieved when equity principles underpin service access and service provision. Building equity principles into political practice and institutions such as the health system can yield tremendous positive social and health consequences. Policy approaches can provide a context for people to achieve equality of capabilities, a social system where people have the capability and freedom to choose one type of life rather than another (Public Health Agency of Canada [PHAC] & WHO, 2008; Sen, 1992).

A principle of absolute equality or sameness across a population cannot be an ideal aspiration. While it is desirable for all people to be treated equally, and for all people to have equal opportunities for health gain, it is impossible and undesirable to 'even-out' the natural differences in people's colour, shape, strengths, talents, desires, and physical and mental attributes. Similarly, not all disparities in health status are unfair. For instance, men and women are affected by different diseases such as prostate and breast cancer, and have different rates of heart disease in part based on biological characteristics. Female newborns tend to be a naturally lighter weight at birth. These are inequalities (differences) but they are not necessarily inequities (unfair).

Inequity exists when there is unfairness in the way people are treated based on factors that are socially constructed, such as discrimination based on gender, skin colour, body size, sexuality or religion. For example, the social construction of female gender stereotypes and assumptions leads to unfair unequal access to education, employment opportunities or income. SDG 5 aims to achieve gender equality and empower all women and girls, with targets related to violence, discrimination, recognition of unpaid work, sexual and reproductive health, participation in leadership, and equal rights to economic, natural and technological resources (UN, 2015).

In some countries, males have a much higher rate of death from suicide than females. This is an example of both inequality (different rates) and inequity (unfair) due to the social construction of male gender stereotypes and assumptions. The inequalities in health status between Indigenous Australians and non-Indigenous Australians, or Māori and non-Māori people in New Zealand discussed in Chapter 1 are overwhelmingly a result of socio-ecological determinants of health and wellbeing, and these differences are therefore unfair—that is, inequitable.

SDG 10 aims to reduce inequality within and among countries, and some of its targets focus on the social, economic and political inclusion of all, irrespective of age, sex, disability, race, ethnicity, origin, religion or economic or other status; eliminating discriminatory laws, policies and practices; and assisting with the orderly, safe, regular and responsible migration and mobility of people. The remainder of the targets focus on economic inequality and the structural factors that contribute to the socio-ecological determinants of health and wellbeing (UN, 2015).

One of the major objections to the ideals of equality is that the social pursuit of equality, such as through policy approaches, inevitably violates the personal liberty of some—equality ideals as a basis for resource allocation may impinge on a person's abilities to make individual decisions. It is true that sometimes equality policies, such as the taxation system, will be contrary to personal choice, but a society needs to have a policy which reflects equal concern for its citizens and to create an environment where all citizens have the opportunity to achieve their health and wellbeing goals (Duckett, 2007; Sen, 1992).

Equity, equality and social justice are fundamental values that underpin CPHC philosophy and health promotion practice. Putting these values into practice means working to reduce the systematic disparities in society by providing opportunities for disadvantaged groups to take control over aspects of their lives that would improve their health and wellbeing.

Social justice

Social justice implies a commitment to fairness or equity of access to health opportunities for all members of society. Social justice is the collective expression of equity. In CPHC, social justice or 'equity for all' must supersede individual goals and must inform international health-enhancement goals (UN, 2006).

When we reflect on the socio-ecological determinants of health and wellbeing, it becomes clear that a socially just society is much more likely to be a healthy society. If policy approaches, planning decisions and the strategies that are undertaken constantly seek to enhance access to those factors and situations that support health, then the society is acting in a socially just manner. If policymakers ask themselves 'Will this policy change make society fairer?', the eventual outcomes of adopting a fairer approach will be improved population health. As indicated earlier, the social gradient, even within high-income nations, is a key determinant of health and wellbeing. The link between health and socio-economic status follows the social gradient (Marmot, 2012; Mooney, 2012; Sommeiller & Price, 2015). Countries with more even income distribution have longer life expectancy (Marmot & Wilkinson, 2006; Wilkinson & Pickett, 2009), even in relatively poor nations. States within the United States of America (USA) with greater inequality in income distribution have higher mortality rates, lower birth weight rates, higher crime rates, higher levels of expenditure on medical care, and higher smoking and lower exercise rates than states with more equal income distribution. This association between poor health and income inequality is also associated with poor employment, imprisonment, social services and education levels.

The trends in health inequalities are becoming even more marked (Centers for Disease Control and Prevention, USA, 2013). The health status of Indigenous populations in Australia, New Zealand, Canada and the USA, all countries where original populations were affected by colonisation, has been significantly poorer than that of the dominant white (European) populations. Sustained improvements have been made in New Zealand, USA and Canada, but Australia has lagged behind the other nations in closing the gap in life expectancy (Anderson et al., 2007; AHRC, 2015; Australian Government, 2020; Ministry of Health, 2015). Achievement of a number of other milestones in the Australian Closing the Gap initiative has also lagged significantly behind expectations (AIHW, 2017; Australian Government, 2020). Closing the Gap included seven targets. In 2020, only two targets, early childhood education and Year 12 attainment, were on track to be met (Australian Government, 2020). The *Closing the Gap Report 2020* included the following summary of whether Australia met or is on track to meet the targets or not:

- The target to halve the gap in child mortality rates by 2018 was not met. From the baseline year of 2008, Indigenous child mortality rates declined by 10% but the gap did not narrow as the non-Indigenous mortality rate declined at a faster rate.

- The target to have 95% of Indigenous four-year-olds enrolled in early childhood education by 2025 is on track. In 2017, 95% of Indigenous four-year-olds were enrolled in early childhood education.

- The target to close the gap in school attendance by 2018 was not met. Attendance rates for Indigenous students did not improve between 2014 and 2018 (around 82% in 2018) and remained below the rate for non-Indigenous students (around 93%).

- The target to close the gap in life expectancy by 2031 is not on track. Between 2010 and 2012, and 2015 and 2017, Indigenous life expectancy at birth improved by 2.5 years for Indigenous males and by 1.9 years for Indigenous females (both not statistically significant), which has led to a small reduction in the gap, but not enough to close the gap completely.

- The target to halve the gap in Year 12 attainment or equivalent by 2020 is on track. In 2018–19, 66% of Indigenous Australians had completed Year 12 compared with 91% of non-Indigenous Australians. Between 2008 and 2018, the gap narrowed by 15 percentage points.

- The target to halve the gap in reading and numeracy by 2018 was not met. The proportion of Indigenous students at or above national minimum standards in reading and numeracy improved between 2008 and 2018, with the gap narrowing across all year levels by between 3 and 11 percentage points. However, these improvements were not sufficient to achieve the target to halve the gap.

- The target to halve the gap in employment by 2018 was not met. In 2018, the employment rate for Indigenous Australians was 49% compared with 75% for non-Indigenous Australians.

The effect of the social gradient on health is not explained by effects on health caused by individual behaviours such as smoking. Rather, the death rate pattern across groups with differing income levels seems far stronger than the effect of any individual risk factors for most diseases; socio-economic position and education are key markers of health outcome (Marmot, 2012). Even for diseases regarded as strongly linked to behaviours, such as coronary heart disease, the impact of income inequality is strong (Marmot, 2012; Mooney, 2012). These outcomes highlight the significant impact that inequality and the conditions that encourage it have on health, even in relatively affluent populations (Beaglehole & Bonita, 2004). They highlight the potential for long-term health improvements that could be achieved with policies based on fairer access to the fundamental conditions of living. People who have access to CPHC services are showing evidence of improved health over time in indicators such as infant mortality, making a strong argument that financial investment in CPHC for vulnerable populations does bring improvements (Mooney, 2012; Wiseman, 2014).

Evidence of the impact of inequality on individual health and the wellbeing of populations highlights the importance of applying social justice principles. Inequality affects more than the health of the population—it also affects the economic health of a society. Policies based on social justice or fairness are good for a country's economy. Inequalities in a society have detrimental effects on a country's productivity.

Power and empowerment

The concept of empowerment is fundamental to any social justice strategy. Empowerment of communities, groups, clients, isolated individuals or others is core to all health promotion action, irrespective of the setting. Empowerment is an essential component of structural or social change. It is essential in bringing sustained improvement in the context of people's lives. Empowerment within the community or social setting has been defined as:

> *a social action process that promotes participation of people, organisations, and communities towards the goals of increased individual and community control, political efficacy, improved quality of community life, and social justice.*
> *(Wallerstein, 1992, p. 198)*

The notion of empowerment is at the heart of the Ottawa Charter action area to 'strengthen community action'. Empowerment can be described as both a process and an outcome (Labonté & Laverack, 2008). In health promotion work empowerment describes the processes involved in working with individuals, organisations and communities to identify and achieve their goals. When a community is disempowered and without the capacity to bring about a desired change, empowerment can also be the outcome or goal in itself because increasing individual and community power can influence their health in a positive manner (Labonté & Laverack, 2008). Community powerlessness is a risk factor for poor health and wellbeing (Labonté & Laverack, 2008; Marmot, 2006; Wallerstein, 2006). There are two distinct pathways between community empowerment and health.

1. The processes of generating empowerment bring about changes in communities, which protect the health of residents. This can occur through psychological, social and organisational changes in families and communities.

2. The outcomes or effects of community empowerment reduce health inequities and increase access to services by influencing economic policy, decision-making and program changes (Labonté & Laverack, 2008; Wallerstein, 2006).

Laverack (2007) illustrates how community empowerment brings together a number of related community practice areas: community participation, community capacity building and community development. Equity is used as a principle to guide actions. The goals of community empowerment are the same as CPHC, the goals and strategies of which are described in more detail in the following chapters of this text, including:

- *improving community participation*
- *increasing local leadership*
- *enhancing community assessment capacities*
- *increasing community control over program planning and management*
- *improving collaboration across sectors and organisations.*

(adapted from Laverack, 2007, p. 60)

Empowerment does not mean gaining 'power over' another individual or agency. Three important points about empowerment are worth noting. First, empowerment is a term that is popular and tends to be used frequently, often in a bandaid fashion without consideration of the real implications of the term. Second, empowerment is not about people simply feeling better about themselves, but rather about people improving their control over issues impacting on them (Labonté & Laverack, 2008, Tesoriero, 2010). It is also about organisations working democratically, and communities working constructively to improve the quality of life of the community (Baum, 2016). Third, empowerment is not something that can be 'done to' someone or to a community. Rather, people and communities can only empower themselves in an interactive process (Labonté, 1989; Labonté & Laverack, 2008).

Uneven power differentials can create and maintain disadvantage in a number of ways and, through these, health status is put at risk. Power disparities are summarised from Tesoriero (2010, pp. 72–73) into the three themes below.

1. Structural disadvantage expressed through distinctions made on the basis of gender, race/ethnicity, sexuality, religion and body size. Discrimination occurs in those areas that have the greatest impact on health of populations: income, occupation and educational attainment. Further, mainstream health services are structured in such a way as to provide services that are less appropriate for the healthcare needs of people who are, for example, poor, unemployed, transsexual, from a racial minority, or in a larger body. When these forms of oppression are combined, known as intersectionality (Hancock, 2016), people suffer significant barriers to health and other services. For example, the experiences of poor Aboriginal women with larger bodies are dramatically worsened by multiple intersecting forms of oppression (Anderson et al., 2007; Kelaher et al., 2014).

2. Groups who are oppressed because of other personal characteristics. These groups may be discriminated against because they belong to minority groups, or groups of people that are stigmatised by society. They may include those

who are old, homosexual, physically or intellectually disabled, those who suffer from mental illnesses or who live in isolated rural areas or are people from visible minority groups. They are not necessarily affected by structural disadvantage; however, they are less powerful because of their condition or situation.

3. Individuals who are disadvantaged or disempowered because of their personal circumstances, such as relationship issues, poverty, loneliness or grief. The issues causing disempowerment may be temporary, but they often interact with other forms of structural disadvantage, making it more difficult for those affected to access relevant support (Kelaher et al., 2014; Markwick et al., 2015).

Perspectives on power are explored by social theorists. Power and empowerment literature relevant to health promotion practitioners includes the work of Anderson and colleagues (2007), Baum (2016), Freire (1974), Kelaher and others (2014), Labonté (1989, 1997), Labonté and Laverack (2008), Laverack (2007), Tesoriero (2010), Wallerstein (1992, 2006) and Wallerstein and Bernstein (1994). This text does not provide a sociological analysis. However, it is important to understand the ways that power is exercised in society.

Tesoriero (2010, p. 240) describes the role of practitioners supporting empowerment of a vulnerable group as one of providing people with the resources, opportunities, vocabulary, knowledge and skills to increase their capacity to determine their own future, and to participate in, and affect the life of, their community. Tesoriero (2010, pp. 64–68) offers four perspectives on empowerment.

1. Various groups in society are competing for power (politicians, unionists, lobby groups, professions, media, etc.). Empowerment is a process of helping disadvantaged groups to compete more effectively with other interests.

2. Elite groups have more than their share of power and exercise disproportionate influence over decision making. They control the institutions, media, education, political parties, public policy, the bureaucracy, parliament, professions, etc. Empowerment is learning the ability to compete for political power, to seek alliances with elites, or to limit their power, such as through participation in service clubs, school networks, the Australian Medical Association and other professional associations.

3. Structural inequality and oppression are major forms of power (white, wealthy, men). Empowerment is achieved by challenging structural disadvantage through social change.

4. Power is expressed through the use of language (discourse), which is used as a mechanism of control. Empowerment is achieved through validating voices other than those currently dominating the discourse.

If people are to gain greater power over their lives, they need ready access to information, supportive relationships, decision-making processes and resources (Labonté & Laverack, 2008; Kelaher et al., 2014; Markwick et al., 2015; Tesoriero, 2010). Health practitioners can play an important role in creating a climate for empowerment by enabling access to these things through the community development process. Empowerment needs to occur through both the process and the outcome of community development activity. Working to enable individuals and communities to become empowered requires particular skills in health practitioners. They must be willing to share their skills and time, and relinquish their need to be the 'expert' who holds the wisdom (Gregg & O'Hara, 2007a). That is, it is not acceptable to take over from community members in order to achieve a positive outcome for them, when in the process they are left feeling no more capable, or even less capable, of acting more independently next time. While there may be times when quick action on issues by practitioners is warranted, this action cannot be described as community development.

Two last points are worth emphasising. The first is that empowerment is about increasing people's power over things influencing their lives, but power is rarely a neutral concept. An increase in the power that one person or group has over something in their lives will often result in someone else losing that power. This is extremely important because it reminds us that as long as community development concerns itself with the empowerment of people, those involved in the process risk experiencing conflict. Although consensus building is an important part of community development, conflict may sometimes be an unavoidable consequence (Tesoriero, 2010). The second point is to recognise that the majority of health practitioners generally still work within the traditional culture and organisational power structures that can create and perpetuate circumstances of disempowerment, and they may feel they have little capacity to change this. There is potential for significant philosophical challenges to the health practitioner's values and beliefs that may be very difficult to resolve, at least in the short term.

Social capital

The term 'social capital' has been used a great deal in recent years as a concept which encapsulates social processes at the community level. Social capital is more complex to define and understand than either human (discussed earlier in this chapter) or economic (discussed later in this chapter) capital, probably because its characteristics are less tangible and more subjective. Social capital describes characteristics of social norms and values and the quality of the links and associations between people in different forms of communities. Social capital is important because, where it is stronger, human health and wellbeing is better. Robert Putnam (1993) described social capital as the 'invisible glue' between people that binds a community together. In the context of health promotion, social capital gives rise to a range of strategies for connecting and building communities in line with the Ottawa Charter action are a of strengthening community action (WHO, 1986).

The relationships contributing to social capital reflect mutuality, specifically shared respect and trust, and produce collective benefits when applied to the pursuit of shared goals. Indicators and measures of social capital illustrate the link between social capital and individual and community health and wellbeing. People whose lives and activities are deeply embedded in their communities are healthier and happier and less likely to engage in risk-taking behaviour (Field, 2004). Research has indicated that social capital is also likely to enhance economic productivity and reduce economic and social transaction costs (Field, 2004; Talbot & Walker, 2007). Social capital enables interactions among strangers without expectation of immediate reciprocity or payment. There are clear public benefits in this, and this explains the interest in the concept shown by national policy advisers.

Additional research about the concept of social capital has enabled the definition to be refined to accommodate differences in the patterns of participation in community relationships, thus enabling development of specific approaches to building or maintaining social capital. Three forms of social capital have been described by Woolcock (1998) and refined by Healy and Coté (2001). These three forms are bonding, bridging and linking social capital.

Bonding social capital describes the strong links between a relatively homogeneous group of people such as close friends and family who share identity relations. It is based on the expectation that other members of the group are like oneself and therefore worthy of cooperation and trust. Bonding social capital networks typically exclude people who are perceived as different. There is potential for strong bonding social capital networks, such as religious sects or youth gangs, to be unhealthy in that they deliberately exclude 'outsiders'.

Bridging social capital refers to the links between distant friends, associates and colleagues. Members of bridging networks join together in pursuit of a collective goal that they cannot achieve alone or through their bonding social capital networks. Membership of bridging networks is typically inclusive of diverse people who value and gain benefits from pursuit of a shared goal and is exemplified by the informal networks of association found in volunteer activity within a community.

An individual's access to bonding and bridging social capital is in part a consequence of individual action and in part a consequence of the person's position in the broader social structures of a community. Poor and marginalised people may have strong bonding relationships but little access to bridging networks that may help them escape disadvantage.

Linking social capital refers to the links between individuals and groups in 'different social strata in a hierarchy where power, social status and wealth are accessed by different groups' (Healy & Coté, 2001). Linking social capital describes the formal levels of trust that develop or are assumed between community members and agencies they interact with that may have power, control and decision-making capacity. It is explicitly about creating bridges across social boundaries, such as between the state and civil society, public and private institutions, business organisations and their communities. Where the quality of the relationships are appropriate and respectful and trusting, such as with banks, health organisations, and local government agencies, linking social capital can have a positive influence on the welfare of citizens. Because community members' interactions with these agencies have the potential to be characterised by unequal hierarchies of power, linking social capital is the form of social capital where the context of policy change will be most clearly evident (Talbot & Walker, 2007). Local government has potential to serve as a very valuable conduit for linking social capital between community members and services. When local mechanisms to facilitate access to services are no longer available, people lose their faith that services will be provided equitably or that their voices will be heard in debate about local issues of concern (Talbot & Walker, 2007).

There can be a strong positive interrelationship between human and social capital. Aspects of human capital such as education, learning and skills are associated with strong community links between people. Likewise, accepted values of cooperation and collaboration at community level enhance opportunities for development of human capital (Field, 2004).

The intangible nature of social capital means that the processes of building social capital are more difficult to describe than other types of capital. An important reason that social capital has been difficult to define is because the presence or strength of social capital only becomes evident when it is used. In this respect, social capital is a potential resource. Baum (1999, p. 1) stated that 'social capital's importance lies in the way in which it assists members of society to gain access to other forms of capital', such as economic capital, cultural capital and symbolic capital (legitimation).

The nature and quality of links people have with others and with other communities has a significant impact on their quality of life and sense of wellbeing. While it has been assumed that social isolation relates to a deficit in the number of contacts in a person's network, the rise in use of the internet, especially in social media, has focused on the quality of interactions as a measure of social isolation. Social media is predominantly used as a means of social connection and interaction, and there has been considerable debate about whether this leads to greater social isolation in the usual sense, or whether it is an indicator of effective social connection in a new form (Parigi & Henson, 2014). People who have limited close or community ties may feel isolated and lose hope. However, Parigi and Henson (2014), in their extensive review of the literature, have argued that social isolation can refer to people with few connections or also people with many and diverse connections which have little 'meaning' or 'quality'; people may rarely have the undivided attention of another, and there may be no deep engagement with the other. People who feel socially connected are more able to take part in volunteer community activities and are more inclined to do so (Talbot & Walker, 2007).

Social connectedness is a way of describing the quality of the relationships people have with others and the benefits those relationships bring to the individual as well as to society. It includes informal relationships with family, friends, colleagues and neighbours, as well as relationships people make through participating in sport or other leisure activities, paid work or by contributing to their communities through voluntary work or community service. Social connectedness can also arise in virtual communities through social media platforms, blogs, YouTube and email networks.

The links of community connectedness or community engagement are important at the interpersonal level within families, close friends and community networks, and in the links people have with institutions, business and government (Labonté & Laverack, 2008; Talbot & Walker, 2007). Working to enhance community connectedness provides an alternative framework for working with individuals and institutions to bring about positive social change. Mechanisms to enhance community connectedness are discussed in Chapter 6.

Resilience

Use of the term 'resilience' is now widespread, and it has been used for some time in ecological literature (Brown, 2013). It is portrayed as a positive attribute describing a person's or a community's ability to 'bounce back' after a challenge. For example, a community that is able to rebuild and reconnect after a devastating fire is labelled as resilient, and celebrated because of the characteristics it has demonstrated. Adger (2000, cited in Brown, 2013, p. 111) described social resilience as 'the ability of communities to withstand shocks to their social infrastructure'. The ability to adapt and transform is core to resilience: 'adjustments occur at all (and interlinked) scales—for individuals, society, institutions, technology, economy and ecology—and may involve changes to practices, norms and values' (Brown, 2013, p. 113). Taylor and Guerin (2014) emphasise that adversity has effects, even if a community or person is resilient and is able to 'bounce back'. If there is constant adversity over a long period, resilience is eventually lost. Resilience is being used as a local organising principle to build activism and as a policy aspiration in local and regional government. Resilient communities are portrayed as those that are able to recognise and build on their assets to bring about change that meets their needs (Hall & Lamont, 2013). Community development approaches are used to build local action, value diverse approaches and make local changes; achieving social justice and building social capital are core values (Brown, 2013). Okvat and Zautra (2011) make the argument that community gardening has the potential to strengthen community resilience and build social capital, and reduce the impacts of climate change through sustained local action. This is also the philosophy behind the Transition Towns movement, which originated in Totnes, Devon, in England as a local community action response to peak oil and climate change, and that has now become a global movement (Transition Town Totnes, n.d.).

Taylor and Guerin (2014), reflecting on the continuing experiences of Indigenous Australians, argue that greater emphasis needs to be placed on reducing adversity rather than expecting communities to be resilient. Brown (2013) and Hall and Lamont (2013) also emphasise caution in unquestioned use of the term, firstly because it is insufficiently theorised, but especially because it fails to take account of the influence of neoliberal politics and power relations; it is an inherently conservative term. In this context, there is a danger of romanticising the seeming capacity of communities to cope with significant challenge or change, and this undermines their access to support and recovery services or their ability to have influence in local democratic processes.

Cultural environment

Culture

Health practitioners may not be conscious of the norms and values of their own culture, especially when they are part of the dominant society. They may not consider that their worldview is different from that of some of the people that they work with. Culture has been defined as:

> *... a set of guidelines ... which an individual inherits as a member of a particular society and which tells him how to view the world and learn how to behave in relation to other people. It also provides him with a way of transmitting these guidelines to the next generation.*
> **(Helman, 2007, cited in De & Richardson, 2015, p. 17)**

Culture develops within a social, political and historical context and expresses a group's preferred ways of thinking about the world. These worldviews permeate all social structures, and are reflected in the policies and procedures that govern the system itself. Culture defines relationships and roles within society by describing rights and obligations. In some instances, culture constrains individual behaviour, while in others it results in shared meanings and understandings, leaving room for the beliefs and interpretations of individuals. As a result, the culture of the dominant group in a society, community or group is largely taken for granted by them.

The interrelationship between culture and history is reflected in the shared meanings that make up a culture. The meanings have developed from the history of that cultural group. While some of that history may be in the distant past, other history may be relatively recent and very much alive for the people concerned. The history of European treatment of Indigenous peoples across the world including in Australia, New Zealand, the USA and Canada is a stark example of this point, and this history remains significant in determining their attitudes to services and staff that represent the colonising powers, including wariness of mainstream health systems (Anderson et al., 2007). Recognition and public acknowledgement of past cultural oppression, and in the case of New Zealand, enshrining this in the national constitution, has been significant in overcoming the wariness that characterises much Indigenous–non-Indigenous communication. Australia has lagged behind the other nations on this matter, to the clear detriment of the wellbeing of the Aboriginal peoples (Eckermann et al., 2010).

Because culturally driven beliefs and practices are so unconscious, many people are often unable, unless they make a conscious effort, to recognise the culturally influenced values and behaviours they portray to others (Anderson et al., 2007). Furthermore, because the 'mainstream' or dominant culture is so familiar to most people, they assume their values are 'normal' and only others have culture. They tend to believe that their way of thinking, acting and judging should be shared by others, and they tend to unfavourably judge others who do not have similar values. Consider how traditional British culture and values have underpinned the whole structure and processes of the medical care system in Australia, New Zealand and Canada. This culture and its associated values continue to influence the perceptions of appropriate 'patient role' behaviour and how health practitioners react and treat people who appear not to fit with traditional expectations (Anderson et al., 2007).

An individual's upbringing, their education and their own 'enculturation' may make it difficult to reflect on and challenge notions that are considered commonsense or traditional in their own culture, but being willing and able to do this is at the basis of ensuring 'cultural safety' in professional practice and personal life (Harris et al., 2006). If health practitioners are to work effectively with others, they must ensure that they are able to critically reflect on their own beliefs and values that are taken for granted, so they can respond effectively in the face of differing cultures and values.

Language plays a key role in transmitting and reproducing the dominant culture, and can be a major barrier to effective communication. This can be the case even when communicating in English with people from another culture, as meanings and nuances can be culturally specific even when the same language is apparently being spoken. In addition, non-verbal communication is just as much culturally driven as verbal communication and so greater awareness of non-verbal communication is vital. Being mindful that other people's non-verbal communication may not mean what it appears to, and that one's own non-verbal communication may be misinterpreted, is essential.

Fear and alienation stem from different definitions and understanding of 'health' derived from cultural and spiritual backgrounds (Naidoo & Wills, 2011). Healthcare settings have been places of overt or covert discrimination, stereotyping, prejudice and racism (Gallaher et al., 2009; Jeffreys, 2010). Culturally inappropriate health services can contribute to or maintain inequalities (Downing et al., 2011). Minority groups, including homeless people and immigrants, may also challenge providers' attitudes because of the provider's lack of awareness about illiteracy, poverty and fear. Ongoing economic and social uncertainty, perhaps created by 'illegal' immigration or refugee status, creates greater numbers needing acute mental health services, which in turn demands great sensitivity by healthcare providers. For Indigenous peoples in particular, health is a spiritual concept. To maintain health means sustaining links with all forms of cultural expression; through one's language, family ties and links to the land. Conversely, when cultural worth is not recognised, when one cultural system restricts the level of choice of healthcare facilities or fails to respect health values and attitudes, clients find themselves in a position of 'cultural danger' (Eckermann et al., 2010).

When people find they need to work with someone from another culture, their initial reaction is often to find out about the other culture by reading. However, books and articles are a limited way of finding out about another culture. First, they tend to portray a static picture of a culture, when in fact culture is dynamic and constantly changing. Second, because they provide little or no room to individualise cultural beliefs and interpretation, an image of a culture as uniformly shared by all its members is presented. Just as members of our own culture vary widely in the acceptance of its values, so too do members of other cultures. Third, books often represent a very limited view of the cultures they discuss. For example, many anthropological accounts of cultures ignore women's roles, and present a one-sided picture of cultural life. While reading about other cultures may be useful, understanding them will be strengthened by getting to know people who represent the foreign culture on a personal level, listening to these people and coming to conclusions tentatively (Giles et al., 2015; Harris et al., 2006; Robson & Harris, 2005). Living in a foreign culture and becoming immersed in the daily lives of the people can provide greater cultural understanding.

Particular cultural 'ways of being' will vary between different cultures and communities and according to current situations. Common differences between cultures that health practitioners need to understand are time orientation, personal space, the interrelationship between culture and religion, family practices (such as avoidance relationships), status rules according to gender and age, philosophies and beliefs about health and wellbeing and illness, and forms of non-verbal communication (Robson & Harris, 2005).

Cultural safety and competence

The concept of a cultural safety approach was developed in Indigenous health care in New Zealand (Papps & Ramsden, 1996; Ramsden, 2002). It is widely used in New Zealand, where it is a core component of the nursing and midwifery curricula, and by health professionals working particularly with Indigenous populations in Australia, and in Canada (Eckermann et al., 2010; Johnstone & Kanitsaki, 2007; Taylor & Guerin, 2014). The term emerged from expressions of oppression experienced by people in their interactions within the health sector (Eckermann et al., 2010; Ramsden, 2002).

> Cultural safety ... investigates setting up systems which enable the less powerful to genuinely monitor the attitudes and services of the powerful, to comment with safety, and ultimately, to create useful and positive change which can only be of benefit to nursing and to all the people with whom nurses and midwives serve.
>
> *(Ramsden, 2002, cited in Eckermann et al., 2010, p. 183)*

There is growing literature on a range of concepts related to culturally appropriate professional practice, and a number of related terms (see Australian Indigenous Doctors Association, 2017; Downing et al., 2011; Gallaher et al., 2009; Giles et al., 2015; Jeffreys, 2010; Johnstone & Kanitsaki, 2007; Taylor & Guerin, 2014; Woods, 2010). Table 2.1 provides a summary of the main terms, their differences and some critique of the strengths and limitations of each. Of these terms, cultural safety and cultural competence appear most commonly in health and health-related professional policy, competency standards and professional training initiatives. In short, cultural safety is an 'outcome experienced by the recipient of health care' (Eckermann et al., 2010, p. 185). Cultural competence refers to the capabilities (awareness, knowledge and skills) of, in this case, health practitioners to practise in a culturally safe and respectful way. Cultural humility is an important cultural capability that requires 'self-humility', or the ability to reflect on one's own values, biases and stereotypes about one's own and the cultures of others, and cognisant of power imbalances in all interactions, achieved through ongoing lifelong self-reflection (Foronda et al., 2016; Greene-Moton & Minkler, 2020).

There has, however, been inadequate progress in recognising the unique voices of Indigenous and minority groups in defining culturally safe care, and in the development of cultural competency across society, not only in the health workforce (Eckermann et al., 2010). Together, cultural safety and CPHC principles require people to reflect on their practice, and potentially provide solutions to significant imbalances of power in health systems and processes (Eckermann et al., 2010, p. 188; Taylor & Guerin, 2014). The Mahitahi Trust (Insight 2.2) is an example where the services that the Trust delivers are based on nga Tikanga Māori (Māori cultural beliefs and practices, or general behaviour guidelines). Tikanga Māori philosophy is guided by the Te Whare Tapa Whā (the Māori Health Models) which form the four cornerstones of Māori Health and which are embedded in New Zealand training programs for all health professionals. These are taha tinana (physical health: the capacity for physical growth and development), taha wairua (spiritual health: the capacity for faith and wider communication), taha whanau (family health: the capacity to belong, to care and to share where individuals are part of wider social systems) and

TABLE 2.1 Terms relating to culturally appropriate professional practice

Term	Description	Critique

Cultural competency	• The development of awareness, knowledge and skills to provide care and services that fit with the person's own values, beliefs, traditions and practices.
	• Cultural competence is developed through two processes:
	  1. diversity self-awareness—'active reflection about one's own cultural identity' (Jeffreys, 2010, p. 28)
	  2. diversity awareness—'one becomes proactively aware of similarities and differences within and between various cultural groups' (Jeffreys, 2010, p. 28).
	• Should occur within an organisational setting that embraces diversity and seeks to promote multicultural harmony.
	• The culturally competent practitioner has the ability to work in the context of (another) set of cultural beliefs (working in partnership, rather than as the expert).
	• Community consultation around decision making.
	• Drawing on the wisdom of the cultural groups for whom the service is being planned or provided (as translators, advisers, peer educators).
		• Culture is understood as a static variable. Race is often assumed to be the same as ethnicity without reference to within-group differences.
		• It focuses on the individual carer having the competency, rather than a system-wide set of values and expectations.
		• Ignoring relations of power (the practitioner may never have to examine their own cultural values and how they may influence the health promotion action), it portrays the clients' culture as 'different' from the 'normal' of the practitioner, and thus fails to adequately address power differentials inherent in many health services (Woods, 2010).

Cultural appropriateness	• Creation and delivery of programs that reflect the diversity within a racial or ethnic group. • The program elements are situated within the cultural and geographic context of the intended audience: it reflects their cultural values; the strategies reflect the social and behavioural norms of the intended audience; and, the activities reflect the behavioural preferences of the group.	• The (different) cultural origins of the person delivering the program influences the uptake of the strategies and the effectiveness of the outcomes.

Cultural sensitivity	• Recognition of the value base of our own and others' cultures.
	• The program designer or practitioners would need to adapt four concepts to the culture of the target group/audience:
	  o knowledge—reflected by practitioners' preparedness to listen and to learn from those with whom they are working. Recognising that there is scope within culture for individual difference; indeed, there is as much variety and conflict within communities from other cultures as there is within communities generally
	  o making consideration of the cultural context—canvass the perspectives of as many people as possible, rather than assuming one small group reflects the opinions of the community overall
	  o understanding the perspective and priorities of the cultural group—building on what is known within the cultural group and what is possible economically, socially, environmentally
	  o respect and tailoring—being willing to make changes to get greater buy-in.
		• The criteria can lead to stereotyping—the planner learns some general cultural characteristics and applies these uncritically to all people from that cultural group.
		• The provider is not obliged to reflect on his or her cultural values, or on the variances within the cultural group of the audience.
		• It perpetuates the perspective of cultural superiority and power-over of the provider—it renders the culture of the practitioner as invisible in the planning and delivery of programs.
		• Fails to attend to the relations of power inherent in the interactions (cultural disempowerment).

Continued

TABLE 2.1 Terms relating to culturally appropriate professional practice—cont'd

Term	Description	Critique

Cultural safety	• Cultural safety encourages the practitioner to reflect on their own cultural history, values and cultural power, as a tool to shift interactions to be representative of non-dominant knowledge and cultures. It builds on the concepts above, especially the need for reflective self-awareness. In order to understand and meet the participants' needs, cultural safety challenges the view of the dominant group as being 'normal'.
	• Principles:
	  1. Recognise the health perceptions of the client group that are different from those of the practitioner in any way. This includes ensuring a systemic awareness of the historical, political and social processes that influence their practice, and the values of those in their care, including why they may feel unsafe in the care setting.
	  2. The practitioner acknowledges ways in which these differences can influence the power dynamics involved in the relationship between service providers and service users, and the institutional structures and policies that contribute to these relationships of power.
	  3. Acknowledge that power imbalances in the healthcare field reflects broader inequalities, and thus requires that the practitioner acknowledge the historical, social and political systems that have influenced this dynamic.
	  4. Focus on the practitioner's ability to examine his/her own culture and practice to address the potential to further contribute to unequal power relationships. Cultural safety is achieved through mutual respect for another's worldview and development of shared understanding of socio-cultural practices. The vulnerable recipient of care defines what culturally safe care is, and the health practitioners seek guidance where necessary.
		• The responsibility to protect cultural safety rests with the health service, not only with the practitioner.
		• Cultural safety in practice allows health practitioners to better respond to unequal relations of power, and thus is more socially just.
		• Individuals, communities and health agencies become partners in planning and delivering health care, drawing on the wisdom of the experts whose culture is different from the 'norm'.

INSIGHT 2.2 The Mahitahi Trust

Mahitahi Trust (2019) is a Māori organisation that provides support services within a Kaupapa Māori framework. The Trust aims to assist people to regain mental wellness through the delivery of community, education, employment and housing services. The Trust aims to decrease prevalence of mental illness in the community, while at the same time, increasing the health status, and reducing the impact of mental disorders on tangata whaiora (those who use their services) and the impact upon whānau (family), hapū (subtribe) and iwi (tribe).

All of the services that the Trust delivers are based on Nga Tikanga Māori (Māori cultural beliefs and practices). The work of the Trust often starts with assisting tangata whaiora to reconnect culturally and learn about their whakapapa. This preparatory work assists tangata whaiora to improve their life skills and strengthen their sense of identity, knowledge and understanding of their Māoritanga (Māori practices and beliefs).

Staff demonstrate eight guiding values, known as Nga Pou e Waru, in their day-to-day work. These are eight carefully selected values that cement Tikanga into every aspect of the work and care that Mahitahi Trust performs.

CEO Raewyn Allan sums up the work of Mahitahi by saying, 'Everything we do is steeped in Māori.'

Source: Mahitahi Trust, 2019.

taha hinengaro (mental health: the capacity to communicate, to think and to feel mind and body are inseparable). They are seen as equally important pillars of wellbeing (Ministry of Health, 2017).

Another example is the *Cultural Respect Framework for Aboriginal and Torres Strait Islander Health 2016–2026* (Australian Health Ministers' Advisory Council, 2016) which provides national guidance on how to build a health system that is culturally respectful. Cultural respect is defined in the framework as 'recognition, protection and continued advancement of the inherent rights, cultures and traditions of Aboriginal and Torres Strait Islander people' (p. 5). It is premised on an understanding that cultural respect leads to better health outcomes and aims 'to support the corporate health governance, organisational management and delivery of the Australian health system to further embed safe, accessible and culturally responsive services' (p. 4). Guiding principles underpin six domains for action with focus areas for each domain. For each focus area there is a set of elements that jurisdictions and organisations need to consider to ensure cultural respect. The framework is also linked to other national-level policy documents including the National Aboriginal and Torres Strait Islander 2013–2023 Health Plan (Australian Government, 2013) and the Implementation Plan for the National Aboriginal and Torres Strait Islander Health Plan 2013–2023 (Australian Government, 2015).

Professional competency or standards frameworks, including the Core Competencies and Professional Standards for Health Promotion (Barry et al., 2012), specify competencies related to the cultural capability of practitioners. We suggest that you identify specific cultural competencies in the competency framework relevant to your profession. Tertiary training programs also play an important role in ensuring health professional graduates have the cultural capabilities to work effectively and respectfully in cultural contexts different from their own. Many universities have frameworks to guide the embedding of Aboriginal and Torres Strait Islander knowledges and perspectives into the curriculum. In Australia, the Aboriginal and Torres Strait Islander Health Curriculum Framework

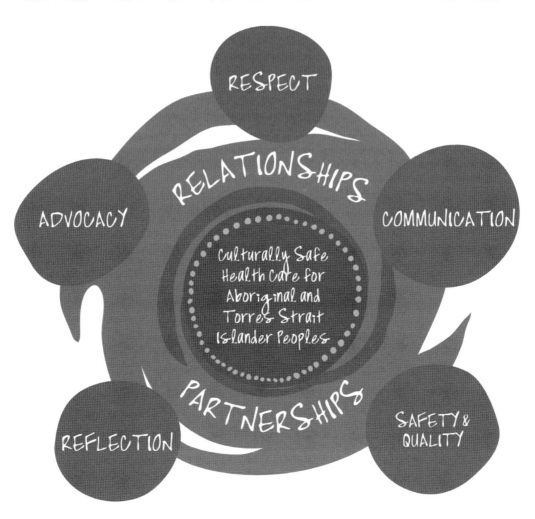

FIGURE 2.2 Graduate Cultural Capability Model
Source: Australian Government, 2014.

(Australian Government, 2014) was developed as a resource to support tertiary institutions to integrate cultural capability attitudes, knowledge and skills into an Aboriginal and Torres Strait Islander health curriculum. The framework presents a 'Graduate Cultural Capability Model' (Fig. 2.2) for 'Culturally safe health care for Aboriginal and Torres Strait Islander Peoples'. It comprises the following five interrelated cultural capabilities, each with a set of descriptors that specify what students need to demonstrate cultural competence:

1. Respect—historical context, cultural knowledge, diversity, and humility and lifelong learning.
2. Communication—culturally safe communication, partnerships.
3. Safety and quality—clinical presentation, population health.
4. Reflection—cultural self and health care, racism, white privilege.
5. Advocacy—equity and human rights, leadership.

The Public Health Indigenous Leadership in Education (PHILE) Network (2016) developed the National Aboriginal and Torres Strait Islander Public Health Curriculum Framework to assist universities offering Master of Public Health programs to achieve effective integration of Aboriginal and Torres Strait Islander health concepts within their programs. The first five of the six competencies included in the Framework refer to content, which is important for ensuring the embedding of Indigenous knowledges and perspectives into curricula. The sixth competency is that MPH graduates should 'demonstrate a reflexive public health practice for Aboriginal and Torres Strait Islander health contexts'. Reflexive practice is essential to the development of cultural competence.

Economic and political environment
Health services
Access to health services

People's access to health services is greatly influenced by the overall quality and philosophy of the health system of the nation. People may experience structural and personal barriers in accessing the health services they need because of the political philosophy and level of funding to the health system in their country. National funding for health services reflects national policy and/or the political philosophy of the government, and this determines the range and quality of services available to the ordinary population. Structural barriers in particular relate to cost and geography. Cost can be a barrier, even when health services are provided 'free' through a national health service, or the usual cost of the service is subsidised, such as the cost of medicines provided through the Pharmaceutical Benefits Scheme in Australia and the Pharmaceutical Management Agency in New Zealand. Geography can be a structural barrier to equitable access to services because there are fewer services, which are more sparsely spread in rural areas, and because the costs of travel to access those services must be borne by the individual. In nations with less well-developed health systems, the problems of inequitable access are even greater, and, in these situations, international political philosophy, such as neoliberalism, has made accessing services more difficult and with increased inequalities (Mooney, 2012; Verrinder & Talbot, 2015).

Personal barriers that limit access to or uptake of services may relate to poorer education and health literacy or the competency of the person seeking the care, which, as the discussions earlier have set out, are usually a product of the person's experience of the socio-ecological determinants of health and wellbeing (Verrinder & Talbot, 2015).

Health system expenditure

A number of factors at a national level are combined to influence the relationship between health system expenditure and health status in a country. Some of them are summarised here.

- *Taxation system.* This relates to the level of taxation and the redistributive nature of taxation. When wealthy people are taxed at higher levels than those on modest incomes, and the funds are used to pay for universal access to public health measures, health equity is improved.
- *Social welfare philosophy.* This may be enshrined in legislation or the national/state constitution. A nation or government may see it as a public duty to provide some health-related services to all people to protect their health. Nations with an individualistic political philosophy (such as the USA) expect people to make provision for most of their own healthcare costs. Poorer people and those with poor health are disadvantaged with this approach. Social

welfare can include services from a range of sectors that are not traditionally considered to be 'health', including housing assistance, unemployment benefits, employment assistance, transport and so on.

- *Proportion of the GDP spent on the health system.* This is the proportion of money drawn from the total national productivity that is allocated to the health system, compared with competing demands, such as spending on warfare. When this proportion is low, fewer services are available, and/or costs to the individual tend to be higher. This is greatly influenced by the social philosophy of the nation, the range of other 'non-health' services provided by the government, and whether there is a universal health system or a private health insurance program.

- *The public/private mix in service provision.* Private health insurance effectively means a two-tier system is created, which results in increasing costs and increasing inequities in access.

Refer also to the European Observatory on Health Systems and Policies (2016), which supports and promotes evidence-based health policymaking in Europe and provides a detailed analysis of various health systems.

If a nation adopts social justice philosophy in its constitution, or the principle is supported by an elected government, the government is philosophically obliged to enact policy for the benefit of the entire population. Governments that fail to provide health policy and funding that safeguards the welfare of their citizens are failing to uphold their part in the social contract and are, therefore, unjust. Unjust societies have poorer population health than just societies. Use of the taxation system to redistribute resources conducive to health is an equity-based approach, which can have a significant impact on the health status of populations.

It is evident that economic growth will not be sufficient by itself to further improve health status in the majority low-income world, and since the global financial crisis, sustaining previous levels of financial growth is no longer ensured (Mooney, 2012; Scott, 2012; UN, 2014). High levels of funding for a health system does not guarantee equitable access to its resources; appropriate political will and policy are essential. Likewise, the proportion of GDP spent on the health system in a nation does not necessarily reflect the quality of access for all people, or the quality of CPHC services in a country. Vulnerable groups, including the poor, women, religious and sexual minority groups, Indigenous populations and people living in isolated areas, will face increased barriers to accessing their rights to equitable services (UN, 2014). However, on an international level, there are clear positive health outcomes from increased funding of CPHC services (as distinct from medical services) as a proportion of total health system expenditure. In addition, spending money on CPHC tends to reduce overall healthcare costs, particularly because of the multidimensional health impacts of the socio-ecological determinants of health and wellbeing and the potential impacts of CPHC on avoidable mortality (UN, 2014).

International comparisons

Total health expenditure in a nation is the total of public and private health expenditure. It covers the provision of health promotion, prevention, treatment and rehabilitation, but not other public health measures such as water and sanitation. The Global Health Expenditure Database (WHO, 2019a) shows that in 2016 total health spending accounted for 9.25% of GDP in Australia and 9.22% of GDP in New Zealand, with both countries slightly lower than the global average of 10.02% and well below the OECD average of 12.59% (WHO, 2019b). The level of expenditure in Australia has continued to steadily increase over time

(AIHW, 2018). Globally, as the health sector has grown, it has become less reliant on out-of-pocket spending by individuals. Total out-of-pocket spending has grown more slowly than public spending across low- middle- and high-income countries (WHO, 2019b).

Norway is one of the richest countries in the world and ranks highly in the Human Development Index; however, it spends considerably less of its GDP (10.5%) on its health system than the OECD average (WHO, 2019a). The general trends in health reform in Norway over the past few decades have been a focus on reducing inequities in the 1970s, cost containment and decentralisation in the 1980s, efficiency and leadership in the 1990s, and structural changes in delivery and organisation to reduce inequalities in the 2000s. Although health spending as a proportion of GDP in Norway is similar to that of Australia, there is a high general taxation rate which provides a considerable range of other socio-ecological determinants of health and wellbeing, including child care, dental care, education, employment assistance, social support and transport assistance, almost all (85%) of which is funded from tax revenue (European Observatory on Health Systems and Policies, 2016). Japan also ranks high in the Human Development Index and has one of the highest life expectancies in the world. Health expenditure in Japan was 11% of GDP in 2016 (WHO, 2019a).

The health of Australians and New Zealanders generally compares well with comparable countries in the OECD. Despite the improvements to economic stability, sanitation, water supply and nutrition that have been achieved in many nations in the Asia-Pacific region in the last two decades, numerous countries still have life expectancies of less than 70 years. In Papua New Guinea, Cambodia, Myanmar and India, a child born in 2010 can expect to live an average of less than 65 years. Mortality from some conditions, including cardiovascular disease and injuries, is lower than the OECD average for both Australia and New Zealand. Deaths from avoidable mortality tend to be slightly higher in New Zealand than Australia, perhaps indicating the higher ratio of medical doctors and other health professionals per head of population in Australia (OECD, 2016). By comparison, New Zealand cancer mortality tends to be lower than the OECD average and significantly better than that of Australia. Australia and New Zealand rank highly within the OECD for self-rated health and low rates of all-cause mortality, but are lower than the OECD average for infant mortality, alcohol consumption and vegetable intake. While there have been significant improvements in a number of areas in the past 20 years, in areas such as coronary heart disease, there are also significant causes of mortality and morbidity that would be amenable to change, especially in areas such as smoking, type 2 diabetes mellitus, and mental health (AIHW, 2018; Ministry of Health, 2016).

Australia and New Zealand maintain predominantly publicly funded healthcare systems, which provide equal access to public health services. In 2010, the proportion spent on public healthcare services was higher in New Zealand (79.8%) than in Australia (68%). In countries such as Australia that have continued to actively support private health services, the public sector proportion of total expenditure is lower than in other OECD countries (OECD average 72.7%). This compares with 48.2% public funding in the USA, which has a large private health sector (OECD, 2016). Publicly funded healthcare systems have been better able to contain costs while generating universal cover compared with more privatised systems (Figueras & McKee, 2012). Britain was the first Western nation to introduce a national universal health system in 1946, but many would argue that this system now urgently needs higher funding and the support of national public health measures funded through the taxation system (European Observatory on Health Systems and Policies, 2016; Figueras & McKee, 2012). Some high-taxing nations that have redistributive tax regulations are able to improve population health status through these measures.

Traditionally, the USA has spent a considerably higher proportion of GDP on health than any other country; 17% in 2016. The US health system has been predominantly managed by private health insurance companies linked to a person's employment contract. A very high proportion of funds is spent on administration, and access to services has been highly inequitable, depending on the agreement between the worker, employer and provider. Workers on lower wages get much less in their package of benefits. The government has provided access to basic medical services for the very poor through Medicaid, but it is estimated that close to 10% of Americans, mostly in low-paid casual employment, have no health insurance, and are not able to pay the cost of hospital care when needed (European Observatory on Health Systems and Policies, 2016). The healthcare reform bill introduced by President Obama ('Obamacare') had a difficult passage through Congress. It is designed to introduce equity-based reforms that allow Americans not wishing or able to purchase health insurance from a private provider to be able to purchase health insurance cover under the Health Care for America Plan, meaning that for the first time, access to health insurance cover is now available for low-paid workers (Waitzkin & Hellander, 2016). However, with the election of Donald Trump as US president, and his strong individualist philosophy, the strength of the Health Care for America Plan reforms introduced by President Obama has already been undermined and the longer-term policy impact is unclear.

Positive outcomes of a state-funded equity-based primary health care approach can be seen in Kerala, India, which has better population health status and life expectancy than the majority of India, despite spending a very low proportion of GDP on health. Life expectancy at birth in Kerala in 2010–14 was 74.9 years, the highest in the country (Government of India, n.d.), compared with 68.8 years for the whole of India (WHO, 2019a), where health spending is 3.66% of GDP. Likewise, Cuba has managed to achieve high levels of health status on a limited budget. In 2018, life expectancy at birth in Cuba was 79 years, ranking it one position higher than the USA with a life expectancy at birth of 78.5 years, but on a low-income budget (Mooney, 2012). Annual per capita expenditure on health in 2013 in Cuba was US$707 (Mooney, 2012) whereas in the USA it was US$8713 (OECD, 2016). Clearly, achieving good population health outcomes is not just reliant on the amount of money in the health budget, but how the resources are used. Although health services are not the major determinant of population health outcomes, Mooney (2012) argues that a key factor in the remarkably good health status of people in Kerala and Cuba is the significant power of local community members in decision making about the range of services provided by community-level public health and comprehensive primary health care services. Other major contributors to these remarkable health and wellbeing success stories in Kerala and Cuba are population-wide social and public health measures such as access to education (especially for girls and women), clean water, sanitation, childhood nutrition, and immunisation programs. The economic environment also plays a significant role.

Economic capital

Economic capital encompasses the monetary system and assets of commercial value and the series of financial processes that make up commercial transactions between individuals, trading partners and nations. It often refers to the amount of accessible money a country, company or person requires to remain solvent. Usual use of the term refers to the accumulation of wealth.

National success and strength are generally interpreted through measures of economic activity, such as the GDP. Economic growth has been seen as the ultimate aim for nations and this aim underpins trade policy, economic primary production and industrial activities. In the period from the 1970s until recently, economic capital processes in high-income countries such as the United Kingdom, USA, Australia and New Zealand were underpinned by the neoliberal or economic rationalist philosophy. A key assumption inherent in this approach is that economic growth provides a foundation for 'development'. The market is regarded as the source of social and economic wellbeing due to the 'trickle-down' effect, whereby the economic success of the richest and most powerful is assumed to benefit all, even those at the bottom of the socio-economic hierarchy in society. Health enhancement is assumed to occur as a product of continued economic growth. While there is evidence that improved economic prosperity can improve overall population health (OECD, 2016), there is also evidence that internal economic rationalist policies can undermine the health status of the most vulnerable community members. For example, there was an increase in avoidable mortality in New Zealand in the 1990s that occurred in parallel with the introduction of a range of user-pays obligations for a range of health services (Tobias & Yeh, 2007). The global financial crisis (GFC), commencing in 2008, slowed economic activity dramatically in some nations, and as a result there was higher unemployment, increased social dislocation and poverty. A number of population health theorists (Labonté & Laverack, 2008; Labonté & Schrecker, 2006; Mooney, 2012; Navarro, 2011; Scott, 2012) have argued that neoliberalism has produced greater income and social inequality, with negative health implications. Within nations severely affected by the GFC, people have sought alternative political perspectives; political unrest, change and turmoil have been ongoing outcomes.

Economic capital is used to describe financial transactions at national as well as personal or family level; the ability to take part in fair financial exchange is fundamental to population wellbeing. When unequal economic power relations exist between trading nations, the health of a nation may be undermined; when people are unemployed and unable to take part in the economic system, every dimension of their health is undermined (Navarro, 2011).

Economic globalisation and neoliberalism

In 2018, according to the *Public Good or Private Wealth* report published by Oxfam (Lawson et al., 2019), the 26 richest people in the world had the same amount of net wealth as the bottom half of the world's population, down from 85 people in 2014, and 388 people in 2010, indicating that extreme wealth is progressively becoming more concentrated. Almost half of the world's population live on less than US$5.50 per day. In 2018, the world's 2208 billionaires saw their wealth grow by 12%, with a new billionaire created every two days between 2017 and 2018, and the number of billionaires almost doubling since the global financial crisis. The wealth of the world's billionaires increased by US$2.5 billion per day in 2018 (Lawson et al., 2019). The human brain has a difficult time conceptualising the scale of the difference between a million and a billion. To get a sense of this scale, a million seconds is equal to 11.6 days, whereas a billion seconds is equal to 31.7 years. Billionaires are extremely rich, and getting richer by the day.

Neoliberalism is a policy model that transfers control of economic factors to the private sector from the public sector. This model has had a profound effect on health. PHM and others (2011) argue that:

> The [global] financial system is profoundly dysfunctional, triggering economic crises, increasing inequality, and generating potentially disastrous environmental impacts, while conspicuously failing to meet social goals such as poverty eradication, 'health for all', access to education, and the fulfilment of basic needs for the majority of humanity. It is at least arguable that it is doing more harm than good.

(p. 24)

The inequality gap is widening and probably 'locking billions of people into a cycle of poverty and there aren't the mechanisms there to pull them out of that' (Szoke, 2016, cited in Pett, 2016). This is a significant factor influencing health, education, living conditions, the functioning of the Earth's ecosystem and thus quality of life and, in some cases, life expectancy. The quality of health care available to people within nations also influences health, especially the degree to which equity underpins access to services (PHM et al., 2014; Wilkinson & Pickett, 2009). A major factor influencing access has been this rise of global neoliberalism and the adoption of economic policy decisions in line with that ideology (Labonté & Schrecker, 2007; Mooney, 2012; PHM et al., 2014). Neoliberalism is built around the belief that as much of national and international life as possible should be left in the hands of the market, and that governments should minimise their involvement in public life. The beliefs support sovereign individuals and strong property rights (PHM et al., 2014). The 1970s commenced a significant period of social and political change internationally, which brought about changes in fiscal policies that continue to underpin international trade decisions and internal political policies. These policies include 'public goods', such as provision of universal health care, education and social welfare provisions (Labonté & Schrecker, 2007; PHM et al., 2014).

Internationally, liberalisation of trade continues, particularly within the development of regional arrangements, such as the European Community (EC), the trade agreement between the USA and Canada, similar agreements between Australia and New Zealand, and other agreements such as the ASEAN–Australia–New Zealand Free Trade Area (AANZFTA), and the Trans-Pacific Partnership Agreement (TPPA). Governments open up their economies to global markets and liberalised market processes, especially reducing export barriers and import taxes, which purportedly increases competition in global markets for all commodities.

The twin policy agendas of liberalisation of trade and privatisation of government assets have been adopted by many high-income nations and, in some cases, imposed on low-income nations since the early 1980s. Using commercial principles for services that are not based on discretionary decisions contradicts the philosophical assumption that 'public goods' are distributed as a part of a national ethos of rights and fairness, and should not be purely profit-driven (Leeder, 2003). The negative health consequences of neoliberalism have arisen from a set of values fundamentally at odds with the comprehensive primary health care approach.

When a neoliberal ideology underpins national policy, economic exchange figures are almost the only criterion by which government policy success is measured (Hancock, 1999; Labonté & Schrecker, 2007). The socio-ecological impacts of these influences on national policy have been clearly articulated (e.g. Labonté & Schrecker, 2006; Mooney, 2012; PHM et al., 2014). Researchers and social commentators have argued that globalised economic processes are having widespread and sustained social policy effects within nations, leading to the end of social welfare programs that are underpinned by taxation and wealth distribution policies and which support the philosophy of equality of opportunity (e.g. Beresford, 2000; Lawson et al., 2019; Mooney, 2012; PHM et al., 2014). The Trans-Pacific Partnership Agreement is an example of a policy that is of significant concern for many health practitioners in Australia. The TPPA includes investor-state dispute settlement mechanisms that will enable foreign corporations to bring claims against Australian governments over health and environment policies (Gleeson, 2015).

The adoption of neoliberalism within nations has supported the burgeoning development of globalised economic business. According to Labonté and Schrecker (2006), globalisation 'describes the ways in which nations, businesses and people are becoming more connected and interdependent across national borders through increased economic integration, communication, cultural diffusion and travel' (p. 3). Globalised neoliberal-inspired policies have been the driving force of other dimensions of globalisation, such as developments in communications technologies and cultural homogenisation. Globalised economic changes have local, social, environmental and health impacts.

Transnational corporations

The influence of transnational corporations (TNCs) on the world economy is significant. Many have annual profits that exceed the GDPs of low- and middle-income countries and seek to exert a great deal of power in monetary regulations. TNCs use their profits and power to lobby governments to create a policy environment that protects and enhances their interests further (Hardoon, 2015). This, in turn, reflects the diminished relative power of individual nations to influence trade decisions made by global corporations. They are relatively powerless to achieve an equitable price when they must compete in price negotiations between the multinational corporations and powerful trading blocs and nations, such as the USA, EC and TPPA, which are able to directly subsidise producers, so market prices are artificially low but good producer returns are safeguarded (Institute for Agriculture and Trade Policy [IATP], 2004). When the small nations are unable to compete in trade, they go into debt and internal political systems become unstable.

Role of global organisations

International organisations such as the WHO, the International Monetary Fund (IMF), the World Bank and the World Trade Organization (WTO) have also been substantially powerful in structuring the global marketplace, and the decisions they make are controlled to a significant extent by the rich and powerful countries. Within these organisations there is an 'economically weighted' voting system; that is, the high-income nations (amounting to 14% of the world population), dominate the global decision-making processes, and the USA alone has a veto on all major policy decisions in the IMF and WHO (PHM et al., 2011).

Overall, economic globalisation has led to a number of developments that have had a grave impact on the health of people in the least powerful nations and on vulnerable groups within affluent nations. Inequality has risen, with marked growth in the concentration of wealth in the hands of a few. As a consequence, health inequalities between rich and poor have been exacerbated (Lawson et al., 2019; Mooney, 2012; PHM et al., 2014).

Globalisation has negative impacts on socio-ecological determinants of health through both direct means (by influencing health system structures, funding and health policy) and indirect means (where the impacts of global trade competition on national economies have flow-on effects to the health sector). A series of guidelines for 'making globalization work for the benefit of health' (Woodward et al., 2001, p. 879) will require new economic policies with population wellbeing at their core (Lawson et al., 2019; PHM et al., 2014). Oxfam (Hardoon, 2015; Lawson et al., 2019) has repeatedly called on governments to adopt a seven-point plan to tackle inequality.

1. Clamp down on tax dodging by corporations and rich individuals.
2. Invest in universal, free public services such as health and education.
3. Share the tax burden fairly, shifting taxation from labour and consumption towards capital and wealth.
4. Introduce minimum wages and move towards a living wage for all workers.
5. Introduce equal pay legislation and promote economic policies to give women a fair deal.

6. Ensure adequate safety nets for the poorest, including a minimum income guarantee.

7. Agree on a global goal to tackle inequality.

Phases of neoliberalism

There have been three major phases of neoliberalism globally—structural adjustment, financialisation and austerity—all of which have impacted negatively on population health (PHM et al., 2014). Throughout the 1970s, a number of nations accumulated severe trade deficits after having been encouraged to borrow large amounts of money from the major banks. With changes to the international financial situation, interest rates 'skyrocketed' in the 1980s, resulting in those countries owing huge debts that they could not pay (Labonté & Schrecker, 2006; PHM et al., 2014). Almost all countries in Latin America and sub-Saharan Africa, and a considerable number of Asian and Eastern European countries, faced acute debt problems by 1983 (PHM et al., 2014).

The banks were concerned that these countries would not be able to repay their loans, and their political systems would become unstable; as a result, the IMF and the World Bank stepped in. They offered to refinance the loans on the proviso that countries accepted 'structural adjustment programs', designed to ensure that countries serviced the debt owed. However, there were major consequences for their internal policies.

There were four main tenets of the structural adjustment programs which debt-ridden countries agreed to in order to qualify for loans. First, countries had to agree to the devaluation of the local currency, which immediately decreased the purchasing power of individuals. Devaluing of the currency made exports cheaper for the nations they sold to, and therefore more competitive, and imports more expensive, and therefore less desirable. Second, governments were required to make drastic cuts to public spending, such as health, education and other social services. Third, exports were promoted through, for instance, a move away from domestic food production to production of export goods and putting a freeze on local wages to ensure low-cost tradeable items. Fourth, countries were required to open up their economy for overseas goods and investment, such as through easing rules for foreign investment or bypassing environment legislation (Bello et al., 1994; Labonté & Schrecker, 2006). These changes have increased socio-economic inequalities within and between nations and impacted seriously on the poorest of the poor. For example, the reduction in land for family food production and subsistence farming has meant that many of the poor can no longer get enough food to eat.

In the face of criticism that the impacts of structural adjustment packages benefited the loan agencies of the IMF and World Bank, but consigned the recipient nations to overwhelming debt, some reform of the programs and debt-forgiveness were implemented. In recent years, poverty reduction rhetoric has replaced structural adjustment in the language of the World Bank and IMF; however, the impacts on low-income countries are very similar. Vast quantities of money are being moved each year from poor countries to rich countries, in order to service debt repayments. The impact of this drain on resources is experienced most heavily by the poor, especially children (Stallings, 2003, cited in Labonté & Schrecker, 2006, p. 17; PHM et al., 2011).

Many affluent industrialised countries have undergone their own self-imposed structural adjustment programs, including Australia and New Zealand. The gap between rich and poor has increased, as it has globally. Structural adjustment, financialisation and austerity continue globally. Following the global financial crisis, the PHM and others (2014, p. 2) argue that public investment in education, health care and infrastructure were attacked.

This highlights the inextricable link between the political philosophy of an elite and the social impacts felt worldwide.

According to the PHM and others 'neoliberal globalisation has produced a global health crisis' (2014, p. 2). Currently, the world is facing five acute major crises: food, fuel, financial, development, and environmental degradation, leading to Earth system changes such as climate change (PHM et al., 2011). The five crises are each connected to the other and each impact on the health of populations. The causes of these crises are said to be:

- global economic inequality
- the dominant role of the financial sector
- unequal global economic integration, and
- ineffective and undemocratic global governance.

Structural adjustment, financialisation and austerity packages following the 2007–08 GFC have affected high- and low-income countries. The austerity created by these packages is not only increasing inequalities within nations, but is also causing some nations to lose any sense of hope for the future (Mooney, 2012). The bank write-downs for the 2007–08 GFC alone are estimated as 'broadly equivalent in purchasing power terms to the annual income of the poorer half of the world population' (PHM et al., 2011, p. 9) and this approach to financial crises continues. The globalised trade processes described earlier are having a drastic effect on food availability and prices, for example, which is of particular concern to low-income countries. Producers often receive better returns for fuel oil crops, such as canola, than for food crops, such as grains. Grain shortages cause dramatic price rises over a short period and the number of starving people in poor nations increases proportionately (PHM et al., 2011). According to De Schutter (2010), after the GFC 'the food price crisis arose because a deeply flawed global financial system exacerbated the impacts of supply and demand' (cited in PHM et al., 2011, p. 12). Further, climate change contributed to the food crisis as major cereal producers such as Australia experienced drought and other exceptional weather patterns. Some 'emerging market' countries have been less affected by the food and fuel crises overall but are vulnerable to the financial crisis because of their reliance on commercial capital. As we have discussed earlier, the gap between rich countries and poor countries is widening, with very poor countries unable to provide the infrastructure and public goods for living conditions for health (PHM et al., 2011). Their capacity for adaptation to climate change is also compromised.

Physical environment

The physical environment includes the natural environment and the built environment. These environments are usually what are being referred to when we use the term 'the environment'. The natural environment refers to the land, air, fresh water, oceans, fish, forests, etc. Our lives all depend on the natural environment. We have abundant evidence of the importance of the natural environment to the health and wellbeing of humans and other species (Whitmee et al., 2015). These issues will be covered in more depth in Chapter 3. The built environment refers to things that are built or created by humans, such as buildings, furniture, lighting, roads, footpaths, drainage, sanitation systems, waste products, etc. The natural and built environments include factors that promote and protect health and wellbeing, as well as factors that have the potential to harm us.

Environmental justice

Environmental justice refers specifically to the natural and built environments, and is a major determinant of health. Environmental discrimination occurs in two ways: when people are disproportionately exposed to environmental hazards; and when people are denied access to environments required for their health and wellbeing. Environmental hazards include biological, chemical, radiological, nuclear and physical dangers, and can be present in homes, communities, workplaces and schools. As a result of exposure to environmental hazards, people may suffer loss of quality of life, lower self-rated health and higher levels of morbidity and mortality. The people most exposed to and affected by environmental hazards are those who are poor. Many poor communities are exposed to multiple sources of environmental hazards while others lack the most basic environmental health infrastructure.

The communities of course include children, who have little control over their own lives, where they live and play, and what they eat, and their financial circumstances are determined by others. Children of socio-economically disadvantaged families are exposed more frequently than other children to potentially dangerous chemicals and other environmental hazards that can affect health. Further, in-utero exposures to environmental health hazards may constitute a source of inequity between generations. A study in the Kimberley region sought to quantify for the first time in Australia, the proportion of primary health care encounters that could be directly attributed to the physical environment. The Kimberley is a remote area in Western Australia with a predominantly Aboriginal Australian population that has among the worst health statuses in Australia. The study found that the proportion of encounters directly due to the physical environment was significantly higher for Aboriginal children aged 0–4 years than non-Aboriginal children (25.6% v. 18.6%) (McMullen et al., 2016). Such disproportionate impact on Aboriginal children is evidence of environmental discrimination and injustice.

Environmental discrimination also occurs when people are denied access to natural environments required for their health and wellbeing. There are significant physical and mental health and wellbeing benefits from accessing natural environments such as oceans, lakes or green spaces. For example, a short walk in a forest can reduce stress levels and decrease the heart rate (Kobayashi et al., 2018). Even the simple act of paying more attention to nature in everyday surroundings and reflecting on one's emotional response to nature can result in a net positive effect, with a greater general sense of connectedness (to other people, to nature and to life as a whole) and prosocial orientation (Passmore & Holder, 2017).

At a much more fundamental level, for Indigenous peoples in many parts of the world, connection with the natural environment is integral to their entire concept of life and wellbeing. The interconnection between people, the land and place-specific practices is central to their consciousness, sense of place, agency, responsibility and wellbeing with the world (Freeman, 2019). Māori use the term 'tangata whenua', to describe themselves as Indigenous people, which means 'people of their land' in the sense of 'belonging' to the land, rather than 'owning' it (Hond et al., 2019). The Māori health promotion model (see Insight 2.1 on page 51) includes the physical environment as one of four areas of health (Durie, 2004). To Māori, land is 'a fundamental source of identity and spiritual connection that establishes a grounding for wellbeing beyond individual aspirations and needs' (Hond et al., 2019, p. 45). As a result of colonisation and the subsequent commodification of land, many Indigenous peoples have become disenfranchised from ancestral lands. This has resulted in significant negative effects on physical, mental, social and spiritual health and wellbeing (Freeman, 2019; Ho-Lastimosa et al., 2019; Hond et al., 2019). Just one of the many consequences of settler colonisation has been the loss of traditional food sources and the abandonment of many traditional practices related to food production

(Ho-Lastimosa et al., 2019; Hond et al., 2019). These are all forms of environmental discrimination.

Environmental health justice demands action to address environmental discrimination. Boyden (1987) suggested that for change to take place, first we need to recognise that an undesirable state exists. Second, we need knowledge of the cause of the threat or the ways and means of overcoming it. Third, we need the means to do something about it. And finally, we need the motivation, or political will, to take action. Action must ensure that natural and built environments contribute to enhanced health and wellbeing now and for future generations.

Liveability

The concept of 'liveability' is being increasingly used to describe and define the quality-of-life infrastructure of geographic locations. Liveability has been defined as:

> *the degree to which a place supports quality of life, health and wellbeing. In broad terms, liveable cities are healthy, safe, harmonious, attractive and affordable. They have high amenity, provide good accessibility and are environmentally sustainable.*
>
> *(Major Cities Unit, 2012, p. 139)*

Several different national and international organisations have published liveability ratings and there is substantial research being undertaken in Australia regarding use of the concept, especially in local government settings, as the basis for decision making about strategies to enhance community wellbeing over time (Lowe et al., 2013, 2014, 2015). Overall positive ratings, or comparatively good scores on certain items, are used increasingly as a way of ranking cities, as points to encourage new residents to settle in a location, or as a real estate selling point.

The concept of being the 'most liveable' implies that a place needs to have a range of assets or characteristics that define it more positively in comparison with other places. These attributes produce a high degree of satisfaction for the people who live there. Liveability is about the way that a place enables and assists people to achieve the quality of life they desire to be healthy and fulfilled. A liveable city is one where people can be healthy, safe and live in harmony; one that is attractive and provides affordable living, transport and good education and employment opportunities in a sustainable environment.

Measuring liveability involves using a set of indicators. Indicators may be numerical values or particular items where the city's record or performance can be directly compared with other cities and where the progress of the city can be measured both for external and internal audiences (Giles-Corti et al., 2014). The range of possible liveability themes is broad but may include measures reflecting the following:

- public and community amenity
- access to public open space
- celebrations of culture and heritage
- wellbeing and health
- housing
- infrastructure and transportation
- economic diversity
- lifelong learning
- social and civic capital

INSIGHT 2.3 City of Melbourne liveability and quality of life

The City of Melbourne is Australia's second largest city with a population of approximately 170,000 people and the fastest growing municipality in Australia with a projected population of approximately 384,000 by 2041. The City of Melbourne is a member of the global 100 Resilient Cities Network, an initiative of the Rockefeller Foundation to support cities across the world to become more resilient to future economic, social and physical environmental challenges. In 2015 the City of Melbourne along with 32 metropolitan councils and other stakeholders came together to develop Melbourne's first resilience strategy, endorsed in 2016. The primary purpose of the strategy was to chart action to ensure Melbourne is a 'viable, sustainable, liveable and prosperous city, today and long into the future'. The broad action areas of the strategy are to:

- adapt—reduce exposure to future shocks and stresses
- survive—withstand disruptions and bounce back better than before
- thrive—significantly improve people's quality of life
- embed—build resilience thinking into institutions and ways of working.

The City of Melbourne also collects and monitors a range of liveability and quality-of-life data to assess progress, compare their progress with other cities, and inform future city development planning. Liveability indicators are drawn from the *ISO 37120 Sustainable Development of Communities: Indicators for City Services and Quality of Life* developed by the World Council on City Data. These data provide standardised urban metrics that cities can use to plan for resilience and build more liveable cities into the future. The City of Melbourne liveability indicators are organised according to the following 10 themes: Profile—people; Profile—housing, government and economy; Economy; Finance; Fire, safety and shelter; Governance; Health and education; Recreation and urban planning; Transportation; and Water, energy and environment. Quality-of-life indicators are drawn from the *City of Melbourne Social Indicator Survey* and are organised according to the following five themes: Health and physical activity; Wellbeing; Food security and production; Culture, diversity and safety; and Participation in activities. A dashboard is available for each indicator theme on the City of Melbourne website. A description of each indicator and the status for each indicator compared with selected benchmarks are provided.

Sources: City of Melbourne, n.d.a, n.d.b.

- ecological sustainability
- leadership and decision making.

Aspects of liveability such as these are being increasingly used by local governments as a basis for planning, setting priorities, making financial decisions and evaluating the effectiveness of previous strategies. Local government is an important setting where liveability can be set as an aspiration because of the potential to enhance the wellbeing of the entire population over time, provided the commitment is sustained. For example, in Australia, the Environment and Liveability Strategy 2017, developed by the Sunshine Coast Council, Queensland, provides strategic direction for the local government and their partners for a healthy and liveable environment up to 2041 (Sunshine Coast Council, 2017). The City of Melbourne Council has also made considerable progress in initiatives to plan for and create a resilient and liveable city into the future (Insight 2.3) (City of Melbourne, n.d.a). This concept is discussed in Chapter 3 in more detail, with specific reference to ecological sustainability.

COMMUNITY AS A FOCUS OF HEALTH PROMOTION PRACTICE

Defining community

'Community' has been defined in various ways but is usually characterised by either geographical communities, based on location, or functional communities, based on a common element providing a sense of identity. Within the geographic or functional elements of community, multiple communities exist, and individuals may belong to several different communities at the same time.

Two major characteristics of community are identified: social interactions that are dynamic and enable relationships to occur, and through these relationships, the identification of shared needs and concerns that occur (Laverack, 2007). Tesoriero (2010) goes further and describes five interrelated characteristics of community as follows (pp. 96–98).

1. *Human scale*. This is where people know each other or can get to know each other relatively easily and as needed. Structures are small enough for people to be able to control them, facilitating genuine empowerment. There is no magic number, but it could mean several thousand.

2. *Identity and belonging*. This implies acceptance by others and allegiance or loyalty to the aims of the group. Belonging to a community gives one a sense of identity.

3. *Obligations*. The responsibility for survival lies with the members and so membership is supposedly an active experience. It carries both rights and responsibilities.

4. *'Gemeinschaft'*. People interact with a relatively small number of people, whom they know well, in many different roles. Members develop and contribute a wide range of talents for the benefit of themselves and the wider community. This is different to 'Gesellschaft', where we don't know the people we have contact with except for the roles they have; for example, teacher, bus driver, shop assistant, and so on.

5. *Culture*. The valuing of locally based culture rather than the mass culture of the wider society. Members are producers of the culture rather than consumers.

People form communities by virtue of facing common sets of issues in their daily lives that create interactive webs of ties among organisations, neighbourhoods, families and friends (DeFilippis & Saegert, 2013). Communities are social systems bound together by geography, shared values or shared interests. Participation in the life of the community and identification as a member of the community are important and result in a sense of belonging. This sense of belonging may also be described as a 'sense of community'.

A community of interest or 'community-of-common-purpose' (Falk & Kilpatrick, 2000, p. 103) has been described as a group of people who share beliefs, values or interests on a particular issue. For example, communities of interest may include residents of a housing estate, groups of single parents or unemployed people, members of particular ethnic groups, and global communities, such as religious groups that span nations, or social movements, such as the women's movement or the environmental movement. Defining a community of interest around a shared perspective on a particular issue, recognises heterogeneity among people and the fact that those who share an interest in one issue may have few other shared interests or beliefs, and may even be divided on other issues. Examples of the way the term 'community' is currently used include the following.

- *Global community* with interdependent networks of trade, communication and travel and with global commons such as clean air and water and the protection of biodiversity. These are important issues facing the global community, given the health impacts of insufficient fresh water and climate change from greenhouse gas emissions.

- *National community* where people identify with a range of potent symbols such as Australia and the kangaroo, or Australia and the idea of giving people 'a fair go'.

- *Loyal community* where people identify with a city or region or identify themselves as other; for example, some people in Australia identify with 'the bush'. This is a mixture of geography and emotional attachment.

- *Community of identity* that binds people through beliefs such as culture and religion. A local community that shares a range of living and working conditions such as climate, access to services and morale. This is often a combination of geography and interest.

- *Community of interest* where people share attitudes, enthusiasm, need and activities around a particular issue.

- *Virtual community* where people communicate online. With recent rapid advances in internet communications, virtual communities can develop overnight as followers of an idea, issue or a person.

- *Intimate community* comprising family and friends.

The term 'community' is often romanticised, described in a way that assumes communities are made up of close-knit groups of people who care for one another and experience little conflict (DeFilippis & Saegert, 2013; Labonté, 1989). Such an impression is far from the truth. Communities are very often not characterised by harmony and shared values on all issues and are likely to reflect elements of conflict and competing interests. Communities may be strongly divided by opposing values, and may even be built on attitudes that reflect racism, sexism or ageism, for example, rather than mutual care and concern (DeFilippis & Saegert, 2013). In addition, the term 'community' may often be deliberately used to take advantage of its romantic connotations, such as when governments use terms like 'community care' or 'community programs'. Such programs may be seen positively because they are described in this way, yet such programs are often underfunded or reliant on volunteer labour that, in the case of community care, is usually provided by women, with negative impacts on their own health and wellbeing (Talbot & Walker, 2007).

Health promotion practice will be influenced differently by geographic, demographic and social communities, and by the policy and political context (DeFilippis & Saegert, 2013). Demographic or population communities such as men, women or children and geographic settings such as neighbourhoods, schools or workplaces have tended to focus on 'top-down' approaches to health promotion, especially where there is national or state/regional government funding tied to the policy action or health promotion initiative. However, strategies supported for social communities have been more likely to provide opportunities for 'bottom-up' approaches to health promotion; for example, through various 'neighbourhood renewal' initiatives (DeFilippis & Saegert, 2013; Labonté & Laverack, 2008).

Community participation in health promotion

Community participation in all stages of planning, implementing and evaluating policies and services that impact on people's health and wellbeing is recognised in the Universal Declaration of Human Rights (UN, 1948), the Declaration of Alma-Ata (WHO, 1978), the

Ottawa Charter for Health Promotion (WHO, 1986), and the other documents in the appendices of this book. Community participation has been increasingly reflected in the rhetoric of health policy documents and health practitioners are urged to incorporate strategies to engage the participation of the communities that they work with into their practice. As the health and economic benefits of connected communities are increasingly recognised, more funding has been made available for these long-term approaches. Accompanying this has been the development of related evaluation indicators. As Farmer and colleagues (2015) have illustrated in their research, moving past the rhetoric to embedding community participation in agency strategic plans and best practice continues to be a challenge. Health practitioners provide an important conduit in ensuring ongoing and effective community participation. Discussion of the different approaches to participation is therefore valuable and presented in more detail in Chapter 6. Arnstein's (1971) Ladder of Citizen Participation (Fig. 6.1) continues to be a relevant diagrammatic illustration of the different forms of participation.

In many respects, community members may not be adequately prepared to participate effectively in decision making about their health and wellbeing. Even in democratic societies such as Australia and New Zealand, we do not necessarily learn how to participate. Therefore, if people are to be encouraged to participate, they need to be provided with an opportunity to develop the skills and resources to do so. Effective participation and decision-making processes need to be established so they can enable people to participate meaningfully in the decisions that affect their lives (Farmer et al., 2015). Health practitioners are currently endeavouring to develop more innovative participation strategies. Using a diverse range of creative strategies to enhance community participation that meets the needs and characteristics of the community has the potential to create lasting positive changes in local communities.

Unless people feel that they are likely to have an impact, they may decide that it is not worth the effort of trying to participate. Organisations that decide they want to encourage participation must therefore decide to prevent manipulative tactics that exclude community members from effective decision making, and instigate affirmative action techniques in meetings and decision making so that all potential participants have a fair say. Otherwise, only those people who are most comfortable with meeting procedures, and are therefore the most dominant within the group, may have their voices heard and their ideas acted upon (Farmer et al., 2015). As Arnstein (1971, p. 72) has said, 'participation without redistribution of power is an empty and frustrating process for the powerless'. Questions that need to be asked here include who decides what is for the good of the community, and on what basis? Imposition of decisions by others can be problematic for community members, unless they are decisions related to policies that reverse disadvantage. However, it is not always practical or possible to involve the whole community in decision making and assist them in developing all of the knowledge and skills to make informed decisions. When is it acceptable for decisions to be made on behalf of the community? Do health practitioners have the right to manipulate the environment 'for the good of the community'? When different parts of the community have conflicts of interest on particular issues, whose interests should take precedence? These are just some of the ethical questions raised in health promotion practice.

If people are going to participate, then obviously the agendas of the organisations concerned must be relevant to them. This has an added advantage; if organisations adjust their agendas so that they are more relevant to the community and people are therefore more willing to participate, it is likely that their activities will more effectively meet the priorities of their community. Consequently, organisations are made increasingly accountable to the public, which goes hand in hand with the power sharing discussed above.

CONCLUSION

This chapter has explored a number of core concepts informing health promotion practice within a CPHC context and which provide a foundation for following chapters. Concepts of health, wellbeing, quality of life and salutogenesis were introduced, with particular attention to the fact that health and wellbeing is more than a physical state, and is an individual phenomenon. The characteristics of people, including their values, attitudes and beliefs, affect their likelihood to adopt particular health promoting or risk behaviours. These factors are entwined with factors within the social, cultural, economic, political and physical environments in which people live.

Resilience and liveability are emerging concepts in health promotion and reflect the importance of local action that builds the strength and control of local communities, and their ability to work together to enhance the health and wellbeing of people at individual and population levels. Continuing to examine concepts presented in this chapter is important as readers review the range of health promotion priorities and strategies introduced throughout the remainder of this book.

MORE TO EXPLORE

USEFUL RESOURCES TO PROVIDE DEEPER UNDERSTANDING OF CORE CONCEPTS

- ABC Radio National (2016, September 3) The 56th Boyer Lecture Series by Sir Michael Marmot on health inequalities and the causes of the causes: http://www. abc.net.au/radionational/programs/boyerlectures/ boyer-lecture-health-inequality-and-the-causes-of-the-causes/7763106

- Māori health models – Te Whare Tapa Whā: http://www.health.govt.nz/our-work/ populations/maori-health/maori-health-models/ maori-health-models-te-whare-tapa-wha

- Melbourne liveability and quality of life: https://www.melbourne.vic.gov.au/ about-melbourne/research-and-statistics/Pages/liveability.aspx

- Sunshine Coast Council Environment and Liveability Strategy 2017: https://www. sunshinecoast.qld.gov.au/Council/Planning-and-Projects/Regional-Strategies/ Environment-and-Liveability-Strategy-2017

- Transition Town Totnes: https://www.transitiontowntotnes.org/.

IUHPE Core Competencies for Health Promotion

The IUHPE Core Competencies for Health Promotion comprises nine domains of action. Each domain has a series of core competency statements and a detailed outline of the knowledge and skills that contribute to competency in that domain.

The content of this chapter relates especially to the achievement of competency in the health promotion domains outlined below.

1. Enable change	*1.2 Use health promotion approaches which support empowerment, participation, partnership and equity to create environments and settings which promote health*
	Understanding of social and cultural diversity
2. Advocate for health	*2.4 Advocate for the development of policies, guidelines and procedures across all sectors which impact positively on health and reduce health inequities*
	Health and wellbeing issues relating to a specified population or group
3. Mediate through partnership	*3.2 Facilitate effective partnership working which reflects health promotion values and principles*
	Theory and practice of collaborative working
4. Communication	*4.3 Use culturally appropriate communication methods and techniques for specific groups and settings*
	Understanding of social and cultural diversity
5. Leadership	*5.2 Use leadership skills which facilitate empowerment and participation (including teamwork, negotiation, motivation, conflict resolution, decision making, facilitation and problem solving)*
	Theory and practice of collaborative working
	5.6 Contribute to team and organisational learning to advance health promotion action
	Emerging challenges in health and health promotion
6. Assessment	*6.4 Identify the determinants of health which impact on health promotion action*
	Social determinants of health
	Health inequalities
	Evidence base for health promotion action and priority setting
	6.6 Use culturally and ethically appropriate assessment approaches
	Understanding social and cultural diversity
7. Planning	*7.2 Use current models and systematic approaches for planning health promotion action*
	Use and effectiveness of current health promotion planning models and theories
8. Implementation	*8.1 Use ethical, empowering, culturally appropriate and participatory processes to implement health promotion action*
	Understanding social and cultural diversity

In addition, IUHPE specifies knowledge, skills and performance criteria essential for health promotion practitioners to act professionally and ethically, including having knowledge of ethical and legal issues, behaving in an ethical and respectful manner and working in ways that review and improve practice. Full details are available at: http://www.iuhpe.org/index.php/en/the-accreditation-system.

Reflective Questions

1. Consider the Māori health and wellbeing models and health promotion model presented in Insight 2.1. What constructions of health and wellbeing are evident in these models? What implications do these models have for health promotion action that you are or might be involved in in the future if you were to adopt them in your professional practice?

2. Access the Health Equity Monitor from the WHO (http://www.who.int/gho/ health_equity/en/). With reference to specific population subgroups, such as women and children, explore some examples where inequitable access to services or life chances, or where unequal treatment, has a profound and lifelong impact on health and wellbeing. What structural determinants need to be challenged to improve the situation?

3. Cultural safety is a philosophical commitment which should underpin all professional practice. Identify a particular cultural community that you have interacted with either in the past or currently. Explore the differences in cultural 'ways of being' between your own and the cultural community you have chosen. You will need to talk with people from the cultural community that you have identified to explore these differences in depth.

4. Critical reflection is a core skill for ethical health promotion practice. This chapter has presented a number of concepts and personal characteristics which should form the basis of critical reflection, such as personal values around race, culture and ability, or the challenge of empowering community members and the threat this may mean to one's professional standing. Think of an experience in your professional practice or personal life where your values were challenged. Write a personal critique of the experience. Begin by describing the incident or experience. Describe what it was about that experience that made you feel uneasy and why. Reflect on what you have learned from the experience. What would you do differently next time?

5. Identify three population groups who experience inequity. For each group, provide an example of a social injustice experienced by the equity group and discuss how economic, social, cultural and political factors contribute to the social injustice.

6. A major focus of many local governments globally and locally is planning for and creating resilient and liveable communities for the future. Review the range of liveability and quality-of-life indicators presented in Insight 2.3 (City of Melbourne, n.d.b). Identify and discuss the range of socio-ecological determinants of health and wellbeing reflected in the liveability and social indicators. Review the local government website for the geographical region in

which you live. What is your local government doing to plan for and create a resilient and liveable future for your local community?

REFERENCES

Aboriginal and Torres Strait Islander Social Justice Commissioner. (2015). Social justice and native title report 2015. Australian Human Rights Commission. Retrieved from https://www.humanrights.gov.au/sites/default/files/document/publication/SJRNTR2015.pdf.

Ajzen, I., & Fishbein, M. (1991). Understanding attitudes and predicting social behavior. New Jersey: Prentice-Hall.

Allen, C., Boddy, J., & Kendall, E. (2018). An experiential learning theory of high level wellness: Australian salutogenic research. Health Promotion International, 34(5), 1045–1054. doi:10.1093/heapro/day051

Anderson, I., Baum, F., & Bentley, M. (Eds.). (2007). Beyond bandaids: exploring the underlying social determinants of Aboriginal health. Papers from the Social Determinants of Aboriginal Health Workshop, Adelaide, July 2004. Cooperative Research Centre for Aboriginal Health, Darwin. Retrieved from https://www.lowitja.org.au/content/Document/Lowitja-Publishing/BeyondBandaidsText.pdf.

Antonovsky, A. (1996). The salutogenic model as a theory to guide health promotion. Health Promotion International, 11(1), 11–18. https://doi.org/10.1093/heapro/11.1.11.

Arnstein, S. (1971). Eight rungs on the ladder of citizen participation. In E. S. Cahn & B. A. Passett (Eds.), Citizen participation: effecting community changes. New York: Praeger Publishers.

Australian Government. (2013). National Aboriginal and Torres Strait Islander health plan 2013–2023. Retrieved from https://www1.health.gov.au/internet/main/publishing.nsf/Content/natsih-plan.

Australian Government. (2014). Aboriginal and Torres Strait Islander health curriculum framework. Retrieved from https://www1.health.gov.au/internet/main/publishing.nsf/Content/72C7E23E1BD5E9CFCA257F640082CD48/$File/Health%20Curriculum%20Framework.pdf

Australian Government. (2015). Implementation plan for the National Aboriginal and Torres Strait Islander Health Plan. Retrieved from https://www1.health.gov.au/internet/main/publishing.nsf/Content/indigenous-implementation-plan.

Australian Government. (2020). Closing the gap report 2020. Retrieved from https://ctgreport.niaa.gov.au/.

Australian Health Ministers' Advisory Council. (2016). Cultural respect framework 2016–2026 for Aboriginal and Torres Strait Islander Health. Retrieved from http://www.coaghealthcouncil.gov.au/Portals/0/National%20Cultural%20Respect%20Framework%20for%20Aboriginal%20and%20Torres%20Strait%20Islander%20Health%202016_2026_2.pdf.

Australian Human Rights Commission (AHRC). (2015). Social justice and native title report 2015. Retrieved from https://www.humanrights.gov.au/sites/default/files/document/publication/SJRNTR2015.pdf.

Australian Indigenous Doctors Association. (2017). Position paper: cultural safety for Aboriginal and Torres Strait Islander doctors, medical students and patients. Canberra: Australian Indigenous Doctors Association. Retrieved from https://www.aida.org.au/wp-content/uploads/2017/06/Cultural_Safety.pdf.

Australian Institute of Health and Welfare (AIHW). (2017). Aboriginal and Torres Strait Islander health performance framework (HPF) report 2017. Retrieved from https://www.aihw.gov.au/reports/indigenous-australians/health-performance-framework/report-editions.

Australian Institute of Health and Welfare (AIHW). (2018). Australia's health 2018. Retrieved from https://www.aihw.gov.au/reports-data/health-welfare-overview/australias-health/reports.

Bandura, A. (1986). Social foundations of thought and action: a social cognitive theory. Englewood Cliffs, NJ. Prentice Hall.

Barry, M. M., Battel-Kirk, B., Davison, H., et al. (2012). The CompHP project handbooks (2012). International Union for Health Promotion and Education (IUHPE), Paris. Retrieved from: http://www.iuhpe.org/images/PROJECTS/ACCREDITATION/CompHP_Project_Handbooks.pdf.

Baum, F. (1999). The role of social capital in health promotion: Australian perspectives. Proceedings of the 11th National Health Promotion Conference, Perth.

Baum, F. (2016). The new public health (4th ed.). Melbourne: Oxford University Press.

Beaglehole, R., & Bonita, R. (2004). Public health at the crossroads: achievements and prospects (2nd ed.). New York: Cambridge University Press.

Becker, M. H. (Ed.). (1974). The health belief model and personal health behaviour. Thorofare, NJ: Charles B Slack.

Bello, W. S., Cunningham, A., & Rau, B. (1994). Dark victory: the United States, structural adjustment and global poverty. London: Pluto Press.

Beresford, Q. (2000). Governments, markets and globalization: Australian public policy in context, pp. 58–59. Sydney: Allen & Unwin.

Boyden, S. (1987). Western civilisation in biological perspective. Oxford: Oxford University Press.

Braveman, P. (2014). What is health equity: how does a life-course approach take us further toward it? Maternal and Child Health Journal, 18, 362–372. https://doi.org/10.1007/s10995-013-1226-9.

Brown, K. (2013). Global environmental change 1: a social turn for resilience? Progress in Human Geography, 38(1), 107–117. https://doi.org/10.1177/0309132513498837.

Brown, L., Thurecht, L., & Nepal, B. (2012). The cost of inaction on the social determinants of health, Report no, 2/2012. Canberra: National Centre for Social and Economic Modelling, University of Canberra.

Carter, S., Rychetnik, L., Lloyd, B., et al. (2011). Evidence, ethics and values: a framework for health promotion. American Journal of Public Health, 101(3), 465–472. https://doi.org/10.2105/AJPH.2010.195545.

Centers for Disease Control and Prevention, USA. (2013). Health disparities and inequalities report—United States, 2013. MMWR Supplements, 62(Suppl. 3), 1–187. Retrieved from http://www.cdc.gov/minorityhealth/CHDIReport.html.

City of Melbourne. (n.d.a). 100 resilient cities. Retrieved from https://www.melbourne.vic.gov.au/about-melbourne/melbourne-profile/pages/100-resilient-cities.aspx.

City of Melbourne. (n.d.b). Liveability and quality of life. Retrieved from https://www.melbourne.vic.gov.au/about-melbourne/research-and-statistics/Pages/liveability.aspx.

Cummins, R., Eckersley, R., Pallant, J., et al. (2003). Developing a national index of subjective wellbeing: The Australian Unity Wellbeing Index. Social Indicators Research, 64(2), 159–190. https://doi.org/10.1023/A:1024704320683.

De, D., & Richardson, J. (2015). Ensuring cultural safety in nurse education. Nursing Times, 111(39), 17–19.

DeFilippis, J., & Saegert, S. (2013). The community development reader (2nd ed.). New York: Taylor and Francis.

De Schutter, O. (2010). Food commodities speculation and food price crises: regulation to reduce the risks of price volatility: Briefing note 2 September 2010. United Nations special rapporteur on the right to food. Retrieved from http://www2.ohchr.org/english/issues/food/docs/Briefing_Note_02_September_2010_EN.pdf.

de Vries, M. J. (1993). Theoretical model for healing processes: rediscovering the dynamic nature of health and disease. In R. LaFaille & S. Fulder (Eds.), Towards a new science of health. London and New York: Routledge.

Downing, R., Kowal, E., & Paradies, A. (2011). Indigenous cultural training for health workers in Australia. International Journal for Quality in Health Care, 23(3), 247–257. https://doi.org/10.1093/intqhc/mzr008.

Duckett, S. (2007). The Australian health care system (3rd ed.). South Melbourne: Oxford University Press.

Durie, M. H. (1985). A Maori perspective of health. Social Science & Medicine, 20(5), 483–486. https://doi.org/10.1016/0277-9536(85)90363-6.

Durie, M. H. (2004). An Indigenous model of health promotion. Health Promotion Journal of Australia, 15(3), 181–185. https://doi.org/10.1071/HE04181.

Eckermann, A. K., Dowd, T., Chong, E., et al. (2010). Binan goonj: bridging cultures in Aboriginal health (3rd ed.). Sydney: Churchill Livingstone/Elsevier.

European Observatory on Health Systems and Policies. (2016). Health system reviews (HiT series). Retrieved from http://www.euro.who.int/en/about-us/partners/observatory.

Falk, I., & Kilpatrick, S. (2000). What is social capital? A study of interaction in a rural community. Sociologica Ruralis, 40(1), 87–110. https://doi.org/10.1111/1467-9523.00133.

Farmer, J., Currie, M., Kenny, A., & Munoz, S.-A. (2015). An exploration of the longer-term impacts of community participation in rural health services design. Social Science & Medicine, 141, 64–71. https://doi.org/10.1016/j.socscimed.2015.07.021.

Field, J. (2004). Social capital. London: Taylor and Francis.

Figueras, J., & McKee, M. (Eds.). (2012). Health systems, health, wealth and societal well-being: assessing the case for investing in health systems. Geneva: McGraw-Hill, European Observatory on Health Systems and Policies and World Health Organization. Retrieved from http://www.euro.who.int/__data/assets/pdf_file/0007/164383/e96159.pdf.

Forgas, J., Cooper, J., & Crano, W. (Eds.). (2011). The psychology of attitudes and attitude change. New York: Taylor and Francis.

Foronda, C., Baptiste, D., Reinholdt, M., & Ousman, K. (2016). Cultural humility: a concept analysis. Journal of Transcultural Nursing, 27(3), 210–217. https://doi.org/10.1177/1043659615592677.

Freeman, B. M. (2019). Promoting global health and well-being of Indigenous youth through the connection of land and culture-based activism. Global Health Promotion, 26(Supp. 3), 17–25. https://doi.org/10.1177/1757975919831253.

Freire, P. (1974). Education for critical consciousness. London: Sheed & Ward.

Fritzell, J., Rehnberg, J., Hertzman, J., & Blomgren, J. (2015). Absolute or relative? A comparative analysis of the relationship between poverty and mortality. International Journal of Public Health, 60, 101–110. https://doi.org/10.1007/s00038-014-0614-2.

Gallaher, V., Dahlman, C., Gilmartin, M., et al. (2009). Key concepts in political geography. Thousand Oaks CA: Sage.

Gerrig, R., & Zimbardo, P. (2010). Psychology and life (19th ed.). Boston: Allyn and Bacon.

Giles, A. R., Hognestad, S., & Brooks, L. A. (2015). The need for cultural safety in injury prevention. Public Health Nursing, 32, 543–549. https://doi.org/10.1111/phn.12210.

Giles-Corti, B., Badland, H., Mavoa, S., et al. (2014). Reconnecting urban planning with health: a protocol for the development and validation of national liveability indicators associated with noncommunicable disease risk behaviours and health outcomes. Public Health Research Practice, 25(1), e2511405. Retrieved from https://ro.uow.edu.au/cgi/viewcontent.cgi?article=2600&context=sspapers.

Gleeson, D. (2015, November 6). TPP final text shows cause for concern. PHAA Media Release. Canberra: Public Health Association.

Government of India. (n.d.). Life expectancy. Retrieved from http://niti.gov.in/content/life-expectancy.

Green, J., & Tones, K. (2010). Health promotion: planning and strategies. California: Sage.

Greene-Moton, E., & Minkler, M. 2020. Cultural competence or cultural humility? Moving beyond the debate. Health Promotion Practice, 21(1), 142–145. https://doi.org/10.1177/1524839919884912.

Gregg, J., & O'Hara, L. (2007a). The Red Lotus Health Promotion Model: a new model for holistic, ecological, salutogenic health promotion practice. Health Promotion Journal of Australia, 18(1), 12–19. https://doi.org/10.1071/HE07012.

Gregg, J., & O'Hara, L. (2007b). Values and principles evident in current health promotion practice. Health Promotion Journal of Australia, 18, 7–11. https://doi.org/10.1071/HE07007.

Hall, P., & Lamont, M. (2013). Social resilience in the neoliberal era. Cambridge: Cambridge University Press.

Hancock, A. M. (2016). Intersectionality: an intellectual history. New York: Oxford University Press.

Hancock, L. (1999). Health, public sector restructuring and the market state. In L. Hancock (Ed.), Health policy in the market state (pp. 48–68). Sydney: Allen and Unwin.

Hardoon, D. (2015). Wealth: having it all and wanting more. Oxford: Oxfam. Retrieved from https://www.oxfam.org/en/research/wealth-having-it-all-and-wanting-more.

Harris, J., & White, V. (Eds.). (2013). A dictionary of social work and social care. Oxford, UK: Oxford University Press.

Harris, R., Tobias, M., Jeffreys, M., et al. (2006). Racism and health: the relationship between experience of racial discrimination and health in New Zealand. Social Science and Medicine, 63(6), 1428–1441. https://doi.org/10.1016/j.socscimed.2006.04.009.

Healy, T., & Coté, S. (2001). The well-being of nations: the role of human and social capital. Paris: Centre for Educational Research and Innovation, OECD.

Ho-Lastimosa, I., Chung-Do, J. J., Hwang, P. W., et al. (2019). Integrating native Hawaiian tradition with the modern technology of aquaponics. Global Health Promotion, 26(Supp. 3), 87–92. https://doi.org/10.1177/1757975919831241.

Honari, M., & Boleyn, T. (Eds.). (1999). Health ecology: health, culture and human-environment interaction. London: Routledge.

Hond, R., Ratima, M., & Edwards, W. (2019). The role of Māori community gardens in health promotion: a land-based community development response by tangata whenua, people of their land. Global Health Promotion, 26(Supp.3), 44–53. https://doi.org/10.1177/1757975919831603.

Human Rights and Equal Opportunity Commission. (2003). Social justice and human rights for Aboriginal and Torres Strait Islander people. Retrieved from https://www.humanrights.gov.au/sites/default/files/content/social_justice/infosheet/infosheet_sj.pdf.

International Monetary Fund. (2016). Poverty reduction strategy papers. Retrieved from http://www.imf.org/external/np/prsp/prsp.aspx.

International Union for Health Promotion and Education (IUHPE). (2016). Core competencies and professional standards for health promotion 2016. Retrieved from https://www.iuhpe.org/images/JC-Accreditation/Core_Competencies_Standards_linkE.pdf.

Institute for Agriculture and Trade Policy (IATP). (2004). United States dumping on world agricultural markets. Minneapolis: Institute for Agriculture and Trade Policy.

Jeffreys, M. (2010). Teaching cultural competence in nursing and health care (2nd ed.). New York: Springer Publishing Co.

Johnstone, M. J., & Kanitsaki, O. (2007). An exploration of the notion and nature of the construct cultural safety and its applicability to the Australian health care context. Journal of Transcultural Nursing, 18, 247–256. https://doi.org/10.1177/1043659607301304.

Jonas, W., Chez, R., Smith, K., & Sakallaris, B. (2014). Salutogenesis: the defining concept for a new healthcare system. Global Advances in Health and Medicine, 3(3), 82–91. https://doi.org/10.7453/gahmj.2014.005.

Kelaher, M., Sabanovic, H., La Brooy, C., et al. (2014). Does more equitable governance lead to more equitable health care? A case study based on the implementation of health reform in Aboriginal health Australia. Social Science & Medicine, 123(2014), 278–286. https://doi.org/10.1016/j.socscimed.2014.07.032.

Kirschenbaum, H. (2013). Values clarification in counselling and psychotherapy. Practical strategies for individual and group settings. New York: Oxford University Press.

Kobayashi, H., Song, C., Ikei, H., et al. (2018). Forest walking affects autonomic nervous activity: a population-based study. Frontiers in Public Health, 6(278). https://doi.org/10.3389/fpubh.2018.00278.

Labonté, R. (1989). Community empowerment: the need for political analysis. Canadian Journal of Public Health, 80(March/April), 87–88.

Labonté, R. (1997). Power participation and partnerships for health promotion. Melbourne: VicHealth.

Labonté, R. (2014). Development goals in the post-2015 world: whither Canada? Canadian Journal of Public Health, 205(3), e224–e228. https://doi.org/10.17269/cjph.105.4399.

Labonté, R., Blouin, C., Chopra, M., et al. (2007). Towards health equitable globalization: rights, regulation and redistribution. Final Report of the Globalization Knowledge Network to the Commission on Social Determinants of Health. Geneva, WHO. Retrieved from https://www.who.int/social_determinants/resources/gkn_report_06_2007.pdf.

Labonté, R., & Laverack, G. (2008). Health promotion in action: from local to global empowerment. The University of Michigan: Palgrave Macmillan.

Labonté, R., & Schrecker, T. (2006). Globalization and social determinants of health: analytic and strategic review paper. On behalf of the Globalization Knowledge Network. Institute of Population Health. University of Ottawa. Retrieved from http://www.who.int/social_determinants/resources/globalization.pdf.

Labonté, R., & Schrecker, T. (2007). Globalization and social determinants of health: the role of the global marketplace (part 2 of 3). Globalization and Health, 3, 6. https://doi.org/10.1186/1744-8603-3-6.

Laverack, G. (2007). Health promotion practice: building empowered communities. London: McGraw-Hill, Open University Press.

Laverack, G. (2012). Health activism. Health Promotion International, 27(4), 429–434. https://doi.org/10.1093/heapro/das044.

Lawson, M., Chan, M. K., Rhodes, F., et al. (2019). Public good or private wealth? Oxford: Oxfam. Retrieved from https://indepth.oxfam.org.uk/public-good-private-wealth/.

Leeder, S. R. (2003). Achieving equity in the Australian healthcare system. Medical Journal of Australia, 179(9), 475–478. Retrieved from https://www.mja.com.au/system/files/issues/179_09_031103/lee10203_fm.pdf.

Lowe, M., Boulange, C., & Giles-Corti, B. (2015). Urban design and health: progress to date and future challenges. Health Promotion Journal of Australia, 25, 14–18. https://doi.org/10.1071/HE13072.

Lowe, M., Whitzman, C., Badland, H., et al. (2013). Liveable, healthy, sustainable: what are the key indicators for Melbourne neighbourhoods? Research Paper 1, Place, Health and Liveability Research Program, University of Melbourne. Retrieved from https://socialequity.unimelb.edu.au/__data/assets/pdf_file/0006/1979574/Liveability-Indicators-report.pdf.

Lowe, M., Whitzman, C., Badland, H., et al. (2014). Planning healthy, liveable and sustainable cities: how can indicators inform policy? Urban Policy and Research, 33(2), 131–144. https://doi.org/10.1080/08111146.2014.1002606.

McMullen, C., Eastwood, A., & Ward, J. (2016). Environmental attributable fractions in remote Australia: the potential of a new approach for local public health action. Australian and New Zealand Journal of Public Health, 40(2), 174–180. https://doi.org/10.1111/1753-6405.12425.

Mahitahi Trust. (2019). Mahitahi Trust. Retrieved from http://www.mahitahi.co.nz/.

Major Cities Unit. (2012). State of Australian cities 2012. Canberra: Department of Infrastructure and Transport, Australian Government. Retrieved from https://infrastructure.gov.au/infrastructure/pab/soac/2012.aspx.

Markwick, A., Ansari, Z., Sullivan, M., & McNeil, J. (2015). Social determinants and psychological distress among Aboriginal and Torres Strait Islander adults in the Australian state of Victoria: a cross-sectional population based study. Social Science and Medicine, 128, 178–187. https://doi.org/10.1016/j.socscimed.2015.01.014.

Marmot, M. (2006). Health in an unequal world: social circumstances, biology and disease. Presented at: Royal College of Physicians Harveian Oration, London, UK. Retrieved from http://discovery.ucl.ac.uk/4511/.

Marmot, M. (2012). Fair society, healthy lives; the Marmot review: Strategic review of health inequalities in England post-2010. UK Department of Health. Retrieved from http://www.instituteofhealthequity.org/resources-reports/fair-society-healthy-lives-the-marmot-review.

Marmot, M., & Wilkinson, R. (Eds.). (2006). Social determinants of health (2nd ed.). Oxford: Oxford University Press.

Miller, G., & Foster, L. T. (2010). Critical synthesis of wellness literature. Victoria, Canada: University of Victoria.

Ministry of Health. (2015). Annual update of key results 2014/15. New Zealand Government. Retrieved from https://www.moh.govt.nz/notebook/nbbooks.nsf/0/997AF4E3AAE9A767CC257F4C007DDD84/$file/annual-update-key-results-2014-15-nzhs-dec15-1.pdf.

Ministry of Health. (2016). Health loss in New Zealand: a report from the New Zealand burden of diseases, injuries and risk factors study, 2006–2016. New Zealand Government. Retrieved from https://www.moh.govt.nz/notebook/nbbooks.nsf/0/F85C39E4495B9684CC257BD3006F6299/$file/health-loss-in-new-zealand-final.pdf.

Ministry of Health. (2017). Māori health models – Te Whare Tapa Whā. New Zealand Government. Retrieved from: http://www.health.govt.nz/our-work/populations/maori-health/maori-health-models/maori-health-models-te-whare-tapa-wha.

Mittelmark, M. B., & Bull, T. (2013). The salutogenic model of health in health promotion research. Global Health Promotion, 20(2), 30–38. https://doi.org/10.1177/1757975913486684.

Moncrieffe, J., & Eyben, R. (2013). The power of labelling: how people are categorized and why it matters. London: Taylor and Francis.

Mooney, G. (2012). Health of nations: towards a new political economy. London: Zed Books.

Naidoo, J., & Wills, J. (2011). Developing practice for public health and health promotion. Edinburgh; New York: Bailliere Tindall/Elsevier.

National Aboriginal Community Controlled Health Organisations (NACCHO). (2011). NACCHO Constitution. Ratified NACCHO AGM 15 November 2011. Retrieved from https://www.naccho.org.au/about/governance/.

Navarro, V. (2011). The importance of politics in policy. Australian and New Zealand Journal of Public Health, 35(4), 313. https://doi.org/10.1111/j.1753-6405.2011.00715.x.

Norman, E. (Ed.). (2012). Resiliency enhancement: putting the strength perspective into social work practice. Columbia: Columbia University Press.

Office of the United Nations High Commissioner for Human Rights (OHCHR). (2008). Human rights, health and poverty reduction strategies. With the Department of Health Policy, Development and Services, and the Health & Human Rights Team of the Department of Ethics, Equity, Trade & Human Rights, of the World Health Organization (WHO). Retrieved from http://www.ohchr.org/Documents/Publications/HHR_PovertyReductionsStrategies_WHO_EN.pdf.

O'Hara, L., & Gregg, J. (2012). Human rights casualties from the 'war on obesity': why focusing on body weight is inconsistent with a human rights approach to health. Fat Studies, 1(1), 32–46. https://doi.org/10.1080/21604851.2012.627790.

O'Hara, L., & Taylor, J. (2018). What's wrong with the 'war on obesity?' A narrative review of the weight-centered health paradigm and development of the 3C framework to build critical competency for a paradigm shift. SAGE Open, 8(2), 1–28. https://doi.org/10.1177/2158244018772888.

Okvat, H., & Zautra, A. (2011). Community gardening: a parsimonious path to individual, community, and environmental resilience. American Journal of Community Psychology, 47(3), 374–387. https://doi.org/10.1007/s10464-010-9404-z.

Organisation for Economic Cooperation and Development (OECD). (2015). How's Life? 2015. Measuring Well-being. Retrieved from https://www.oecd.org/statistics/How-s-life-2015-60-seconde-guide.pdf.

Organisation for Economic Cooperation and Development (OECD). (2016). Health statistics 2016. Retrieved from https://www.oecd.org/els/health-systems/Table-of-Content-Metadata-OECD-Health-Statistics-2016.pdf.

Papps, E., & Ramsden, I. (1996). Cultural safety in nursing: the New Zealand experience. International Journal of Quality Health Care, 8(5), 491–497. https://doi.org/10.1093/intqhc/8.5.491.

Parigi, P., & Henson, W. (2014). Social isolation in America. Annual Review of Sociology, 40, 153–171. https://doi.org/10.1146/annurev-soc-071312-145646.

Passmore, H.-A., & Holder, M. D. (2017). Noticing nature: individual and social benefits of a two-week intervention. The Journal of Positive Psychology, 12(6), 537–546. https://doi.org/10.1080/17439760.2016.1221126.

People's Health Movement, Medact, Medico International, Third World Network, Health Action International and Asociación Latinoamericana de Medicina Social. (2011). Global health watch 3: an alternative world health report. London: Zed Books.

People's Health Movement, Medact, Medico International, Third World Network, Health Action International and Asociación Latinoamericana de Medicina Social. (2014). Global health watch 4: an alternative world health report. London: Zed Books.

Pere, R. & Nicholson, N. (1991). Te wheke: a celebration of infinite wisdom. Gisborne: Ao Ako Global Learning New Zealand.

Pett, H. (2016). Richest 62 people own as much as half the world's population: Oxfam. ABC News, January. Retrieved from http://www.abc.net.au/news/2016-01-18/oxfam-uses-global-wealth-report-to-highlight-inequlity/7096688.

Prochaska, J. O., & Di Clementi, C. C. (1984). The transtheoretical approach: crossing traditional boundaries of therapy. Homeward Illinois: Down Jones, Irwin.

Productivity Commission. (2012). Schools workforce, research report. Canberra: Australian Government Productivity Commission. Retrieved from https://www.pc.gov.au/inquiries/completed/education-workforce-schools/report.

Public Health Agency of Canada (PHAC) and World Health Organization. (2008). Health equity through intersectoral action: an analysis of 18 country case studies. Ottawa: PHAC.

Public Health Indigenous Leadership in Education (PHILE) Network. (2016). National Aboriginal and Torres Strait islander public health curriculum framework: 2nd ed. Retrieved from http://caphia.com.au/testsite/wp-content/uploads/2016/07/Curriculum-Framework-2nd-Edition.pdf.

Putnam, R. (1993). Making democracy work: civic traditions in modern Italy. Princeton, NJ: Princeton University Press.

Raeburn, J., & Rootman, I. (1998). People-centred health promotion. Chichester: John Wiley and Sons.

Ramsden, I. (2002). Cultural safety and nursing education in Aotearoa and Te Waipounamu. New Zealand: University of Wellington.

Robson, B., & Harris, R. (Eds.). (2005). Hauora: Māori standards of health IV: a study of the years 2000–2005. Wellington: Te Rōpù Rangahau Hauora a Eru Pòmare.

Ryan, W. (1976). Blaming the victim. New York: Vintage Books.

Scott, K. (2012). Measuring wellbeing: towards sustainability? London: Taylor and Francis.

Sen, A. (1992). Inequality re-examined. New York: Russell Sage Foundation.

Sommeiller, E., & Price, M. (2015). The increasingly unequal states of America: income inequality by state, 1917 to 2012. Washington: Economic Analysis and Research Network. Retrieved from http://www.epi.org/files/2014/IncreasinglyUnequalStatesofAmerica1917to2012.pdf.

Stallings, B. (2003). Globalization and liberalization: the impact on developing countries. In A. Kohli, C. Moon, & G. Sørensen (Eds.), States, markets, and just growth: development in the twenty-first century (pp. 9–38). Tokyo: United Nations University Press.

Sunshine Coast Council. (2017). Environment and liveability strategy 2017. Retrieved from https://www.sunshinecoast.qld.gov.au/Council/Planning-and-Projects/Regional-Strategies/Environment-and-Liveability-Strategy-2017.

Svalastog, A. L., Donev, D., Jahren Kristoffersen, N., & Gajović, S. (2017). Concepts and definitions of health and health-related values in the knowledge landscapes of the digital society. Croatian Medical Journal 58(6), 431–435. https://doi.org/10.3325/cmj.2017.58.431.

Talbot, L., & Walker, R. (2007). Community perspectives on the impact of policy change on linking social capital in a rural community. Health and Place, 13(2), 482–492. https://doi.org/10.1016/j.healthplace.2006.05.007.

Taylor, K., & Guerin, P. (2014). Health care and indigenous Australians: cultural safety in practice (2nd ed.). Melbourne: Palgrave Macmillan.

Teshuva, K., Kendig, H., & Stacey, B. (1997). Spirituality, health and health promotion in older Australians. Health Promotion Journal of Australia, 7(3), 180–184.

Tesoriero, F. (2010). Community development: community-based alternatives in an age of globalization (4th ed.). Frenchs Forest, NSW: Pearson Australia.

Tobias, M., & Yeh, L. C. (2007). How much does health care contribute to health inequality in New Zealand? Australia and New Zealand Journal of Public Health, 31(3), 207–210. https://doi.org/10.1111/j.1753-6405.2007.00049.x.

Transition Town Totnes. (n.d.). Transition Town Totnes. Retrieved from https://www.transitiontowntotnes.org/.

United Nations. (1948). The universal declaration of human rights. Retrieved from http://www.un.org/en/universal-declaration-human-rights/index.html.

United Nations. (2006). The International Forum for Social Development: Social justice in an open world: the role of the United Nations. Retrieved from http://www.un.org/esa/socdev/documents/ifsd/SocialJustice.pdf.

United Nations (UN). (2007). United Nations declaration on the rights of Indigenous people. Retrieved from https://www.un.org/development/desa/indigenouspeoples/wp-content/uploads/sites/19/2018/11/UNDRIP_E_web.pdf

United Nations. (2014). Human development report 2014: Sustaining human progress: reducing vulnerabilities and building resilience. New York: United Nations Development Program. Retrieved from http://hdr.undp.org/sites/default/files/hdr14-report-en-1.pdf.

United Nations (UN). (2015). Transforming our world: the 2030 agenda for sustainable development. Retrieved from https://sustainabledevelopment.un.org/post2015/transformingourworld.

United Nations (UN). (n.d.). Sustainable development goals. Retrieved from https://www.un.org/sustainabledevelopment/sustainable-development-goals/.

Verrinder, G., & Talbot, L. (2015). Rural communities experiencing climate change: a systems approach to adaptation. In R. Walker & W. Mason (Eds.), Climate change adaptation for health and social services. Melbourne: CSIRO Publishing.

Waitzkin, H., & Hellander, I. (2016). The history and future of neoliberal health reform: Obamacare and its predecessors. International Journal of Health Services, 46(4), 747–766. https://doi.org/10.1177/0020731416661645.

Wallerstein, N. (1992). Powerlessness, empowerment and health: implications for health promotion programs. American Journal of Public Health, 6(3), 197–205. https://doi.org/10.4278/0890-1171-6.3.197.

Wallerstein, N. (2006). What is the evidence on effectiveness of empowerment to improve health? WHO Regional Office for Europe, Copenhagen, Health Evidence Network Report. Retrieved from http://www.euro.who.int/__data/assets/pdf_file/0010/74656/E88086.pdf.

Wallerstein, N., & Bernstein, E. (1994). Introduction to community empowerment, participatory action and health. Health Education Quarterly, 21(2), 141–148. https://doi.org/10.1177/109019819402100202.

Whitmee, S., Haines, A., Beyrer, C., et al. (2015). Safeguarding human health in the Anthropocene epoch: report of The Rockefeller Foundation–Lancet Commission on planetary health. Lancet, 386(10007), 1973–2028. http://dx.doi.org/10.1016/S0140-6736(15)60901-1.

Wilkinson, R., & Pickett, K. (2009). The spirit level: why more equal societies almost always do better. London: Allen Lane.

Wiseman, V. (2014). Inclusiveness in the value base for health care resource allocation. Social Science & Medicine, 108, 252–256. https://doi.org/10.1016/j.socscimed.2014.01.028.

Woods, M. (2010). Cultural safety and the socioethical nurse. Nursing Ethics, 17(6), 715–725. https://doi.org/10.1177/0969733010379296.

Woodward, D., Drager, N., Beaglehole, R., & Lipson, D. (2001). WHO globalization and health: a framework for analysis and action. Bulletin of the World Health Organization, 79(9), 875–881. Retrieved from http://www.who.int/bulletin/archives/79(9)875.pdf.

Woolcock, M. (1998). Social capital and economic development: toward a theoretical synthesis and policy framework. Theory and Society, 27, 151–208.

World Health Organization. (1948). World Health Organization Constitution. Retrieved from https://www.who.int/about/who-we-are/constitution.

World Health Organization. (1978). Declaration of Alma-Ata. Retrieved from http://www.who.int/publications/almaata_declaration_en.pdf.

World Health Organization. (1986). The Ottawa charter for health promotion. Retrieved from http://www.who.int/healthpromotion/conferences/previous/ottawa/en.

World Health Organization. (2010). Equity, social determinants and public health programmes. Retrieved from http://apps.who.int/iris/handle/10665/44289.

World Health Organization. (2019a). Global health expenditure database. Retrieved from http://apps.who.int/nha/database/.

World Health Organization. (2019b). Global spending on health: a world in transition. Geneva: World Health Organization (WHO/HIS/HGF/HF Working Paper/19.4). Licence: CC BY-NC-SA 3.0 IGO. Retrieved from https://www.who.int/health_financing/documents/health-expenditure-report-2019.pdf?ua=1.

World Health Organization. (n.d.) Equity. Retrieved from https://www.who.int/healthsystems/topics/equity/en/.

World Health Organization and World Bank. (2005). Dying for change: poor people's experience of health and ill-health. Retrieved from http://www.who.int/hdp/publications/dying_change.pdf.

3 Ecological sustainability and human health and wellbeing

INTRODUCTION

Human health and wellbeing is a function of the relationship between people and their social, economic, political, built and natural environments. This knowledge, and the identification of the need for health practitioners to work within a socio-ecological approach to health and wellbeing that conserves the natural environment for human health and wellbeing and survival of our species, spans decades (e.g. McMichael, 1993; Smith et al., 2014). Natural ecosystems are inextricably linked to all other types of environments and tackling the interrelated issues of social inequality and degradation of the natural environment presents humanity with unprecedented challenges. Scientific evidence indicates that the global natural ecosystem and thus the future of humanity is in a critical period (e.g. Homer-Dixon et al., 2015; Horton et al., 2014; Lenton et al., 2019; Rockström et al., 2009; Steffen et al., 2015). The Rockefeller Foundation–*Lancet* Commission's report states:

> *The degradation of nature's ecological systems [is on] a scale never seen in human history. A growing body of evidence shows that the health of humanity is intrinsically linked to the health of the environment, but by its actions humanity now threatens to destabilise the Earth's key life-support systems.*
>
> *(Whitmee et al., 2015)*

Innovative intersectoral responses are required to mitigate the current and projected health- and wellbeing-related consequences of natural resource depletion, pollution of air, water and soil, climate change, food shortages and changing disease patterns. Health practitioners need to take a leading role and both 'top-down' and 'bottom-up' approaches are required.

A healthy ecosystem is a principal determinant of human health and wellbeing. On the health iceberg, presented in Chapter 1, the health of the natural environment is positioned well below the waterline. In Labonté's 1997 framework of the determinants of health (presented in Chapter 1), ecosystem viability, sustainable development and convivial communities are outlined as health promoting conditions, while natural resource depletion, the enhanced greenhouse effect and polluted environments are located in the risk conditions, along with poverty, low social status and discrimination.

Chapter 3 focuses specifically on the natural environment, and builds on the ideas presented about the socio-ecological determinants of health and wellbeing in Chapter 1 and the core concepts discussed in Chapter 2. An introduction to ecological sustainability for health practitioners is presented by: providing definitions and principles of ecological sustainability; introducing the concepts of systems and resilience thinking; presenting a rationale for the engagement of health practitioners in sustainability; and case studies for health workers working with individuals, in community settings and as citizens playing a leading role in ensuring ecosystem viability and, consequently, healthy humans. Links between the health and wellbeing of people, the health of the natural environment and the implications for practice are made. Before starting the chapter, take some time to review 'Putting the Ottawa Charter into Practice' on pages 115–116.

ECOLOGICAL SUSTAINABILITY CONCEPTS

There is substantial evidence that human life as we know it is under threat due to rapid changes in the global ecology. A manifesto for transforming public health to meet these challenges states that:

PUTTING THE OTTAWA CHARTER INTO PRACTICE

The following reflective questions, arranged in the Ottawa Charter action areas, are presented to guide health practitioners to critically evaluate their professional role and practice, and the health promotion philosophy of their organisation. Content of this chapter will assist practitioners to develop the necessary knowledge and skills to advocate for and contribute to ecological sustainability in their professional roles.

PUTTING THE OTTAWA CHARTER INTO PRACTICE TO BUILD RESILIENCE FOR ECOLOGICAL SUSTAINABILITY

Build healthy public policy

- Are organisational vision or mission statements underpinned by sustainability principles?
- Do strategic plans incorporate the Sustainable Development Goals?
- Do strategic plans have policies to reduce their ecological footprint?
- Are plans and criteria in place to monitor progress?
- Are there plans for organisational adaptation to climate change?

Create supportive environments

- Are workplace health promotion programs in place within the organisation?
- Has 'reduce, reuse, recycle' become part of the culture and activities of the organisation?
- Are green spaces being established locally?
- Has a health impact assessment of, and plans for, climate change been conducted for vulnerable populations within the catchment area of the organisation?
- Have organisational impact assessments been conducted for extreme weather events (power, staffing, volunteers)?

Strengthen community action

- Have interagency partnerships been established to plan for ecologically sustainable development locally?
- Have community leaders from all sectors been involved in the development of policy and program plans for ecologically sustainable development locally?
- Have interagency partnerships been established to manage extreme weather events?
- Has the wider community been involved in the development of policy and program plans for ecologically sustainable development locally?
- Have interagency plans been developed with clear roles and responsibilities for extreme events?

Develop personal skills

- Are training plans in place for staff and volunteers to increase knowledge of the health impacts of sustainability and of degraded environments?

Continued

PUTTING THE OTTAWA CHARTER INTO PRACTICE Cont.

- Are training plans in place for staff and volunteers to increase knowledge of the health impacts of climate change and the impact of extreme weather events on organisations and vulnerable communities?
- Are messages consistent with health literacy principles?
- Are the communication strategies for vulnerable groups culturally and age appropriate?

Reorient services

- Are all sectors represented in partnership plans?

... public health is critical to this vision because of its values of social justice and fairness for all, and its focus on the collective actions of interdependent and empowered peoples and their communities. Our objectives are to protect and promote health and wellbeing, to prevent disease and disability, to eliminate conditions that harm health and wellbeing, and to foster resilience and adaptation. In achieving these objectives, our actions must respond to the fragility of our planet and our obligation to safeguard the physical and human environments within which we exist.

(Horton et al., 2014, p. 847)

Degradation of ecosystems on which all life depends is having, and will increasingly have, an impact on human health, wellbeing and survival. There are five major tenets for consideration that will be discussed throughout this chapter.

1. There are global and local, direct and indirect, short- and long-term, negligible and devastating effects of degraded ecosystems on human health and wellbeing.
2. The effects of degraded ecosystems on health and wellbeing are already being experienced globally.
3. The associated burden on health and wellbeing is borne by individuals and communities unequally.
4. The strain on the resources of the health sector is mounting and it is important to build resilience for predicted changes and challenges to health and wellbeing and health care.
5. Health promotion approaches can guide health practitioners in their thinking and actions in achieving ecological sustainability.

Ecological sustainability

Ecological sustainability is both a process and an outcome. It is a process of change that improves the long-term health and wellbeing of humans and ecological systems. We can promote sustainability and consequently human health and wellbeing by 'using, conserving and enhancing the community's resources so that ecological processes, on which life depends, are maintained, and the total quality of life, now and in the future, can be increased' (Department of Environment, Water, Heritage and the Arts, 1992). The Convention on Biological Diversity defined an ecosystem as a 'dynamic complex of plant, animal and micro-organism communities and their non-living environment interacting as a functional unit' (United Nations [UN], 1992c).

In the 1970s, the concept of sustainability and the practice of sustainable development emerged when concerned citizens who belonged to a 'think tank' called the Club of Rome commissioned research to examine trends in consumption patterns and population growth. Their hypothesis was that if these trends continued at the same rate as they were at that time, the Earth would reach its limits within a short time. The resulting report *Limits to Growth* (Meadows et al., 1972) provided scientific evidence and impetus for global action. In 1987, the World Commission on Environment and Development (WCED), more commonly known as the Brundtland Commission, defined sustainable development as 'development that meets the needs of the present without compromising the ability of future generations to meet their own needs' (WCED, 1987, p. 43). Sustainable development is also referred to as sustainability, ecological sustainability or ecologically sustainable development. The debate continues about which is the best term to use when discussing human health and wellbeing. In this text we use the terms interchangeably. The critical importance of ecologically sustainable development was further evidenced in the establishment of the internationally agreed 2015 Sustainable Development Goals (SDGs) introduced in Chapter 1 (UN, 2015b).

Ecological sustainability will be achieved with consequent improvement in the quality of life of humans through social justice, intergenerational equity, employing the precautionary principle and conserving biological and cultural diversity. Working towards ecological sustainability is consistent with health promotion and CPHC principles. These principles enable us to prevent and reverse adverse impacts of human activities on the ecosystem, while continuing to allow the sustainable, equitable development of societies (see Insight 3.1). The philosophy and actions of health promotion in a CPHC context, as presented throughout this book, are entirely consistent with working towards sustainability.

Global responses to sustainable development

In 1972, the first UN Conference on the Human Environment was convened in Stockholm, Sweden, to address issues concerning the environment and sustainable development (UN, 1972). The conference declaration and action plan included specific strategies for preserving and enhancing the human environment. The concepts and plans developed by this groundbreaking conference have shaped every subsequent international conference and treaty on the environment. In the decades since that first conference on the human environment, many global conferences have been held and documents produced focusing directly or indirectly on sustainable development. Table 3.1 provides a reference for major global declarations, charters and conventions that acknowledge the interdependence of socio-ecological systems and the rights and responsibilities for global, national and local governance.

The SDGs are the current framework for action across all of the determinants of sustainable development (UN, 2015a). The Preamble of *Transforming Our World: The 2030 Agenda for Sustainable Development* (UN, 2015b) states that the members 'are resolved to free the human race from the tyranny of poverty and want to heal and secure our planet' which indicates that there is a recognition by the signatories that the burden of poor health due to environmental degradation is not shared equally. The SDGs (UN, 2015b) were timely given that inequalities in health and wellbeing are increasing, and further environmental degradation is inevitable if the political and economic conditions discussed in Chapters 1 and 2 continue. Add a burgeoning population and overconsumption to this and the

INSIGHT 3.1 Principles of ecological sustainability

These overarching principles reflect the predominant spirit and intent of sustainable development as advocated by the Rio de Janeiro Declaration on Environment and Development
(UN, 1992b) and reaffirmed at the Earth Summit 2012 (http://www.slideshare.net/uncsd2012/
the-future-we-want-rio20-outcome-document).

- *Precautionary principle*: 'Where there are threats of serious or irreversible environmental damage, lack of full scientific certainty should not be used as a reason for
  postponing measures to prevent environmental degradation. In the application of
  the precautionary principle, public and private decisions should be guided by
  careful evaluation to avoid, wherever practicable, serious or irreversible damage to
  the environment and an assessment of the risk-weighted consequences of various
  options' (Deville & Harding, 1997, p. 13).
- *Intergenerational equity*: Extends the principle of fairness and justice to future
  generations. The principle holds that the present generation has a stewardship role
  in conserving the natural and cultural resources of the Earth and all species so
  that future generations may live healthy lives.
- *Biodiversity conservation*: The 'protection of ecosystems, natural habitats and the
  maintenance of viable populations of species in natural surroundings' (Convention
  on Biological Diversity) (UN, 1992b). Biodiversity refers to the variety of all life on
  Earth—plants, animals and microorganisms, as well as the genetic material they
  contain and the ecological systems in which they occur. Biodiversity is necessary
  to maintain our atmosphere, climate, water and soils in a healthy state. There are
  aesthetic, cultural and ethical reasons for maintaining biodiversity. Humans define
  themselves through their ecosystems. It is an essential element of intergenerational
  equity and, in addition, other species have as much right to the Earth as humans.
- *Environmental resource accounting*: A means of benchmarking the current usage
  against ideal usage and then, for the future, reporting on the progress.
- *Community participation*: Acknowledges that the practice of sustainable development
  is dependent upon the involvement of communities in decision making at the local
  level.

TABLE 3.1 Global watershed developments linking health and the environment

Year	Organisation	Event and/or document
1972	United Nations (UN)	United Nations Conference on the Human Environment, Stockholm, Sweden Declaration of the United Nations Conference on the Human Environment (UN, 1972)
1978	World Health Organization (WHO)	International Conference on Primary Health Care, Alma-Ata, USSR The Declaration of Alma-Ata (WHO, 1978)
1985	UN	Vienna Convention for the Protection of the Ozone Layer (UN, 1985)
1986	WHO	1st Global Conference on Health Promotion, Ottawa, Canada The Ottawa Charter for Health Promotion (WHO, 1986)

TABLE 3.1 Global watershed developments linking health and the environment—cont'd

Year	Organisation	Event and/or document
1987	UN	World Commission on Environment and Development (informally known as the Brundtland Commission) Our Common Future (UN, 1987b)
1987	UN	Montreal Protocol on Substances that Deplete the Ozone Layer (UN, 1987a)
1992	UN	United Nations Conference on Environment and Development, Rio de Janeiro, Brazil (informally known as the Rio Earth Summit) Rio Declaration on Environment and Development (UN, 1992b)
1992	UN	Agenda 21, companion document to Rio Declaration on Environment and Development, adopted at the Rio Earth Summit (UN, 1992a)
1992	UN	United Nations Framework Convention on Climate Change, opened for signature at the Rio Earth Summit (UN, 1992d)
1992	UN	United Nations Convention on Biological Diversity (UN, 1992c)
1997	UN	United Nations Framework Convention on Climate Change Kyoto Protocol (UN, 1997)
2001	UN	Stockholm Convention on Persistent Organic Pollutants (UN, 2001)
2012	Global Health and Climate Alliance	Doha Declaration on Climate Health and Wellbeing (Global Health and Climate Alliance, 2012)
2015	UN	Transforming Our World: The 2030 Agenda for Sustainable Development (UN, 2015b)
2015	UN	United Nations Framework Convention on Climate Change Paris Agreement (UN, 2015c)
2016	WHO	9th Global Conference on Health Promotion Shanghai Declaration on promoting health in the 2030 Agenda for Sustainable Development (WHO, 2016)
2018	WHO	Global Conference on Primary Health Care, Astana, Kazakhstan Declaration of Astana (WHO, 2018b)
2019	UN	United Nations Climate Change Conference (UN, 2019a)

outlook to reduce inequalities in health and environmental degradation is poor. The OECD (n.d.) reports that most countries will fall short of their adaptation goals for climate change (a planetary boundary that has already been transgressed) and governments need to significantly accelerate their efforts. Furthermore, the OECD reports child poverty (SDG 1) has risen in 16 OECD countries since the world economic crisis in 2007 and that children and young people are the groups most at risk of income poverty (OECD, 2019).

While the monitoring indicators of the SDGs have been set and many have expressed enthusiasm for the goals, there have also been criticisms that they are too broad (Horton, 2014; WHO, 2018a). In the proposed but never ratified Trans-Pacific Partnership Agreement (TPPA), some of the goals were threatened to be undermined. Gleeson (2015) reports the investor-state dispute settlement (ISDS) mechanisms in the TPPA would have enabled foreign corporations to bring claims against governments over health and environmental policies, thereby weakening the state's right to enact high standards of health and environmental legislation. The subsequent Comprehensive and Progressive Agreement for Trans-Pacific Partnership (CPTPP) (a free trade agreement to which Australia is a signatory) may enable similar claims that reduce the state's capacity to protect its citizens from health and environmental risks.

The SDGs support action for protection of the environment and promoting human health and wellbeing. The international health sector is an important partner in the efforts to achieve the SDGs, and has been active in articulating the relationship between the environment and human health and wellbeing. The Declaration of Alma-Ata (WHO, 1978), Ottawa Charter for Health Promotion (WHO, 1986), and Sundsvall Statement on Supportive Environments for Health (WHO, 1991) all elucidated the importance of the environment in creating health and wellbeing. The Shanghai Declaration on Promoting Health in the 2030 Agenda for Sustainable Development (WHO, 2016) and Declaration of Astana (WHO, 2018b) commit to action on the SDGs. With respect to climate change specifically, in the lead-up to the UN Climate Change Conference in Paris, the World Health Organization (WHO) (2015c) called for urgent action to protect human health from climate change, including:

- strong and effective action to limit climate change, and avoid unacceptable risks to global health

- scaling up of financing for adaptation to climate change including public health measures to reduce the risks from extreme weather events, infectious disease, diminishing water supplies and food insecurity

- actions that both reduce climate change and improve health, including reducing the number of deaths from cancer and from respiratory and cardiovascular diseases that are caused by air pollution

- raising awareness of the health effects of climate change and the potential health co-benefits of low carbon pathways, among health professionals and the general public

- contributing to the development and implementation of measures to limit climate change and protect our countries, workplaces and communities

- working to minimise the environmental impacts of our own health systems, at the same time as improving health services.

The resulting *Climate Agreement—Moving towards healthier people and a healthier planet* (WHO, 2015a), officially known as the UN Framework Convention on Climate Change Paris Agreement (UN, 2015c) entered into force in 2016 and took effect from 2020.

In addition to commitments from global agencies and nation states, international health-related organisations have been active in responding to sustainable development issues. For example, signatories to the 2012 Doha Declaration on Climate Health and Wellbeing included a significant number of professional health bodies such as the World Medical Association, the International Council of Nurses, the Climate and Health Alliance, the Public Health Association of Australia, the Climate and Health Council, OraTaiao: New Zealand Climate and Health Council, International Federation of Medical Students, Health Care Without Harm, European Public Health Association, and many others (Global Health and Climate Alliance, 2012).

All of the international declarations, charters, conventions and agreements that address ecological sustainability directly or indirectly reflect a systems approach to improving health and wellbeing, and provide a guide for policy development at the national level. However, evaluation of the actions of national governments does not give cause for optimism. For example, a study on national responses to climate change by the World Federation of Public Health Associations (WFPHA) found that only 17 of the 35 national governments that responded reported that they considered the public health impacts of climate change in their mitigation and adaptation plans (WFPHA, 2015). Developing healthy public policy is discussed in depth in Chapter 5.

Many cultural attitudes, as well as government policies, are the cause of the damage in the past and are continuing to cause damage (AtKisson, 2010; Brown, 2009; Diamond, 2005). The impact of neoliberalism, discussed in Chapters 1 and 2, has been bad news for the environment and consequently our health (Labonté & Schrecker, 2006). There has been neglect of public goods in favour of private goods. On the one hand, environmental problems are accelerating exponentially; on the other hand, public concern for the environment is also accelerating exponentially. Examination of our values is critically important.

Look forward 20 years from now. What do you see? What is the legacy of today's policymakers? Is the ecosystem still viable? Are there public institutions that support social capital, convivial communities, 'green' town-planning policies? Is there enough clean water and food for people the world over, or

> *... are you shaking your head at the feeble attempts at mitigation by the present generation, the endless dithering over the reality of climate change, and the head-in-the-sand policies that assumed addressing the problem could be put off for another day and that the future would be clever enough and rich enough to take care of itself.*
>
> *(Scientific American Editorial, 2008)*

This major ecological transition requires us to search for new ways of thinking about our relationship with the planet. This transition is having a profound effect on the health of the planet and, consequently, humans. In light of this, a great deal has been written about the need to explore Indigenous knowledges (e.g. Arabena, 2010; Arabena & Kingsley, 2015). Arabena (2010, pp. 260–267) reminds us that many Indigenous peoples, for example in Australia, New Zealand, Canada, Africa, India and the Americas, do not see the universe in merely physical terms or as an external, separate entity but rather 'humanity as fused with the universe' (p. 262). She reminds us that the understanding Indigenous people have of the universe has ensured sustainability throughout thousands of generations. She suggests that 'perhaps by approaching all knowledges with Indigenous spatial references we would not see ourselves as separate from anything' (p. 265). She argues that we need to transcend various worldviews and explores the notion of synthesising the knowledge of Indigenous peoples, deep ecologists and ethicists. Arabena argues that there are unifying themes in terms of understanding the universe within these different traditions that are integral to sustainability. *Strong Sustainability for New Zealand: Principles and Scenarios* (Sustainable Aotearoa New Zealand [SANZ], 2009) is a good example of this. Furthermore, each of the appendices in this book—the Declaration of Alma-Ata (WHO, 1978), the Ottawa Charter for Health Promotion (WHO, 1986), the Universal Declaration of Human Rights (UN, 1948), the Earth Charter (Earth Charter, 2000), and Declaration of Astana (WHO, 2018b)—have all been agreed to by hundreds of countries throughout the world. They all make links in some way to the importance of the health of the natural environment to human health and wellbeing. The Earth Charter in particular draws together the social and natural environmental elements needed for ecological sustainability and health. All provide the principles upon which to base healthy public policies and action. They are all based on systems and resilience thinking as a process and sustainability as a process and outcome.

Working towards sustainability will result in positive health and wellbeing outcomes. For example, clean energy will protect biodiversity by reducing the need to clear forests and so the integrity of the soil and water will be maintained. Local food production and economies will feed local communities instead of being subject to the vicissitudes of a global fossil fuel-based economy. Improved agricultural practices will reduce exposure to animal-to-human infections associated with land clearing. Better economic and social opportunities for vulnerable communities will reduce inequalities, the number of social and environmental refugees, and pressure on overburdened health resources.

Planetary health

One approach to understanding and managing sustainability has been the concept of planetary boundaries, where scientists have identified and quantified boundaries within which humanity can continue to develop and thrive for generations to come (Rockström et al., 2009; Steffen et al., 2015; Stockholm Resilience Centre, 2015). The Stockholm Resilience Centre is internationally recognised for its transdisciplinary research in this field. It advances the understanding of complex social-ecological systems and generates new insights and developments to improve ecosystem management practices and long-term sustainability. It proposes that respecting planetary boundaries reduces the risks to human society of crossing environmental thresholds, and not respecting them could generate abrupt or irreversible changes (Stockholm Resilience Centre, 2015). The nine planetary boundaries are:

- climate change
- biosphere integrity
- land-system change
- freshwater use
- biogeochemical flows (nitrogen and phosphorus cycles)
- atmospheric aerosol loading (no global quantification)
- stratospheric ozone depletion
- ocean acidification
- novel entities (no global quantification).

In 2009, Rockström and colleagues estimated that humanity had already transgressed three planetary boundaries: climate change, rate of biodiversity loss, and changes to the global nitrogen. Six years on, Steffen and others (2015) reported the transgression of four planetary boundaries: climate change, biodiversity integrity (previously referred to as biodiversity loss), altered biochemical cycles and land-system changes. They highlighted the issue that because the boundaries are interdependent systems, transgressing one may both shift the position of other boundaries and also cause them to be transgressed.

Planetary health recognises the relationship between humanity and the natural environment, now a global health and wellbeing priority (Almada et al., 2017). Crises are becoming more global, rather than being localised. They are affecting more people and wider systems. In a joint report (2012), the UN Environment Program (UNEP) and UN International Human Dimensions Program on Global Environmental Change (UN-IHDP) predicted that by 2030 'the world will need at least 50% more food, 45% more energy and 30% more water, all at a time when environmental limits are threatening supply' (p. xiii). Homer-Dixon and colleagues (2015) argue that future crises will increasingly result from long-term global trends: an increase in human economic activity and connectivity across the globe; and a decrease in the diversity of human cultures, institutions, practices and technologies. These trends will further reduce the capacity of socio-ecological systems to deal with natural disturbances. These authors illustrate these using case studies from the food-energy crises in 2008 when four stressors affected socio-ecological systems simultaneously, diminishing supply of good-quality agricultural land; declining returns on industrial agriculture; climate-change-related extreme weather such as droughts; and consistent high demand for food in a growing population. The authors identify three processes that occur in such a crisis: tipping points and sudden shifts; the combined effect of stresses such as drought, poverty and social conflict; and 'ramifying cascade' when sudden and severe disturbances spread through tightly connected networks. They argue that these processes may result in synchronous, unexpected and irreversible failures of socio-ecological systems at a global scale.

Systems thinking

The evidence encapsulated in the planetary boundaries theory (Rockström et al., 2009; Steffen et al., 2015) and the work of Homer-Dixon and colleagues (2015) highlights the importance of systems thinking. The health of the environment and thus the health and wellbeing of people is influenced by multiple, interacting and interdependent elements of the natural, built, economic, political and social environments. Systems thinking has been defined as 'the understanding of a phenomenon within the context of a larger whole' (Keen et al., 2005, p. 12). Humans are now influencing every aspect of the earth and the biosphere; that is, the social systems are affecting the natural systems and, in turn, these natural systems are affecting social systems. Changes to the relationship over time bring changes in human health and wellbeing. Societies have responded to these environmental and human health and wellbeing changes in different ways and on various scales. We need a systems approach to tackling emergent health and wellbeing issues in global and local ecosystems. Using the socio-ecological model of health and wellbeing approach we:

- acknowledge the interdependence of the natural and social environments
- consider the environment is made up of different subsystems (e.g. the biosphere and geography, and the cultural, economic, political and built systems); these may be local or global systems
- emphasise the relationships and dependencies between these subsystems.

The Mandala of Health (Fig. 3.1) is an example of a model that depicts the human ecosystem as a system of interrelationships, each component of which has the potential to

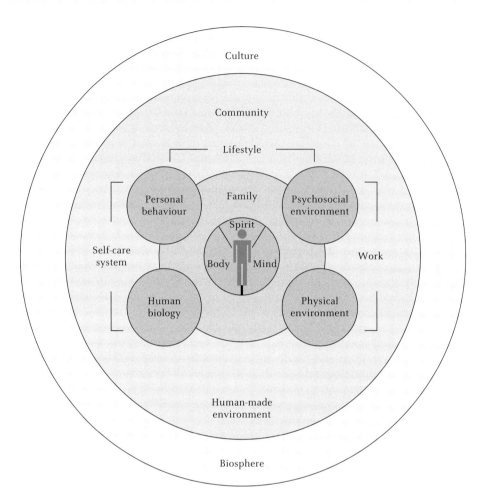

FIGURE 3.1 Mandala of Health
Source: Hancock, 1985.

affect human health (Hancock, 1985). Brown and colleagues (2005) describe the Mandala as a model in which the social unit (individual or family) is placed at the centre of concentric circles, which expand out to the biosphere. Within the circles are four key factors that determine health. The form the Mandala takes serves first to illustrate that the impacts of change in one part of the ecosystem of relationships are not restricted to that part and instead are likely to make an impact across the entire system. The model makes clear that there is a very tight relationship between natural and social systems, thus emphasising the risks of this tightening relationship as humans have learned to manipulate the planet. The Mandala serves as a framework for understanding socio-ecological systems in which systems thinking and sustainability thinking are encapsulated in a socio-ecological approach to health and wellbeing. The Mandala demonstrates that to understand things systemically means to put them into a context and establish the nature of their relationships.

It is important to realise that elements of a system first interact with their neighbours. This law applies 'equally to the weather, society, and life itself' (Finnegan, 2005, cited in

INSIGHT 3.2 Individual action for sustainability

1. Make sure your superannuation is not invested in fossil fuels.
2. Take your mortgage away from the big 4 banks because they support fossil fuel industries.
3. Divest yourself of shares in fossil fuel companies and banks that invest in them.
4. Use an energy company that supports renewable energy.
5. Install solar panels and use solar hot water.
6. Ensure energy conservation and efficiency in your home.
7. Have the smallest, most efficient car you can manage, and switch to cycling, public transport and car-sharing.
8. Don't buy 'stuff' you don't need or will rarely use.
9. Eat mostly plants, and not too much meat.
10. Reconnect—share the progress with others.

Adapted from Ian McBurney Life @ Live ecological 'Imagine Meeting Your Financial Carbon Broker': http://ianmcburney.com/blog/2014/9/19/meet-your-financial-carbon-broker-today.

Verrinder, 2012, p. 198). Applying this law means that 'bottom-up' and local decision making is as important as 'top-down' and global decision making to promote health and wellbeing. 'Bottom-up' decision making means community involvement in planning, implementing and evaluating local solutions to priorities that the community has identified, for example in urban planning (Webb et al., 2018). These approaches are discussed in Chapters 4 to 9.

One of the barriers to systems thinking is that most humans see themselves as separate entities. The notion of interdependence is acknowledged within human systems, but our evolutionary path has resulted in most humans thinking we are separate from the environment when in fact we have co-evolved with plants and other animals and are inseparable from the global ecosystem. The planetary boundary framework, the Mandala of Health, and health promotion and CPHC principles can guide intersectoral action at local and global scales. The health impacts of transgressing planetary boundaries as discussed above will also be a function of building the resilience of both local and global socio-ecological systems. What then can individuals do to be part of the solution to a sustainable future on a daily basis? The UN has published *The Lazy Person's Guide to Saving the World* which specifies some actions for individuals 'from your couch', 'at home' and 'outside your house' (UN, n.d.b). Ecological sustainability campaigner and educator Ian McBurney has also documented a scenario that gives guidance to people to manage their carbon emissions to a level that will possibly keep global warming to below 2°C. His argument is that individual action is essential, and there are things that each of us can do to make a difference to the whole system (see Insight 3.2).

Resilience thinking

Resilience thinking, systems thinking and sustainability thinking are all part of the same worldview (Verrinder, 2012). Resilience is the long-term capacity of a system to deal with change and continue to develop. In resilience thinking there is recognition that systems are dynamic interactions between people and their environments (Folke, 2011). The concept of resilience thinking has been used in research and practice to understand and strengthen socio-ecological systems. For example, natural disasters such as fire, flood, drought or heatwaves have implications for the management of natural, built and social environments and the health and wellbeing of humans. Resilience thinking can be seen as 'insurance against future shocks' (Folke, 2011, p. 6) and it is often referred to as building community resilience by building social capital. As discussed in Chapter 2, the approach builds in flexibility and adaptive capacity. Folke states that 'we know the Earth's resilience and resource base cannot be stretched indefinitely and we are uncomfortably aware that we are heading in the wrong direction' (2011, p. 11). This emphasises the importance for health practitioners in understanding the emergent socio-ecological challenges, bringing their knowledge and skills in environmental stewardship and governance, and as we have argued in Chapter 2 and throughout the book, building social capital through citizen participation.

Climate change

Climate change is one of the global boundaries that have been transgressed (Rockström et al., 2009; Steffen et al., 2015). There is a significant body of evidence about the contributing factors and the health and wellbeing impacts (Zhang et al., 2018). Climate change has been identified as the most pressing SDG due to the potential catastrophic impact on the health and wellbeing of the environment and, in turn, that of the population (UN, 2019b). A rise in greenhouse gas emissions due to human activity is a significant contributing factor. The Intergovernmental Panel on Climate Change (IPCC) (2014b) defines climate change as 'a change in the state of the climate that can be identified by changes in the mean and/or the variability of its properties and that persists for an extended period, typically decades or longer'. The Synthesis Report of the IPCC states:

> Climate change will amplify existing risks and create new risks for natural and human systems. Risks are unevenly distributed and are generally greater for disadvantaged people and communities in countries at all levels of development. Increasing magnitudes of warming increase the likelihood of severe, pervasive and irreversible impacts for people, species and ecosystems. Continued high emissions would lead to mostly negative impacts for biodiversity, ecosystem services and economic development and amplify risks for livelihoods and for food and human security.
>
> *(IPCC, 2014a, p. 64)*

With climate change comes increased risk to the health and wellbeing of individuals and populations. In Australia, for example, health risks associated with climate change include the following (Climate Council, 2018; Horton & McMichael, 2008):

- Accidental death in extreme weather events (floods, storms, cyclones, bushfires, etc.)
- Homelessness due to extreme weather events (floods, storms, cyclones, bushfires, etc.)
- Social dislocation due to homelessness and involuntary separation
- Poverty due to loss of income
- Heat stress from rise of average temperature, heatwaves, spikes in daily temperature
- Dehydration due to heat

- Vector-borne diseases due to habitat expansion resulting from temperature change
- Water-borne infections from poor water quality
- Food-borne infections due to changes in bacterial and viral reproduction resulting from change in weather
- Malnutrition due to reduced food security
- Respiratory diseases due to air pollution
- Mental illnesses due to social dislocation
- Violence due to competition for scarce resources.

The health and social impacts of climate change are widespread, but the impacts are felt most by vulnerable people such as the elderly, children and people with disabilities or chronic diseases. Climate change is experienced differently by men and women and by culturally and linguistically diverse communities and Indigenous communities (e.g. Walker & Mason, 2015). Urban and rural communities also experience climate change in different ways (Verrinder & Talbot, 2015).

Climate change is both an indicator and outcome of widespread degradation of the environment. There is growing certainty about the details, magnitude, timing and health consequences for the future (Smith et al., 2014). Until now, the effects from climate change have been largely indirect. Climate change is altering ecosystems, agricultural productivity and food supply (IPCC, 2014a), and civil war becomes more likely (Collier, 2003; Holland, 2016). The rising salinity of water tables is damaging farmland. Inappropriate adaptation and mitigation strategies to climate change will give rise to further population displacement and livelihood loss. Heat increases due to global warming affect children, the elderly, the frail, those working in high-heat jobs and socio-economically disadvantaged people the most. Heat-related deaths result from increased strain on the cardiovascular system, industrial accidents, behavioural disruption and heat stroke. Rising sea levels cause added exposure to toxic and infectious agents due to disruption of waste disposal. The impact of climate change on diseases such as malaria, dengue fever, Murray Valley encephalitis, Ross River and Barmah Forest virus is already evident. Dengue fever affects 10 million people annually and this number is rising (WHO, n.d.b). Global warming is expected to change human exposure to infectious disease agents further—both vector-borne and microbes (Smith et al., 2014; WHO, 2005).

The global and local, direct and indirect, short- and long-term, negligible and devastating effects of degraded ecosystems on human health are manifest in climate change in a number of key areas, but not confined to, natural disasters, rising temperatures, the quantity and quality of water, air pollution, food security, mental illness and societal stress. The response to climate change could be 'the greatest global health opportunity of the 21st century' (The Lancet, 2019).

IMPACT OF ECOLOGICAL SUSTAINABILITY ON HEALTH AND WELLBEING

A healthy ecosystem comprises: clean air, water and soil; nutrition and food sovereignty; and cultural and spiritual nourishment. It contributes to our individual and collective health and wellbeing, our global and local economies and provides us with medicines. A healthy ecosystem also limits disease in humans. The evidence shows that environmental risk factors play a role in more than 80% of the diseases regularly reported by the WHO (2006).

A mutually reinforcing system of global ecological changes including pollution, ecotoxicity, resource depletion, and loss of habitat, species and biodiversity is threatening human health on a scale not known before. Water, soil and air have been degraded. Exposure to pollutants contributes to cancer, respiratory, cardiovascular and communicable diseases as well as neuropsychiatric disorders (Organisation for Economic Co-operation and Development [OECD], 2012). For example, persistent organic pollutants have been recognised as having adverse effects on humans and ecosystems. There are three broad categories of organic chemicals that are problematic: pesticides, industrial chemicals and by-products. Exposure to these may be direct or indirect. Exposure to pesticides such as Aldrin can kill people directly (a fatal dose is about 5 grams) but it enters the food chain at lower levels through dairy products and meat (UN, n.d.a). Infectious diseases such as SARS, plague, avian (bird) flu, and diseases due to Ebola virus, Nipah virus, hantavirus and Hendra virus all result from ecosystem change created by humans. When diseases emerge or re-emerge after a long time, they usually have high death rates and few effective therapies.

Health practitioners need to contribute to equitable local and global solutions that transcend national boundaries and cultural divides (Folke, 2011, p. 11). We need to make a long-term commitment to integrated action to enhance resilience by developing systems and programs based on the sustainability principle.

(Un)sustainability

Changes to natural ecosystems worldwide have been more rapid over the past 50 years than any other comparable time in history (WHO, 2005). We are now operating in an ecological deficit. The Ecological Footprint (Rees & Wackernagal, 1995) illustrates that, as a global community, we need about 1.5 planets to meet our average resource consumption levels (World Wildlife Fund [WWF], n.d.). These changes are primarily attributed to human activity.

The combination of a burgeoning population, overconsumption and neoliberal economic policies has contributed to socio-ecological degradation including enhanced greenhouse effect (and so climate change), resource wars and pollution. This is unsustainable. *Ecosystems and Human Well-being: Health Synthesis* (WHO, 2005) was produced as a result of the Millennium Ecosystem Assessment (MEA). The report is a synthesis of the evidence produced by the MEA about how ecosystem changes do or could affect human health and wellbeing (WHO, 2005). Fig. 3.2 encapsulates those impacts. The figure describes the causal pathway from escalating human pressures on the environment through to ecosystem changes resulting in diverse health consequences. As we have said, the effects may be direct or indirect, local and global, short and long term, negligible or devastating.

Human health and wellbeing are directly affected by ecosystem degradation by way of extremes of weather: storms, floods, bushfires, landslides, heatwaves, water shortages and exposure to toxic chemical pollutants (e.g. Hughes & McMichael, 2011; McMichael et al., 2015). Storms, floods, heatwaves and landslides are widely reported by the media because they are sporadic and usually cause large-scale disruption and death. There are relatively direct impacts that flow a short time after these events occur, such as mental illness and loss of property, employment and community morale (McMichael et al., 2015). These direct impacts are additional to ongoing socio-ecological problems. Worldwide, 3% of all deaths and 4.4% of all years of life lost are attributed to water-related disease (OECD,

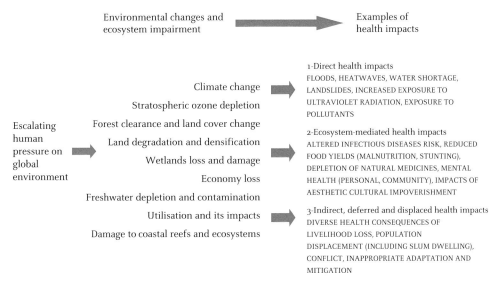

This figure describes the causal pathway from escalating human pressures on the environment through to ecosystem changes resulting in diverse health consequences. Not all ecosystem changes are included. Some changes can have positive effects (e.g. food productions).

FIGURE 3.2 Why do ecosystems matter to human health?
Source: Corvalan, 2005. Reproduced with the permission of the World Health Organization.

2012). The WHO (2015c) estimates that by 2025, half of the world's population will be living in water-stressed areas.

Beyond the challenge of maintaining equitable water supply, in the face of population growth, there is a global deterioration in the quality of drinking water (McMichael, 2001). Polluted drinking water and food contribute to infectious diseases and poisoning (WHO, 2015b). Coastlines are increasingly under pressure from human waste disposal and other human activities. The spread of enteric viruses and bacteria caused by sewage disposal is now a major worldwide problem. Toxic chemicals cause accidental acute poisoning or long-term poisoning from the residues in food. Contamination is accelerating from industrial, agricultural and domestic wastes. Chemicals produced for industrial and agricultural processes may cause cancer and damage nervous, reproductive and immune systems (UN, 2001). Air pollution is also a problem in many cities, particularly in poor countries, because even if health policies exist, they do not have the resources for the infrastructure required to prevent pollution. Respiratory disorders, including asthma, bronchitis and lung cancer, are the result. Around 8.8 million premature deaths a year are linked to air pollution (Burnett et al., 2018). Heatwaves lead to exhaustion and heart failure (Toloo et al., 2014); bushfires exacerbate asthma; and droughts, floods and natural disasters lead to mental illness, post-traumatic stress disorder and social dislocation. All contribute to premature deaths (Hughes & McMichael, 2011). These examples of the health impacts of degraded ecosystems are so constant that they often do not make the daily news.

Natural disasters

The frequency, duration and intensity of extreme weather events is increasing (IPCC, 2014a; NASA, n.d.) and this in turn has led to injury, death and massive social disruption;

for example, Hurricane Katrina in the United States of America (USA) in 2005, Cyclone Yasi in Australia in 2011, Super Typhoon Haiyan in 2013, Hurricane Matthew in 2016 and the 2019 Australian bushfires. Air quality from the bushfires was categorised as hazardous and the smoke was predicted to move around the globe. At the height of the fires, calls to emergency services for respiratory distress alone were significantly higher than usual. Super Typhoon Haiyan was the strongest typhoon ever recorded and caused catastrophic destruction across South-East Asia (NASA, n.d.). NASA reports that 9 million people in the Philippines were affected. In 2011, 78% of Queensland was declared a disaster zone due to flooding—this demonstrated clearly the devastation experienced by 2.5 million people. The impact on health services was enormous (Hughes & McMichael, 2011). Natural disasters cause major disruption to infrastructure, including those services communities need most in a time of crisis. Mallon and Hamilton (2015) report that the health and social services sector in Australia (a comparatively rich country) is underprepared for adaptation to climate change. Only 25% of organisations reported that they could have alternative arrangements for services in place within one week after a natural disaster. Sixty per cent reported they would need a month to recover operations if their premises were damaged, and 25% reported they would no longer operate, which is similar to the statistics for small to medium businesses in the private sector. Services in poor countries fare worse.

Natural disasters from extreme weather events such as bushfires, cyclones and rain and dust storms are expected to intensify due to climate change (IPCC, 2014a). On the *2016 International Day for Disaster Reduction*, UN Secretary-General Ban Ki-moon stated:

> We can replace material possessions, but we cannot replace people. I am repeatedly appalled at how many people die in disasters. The majority of victims are invariably the poor and vulnerable. [...] Let us move from a culture of reaction to one of prevention and build resilience by reducing loss of life.
>
> *(UN, 2016)*

Rising temperatures

There is no doubt that the Earth is warming and temperatures are rising (CSIRO, 2018; NASA, n.d.). Extreme temperatures are being experienced globally, and in Australia there have been record-breaking temperatures since 2012 (CSIRO, 2018). Thermal stress is causing an increase in hospital admissions and premature deaths (Hughes & McMichael, 2011). The heatwaves in August 2003 in Europe contributed to over 35,000 premature deaths (Wibulpolprasert et al., 2005). Rahmstorf and Coumou (2011) report estimates of thousands of deaths due to the heatwave in Moscow in July 2010. Hughes and McMichael's (2011) review of Australian research paints a similar picture. For example, in Brisbane in 2004, overall deaths increased by 23% (excluding injury and suicide) compared with the same period in the previous two years with the temperatures between 22°C and 34°C (Tong et al., 2010). The heatwave in Victoria in 2009 resulted in 374 more deaths than expected (Department of Human Services, 2009), and in Adelaide the reports are similar (Nitschke et al., 2007). Toloo and colleagues (2014) report that heat-related visits to emergency departments in Brisbane increased during heatwaves. All these events strained health services and health practitioners.

The Bureau of Meteorology (2010, cited in Hanna et al., 2011) reports that 'heatwaves are the most underrated weather hazard in Australia and have killed more people than any other natural hazard'. Those who are most vulnerable to heatwaves include infants, older people, people with chronic ill health, and people who are socio-economically disadvantaged. The term 'thermal inequity' is now used to describe the unfair impact of climate change on low socio-economic populations living in urban environments (Mitchell & Chakraborty, 2014). Heatwaves are expected to increase and are predicted to be longer and hotter (IPCC, 2014b).

Water security

The health and wellbeing of societies is inextricably linked to the quality, quantity and management of water. Functioning ecosystems are essential for availability of water but rainfall, snowmelt, river flows and groundwater are all being affected by climate change. Water stress is already high in many parts of the world and food production (and therefore food security) is affected. The aim of land and water management practices needs to be to create resilience in the face of climate change to ensure food production. Furthermore, the IPCC (2014a) predicts worsening risks to health and wellbeing from storm surges, sea-level rise and coastal flooding, and inland flooding. Worldwide, half the victims of all global disasters are due to floods (Alderman et al., 2012). The flow-on effects of extreme events have led to a breakdown of infrastructure networks and critical services. Water security is therefore threatened and those who are poorest will be affected the most. Ecosystem resilience will be compromised further.

Population increases will demand more water supplies, more waste disposal and more energy supplies. Pollution of water can occur so easily. Water supplies can be contaminated and sewerage systems damaged or shut down in natural disasters such as flooding, bushfires and cyclones. Temperature change, heavy rainfall and drought bring different waterborne diseases. For example, cyanobacteria (blue-green algae) blooms occur frequently in droughts and are toxic to humans. Giardiasis and cryptosporidiosis outbreaks occur following floods (Karanis et al., 2007). In Queensland in 2011, councils provided bottled water to residents because of contaminated water following the floods (Hughes & McMichael, 2011).

Air quality

Air quality is closely associated with climate change as climate change concentrates the pollutants in the stratosphere. Air pollutants are on the rise and further increases are expected. According to the World Health Organization, an estimated 4.2 million premature deaths globally are linked to ambient air pollution (WHO, n.d.a). The health effects will vary by population group, region and competency for public health responses. The healthcare costs of air pollution are considerable (Spickett et al., 2011). Scovronick (2015) provides guidance about the health effects of air pollution. The major areas of concern are particulate matter, ozone and airborne allergens. They report that pollutants such as black carbon, methane and ozone not only contribute to climate change, but are responsible for air pollution-related deaths and diseases that kill some 8.8 million people per year. The causes of these deaths include lung cancer, acute lower respiratory infections, ischaemic heart disease and chronic obstructive pulmonary disease. The increases in air pollutants will exacerbate illness in those with respiratory illnesses such as asthma, which is already a common problem in many countries (Hassan et al., 2015).

Air pollution from bushfires is likely to increase with climate change. Bushfires are an increasing problem globally with the bushfire seasons getting longer and the severity increasing (Bowman, 2015), including in Australia (CSIRO, 2018). People are dying in fires and increased hospital admissions for respiratory conditions such as chronic obstructive pulmonary disease and asthma have been reported by comparing smoke and non-smoke event days in New South Wales (Martin et al., 2013). Hospital emergency departments in

New South Wales reported a 25% spike in the number of people presenting with respiratory problems during the 2019 bushfires (Nogrady, 2019).

Food security and sovereignty

Food systems are dependent on a stable biophysical environment. Transgressing the planetary boundaries of climate change, rate of biodiversity loss and changes to the global nitrogen cycle as outlined earlier affects every aspect of food production, food security and food insecurity and therefore human health and wellbeing. Food security exists when all people, at all times, have physical, social and economic access to sufficient, safe and nutritious food which meets their dietary needs and food preferences for an active and healthy life (Food and Agriculture Organization of the UN [FAO], 2003). Household food security is the application of this concept to the family level, with individuals within households as the focus of concern. Food insecurity exists when people do not have adequate physical, social or economic access to food as defined above (FAO, 2003).

The industrial food production system is inextricably linked to the three planetary boundaries that have been transgressed and also land degradation. Food systems are also dependent upon global trade in food commodities (Edwards et al., 2011) and this trade system along with climate change intensifies the existing disparities in availability, accessibility, affordability and acceptability of nutritious food within nations. It is estimated that during the drought of 2005–07 in Australia, the price of vegetables increased by 33% and fruit by 43%. This adds physical and mental stress to all, and in particular to people with low incomes. Climate change has affected the price and availability of food in Australia with the most disadvantaged experiencing the greatest inequality (Barosh et al., 2014). There is also an unequal distribution of food globally.

Climate change also affects food-borne diseases such as salmonella infection. Risk increases with a slight increase in temperature. In Australia, notification of food-borne illness rises with a rise in temperature (D'Souza et al., 2004). Further, chronic under-nutrition weakens immune systems and increases susceptibility to infection (Lloyd et al., 2011). Malnutrition contributes to diabetes, heart disease and bowel cancer.

Mental illness, societal stress and degraded ecosystems

Clear associations have been made between wellbeing, mental illness, societal stress and drought, rising temperatures and other extreme weather events such as flood and fire (Alston, 2012; Dean & Stain, 2010; Hughes & McMichael, 2011; Ng et al., 2015; Nicholls et al., 2006; Nitschke et al., 2007). The incidence of these events is rising due to climate change and so, too, are the associated short- and long-term health consequences. Social disruption due to extreme weather exacerbates displacement within and between countries. 'In 2009, 17 million people around the world were displaced by natural hazards, and 42 million in 2010' (Hughes & McMichael, 2011, p. 27). Mental stress may be increased by a loss of a sense of place following these events (Green et al., 2009; Verrinder & Talbot, 2015). The study of the social impacts of drought conditions in three communities in eastern Australia (Alston & Kent, 2004) provides evidence of the impact of environmental decline on the social fabric and health of communities. Drought is usually protracted and insidious and associated with financial, social and health consequences. Extreme weather events have been an added factor to the environmental, economic and social decline experienced in rural Australia since the 1970s (e.g. Verrinder & Talbot, 2015).

The impact of structural adjustment programs is discussed in Chapter 2. In Australia, these events have contributed to the loss of employment, income, services and population in rural areas. Rural poverty and associated health problems have increased. Chronic conditions such as hypertension and cardiac disease are part of the suite of long-term health consequences. Men, women, children and older people are affected in different ways (Dean & Stain, 2010; Polain et al., 2011). Furthermore, these impacts are gendered because of the different roles of men and women (Alston, 2012). There are also class and sector differences that are magnified because of drought (Alston, 2012; Alston & Kent, 2004).

The impacts of flood and drought on individual wellbeing are associated with feelings of stress, fear and loss. The long-term effects of flood include post-traumatic stress disorder and high levels of chronic anxiety (Ng et al., 2015). The impact of aesthetic and cultural impoverishment due to ecosystem degradation is now clear (Alston & Kent, 2004; Arabena & Kingsley, 2015; WHO, 2005). Social connectedness has been found to buffer the impacts of drought and flood and promote resilience in rural communities in Australia (Ng et al., 2015).

Social and psychological benefits of connection with nature

Involvement in conservation and nature-based activities not only benefits the ecosystems we live in, but also enhances community cohesion and improves individual mental health and wellbeing (Cleary et al., 2017; Frumkin et al., 2017; Markevych et al., 2017). Parks Victoria report that there are economic, environmental and social benefits of parks (Parks Victoria, 2015). Studies examining 'caring for country' as a potential health promoting activity on Indigenous-owned lands found that greater Indigenous participation in 'caring for country' activities is associated with significantly better health (Arabena & Kingsley, 2015; Burgess et al., 2007; Phillips & Kingsley, 2007). Evidence also suggests that contact with nature and volunteering in nature programs may improve human health and wellbeing, including mental health. Improving the health of individuals, communities and ecosystems comes about through developing ongoing social links, learning new land management and personal development skills, increased confidence, reduced stress, increased motivation and interest in life, enjoyment and other benefits from participation in these activities (Ebden & Townsend, 2007).

Over the past decade, there has been growing interest in and evidence about the positive health and wellbeing outcomes of people engaging with the natural environment, particularly green and blue space. For example, BlueHealth (BlueHealth, n.d.), a pan-European research initiative, undertakes extensive research into the links between the environment, climate change and health and wellbeing focusing mainly on blue space in urban settings. Their work in turn informs much policy and health promotion action to create infrastructure and opportunities for urban communities to access blue space.

Vulnerable populations

The burden of disease affects those who are the most socially vulnerable. The iceberg analogy presented in Chapter 1 (Fig. 1.4, page 14) can be used again here. In the bottom part of the iceberg, well below the waterline, are the environmental determinants that underpin the health and wellbeing of entire current and future populations. People living in urban environments (Byrne et al., 2016), children, the frail and aged, and those who are poor, pregnant or have pre-existing diseases, are affected most by environmental degradation (Bennett et al., 2011; OECD, 2012; Smith et al., 2014). For example, metabolic activity in children is higher than in adults and their bodies react differently when exposed to pollutants. Older people do not cope as well with temperature change. Outdoor workers are also vulnerable (Hanna et al., 2011). Overwhelming tiredness, stress and mental illness have been reported. Furthermore, service providers believe people do not attend to their health needs because of the 'misplaced need to be stoic' (Alston & Kent, 2004, p. 56). The key message in The Lancet Countdown report is that climate change will profoundly affect the life of every child born today, and that without accelerated measures to address climate change, it will come to define the health of people at every stage of their lives (Watts et al., 2019).

Rural, regional and remote communities are exposed to greater climate extremes. Rural communities are vulnerable to climate change because of their direct dependence on natural resources, weather-dependent activities and inequitable access to services. Verrinder and Talbot (2015) report that communities are affected in two main ways: first, extreme weather events that impact on infrastructure and cause loss of life; and second, the impact on ecosystems and agriculture. People's health is at greater or lesser risk in different locations but over and above these vulnerabilities, all subgroups of the rural population are influenced by unique characteristics of rural settings. Problems for some communities are aggravated by ongoing difficulties in recruiting and retaining health and other professionals. The impact of environmental changes on communities has seen a loss of people, services, skills and volunteers to run community organisations. Further, studies of the social impacts from extreme weather events can provide health practitioners with important information for the future. Loss of income, high workloads, involuntary separation and loss of educational opportunities have all had an impact on the health of the people in communities affected by a changing rural context (Talbot & Walker, 2007; Verrinder & Talbot, 2015).

The systems and organisations that protect people who are experiencing disadvantage increase resilience; however, in Australia they are failing vulnerable populations during extreme weather events (Mallon & Hamilton, 2015). Planning from now on will need to consider large numbers of environmental refugees. Underpinning health promotion practice with the principles of CPHC and sustainability will be crucial. In relation to climate change, climate justice refers to endeavours to tackle inequities experienced by populations subjected to impacts of climate change and to the responsibilities for mitigation and adaptation (Byrne et al., 2016; Duus-Otterstrom & Jagers, 2012; Mitchell & Chakraborty, 2014).

Social justice and environmental justice have the same goal. One cannot be considered without the other. The principles of CPHC support action to improve the lives of vulnerable people by reducing the risk conditions that contribute to a poor quality of life, such as poverty and environmental degradation. Poverty contributes to environmental degradation and environmental degradation contributes to poverty.

In the extreme, Jared Diamond (2005) provides examples of numerous societies that have collapsed. His thesis describes the 'ecological suicide' of these societies where in the worst cases everybody in the society either emigrated or died (Diamond, 2005, p. 6). The evidence presented in his thesis has been supported by a variety of scientists looking at collapsed societies from different scientific perspectives. Diamond (2005) proposes that:

> ... the processes through which past societies have undermined themselves by damaging their environments fall into eight categories, whose relative importance differs from case to case: deforestation and habitat destruction, soil problems (salinization, erosion and soil fertility losses), water management problems, overhunting, overfishing, effects of introduced species, human population growth, and increased per capita impact of people.
>
> (p. 6)

According to Diamond (2005), Easter Island is an example of societal collapse. There were numerous reasons for its demise, including specific climatic conditions, colonialism and overexploitation of resources. Deforestation resulted in the loss of essential resources for survival including wood and rope (which were essential for shelter and canoe transport), other native plants and birds (affecting food supplies and cloth making) and cultural practices (because there were no means to shift the famous giant moai stone statues). It is a tragic story and as Diamond says, 'if mere thousands of Easter Islanders with just stone tools and their own muscle power sufficed to destroy their environment and thereby destroy their society, how can billions of people with metal tools and machine power fail to do worse?' (2005, p. 119). He not only provides examples of past societies such as the Easter Islanders that have collapsed as a result of a combination of environmental conditions and disastrous decisions, but current societies, including Australia, facing environmental and social challenges that need to be tackled to avoid collapse.

Overexploitation of resources and overconsumption contributing to 'strong' economic growth but ecological degradation is negatively impacting on human health now and will jeopardise the health of future generations. Fairness and sufficiency will improve health now and will ensure the health of populations in the future. A relentless pursuit of economic growth is unsustainable and 'has no moral or ethical compass either' (Soskolne et al., 2008, p. 420). A major challenge is to ensure that economic policies do not enable degradation of the ecological integrity upon which 'geopolitical stability, social order and the economy itself depend' (Soskolne et al., 2008, p. 421). Investment in human capital and protection of natural capital will produce social and environmental justice.

A socially just society is important for maintaining a healthy population. This has been discussed at length in Chapter 2; however, it deserves further discussion here in relation to the interdependence of a healthy natural environment, economy and population. Improvement in life expectancy occurs in poor countries with an increase in gross national product (GNP). However, 'above a GNP per capita of about $5000, the relationship between GNP and life expectancy is weak' (Wilkinson, 1996, cited in Marmot & Wilkinson, 1999, p. 10). That is, life expectancy improves in poor countries when income per capita reaches a certain point that ensures there is sufficient infrastructure. This point is reached when people have sufficient personal resources to be adequately sheltered and well nourished, and have access to education and essential health care to reduce the major killers of infectious diseases and malnutrition. In rich countries, the association between income inequality and poorer health status of a population is strong (Marmot et al., 2010).

In Australia, land degradation has contributed to poverty in some rural areas. Vast tracts of the Australian farming land have succumbed to salinity, for example, due to agricultural practices. Reduced income from this land and reduced worth of the land overall has forced some farmers off the land. A lack of occupational choice, reduced income and changes in community economies and structures have produced environmental refugees and contributed to poor health overall (Pritchard & McManus, 2000; Verrinder & Talbot, 2015). Maintaining a healthy environment is important for human health but this point is often marginalised when discussing social justice.

ECOLOGICAL SUSTAINABILITY AND AUSTRALIA

Countries across the globe have different socio-ecological problems impacting in different ways on human health and wellbeing. Deforestation, ocean acidification and loss of bio-diversity threaten human health on a global scale. Climate change is predicted to produce both winners and losers, and it is argued that in the long term 'Australia will be a loser'

(Diamond, 2005, p. 385). Diamond (2005, Chapter 13) outlined the environmental problems for Australia. Australia has an exceptionally fragile environment that has been damaged in a number of ways. Water availability, soil erosion, soil salinity, disruption of natural nutrient cycles and loss of biodiversity are some of the environmental issues facing Australian communities. The CSIRO (2018) reports that although there are regional variations, the average temperature has increased by 0.7°C since the middle of the 20th century and the frequency of hot days and nights has increased while the frequency of cold days and nights has declined. The decade 2000–09 was the hottest on record. Globally, average temperatures continue to break records year on year. There is also variability in rainfall across Australia, but broadly, the rainfall in south-eastern and south-western Australia has declined substantially, whereas it has increased in the north-west (Cleugh et al., 2011). These problems are interconnected with global environmental problems along with ozone depletion and sea-level rise. Ozone depletion is a global problem being felt in Australia; however, scientists predict that if the international community continues to comply with the Montreal Protocol, the ozone layer should recover to pre-1980 levels between 2050 and 2065 (Department of the Environment and Energy, n.d.). Global sea levels rose by about 17 cm during the 20th century and considerable warming has also occurred in the three oceans surrounding Australia (Cleugh et al., 2011).

More recently and for the first time Zhang and colleagues (2018) reported Australia's progress for climate change and health across the following five areas: 'climate change impacts; exposures and vulnerability; adaptation, planning and resilience for health; mitigation actions and health co-benefits; economics and finance; and public and political engagement' (p. 1). These areas and associated indicators were based on the 2017 Lancet Countdown global assessment. Overall, they found Australia not to be faring so well. They also caution that policy inaction on climate change in Australia to date makes Australia vulnerable to the consequences of the associated impacts on health and wellbeing. At the same time, they emphasise that the means and opportunity to take action exist.

Importance of soil and water

Humans have had impacts on the environment incurring enormous natural and social costs. Two features of the Australian environment are particularly important if we are to understand modern human impacts: soils, especially their nutrient availability and salt levels, and availability of fresh water. Australia is the driest continent on the planet; however, a subtle problem with Australia's rainfall is its unpredictability. Australia's rainfall is unpredictable from year to year within a decade and also from decade to decade. There are technological 'fixes' to support some communities that will suffice for the short term; however, many are beginning to realise that mismanagement of this resource is no longer an option. How this happens is hotly contested. There are some major challenges that need to be considered, not the least of which is that 'given Australia's limited supplies of water … it lacks the capacity to support a significantly larger population' (Diamond, 2005, p. 397).

Australia's other major problem is land degradation and this is the result of several types of damaging environmental impacts: clearance of native vegetation; overgrazing by sheep and rabbits; soil nutrient exhaustion; soil erosion; human-made droughts; weeds; misguided government policies; and salinisation (Diamond, 2005). Low average productivity of Australian soils has had major economic consequences for Australian agriculture. More importantly now is that agricultural practices have, in some parts of the country, caused irreversible damage. These damaging impacts are interrelated and have wider implications. For example, when vegetation is cleared or overgrazed by sheep and rabbits, the soil becomes hotter and drier and leads to human-made drought. Furthermore, clearance of native vegetation and rotting or burning of this vegetation contributes to Australian annual greenhouse gas emissions equal to the country's motor vehicle emissions (Diamond, 2005, p. 399). There is, however, a small but growing movement in Australia towards 'regenerative farming'. Farmers are changing the human-land relationships and improving the health of soil and water. This has a positive impact on the health of animals and crops, which, in turn, benefits humans down the line (Massey, 2017).

Reduce greenhouse gas emissions

It must be emphasised that the enhanced greenhouse effect is largely due to increased levels of carbon dioxide in the atmosphere primarily as a result of burning fossil fuels for energy consumption. According to the Climate Institute (2015a), Australia's greenhouse gas emissions are significant on a global scale and, compared with many countries, Australia can afford to reduce pollution by putting policies in place that will reduce emissions. The OECD countries have agreed to limit subsidies for the export of inefficient coal-fired power technologies. However, Australia and Korea argued successfully for exceptions for developing countries for the construction of smaller less efficient power plants. Still, in the rest of the world, only the most efficient 'ultra-supercritical' technologies will be eligible for credit funding which will limit public financing of coal-fired power generation globally (Kent, 2015).

Australia ratified the Paris Agreement in 2016, and under the Agreement, will reduce greenhouse gas emissions by 26–28% below 2005 levels by 2030. This emissions reduction target is the same as the United States but lower than New Zealand (30%), and has been criticised as being insufficient by both government and independent bodies (Parliament of Australia, 2017).

In Australia, there is increasing awareness of the impacts of climate change. One survey in 2015 found that 70% of respondents believed that climate change was occurring and 59% thought that governments underestimate the seriousness of climate change. Forty-one per cent thought that humans are the main cause and 57% trusted the science of climate change (Climate Institute, 2015b). Talberg and colleagues (2013) suggest that Australia's response has been changeable. On the one hand, the world's first government agency dedicated to reducing greenhouse gas emissions was established in Australia; global climate treaties were signed as soon as they were created; the world's first emissions trading scheme (ETS) was established; and an innovative land-based carbon offset scheme was pioneered. On the other hand, the climate change government agency was disbanded, recreated and disbanded again; the ratification of global treaties was stalled; and legislation to repeal the national ETS was introduced. However, despite the erratic nature of national policy there are many examples of action by state and local governments to reduce carbon emissions. For example, research shows that almost one in five Australian communities and councils have set zero emissions or 100% renewable energy targets (Bygrave, 2016). The Climate and Health Alliance developed the *Framework for a National Strategy for Climate, Health and Wellbeing for Australia* (Horsburgh et al., 2017) which built on earlier work to develop national plans to include a health 'lens' to climate policy decisions. In 2016, the Public Health Association of Australia (PHAA) changed its constitution to recognise:

- *the foundational role of the Earth's ecosystems to human civilisation, prosperity, health and wellbeing, the nature of humanity's inextricable relationships with the ecosystem of which we are a part [and]*

- *in this context, that these ecological determinants of health (an Eco-social viewpoint) are entwined with health and wellbeing along with socially determined influences [furthermore]*

- *will act and call for action for the promotion and protection of the health of the ecosystems in a concerted manner in its policy development and implementation.*

(PHAA, 2016)

ECOLOGICAL SUSTAINABILITY AND NEW ZEALAND

There are similarities and differences in ecological degradation and health impacts within and between countries. The likely health impacts of climate change in New Zealand include higher temperatures, more in the North Island than the South (but still likely to be less than the global average), rising sea levels, more frequent extreme weather events such as droughts (especially in the east of New Zealand) and floods, and a change in rainfall patterns (higher rainfall in the west and less in the east) (Ministry for the Environment [MFE], 2019). All of these have a direct and indirect impact on the health of the population. Higher levels of mortality related to summer heat, for example, are expected, but higher winter temperatures may lead to a reduction in winter-related mortality and illnesses such as colds and influenza. Change driven by global factors in New Zealand include:

- population change
- climate change
- price increases for hydrocarbons
- water
- food
- toxins
- geopolitical shifts
- wide swings in economic activity
- technological advances (SANZ, n.d.).

Strong Sustainability for New Zealand: Principles and Scenarios (SANZ, 2009, p. 12) is a compelling document where core pre-conditions and enabling factors for a sustainable New Zealand are proposed. The core pre-condition is to take an ethical stance of nurturing natural and social capital. The ethical stance is 'a robust sense of mutual respect, fairness, cooperation, gratitude, compassion, forgiveness, humility, courage, mutual aid, charity, confidence, trust, courtesy, integrity, loyalty, and respectful use of resources' (SANZ, 2009). The enabling factors include: investing in natural and social capital through eco-literacy and systems thinking and embedding sustainability in policies; ethical trading; and by limiting emissions (SANZ, 2009). In 2016, New Zealand ratified the UN Framework Convention on Climate Change Paris Agreement. Under the Agreement, New Zealand's commitments to reduce greenhouse gas emissions by 30% below 2005 levels by 2030 will apply from 2021 (MFE, 2018).

LOCAL-LEVEL HEALTH PROMOTION ACTION FOR SUSTAINABILITY

The role of health practitioners in addressing the looming 'public health emergency on planet earth' (Hales & Corvalan, 2006, p. 130) is becoming clearer. McMichael and colleagues (2000, p. 1067) suggested that '... our task in this evolving discourse, as health professionals, is to make clear that population health is a central criterion in the sustainability transition' and Hancock (2000, p. 153) stated that in the 21st century public health 'will be characterised by an ecological approach to the environment; an approach that was first legitimised in the Ottawa Charter for Health Promotion'. Leviston and colleagues (2011) reported that in Australia, health practitioners are among those trusted to provide truthful information. Further, Marmot (2010) proposed that the logical starting point and essential analytical framework for finding ways to reduce health inequalities is a sustainable development lens.

Efforts to effect environmental and social change must be multidimensional and/or multisectoral. For example, mobilising partnerships between health practitioners, urban planners and researchers would assist in planning and policy development in areas such as integrated transport, land use and infrastructure planning and thus create supportive environments for physical activity, social connectedness, air quality, local food security and mental wellbeing. This in turn would contribute to improvements in the health and wellbeing of a population overall (Department of Infrastructure and Transport, Major Cities Unit, 2012). The term 'liveability' is also now used in urban planning and discussed in Chapter 2. Liveable communities can be viewed as addressing the socio-ecological determinants of health and wellbeing and are sustainable communities. Lowe and colleagues (2014) argue that planning liveable communities creates co-benefits across the urban planning, public health and environment sectors. The health promotion program development, implementation and evaluation cycle strengthens the evidence base of action taken for sustainability and enables policymakers and health practitioners to be accountable for their actions. Community engagement in the process is fundamental to success (see Insight 3.3).

The questions posed at the beginning of this chapter under the Ottawa Charter action areas were presented to guide health promotion practitioners to reflect on and critically

INSIGHT 3.3 Place, Health and Liveable Research program

The Place, Health and Liveable Research program (Lowe et al., 2014) is a good example of urban planning, public health researchers, policymakers and practitioner partnerships in planning. The overall aim of the program was to measure the impacts of planning policy on health and wellbeing and part of that was examining liveability indicators, and how they are developed, used and reported to support integrated planning for health, liveability and sustainability. The first step in this planning stage was to conduct an international literature review to identify the types of indicators used for liveability. This resulted in 11 policy domains being developed. This informed part of the community assessment, which was the second step in the planning process involving three workshops conducted with policymakers, planners and practitioners from the public and private sectors. Participants were provided with feedback on the findings of the literature review and then discussion ensued about how liveability indicators informed policy and, therefore, how they could be developed and reported. Indicators were seen by the participants as useful for community assessments, determining policy goals, priority setting and benchmarks and also monitoring progress and outcomes over time. Tools such as *Community Indicators Victoria* (https://communityindicators.net/indicator-projects/community-indicators-victoria/) were regarded as valuable for local government planning, particularly when shared with communities who could then be involved in the planning process. Research was seen by the participants as essential for program and policy development.

Source: Lowe et al., 2014.

evaluate their professional role and practice in relation to ecological sustainability and health and wellbeing. In Chapters 1 and 2 we presented the socio-ecological approach that depicts the multiple individual level and population-wide determinants of health and wellbeing. Using the framework for health promotion practice within a CPHC context (Fig. 1.6) introduced in Chapter 1 will also provide further guidance. This action framework, which is underpinned by the Ottawa Charter action areas, can guide health promotion workers in their thinking about the many opportunities available to work for sustainability and human health and wellbeing.

Healthy public policy for ecological sustainability

The WHO noted that 'healthy public policy is characterised by an explicit concern for health and equity in all areas of policy and by an accountability for health impact' (WHO, 1988). The aim of healthy public policy is to create supportive social and physical environments to enable people to lead healthy lives. Healthy public policy can be very broad and includes national, state and local government policy and strategic plans, regulatory activities including executive orders, local laws, ordinances, organisational position statements and regulations. This is taken up in Chapter 5. However, the global changes require policy links from global through to local settings, which will be briefly discussed here as part of the portfolio of health promotion action to tackling ecological sustainability to promote health and wellbeing.

Policy development process for sustainability

There are numerous ways to look at the aim and the process of policy development. Johnson (2007) suggests that some environmental policies focus on human health and wellbeing, such as regulation of air pollutants and water contaminants. Then there are those policies that focus on environment protections that indirectly affect human health and wellbeing, such as protection of biodiversity in a region. There are policies that focus on neither humans nor environment, but have an impact on the health and wellbeing of both, such as national energy policies, and there are hazards to health and wellbeing that are not regulated. The primary strategy of policymakers may be 'prospective' (e.g. air pollution regulations) or 'retrospective' (such as clean-ups of hazardous wastes). Some policies are developed to provide information about these. International organisations, governments, the private sector, and professional and citizen groups are potential actors in the development of such policies. Citizen groups lobby governments for policy change. Professional bodies such as public health associations develop policies on a range of issues to protect human health. They also provide advice to government.

Strong environmental policies can be a key vehicle for reducing health damage and healthcare costs caused by environmental degradation (OECD, 2012). The benefits of policies that address environmental degradation have been demonstrated in cost–benefit analyses conducted in many OECD countries. Considerable gains can be made with even the least rigorous policies. For example, the benefits outweighed the costs of the European Union Thematic Strategy on Air Pollution by three to one, and in the USA, the Clean Air Act produced a benefit of four dollars for every dollar of cost. With additional control requirements, the projected benefits amounted to US$100 billion compared with US$27 billion of costs (OECD, 2012). These national policies have benefits right down to the local and individual level. The *Transport Integration Act 2010* in Victoria is an example of a policy that has the potential to contribute to a healthy population by guiding communities and all other actors in decision making about transport. Equity, the precautionary principle and community participation are enshrined in the principles of the legislation. The legislation forms the foundation for state and local government planning. Land use, public transport and opportunities for cycling and walking are all considered under the one piece of legislation.

Evidence to support the links between urban planning and chronic disease is growing (Lowe et al., 2015). Diseases such as heart disease, diabetes and depression are associated with poor physical activity, poor nutrition and stress. Social cohesion, personal safety, open space, food supply, air and water quality are all important considerations in policy decisions for urban planning (Capon, 2003; Frumkin et al., 2008). Physical activity is a major contributor to health and wellbeing and a good example of how policies at the local level contribute to population-level health and wellbeing. A study examining barriers, enablers and interventions to cycling (Bauman et al., 2008) provides evidence to support the idea that health practitioners need to work in settings with other sectors, such as urban planning, to promote the health and wellbeing of humans and the environment. The study reveals individual, social and cultural, environmental, safety and policy, and regulation barriers to cycling. Low-density neighbourhoods with poorly connected street networks affect how much time we spend walking and cycling and also our ability to get to and use public transport. Knowing about these barriers provides health promotion practitioners with ample guidance for action. For example, Bauman and colleagues (2008) identified that a lack of skills, confidence and knowledge was one suite of barriers to cycling. They recommended riding skills classes and social marketing campaigns focusing on key motivations such as health and wellbeing.

There are many examples of how local governments and health promotion agencies have taken a strategic approach to creating an environment conducive to promoting the health and wellbeing of humans and the environment. The City of Melbourne's Urban Forest Strategy is an example of this. The aim of this strategy is to increase tree canopy cover from 22% to 40% by 2040. As the infographic of the 202020 Vision policy reveals: 'They're [urban forests] good for cooling, good for water management and good for exercising, relaxing or reading a book' (City of Melbourne, n.d.). The development of this vision and resources for local governments and others to achieve green spaces is the result of collaboration between the public and private sector, non-government organisations, governments and academia. There are supportive protocols, such as the Biosensitive Urban Design protocol, where the primary aim of creating urban environments is that it must be beneficial to biodiversity, which is one of the planetary boundaries identified by Rockström and colleagues (2009). The Biosensitive Urban Design protocol is based on five principles: maintaining or creating habitat for target species; facilitating dispersal of species; minimising disturbance; facilitating natural processes; and facilitating positive human–nature interactions (Kane, 2015). It can be implemented at a range of levels, from individual homeowners to building developers and local and regional authorities. Initiatives such as these create environments and communities that are more resilient.

Community action for ecological sustainability

Community action empowers communities (both geographic areas and communities of interest) to build their capacity to develop and sustain improvements in their social and physical environments. Local groups the world over are working to repair some of the damage done to the environment through unsustainable human activities and, in doing so, have had some positive, unplanned social gains. There are a great many examples of community action that promote the health of populations. The Central Victorian Greenhouse Alliance (CVGA), for instance, comprises a network of alliances including 13 local governments, businesses and community organisations (CVGA, 2019). The aim of the alliance is to reduce the region's emissions by 30% below 1990 levels and zero net emissions by 2020 (Fritz et al., 2009). Strategies of the alliance include leadership, education and facilitation. One of the successes was the facilitation of the Lighting the Regions bulk street lighting upgrade project where 16 municipalities came together in a single funding application to the federal government (CVGA, n.d.). Current projects focus on renewable energy, resilience and heat vulnerability.

Settings

Health promotion action is most often organised around particular settings to bring together groups of people who share common characteristics. The settings approach to health promotion can provide structural and legislative support that cannot be implemented so readily elsewhere. Environmental health and protection strategies within settings can be strengthened by appropriate policy support. For example, in 2019 the CVGA partnered with other greenhouse alliances to form the largest renewable energy buyers group in Australia. Councils from across Victoria committed to a tender process to purchase renewable electricity for council operations through a long-term Power Purchase Agreement. The greenhouse alliances and the City of Darebin facilitated 48 councils to come together to commit to 100% renewable electricity for their own operations including facilities and streetlights from 2021 (CVGA, 2019).

Supporting local communities in their sustainability projects is vital for the community's health. Health practitioners need to understand the key elements of community engagement and local collective action, which supports equitable, innovative and effective responses to environmental degradation. Collective action of this nature also builds personal resilience and mental wellbeing and social cohesion. Insight 3.4 is an example.

Healthcare agencies are major consumers of natural resources and producers of waste, but are also sites for environmental and social gains. Beyond legislative requirements that aim to minimise environmental degradation caused by organisations and create healthy environments, there are many useful guidelines, tools and activities available to assist organisations to assess the environmental impacts of the operations of the organisation, create a healthy space for people who come into contact with the organisation, and plan for the future (Health Care Without Harm, n.d.a). Health Care Without Harm began in 1996 and the The Global Green and Healthy Hospitals network has more than 1000 members in 54 countries who represent the interests of over 32,100 hospitals and health centres. In the USA, Gundersen Health System achieved its first days of energy independence in 2014. Initially, the organisation's goal was to control rising energy costs. There were two main initiatives: reducing consumption by improving efficiency and creating cleaner energy (Envision Gunderson Health System, 2014). Healthcare organisations can reduce their carbon footprints by sourcing and serving healthy food produced by local farmers and donating excess food from the hospital kitchen to local families. In the USA, St Luke's Hospital in Duluth, Minnesota, has provided 1000 meals and composted '40,000 pounds of waste' per year (WHO & Health Care Without Harm, 2009, p. 18). Green transport is an initiative taken in Sweden in The Green Ambulance Project. Drivers receive 'eco-driving' instruction to reduce fuel consumption. This turned out to be a win–win project where fuel consumption was reduced by 10% with no risk to patients and there was less wear and tear on the ambulances (WHO & Health Care Without Harm, 2009). The Royal Children's Hospital in Melbourne is designed to capture and store 85% of the rainfall on the site, and rainwater and wastewater is filtered and reused on the garden and in toilet flushing (WHO & Health Care Without Harm, 2009).

INSIGHT 3.4 Building power from the ground up: the campaign against new coal and gas in Victoria

Environmental campaigners in Australia have long relied on a well-tested formula for winning campaigns. Identify a problem, develop policy and a campaign that targets metro communities, then build enough electoral power to force the government of the day to adopt a particular position.

Over the past decade, the election of highly ideological Liberal–National governments across a number of states and at the federal level has changed the political terrain profoundly in Australia, with traditional avenues of gaining outcomes becoming much more limited. Because of their ideology, these governments have tended to lock out or ignore environmental organisations. As a result, new forms of grassroots organising and campaigning have developed in recent years, which link the environment movement and allies in the broader community.

Many of these have been examples of 'site-based resistance', where environmental groups form alliances with rural communities and often other groups including traditional owners. The most obvious manifestation of this has been the development of the Lock the Gate Alliance (n.d.), which is opposing new coal and gas projects across the country.

In Victoria, groups like Friends of the Earth Australia have been working with more than 70 communities that are at risk from coal or gas mining. It uses a 'gasfield-free' organising model, which sees local community members carry out door knocking to determine if there is broad support for that area to declare itself gasfield free. Once the polling has been completed, the community holds a declaration event, which is a celebration that makes it clear the fossil fuel industry has no social licence to operate locally. While these declarations have no legal power, they have been hugely influential and caused all main political parties to shift their position on the issue of unconventional gas (UCG).

This style of campaigning has mobilised thousands of people who have not previously been active on environmental issues. It is proving to be incredibly successful. For instance, in Victoria the onshore gas-drilling industry has been stopped by community opposition since 2012.

However, there is another way of looking at the benefits of this style of campaigning. The gasfield-free organising model, based on bringing small rural and regional centres together in opposition to a threat, also inherently builds a sense of cohesion and vibrancy in communities. This is because diverse members of the community need to find a common cause and identify viable ways for them to work together. It helps people to articulate their vision for their preferred option for their land, and builds their agency to work towards that outcome. It weaves together a range of concerns, including public health, care for the environment, and the value of activities like farming and tourism, sense of place and appreciation of community, as well as concerns for groundwater and climate change. By virtue of the fact that multiple strands of interest and concern are involved, strong bonds and friendships are able to be built because there are multiple points of commonality.

Source: Written by Cam Walker, Friends of the Earth.

The Green Building Council of Australia and New Zealand Green Building Council operate the Green Star certification program that assists healthcare organisations to enhance their environmental sustainability. Certification is available for new buildings, fit-outs of interiors and operational management of buildings. Application for certification is open to hospitals, community health centres, diagnostic centres, aged care facilities and mental health facilities. Healthcare organisation projects are awarded a Green Star rating based on accumulating credit points in various categories such as energy and water conservation; transport policies and facilities of the organisation; recycling of materials; land use management; patient and staff access to clean and healthy indoor and outdoor areas; and disposal and reduction of trade wastes (Green Building Council of Australia, 2018).

Staff need to be supported through organisational and educational policy change to create a healthy environment. Staff members need to know what to order, what can be reused and what can be recycled. Purchasing decisions are important. Commodities such as paper, cardboard, mattresses, fluorescent light tubes and redundant equipment such as computers can be recycled. It is important to note that recycling needs to be available locally. Transporting recyclable materials long distances defeats the purpose of trying to reduce energy consumption. Retrofitting environmentally friendly equipment such as flow control valves on water taps and dual flush toilets can be done over time. Small changes make a large difference; for example, one healthcare facility bought every staff member a permanent cup and stopped supplying foam cups (McNulty, 2007). The healthcare sector is taking a leadership role in reducing the sector's impact on the environment.

Health education and health literacy for ecological sustainability

It is important to present opportunities for people to enhance their own and collective understanding of the links between health and wellbeing and the environment. Activities may be organised around population groups with the aim of improving knowledge, attitudes, self-efficacy and capacity to change. Health literacy, health education and social marketing are different approaches but there are also crossovers in the intent and purpose of each. Social marketing is used to raise awareness about a priority, often appealing to specific groups at a population level. Health education is provided to individuals and groups to develop knowledge and skills. Nutbeam (2000, pp. 263–264) described three levels of health literacy as outcomes of effective health education: basic/functional literacy; communicative/ interactive literacy; and critical literacy; the latter enabling people to bring about change in wider community and social situations through collective action to address underlying determinants of health. Health education and health literacy are discussed in detail in Chapter 7.

Education and skill development strategies in this context need to encompass everything from emergency management for natural disasters through to association with the environment to prevent further destruction of, and to promote, a healthy environment. Understanding of the links between physical and mental health and wellbeing and the environment needs to be part of that package. Education for health and wellbeing will encompass strategies to build awareness and capacities to deal with and adapt to changing environmental conditions. Disassociation from the natural environment has occurred over time with increasing urbanisation.

All groups need age and culturally specific programs (Hansen et al., 2015). In Australia, there are national curriculum study guides for primary and secondary school children produced by the Meat and Livestock Association (Good Meat, n.d.). The Australian Disaster Resilience Knowledge Hub is another example with the aim to improve disaster resilience in Australia, supporting 'the implementation of the Council of Australian Governments' (COAG) National Strategy for Disaster Resilience, particularly regarding communicating with and educating people about risk' (Australian Institute for Disaster Resilience, n.d.a; b). Consultation with a wide range of organisations, representing practitioners, research, policy, education and information services occurred in the development which provides access to evidence-based research for policy development, decision making and best practice, and education and information about disasters and risk management.

The hub provides opportunities for discussion forums and collaboration between sectors.

There is also increasing interest at the tertiary education level to embed sustainability education into curricula (Australian Education for Sustainability Alliance, 2014). However, there have been barriers to implementation in the university sector (Leihy & Salazar, 2011) with individuals often trying to introduce and sustain education for sustainability without collaboration and cooperation within and across universities or the wider education sector (National Tertiary Education Union, 2011, p. 19). Hanover Research reports that 'while many universities have signed declarations pledging support of sustainability initiatives, most have fallen short in regards to implementation' (2011, p. 2).

Health information, social marketing and ecological sustainability

Social marketing raises public awareness about a health and wellbeing priority through use of mass media, the focus of Chapter 8. Mass media mirrors the dominant culture and all its underlying assumptions, but groups such as the World Watch Institute use social marketing as part of their armoury of strategies to raise awareness of environmental issues. The WHO also has brochures, handbooks, leaflets, posters and video advocacy materials raising awareness of climate change and of means of support for psychological distress. Raising awareness will continue to be part of the health sector's role, but the topics will depend on the location. Information in southern Australia, for example, will include how to dress coolly, drink enough fluids, limit physical activity during the hottest part of the day and keep indoors in the coolest part of the house (Whitmee et al., 2015). Providing information about human health and the health of the environment may extend broader than the health sector. Promoting the use of public transport and physical activity will reduce greenhouse gas emissions and result in a reduction in heart disease, cancer, diabetes, mental illness, road deaths and injuries (Lowe et al., 2014). There are a number of strategies already in place to inform people of potential risks to health, such as high-smog alert days and high-UV times of the day. Water authorities in dry areas assist communities to monitor water consumption levels, organisations exist to help people climate-proof houses, and urban designers are now mindful of green spaces and shade. These facilities will need to extend to early warning systems for heatwaves and other disasters which may stretch the limits of health systems.

Screening, risk assessment, surveillance and ecological sustainability

In high-income countries, the health sector has well-developed disease control and health protection strategies including surveillance for infectious diseases and risk-assessment strategies which extend from individual to community risk-assessment processes. These strategies may have to change with the evolving nature of diseases; for example, 'cases of salmonellosis rise by 5–10% for each 1 degree Celsius increase in weekly temperature when the ambient temperature is at least 5 degrees Celsius' (Wibulpolprasert et al., 2005, p. 1). The problem is caused by a global rise in temperatures, but the risk-assessment measures need to account for local differences. Arbovirus monitoring and surveillance is an example of a well-established program in areas of high mosquito activity in Australia. In states such as Victoria, local governments have specific powers to minimise risks. In regions such as along the Victorian/New South Wales border, environmental health practitioners monitor mosquito populations by setting mosquito traps in breeding seasons and monitoring viruses by blood sample testing of sentinel animals that host disease.

Evaluation of breeding sites and public education form part of the program as well. Mosquito control practices need to be performed in different locations due to the changing patterns of mosquito-borne diseases. Mosquitoes are spreading as the weather warms. Risk assessment for vulnerable populations is important.

Health impact assessment

Health impact assessment (HIA) is a community-based risk-assessment tool that provides practitioners with information about how a policy, program or development project may affect the health of people in that community (WHO, n.d.c). HIAs have emerged from three disciplinary fields: environmental, social and equity perspectives (Harris-Roxas & Harris, 2011). There has been some agreement about the procedural steps of HIA but the different forms are conducted for different purposes. HIAs are applied at the international, national and local levels. The assessments can be narrow or broad in focus. The narrow application produces quantitative retrospective evidence and relies on methods used in epidemiology and toxicology; for example, there is widespread concern over coal seam gas mining and whether the current levels of assessment, monitoring and regulation of exploration and mining activities are adequate to protect people's health. Communities and health practitioners have expressed concerns about the potential for public health to be affected directly and indirectly through contamination of water, air and soil. Adequate clinical and epidemiological assessment and adequate independent environmental monitoring and assessment would be key aspects of any investigation. In another example, the impact of wind farms has been controversial in some countries. Using renewable resources such as wind is seen as necessary action to reduce greenhouse gas emissions; however, some people close to the turbines report that their health has been adversely affected. Researchers are currently assessing whether there is a relationship between human health and exposure to the noise and vibrations of the turbines and wider impacts on health. No connections between wind farms and poor health have been established (Chapman et al., 2013; National Health and Medical Research Council, 2015) but epidemiological assessment would be part of the process.

A wider application of HIA is based on a broad definition of health and uses both qualitative and quantitative methods, including perceptions of health risk (WHO n.d.c). The latter process resonates with CPHC and ecological sustainability principles. It extends particularly to the precautionary principle. Projects that pose an environmental risk need to encompass social and emotional wellbeing aspects. The uptake of the wider application of HIAs is variable. Many countries and organisations have developed guidelines for practitioners; for example, the World Bank uses HIAs as part of their assessment for loans for projects. At all levels the HIA needs to fit into the multi-layered planning processes of local government, rather than allowing separate sectors to continue to plan in silos. In Australia, environmental health practitioners are likely to be involved in all or part of an HIA. The processes are similar to the community assessment processes outlined in Chapter 4 of this book and further discussion of HIAs will be presented in Chapter 9.

CONCLUSION

This chapter has explored key concepts related to ecological sustainability and associated impacts of the physical environment on human health and wellbeing. The unsustainable use and degradation of ecosystems has resulted in irreparable damage to the environment and, in turn, human health and wellbeing. Health practitioners have a role and responsibility to promote the health of the environment to ensure a healthy human population into the future. Many are doing so.

> *Leaders who don't just react passively, who have the courage to anticipate crisis or to act clearly, and who make strong insightful decisions of top-down management really can make a huge difference to their societies. So can similarly courageous, active citizens practicing 'bottom-up' management ...*
> *(Diamond, 2005, p. 306)*

Vulnerable populations depend on action now. Future generations depend on action now. In the remainder of this book, various approaches to promoting health in the CPHC context will be presented.

MORE TO EXPLORE

PLANETARY HEALTH, WELLBEING AND SUSTAINABILITY

- Planetary Health Alliance: https://planetaryhealthalliance.org/planetary-health
- Stockholm Resilience Centre. (2015) Planetary boundaries—an update: www.stockholmresilience.org/research/planetary-boundaries/planetary-boundaries/about-the-research/the-nine-planetary-boundaries.html
- Stockholm Resilience Centre. (2019). Ten years of nine planetary boundaries. Retrieved from https://www.stockholmresilience.org/research/research-news/2019-11-01-ten-years-of-nine-planetary-boundaries.html
- United Nations Sustainable Development Knowledge Platform. (2015a): https://sustainabledevelopment.un.org/topics?utm_source=SDSN&utm_campaign=e9d45f0e02-Sep_Newsletter_2015&utm_medium=email&utm_term=0_2302100059-e9d45f0e02-177873101
- Lock the Gate Alliance: https://www.lockthegate.org.au/
- Friends of the Earth Australia: https://www.foe.org.au/
- United Nations: The lazy person's guide to saving the world (n.d.b): https://www.un.org/sustainabledevelopment/takeaction/

CLIMATE CHANGE

- United Nations: Intergovernmental Panel on Climate Change: https://www.ipcc.ch/event/ipcc-at-cop-25/
- Lancet Countdown: Tracking Progress on Health and Climate Change: http://lancetcountdown.org/
- Global Green and Healthy Hospitals: https://www.greenhospitals.net/
- Australian Association for Environmental Education: http://www.aaee.org.au/
- Australian Government Bureau of Meteorology: State of the Climate 2018: http://www.bom.gov.au/state-of-the-climate/

IUHPE Core Competencies for Health Promotion

The IUHPE Core Competencies for Health Promotion comprises nine domains of action. Each domain has a series of core competency statements and a detailed outline of the knowledge and skills that contribute to competency in that domain.

The content of this chapter relates especially to the achievement of competency in the health promotion domains outlined below.

1. Enable change	*1.5 Work in collaboration with key stakeholders to reorient health and other services to promote health and reduce health inequities*
	Determinants of health and health inequities
2. Advocate for health	*2.2 Engage with and influence key stakeholders to develop and sustain health promotion action*
	Health and wellbeing issues relating to a specified population or group
	2.3 Raise awareness of and influence public opinion on health issues
	Working with a range of stakeholders
	2.4 Advocate for the development of policies, guidelines and procedures across all sectors which impact positively on health and reduce health inequities
	Determinants of health
3. Mediate through partnership	*3.2 Facilitate effective partnership working which reflects health promotion values and principles*
	Systems, structures and functions of different sectors, organisations and agencies
5. Leadership	*5.3 Network with and motivate stakeholders in leading change to improve health and reduce inequities*
	Principles of effective intersectoral partnership working
	Emerging challenges in health and health promotion
6. Assessment	*6.3 Collect, review and appraise relevant data, information and literature to inform health promotion action*
	Social determinants of health
	Health inequalities
	Evidence base for health promotion action and priority setting
7. Planning	*7.1 Mobilise, support and engage the participation of stakeholders in planning health promotion action*
	Use of health promotion planning models
9. Evaluation and research	*9.4 Use research and evidence-based strategies to inform practice*
	Evidence base for health promotion

In addition, IUHPE specifies knowledge, skills and performance criteria essential for health promotion practitioners to act professionally and ethically, including having knowledge of ethical and legal issues, behaving in an ethical and respectful manner and working in ways that review and improve practice. Full details are available at: www.iuhpe.org/index.php/en/the-accreditation-system.

Reflective Questions

1. Review the reflective questions for each of the Ottawa Charter action areas in the Putting the Ottawa Charter into Practice at the beginning of this chapter. Using the questions, undertake an audit for the institution where you are currently working or studying to determine the extent to which ecological sustainability is being addressed within each action area. Discuss the findings of the audit with your peers and make some recommendations on some actions that the organisation could take to enhance ecological sustainability.

2. The Ecological Footprint measures how much nature we use to support our current levels of consumption and waste production. Australia (6.84 global hectares per person) and New Zealand's (4.89 global hectares per person) Ecological Footprints are over the average global footprint of 2.7 global hectares per person (global hectares per capita) and well beyond the level of what the planet can regenerate on an annual basis—an equivalent of about 1.8 global hectares per person per year. Individuals, organisations, cities and countries can measure their footprint. Calculate your footprint by going to: https://www.wwf.org.au/get-involved/change-the-way-you-live/ecological-footprint-calculator#gs.8as1nn. Discuss your footprint results with your peers. Discuss the questions included in the footprint calculator and the extent to which you feel they capture your ecological footprint.

3. Review the individual actions for sustainability listed in Insight 3.2. Discuss with others which actions you are or could potentially act on. Make a plan for enacting three (3) new sustainability actions in the coming year. In your plan, specify your goal and what you will do to achieve that goal for each action. Determine to whom you will be accountable for the changes you plan to make and by when.

4. The Lock the Gate Alliance is an Australian grassroots organisation focused on protecting Australia's resources from inappropriate mining through advocacy and education action. Review the campaigns the alliance is currently involved in and identify any activity that you are particularly passionate about or that is relevant to where you live. Consider actions that you might be able to undertake to support the efforts of the Lock the Gate Alliance. Available at: https://www.lockthegate.org.au/about_us.

REFERENCES

Alderman, K., Turner, L. R., & Tong, S. (2012). Floods and human health: a systematic review. Environmental International, 47, 37–47. doi:10.1016/j.envint.2012.06.003.

Almada, A., Golden, C., Osofsky, S., & Myers, S. (2017). A case for planetary health/GeoHealth. GeoHealth, 1(2), 75–78. https://doi.org/10.1002/2017GH000084.

Alston, M. (2012). Rural male suicide in Australia. Social Science & Medicine, 74(4), 515–522. doi:10.1016/j.socscimed.2010.04.036.

Alston, M., & Kent, J. (2004). Social impact of drought: report to NSW Agriculture. Centre for Rural Social Research. Wagga Wagga, NSW: Charles Sturt University.

Arabena, K. (2010). All knowledge is Indigenous. In V. Brown, J. Harris, & J. Russell (Eds.), Tackling wicked problems: through the transdisciplinary imagination. London: Earthscan.

Arabena, K., & Kingsley, J. (2015). Climate change: impact on country and Aboriginal and Torres Strait Islander culture. In R. Walker & W. Mason (Eds.), Climate change adaptation for health and social services. Clayton South, Victoria: CSIRO Publishing.

AtKisson, A. (2010). Bill McKibben on climate change: the depressing bad news, and the amazing power of people to create good news. Retrieved from http://alanatkisson.wordpress.com/2010/11/01/bill-mckibben-on-climate/.

Australian Education for Sustainability Alliance. (2014). Education for Sustainability and the Australian Curriculum Project: final report for research phases 1 to 3. Melbourne: AESA.

Australian Institute for Disaster Resilience. (n.d.a). Australian Disaster Resilience Knowledge Hub. Retrieved from https://knowledge.aidr.org.au/.

Australian Institute for Disaster Resilience. (n.d.b). The Australian Institute for Disaster Resilience. Retrieved from https://www.aidr.org.au/about-aidr/.

Barosh, L., Friel, S., Englehart, K., & Chan, L. (2014). The cost of a healthy and sustainable diet—who can afford it? Australian and New Zealand Journal of Public Health, 38(1), 7–12.

Bauman, A., Rissel, C., Garard, J., et al. (2008). Getting Australia moving: barriers, facilitators and interventions to get Australians physically active through cycling. Melbourne: Cycling Promotion Fund.

Bennett, C. M., Capon, A. G., & McMichael, A. J. (2011). Climate change and health. Public Health Bulletin SA, 8, 2.

BlueHealth (n.d.). About BlueHealth. Retrieved from https://bluehealth2020.eu/.

Bowman, D. (2015, 20 November). How to prepare your home for a bushfire—and when to leave. The Conversation. Retrieved from https://theconversation.com/how-to-prepare-your-home-for-a-bushfire-and-when-to-leave-50962.

Brown, L. (2009). Could food shortages bring down civilization? Scientific American, May, 38–45.

Brown, V. A., Grootjans, J., Ritchie, J., et al. (Eds.). (2005). Sustainability and health: working together to support global integrity. London: Earthscan.

Burgess, C. P., Johnston, F. H., & Bailie, R. (2007). Healthy country: healthy people: superior Indigenous health outcomes are associated with 'caring for country'. EcoHealth Conference, 30 Nov–3 Dec. Melbourne: Deakin University.

Burnett, R., Chen, H., Szyszkowicz, M., et al. (2018). Global estimates of mortality associated with long-term exposure to outdoor fine particulate matter. Proceedings of the National Academy of Sciences, 115(38), 9592–9597. doi:10.1073/pnas.1803222115.

Bygrave, S. (2016). One in five local councils aiming for zero emissions or 100% renewables. Renew Economy. Retrieved from http://reneweconomy.com.au/2016/one-in-five-local-councils-aiming-for-zero-emissions-or-100-renewables-80850.

Byrne, J., Ambrey, C., Portanger, C., et al. (2016). Could urban greening mitigate suburban thermal inequity? The role of residents' dispositions and household practices. Environmental Research Letters: ERL, 11, 09. Retrieved from http://iopscience.iop.org/article/10.1088/1748-9326/11/9/095014/meta;jsessionid=0DAF9F4A5950AA0C942B7E9A15A74C93.c1.iopscience.cld.iop.org.

Capon, A. (2003). Cities fit to live in. About the House, House of Representatives Magazine, 9, 21–23.

Central Victoria Greenhouse Alliance. (2019). CVGA annual report 2018–19. Retrieved from http://www.cvga.org.au/uploads/9/8/3/8/9838558/cvga-annual_report-2019_final.pdf.

Central Victoria Greenhouse Alliance. (n.d.). Lighting the regions. Retrieved from http://www.cvga.org.au/lighting-the-regions.html.

Chapman, S., St. George, A., Waller, K., & Cakic, V. (2013). The pattern of complaints about Australian wind farms does not match the establishment and distribution of turbines: support for the psychogenic, 'communicated disease' hypothesis. PLoS ONE, 8(10), e76584. doi:10.1371/journal.pone.0076584.

City of Melbourne. (n.d.). How to grow an urban forest. Retrieved from https://www
.greenerspacesbetterplaces.com.au/guides/how-to-grow-an-urban-forest/.

Cleary, A., Fielding, K., Bell, S., et al. (2017). Exploring potential mechanisms involved in the
relationship between eudaimonic wellbeing and nature connection. Landscape and Urban
Planning, 158, 119–128. https://doi.org/10.1016/j.landurbplan.2016.10.003.

Cleugh, H., Stafford Smith, M., Battaglia, M., & Graham, P. (2011). Climate change: science and
solutions for Australia. CSIRO. Retrieved from http://www.publish.csiro.au/pid/6558.htm.

Climate Council. (2018). How could climate change affect me and my family? Retrieved from
https://www.climatecouncil.org.au/resources/?category=health.

Climate Institute. (2015a). Australia's emissions: what do the numbers really mean? Fact Sheet,
July. Retrieved from http://www.climateinstitute.org.au/verve/_resources/TCI_Australias
_Emissions_Factsheet_Final-LR.pdf.

Climate Institute. (2015b). Climate of the nation 2015: Australian attitudes on climate change.
Retrieved from http://www.climateinstitute.org.au/climate-of-the-nation-2015.html.

Collier, P. (2003). Natural resources, development and conflict: channels of causation and policy
interventions. Washington DC: World Bank.

Corvalan, C., Hales, S., & McMichael, A. (2005). Ecosystems and human wellbeing. Health
Synthesis. Geneva: WHO.

CSIRO. (2018). State of the climate 2018. Retrieved from https://www.csiro.au/en/Showcase/
state-of-the-climate.

Dean, J., & Stain, H. (2010). Mental health impact for adolescents living with prolonged drought.
The Australian Journal of Rural Health, 18, 32–37. doi:10.1111/j.1440-1584.2009.01107.x.

Department of the Environment and Energy. (n.d.). The ozone layer. Australian Government.
Retrieved from http://www.environment.gov.au/protection/ozone/ozone-science/ozone-layer.

Department of Environment, Water, Heritage and the Arts. (1992). 1992 National Strategy for
Ecological Sustainable Development. Australian Government. Retrieved from http://www
.environment.gov.au/about-us/esd/publications/national-esd-strategy.

Department of Human Services (DHS). (2009). Heatwave in Victoria: an assessment of health
impacts. Melbourne: Victorian Government Department of Human Services.

Department of Infrastructure and Transport, Major Cities Unit. (2012). State of Australian cities
2012. Australian Government. Retrieved from https://infrastructure.gov.au/infrastructure/pab/
soac/files/2012_00_infra1360_mcu_soac_full_web_fa.pdf.

Deville, A., & Harding, R. (1997). Applying the precautionary principle. Annandale: Federation
Press.

Diamond, J. (2005). Collapse: how societies choose to fail or succeed. USA: Viking Press.

D'Souza, R. M., Becker, N. G., Hall, G., & Moodie, K. (2004). Does ambient temperature affect
food-borne disease. Epidemiology (Cambridge, Mass.), 15, 86–92.

Duus-Otterstrom, G., & Jagers, S. C. (2012). Identifying burdens of coping with climate change:
A typology of the duties of climate justice. Global Environmental Change, 22(3), 746–753.

Earth Charter. (2000). Retrieved from http://www.earthcharter.org/.

Ebden, M., & Townsend, M. (2007). Feeling blue? Then touch green: the benefits of conservation
groups. EcoHealth Conference, 30 Nov–3 Dec. Melbourne: Deakin University.

Edwards, F., Dixon, J., Hall, G., et al. (2011). Climate change adaptation at the intersection of food
and health. Asia-Pacific Journal of Public Health, 23(2 Suppl.), 91S–104S.

Envision Gunderson Health System. (2014). Our envision plan. Retrieved from http://www
.gundersenvision.org/gundersen-reaches-first-days-of-energy-independence.

Folke, C. (Ed.). (2011). Executive summary of scientific background reports: 3rd Nobel Laureate
Symposium on Global Sustainability: transforming the world in an era of global change.
Stockholm, Sweden, May 16–19. Retrieved from http://www.nobel-cause.de/stockholm-2011/
download/Executive_summary.pdf.

Food and Agriculture Organization of the United Nations (FAO). (2003). Trade reforms and food
security: conceptualizing the linkages. FAO corporate document repository, Chapter 2 Food

security: concepts and measurement. Economic and Social Development Department. Retrieved from http://www.fao.org/docrep/005/Y4671e/Y4671e00.Htm#Contents.

Fritz, J., Williamson, L., & Wiseman, J. (2009). Community engagement and climate change: benefits, challenges and strategies. Melbourne: McGaughey Centre, VicHealth Centre for Health Promotion of Mental Health and Community Wellbeing, Melbourne School of Population Health, University of Melbourne.

Frumkin, H., Bratman, G. N., Breslow, S. J., et al. (2017). Nature contact and human health: a research agenda. Environmental Health Perspectives, 125(7), 075001. https://doi.org/10.1289/EHP1663.

Frumkin, H., McMichael, A., & Hess, J. (2008). Climate change and the health of the public. American Journal of Preventive Medicine, 35(5), 405–423.

Gleeson, D. (2015). TPP—final text shows cause for concern. PHAA media release, November 6.

Global Health and Climate Alliance. (2012). Doha declaration on climate, health and wellbeing. Retrieved from http://www.caha.org.au/doha-declaration-on-climate-health-and-wellbeing/.

Good Meat. (n.d.). National curriculum study guides. Retrieved from https://www.goodmeat.com.au/education-resources/national-curriculum-study-guides/

Green Building Council Australia. (2018). Green Star: the case for sustainable healthcare. Retrieved from https://gbca-web.s3.amazonaws.com/media/documents/health-case-short-version-v2-r6-online-nab-14122018.pdf.

Green, D., Jackson, S., & Morrison, J. (2009). Risks from climate change to Indigenous communities in the tropical north of Australia. Canberra: Department of Climate Change.

Hales, S., & Corvalan, C. (2006). Public health emergency on planet earth: insights from the millennium ecosystem assessment: personal commentaries on ecosystems and human well-being: health synthesis—a report of the Millennium Ecosystem Assessment. EcoHealth, 3, 130–135.

Hancock, T. (1985). The Mandala of Health: a model of the human ecosystem. Family and Community Health, 8(3), 1–10.

Hancock, T. (2000). Healthy communities must also be sustainable communities: theory. Public Health Reports, March/April and May/June 2000, 115, 151–156.

Hanna, E. G., Kjellstrom, T., Bennett, C., & Dear, K. (2011). Climate change and rising heat: population health implications for working people in Australia. Asia-Pacific Journal of Public Health, 23, 14S–26S. doi:10.1177/1010539510391457. [Epub 2010 Dec 15].

Hanover Research—Academy Administration Practice. (2011). Embedding sustainability into university curricula. Washington DC: Hanover.

Hansen, A., Hanson-Easey, S., & Bi, P. (2015). Support for adaptation in culturally and linguistically diverse communities. In R. Walker & W. Mason (Eds.), Climate change adaptation for health and social services. Melbourne: CSIRO Publishing.

Harris-Roxas, B., & Harris, E. (2011). Different forms, different purposes: a typology of health impact assessment. Environment Impact Assessment Review, 31, 396–403. doi:10.1016/j.eiar.2010.03.003.

Hassan, N. A., Hashim, Z., & Hashim, J. H. (2015). Impact of climate change on air quality and public health in urban ureas. Asia-Pacific Journal Public Health, 28(2 Suppl), 38S–48S. doi:10.1177/1010539515592951.

Health Care Without Harm. (n.d.a). Global green and healthy hospitals. Retrieved from https://noharm-global.org/issues/global/global-green-and-healthy-hospitals.

Health Care Without Harm. (n.d.b). Health care climate challenge. Retrieved from https://www.greenhospitals.net/about-challenge/.

Holland, A. (2016). Preventing tomorrow's climate wars. Scientific American, June: 53–57.

Homer-Dixon, T., Walker, B., & Biggs, R. (2015). Synchronous failure: the emerging causal architecture of global crisis. Ecology and Society, 20(3), 6. Retrieved from http://dx.doi.org/10.5751/ES-07681-200306.

Horsburg, N., Armsrong, F., & Mulvena, V. (2017). Framework for a national strategy for climate, health and wellbeing for Australia. Climate and Health Alliance. Retrieved from https://

d3n8a8pro7vhmx.cloudfront.net/caha/pages/40/attachments/original/1498008324/CAHA
_Framework_for_a_National_Strategy_on_Climate_Health_and_Well-being_v05_SCREEN
_%28Full_Report%29.pdf?1498008324.

Horton, R. (2014). Offline: why the Sustainable Development Goals will fail: comment. The
Lancet, 383, 2196. Retrieved from http://www.thelancet.com/pdfs/journals/lancet/PIIS0140
-6736(14)61046-1.pdf.

Horton, R., Beaglehole, R., Bonita, R., et al. (2014). From public to planetary health: a manifesto.
The Lancet, 383(9920), 847.

Horton, G., & McMichael, A. (2008). Climate change health check 2020. Climate Institute of
Australia. Retrieved from http://www.climateinstitute.org.au/articles/publications/climat
e-change-health-check-2020—report.html.

Hughes, L., & McMichael, A. J. (2011). The critical decade: climate change and health. Department
of Climate Change and Energy Efficiency. Canberra: Commonwealth of Australia.

Intergovernmental Panel on Climate Change (IPCC). (2014a). Climate change 2014: synthesis
report. Contribution of Working Groups I, II and III to the Fifth Assessment Report of the
Intergovernmental Panel on Climate Change [Core Writing Team, R. K. Pachauri and L. A.
Meyer (Eds.)]. IPCC, Geneva, Switzerland, 151. Retrieved from http://www.ipcc.ch/report/
ar5/syr.

Intergovernmental Panel on Climate Change (IPCC). (2014b). Working group III: climate change
2014: impacts, adaptation and vulnerability: contribution of working group III to the fifth
assessment report of the intergovernmental panel on climate change. Cambridge, UK:
Cambridge University Press.

Johnson, B. (2007). Environmental policy and public health. Boca Raton, FL: Taylor and Francis.

Kane, A. (2015, 19 November). New protocol could help build biodiverse cities. The Fifth Estate.
Retrieved from http://www.thefifthestate.com.au/habitat/environment/new-protocol-could
-help-build-biodiverse-cities/78882.

Karanis, P., Kourenti, C., & Smith, H. (2007). Waterborne transmission of protozoan parasites: a
worldwide review of outbreaks and lessons learnt. Journal of Water and Health, 5(1), 1–38.

Keen, M., Brown, V., & Dyball, R. (2005). Social learning: a new approach to environmental
management. In M. Keen, V. A. Brown, & R. Dyball (Eds.), Social learning in environmental
management: towards a sustainable future. London: Earthscan Publications Ltd.

Kent, L. (2015). Explainer: how the OECD agreement deals another blow to coal worldwide. The
Conversation, November 19. Retrieved from https://theconversation.com/explainer-how
-the-oecd-agreement-deals-another-blow-to-coal-worldwide-50969.

Labonté, R. (1997). Power participation and partnerships for health promotion. Melbourne:
VicHealth.

Labonté, R., & Schrecker, T. (2006). Globalization and social determinants of health: analytic and
strategic review paper: on behalf of the Globalization Knowledge Network. Ottawa: Institute
of Population Health, University of Ottawa.

Leihy, P., & Salazar, J. (2011). Education for sustainability in university curricula: policies and
practice in Victoria. Prepared for Sustainability Victoria, November 2011. Melbourne: Centre
for the Study of Higher Education University of Melbourne.

Lenton, T., Rockström, J., Gaffney, O., et al. (2019). Climate tipping points—too risky to bet
against. Nature, 575(7784), 592–595. https://doi.org/10.1038/d41586-019-03595-0.

Leviston, Z., Leitch, A., Greenhill, M., et al. (2011). Australians' views of climate change. CSIRO
Report. Canberra: CSIRO.

Lloyd, S. J., Kovats, R. S., & Chalabi, Z. (2011). Climate change, crop yields and under nutrition:
development of a model to quantify the impact of climate scenarios on child under nutrition.
Environmental Health Perspectives, 119(12), 1817–1823. doi:10.1289/ehp.1003311.

Lowe, M., Boulange, C., & Giles-Corti, B. (2015). Urban design and health: progress to date and
future challenges. Health Promotion Journal of Australia, 25, 14–18.

Lowe, M., Whitzman, C., Badland, H., et al. (2014). Planning healthy, liveable and sustainable
cities: how can indicators inform policy? Urban Policy and Research, 33(2), 131–144. http://
dx.doi.org/10.1080/08111146.2014.1002606.

Mallon, K., & Hamilton, E. (2015). Community-based health and social services: managing risks from climate change. In R. Walker & W. Mason (Eds.), Climate change adaptation for health and social services. Clayton South: CSIRO Publishing.

Markevych, I., Schoierer, J., Hartig, T., et al. (2017). Exploring pathways linking greenspace to health: theoretical and methodological guidance. Environmental Research, 158, 301–317. https://doi.org/10.1016/j.envres.2017.06.028.

Marmot, M. (2010). Strategic review of health inequalities in England post 2010 (Marmot Review). Retrieved from http://www.instituteofhealthequity.org/resources-reports/strategi c-review-of-health-inequalities-in-england-post-2010-presentation-of-findings.

Marmot, M., Goldblatt, P., Allen, J., et al. (2010). Fair society, healthy lives: the Marmot review: strategic review of health inequalities in England post-2010. Retrieved from http://www .instituteofhealthequity.org/resources-reports/fair-society-healthy-lives-the-marmot-review/ fair-society-healthy-lives-full-report-pdf.pdf.

Marmot, M., & Wilkinson, R. G. (1999). Social determinants of health. Oxford: Oxford University Press.

Martin, K. L., Hanigan, I. C., Morgan, G. G., et al. (2013). Air pollution from fires and their association with hospital admissions in Sydney, Newcastle and Wollongong, Australia 1994–2007. Australian and New Zealand Journal of Public Health, 37(3), 238–249.

Massey, C. (2017). Call of the reed warbler: a new agriculture and new earth. Brisbane: University of Queensland Press.

McMichael, A. (1993). Planetary overload: global environmental change and the health of the human species. Cambridge: Cambridge University Press.

McMichael, A. J. (2001). Human frontiers, environments and disease: past patterns, uncertain futures. Cambridge UK: Cambridge University Press.

McMichael, A., Butler, C., & Dixon, J. (2015). Climate change food systems and population health risks in their eco-social context. Public Health, 129, 1361–1368. The Royal Society of Public Health. Elsevier Ltd. doi:10.1016/j.puhe.2014.11.013.

McMichael, A. J., Smith, K. A., & Corvalan, C. F. (2000). The sustainability transition: a new challenge. Bulletin of the World Health Organization, 78, 1067.

McNulty, S. (2007). Creating a greener environment at Northern Health. Health Issues, 93, 17–20.

Meadows, D. H., Meadows, D. L., Randers, J., & Behrens, W. W., III (1972). The limits to growth. New York: Universe Books.

Ministry for the Environment (MFE). (2018). About the Paris agreement. Retrieved from https:// www.mfe.govt.nz/climate-change/why-climate-change-matters/global-response/ paris-agreement.

Ministry for the Environment (MFE). (2019). How climate affects New Zealand. Retrieved from https://www.mfe.govt.nz/climate-change/likely-impacts-of-climate-change/ likely-climate-change-impacts-nz.

Mitchell, B. C., & Chakraborty, J. (2014). Urban heat and climate justice: a landscape of thermal inequity in Pinellas County, Florida. Geographical Review, 104(4), 459–480. doi:10.1111/ j.1931-0846.2014.12039.x.

NASA. (n.d.). Climate change: How do we know? Retrieved from http://climate.nasa.gov/ evidence/.

National Health and Medical Research Council. (2015). Windfarms. Retrieved from https://www .nhmrc.gov.au/health-advice/environmental-health/wind-farms#.

National Tertiary Education Union. (2011). Pushing the boundaries: NTEU climate change conference pushes the boundaries of the Australian debate. Advocate (Boston, Mass.), 18(2), 16–20. South Melbourne.

Ng, F. Y., Wilson, L. A., & Veitch, C. (2015). Climate adversity and resilience: voice of rural Australia. Rural and Remote Health, 15, 3071.

Nicholls, N., Butler, C. D., & Hanigan, I. (2006). Inter-annual rainfall variations and suicides in NSW, Australia, 1964–2001. International Journal of Biometeorology, 50, 139–143.

Nitschke, M., Tucker, G., & Bi, P. (2007). Morbidity and mortality during the heat waves in Adelaide. Medical Journal of Australia, 187, 662–665.

Nogrady, B. (2019). Bushfires: Australia issues health warnings as Sydney air quality plummets. BMJ, 367. https://doi.org/10.1136/bmj.l6914.

Nutbeam, D. (2000). Health literacy as a public health goal: a challenge for contemporary health education and communication strategies into the 21st century. Health Promotion International, 15(3), 259–267.

Organisation for Economic Cooperation and Development (OECD). (2012). Environmental outlook to 2050. Paris: OECD Publishing.

Organisation for Economic Cooperation and Development (OECD). (2019). OECD work in support of climate action. Retrieved from https://www.oecd.org/env/cc/OECD-work-in-support-of -climate-action.pdf.

Organisation for Economic Cooperation and Development (OECD). (n.d.). Adaptation to climate change. Retrieved from http://www.oecd.org/environment/cc/adaptation.htm.

Parks Victoria. (2015). Valuing Victoria's parks. Retrieved from http://parkweb.vic.gov.au/about-us/ news/valuing-victorias-parks.

Parliament of Australia. (2017). Paris climate agreement: a quick guide. Retrieved from https:// www.aph.gov.au/About_Parliament/Parliamentary_Departments/Parliamentary_Library/pubs/ rp/rp1718/Quick_Guides/ParisAgreement.

Phillips, R., & Kingsley, J. (2007). Healthy country, healthy people. EcoHealth Conference, 30 Nov–3 Dec. Melbourne: Deakin University.

Polain, J., Berry, H., & Hoskin, J. (2011). Rapid change, climate adversity and the next 'big dry': older farmers' mental health. The Australian Journal of Rural Health, 19, 239–243. doi: 10.1111/j.1440-1584.2011.01219.x.

Pritchard, B., & McManus, P. (2000). Land of discontent: the dynamics of change in rural and regional Australia. Sydney: University of New South Wales Press.

Public Health Association of Australia (PHAA). (2016). Proposed constitutional amendments. Retrieved from https://www.phaa.net.au/documents/item/1643.

Rahmstorf, S., & Coumou, D. (2011). Increase of extreme events in a warmer world. Proceedings of the National Academy of Science. doi:10.1073/pnas.1101766108.

Rees, W., & Wackernagal, M. (1995). Our ecological footprint: reducing human impact on the earth. Cabriola Island, BC: New Society Publishers.

Rockström, J., Steffen, W., Noone, K., et al. (2009). Planetary boundaries: exploring the safe operating space for humanity. Ecology and Society, 14(2), 32. Retrieved from http://www .ecologyandsociety.org/vol14/iss2/art32/.

Scientific American Editorial. (2008). Climate fatigue: a grassroots approach alone won't make the Earth stop warming. Scientific American, 298(6), doi:10.1038/scientificamerican0608-39.

Scovronick, N. (2015). Reducing global health risks through mitigation of short-lived climate pollutants: scoping report for policy makers. Geneva: World Health Organization. Retrieved from http://www.who.int/phe/publications/climate-reducing-health-risks/en/.

Smith, K. R., Woodward, A., Campbell-Lendrum, D., et al. (2014). Human health: impacts, adaptation, and co-benefits. In C. B. Field, V. R. Barros, D. J. Dokken, et al. (Eds.), Climate change 2014: impacts, adaptation, and vulnerability. Part A: Global and sectoral aspects Contribution of Working Group II to the Fifth Assessment Report of the Intergovernmental Panel on Climate Change (pp. 709–754). Cambridge, United Kingdom and New York, NY, USA: Cambridge University Press. Retrieved from https://www.ipcc.ch/report/ar5/wg2/.

Soskolne, C., Kotze, L., Mackey, B., & Rees, W. (2008). Challenging our individual and collective thinking about sustainability. In C. Soskolne (Ed.), Sustaining life on earth. Lanham, Maryland: Lexington Books.

Spickett, J. T., Brown, H. L., & Rumchev, K. (2011). Climate change and air quality: the potential impact on health. Asia-Pacific Journal of Public Health, 2, 37S–45S.

Steffen, W., Richardson, K., Rockström, J., et al. (2015). Planetary boundaries: guiding human development on a changing planet. Science, 347(6223). doi:10.1126/science.1259855.

Stockholm Resilience Centre. (2015). Planetary boundaries—an update. Retrieved from https://www.stockholmresilience.org/research/research-news/2015-01-15-planetary-boundaries—an-update.html.

Stockholm Resilience Centre. (2019). Ten years of nine planetary boundaries. Retrieved from https://www.stockholmresilience.org/research/research-news/2019-11-01-ten-years-of-nine-planetary-boundaries.html.

Stockholm Resilience Centre. (n.d.). Tipping points: a new landscape of global crises. Retrieved from https://www.stockholmresilience.org/research/research-news/2015-10-12-a-new-landscape-of-global-crises.html.

Sustainable Aotearoa New Zealand Inc (SANZ). (2009). Strong sustainability for New Zealand: principles and scenarios. Nakedize Limited Publication. Auckland: Nakedize.

Sustainable Aotearoa New Zealand Inc (SANZ). (n.d.). Strong sustainability for New Zealand. Retrieved from http://www.earthslimits.org/strong-sustainability-for-new-zealand.

Talberg, A., Hui, S., & Loynes, K. (2013). Australian climate change policy: a chronology. Research paper series, 2013–14, 2 December. Parliament of Australia, Department of Parliament services, Science, Technology, Environment and Resources Section.

Talbot, L., & Walker, R. (2007). Community perspectives on the impact of policy change on linking social capital in a rural community. Health and Place, 13(2), 482–492.

The Lancet. (2019). Health and climate change. Retrieved from https://www.thelancet.com/climate-and-health.

Toloo, G., Guo, Y., Turner, L., et al. (2014). Socio-demographic vulnerability to heatwave impacts in Brisbane, Australia: a time series analysis. Australian and New Zealand Journal of Public Health, 38(5), 430–435.

Tong, S., Ren, C., & Becker, N. (2010). Excess deaths during the 2004 heatwave in Brisbane Australia. International Journal of Biometeorology, 54, 393–400.

UNEP and UNU-IHDP (2012). Inclusive wealth report 2012: measuring progress towards sustainability. Cambridge: Cambridge University Press.

United Nations. (1948). Universal declaration of human rights. Retrieved from http://www.un.org/en/universal-declaration-human-rights/.

United Nations (UN). (1972). Declaration of the United Nations conference on the human environment. Retrieved from https://www.un.org/ga/search/view_doc.asp?symbol=A/CONF.48/14/REV.1.

United Nations (UN). (1985). Vienna Convention for the Protection of the Ozone Layer. Retrieved from https://ozone.unep.org/treaties/vienna-conventions

United Nations (UN). (1987a). Montreal Protocol on substances that deplete the ozone layer. Retrieved from https://ozone.unep.org/treaties/montreal-protocol.

United Nations (UN). (1987b). Report of the World Commission on Environment and Development: our common future. Retrieved from www.un-documents.net/wced-ocf.htm.

United Nations (UN). (1992a). Agenda 21. Retrieved from https://sustainabledevelopment.un.org/content/documents/Agenda21.pdf.

United Nations (UN). (1992b). Rio declaration on environment and development. Retrieved from https://www.un.org/en/development/desa/population/migration/generalassembly/docs/globalcompact/A_CONF.151_26_Vol.I_Declaration.pdf.

United Nations (UN). (1992c) United Nations convention on biological diversity. Retrieved from www.cbd.int/doc/legal/cbd-en.pdf.

United Nations (UN). (1992d). What is the United Nations Framework Convention on Climate Change? Retrieved from http://unfccc.int/essential_background/convention/items/6036.php.

United Nations (UN). (1997). United Nations framework convention on climate change Kyoto protocol. Retrieved from https://unfccc.int/kyoto_protocol.

United Nations (UN). (2001). Stockholm convention on persistent organic pollutants (POPs). Retrieved from http://chm.pops.int/TheConvention/Overview/tabid/3351/Default.aspx.

United Nations. (2015a). Sustainable Development Knowledge Platform. Retrieved from https:// sustainabledevelopment.un.org/topics?utm_source=SDSN&utm_campaign=e9d45f0e02-Sep _Newsletter_2015&utm_medium=email&utm_term=0_2302100059-e9d45f0e02-177873101

United Nations. (2015b). Transforming our world: the 2030 agenda for sustainable development. Retrieved from http://www.un.org/sustainabledevelopment/sustainable-development-goals/.

United Nations. (2015c). United Nations Framework Convention on Climate Change Paris Agreement. Retrieved from https://sustainabledevelopment.un.org/frameworks/ parisagreement.

United Nations. (2016). 2016 International day for disaster reduction. Retrieved from http:// www.un.org/en/events/disasterreductionday/.

United Nations (UN). (2019a). About the UN Climate change conference 2019. Retrieved from https://unfccc.int/about-the-un-climate-change-conference-december-2019.

United Nations. (2019b). The Sustainable Development Goals Report 2019. Retrieved from https:// unstats.un.org/sdgs/report/2019/The-Sustainable-Development-Goals-Report-2019.pdf.

United Nations. (n.d.a). The 12 initial POPs under the Stockholm Convention. Retrieved from http://chm.pops.int/TheConvention/ThePOPs/The12InitialPOPs/tabid/296/Default.aspx.

United Nations. (n.d.b). The lazy person's guide to saving the world. Retrieved from http://www .un.org/sustainabledevelopment/takeaction.

Verrinder, G. K. (2012). System challenges for public health in a sustainability transition. Unpublished PhD thesis.

Verrinder, G., & Talbot, L. (2015). Rural communities experiencing climate change: a systems approach to adaptation. In R. Walker & W. Mason (Eds.), Climate change adaptation for health and social services (pp. 179–199). Melbourne: CSIRO Publishing.

Walker, R., & Mason, W. (2015). Climate change adaptation for health and social services. Melbourne: CSIRO Publishing.

Watts, N., Amann, M., Arnell, N., et al. (2019). The 2019 report of The Lancet Countdown on health and climate change: ensuring that the health of a child born today is not defined by a changing climate. The Lancet, 394(10211), 1836–1878. doi:10.1016/S0140-6736(19)32596-6.

Webb, R., Bai, X. M., Smith, M. S., et al. (2018). Sustainable urban systems: co-design and framing for transformation. Ambio, 47, 57–77, doi:10.1007/s13280-017-0934-6.

Whitmee, S., Haines, A., Beyrer, C., et al. (2015). Safeguarding human health in the Anthropocene epoch: report of The Rockefeller Foundation–Lancet Commission on planetary health. The Lancet, 386(10007), 1973–2028. http://dx.doi.org/10.1016/S0140-6736(15)60901-1.

Wibulpolprasert, S., Tangcharoensathien, V., Kanchanachitra, C. (2005). Are cost effective interventions enough to achieve the millennium development goals? BMJ (Clinical Research Ed.), 331, 1093–1094.

World Commission on Environment and Development (WCED). (1987). Report of the World Commission on Environment and Development: our common future. Retrieved from http:// www.un-documents.net/wced-ocf.htm.

World Federation of Public Health Associations (WFPHA). (2015). Climate change and health policy assessment project report: a global survey 2015. Retrieved from: http://www .wfpha.org/images/news/WFPHA-Global-Climate-Health-Policy-Survey.FINAL.pdf.

World Health Organization (WHO). (1978). Declaration of Alma-Ata. Retrieved from http:// www.euro.who.int/__data/assets/pdf_file/0009/113877/E93944.pdf.

World Health Organization (WHO). (1986). Ottawa Charter for Health Promotion. Retrieved from http://www.euro.who.int/__data/assets/pdf_file/0004/129532/Ottawa_Charter.pdf.

World Health Organization. (1988). Adelaide recommendations on healthy public policy. Second international conference on health promotion, Adelaide, South Australia, 5–9 April 1988. Retrieved from http://www.who.int/healthpromotion/conferences/previous/adelaide/en/ index1.html.

World Health Organization (WHO). (1991). Sundsvall statement on supportive environments for health. Retrieved from https://www.who.int/healthpromotion/conferences/previous/ sundsvall/en/.

World Health Organization (WHO). (2005). Ecosystems and human well-being health synthesis: Millennium Ecosystem Assessment. Retrieved from http://www.millenniumassessment.org/documents/document.356.aspx.pdf.

World Health Organization (WHO). (2006). Preventing disease through healthy environments: towards an estimate of the environmental burden of disease. Retrieved from https://www.who.int/quantifying_ehimpacts/publications/preventingdisease.pdf.

World Health Organization (WHO). (2015a). COP21 Climate Agreement—moving towards healthier people and a healthier planet. Retrieved from http://www.who.int/globalchange/mediacentre/events/COP21_climateagreement__health/en/.

World Health Organization. (2015b). Drinking-water, Fact sheet No. 391, June. Retrieved from http://www.who.int/mediacentre/factsheets/fs391/en/.

World Health Organization (WHO). (2015c). WHO calls for urgent action to protect health from climate change. Retrieved from http://www.who.int/globalchange/global-campaign/cop21/en/.

World Health Organization (WHO). (2016) Shanghai declaration on promoting health in the 2030 agenda for sustainable development. Retrieved from https://www.who.int/healthpromotion/conferences/9gchp/shanghai-declaration.pdf?ua=1.

World Health Organization (WHO). (2018a). COP24 Special report: health and climate change. Retrieved from https://www.who.int/globalchange/publications/COP24-report-health-climate-change/en/.

World Health Organization (WHO). (2018b). Declaration of Astana, Global Conference on Primary Health Care. Retrieved from https://www.who.int/docs/default-source/primary-health/declaration/gcphc-declaration.pdf.

World Health Organization. (n.d.a). Air pollution. Retrieved from https://www.who.int/health-topics/air-pollution.

World Health Organization (WHO). (n.d.b). Climate change and health. Retrieved from http://www.who.int/globalchange/global-campaign/cop21/en/.

World Health Organization (WHO). (n.d.c). Health impact assessment. Retrieved from https://www.who.int/topics/health_impact_assessment/en/.

World Health Organization & Health Care Without Harm. (2009). Global green and healthy hospitals: a comprehensive environmental health agenda for hospitals and health systems around the world. Retrieved from https://noharm-global.org/issues/global/global-green-and-healthy-hospitals-agenda.

World Wildlife Fund. (n.d.). What is your ecological footprint? Retrieved from http://www.wwf.org.au/get-involved/change-the-way-you-live/ecological-footprint-calculator.

Zhang, Y., Beggs, P. J., Bambrick, H., et al. (2018). The MJA-Lancet Countdown on health and climate change: Australian policy inaction threatens lives. Retrieved from https://www.mja.com.au/system/files/issues/209_11/10.5694mja18.00789.pdf.

PART 2
HEALTH PROMOTION PRACTICE

The socio-ecological determinants of health are the key influences on people's experience of life. There is strong evidence that the inequitable distribution of society's material and social resources is a determinant of poor health, along with racism, poverty and social exclusion. Degradation of the physical environment further exacerbates poor health. These determinants must be addressed if we are to improve the health and wellbeing of the community and reduce health inequities.

In critical health promotion, values of equity and social justice underpin practice. A socially just society is a healthier society, physically, economically, spiritually, emotionally and environmentally. These values are exemplified in concepts such as empowerment and cultural competence; however, these values may not be shared by those in power and may therefore be ignored. Enabling communities to become healthy and stay healthy may become a political activity. International agreements such as the Declaration of Alma-Ata, the Declaration of Human Rights, the Earth Charter and the Ottawa Charter for Health Promotion can provide guidance for practice.

To be effective, health promotion practice requires action across all areas of the Ottawa Charter. Empowerment happens, and social justice is achieved, when people are enabled to make changes in the context of their lives that enhance their health, in its broadest sense. Health practitioners working in a comprehensive primary health care context can be advocates for healthy public policy at all levels. Health promotion work involves advocating on behalf of vulnerable community groups for the desired changes to be enshrined in policy. Policy within government or agencies can be used as 'leverage' to bring about change in the social environment, management systems and structures to provide rationale for actions in support of community. Success in health promotion is dependent upon:

- examining the values that guide the development of healthy public policy
- examining power in communities and challenging the inequitable distribution of power
- raising the consciousness of communities about the socio-ecological determinants of health
- working inclusively, respectfully, collaboratively and flexibly.

At all stages and in all activities, health practitioners who value the wisdom, experience and contributions of community members at all times, will be successful in promoting health.

The second part of this book, Chapters 4 to 9, is practice-based and provides guidance to health practitioners undertaking health promotion practice in a primary health care context. Chapters in Part 2 are underpinned by the principles and concepts fundamental to the health and wellbeing of people and which inform the health promotion practice presented in Part 1. The chapters in Part 2 are presented in reference to the *Framework of health promotion practice in a comprehensive primary health care context* introduced in Chapter 1. Chapter 4 describes the health promotion practice cycle and Chapters 5 to 9 focus on five broad strategy areas of health promotion action. In addition to practice-based content, each chapter includes: putting the Ottawa Charter into action; case examples from Australia and Aotearoa New Zealand; an overview of related IUHPE Core Competencies for Health Promotion; reflective questions; and a More to Explore section.

There are various ways to work in health promotion, and throughout the next six chapters, you will explore many of these, including working:

- *with* individuals, communities and populations
- *in* settings such as workplaces, schools, sporting venues and the arts
- *within* socio-ecological, behavioural and biomedical models
- *on* issues such as discrimination, poverty and natural resource depletion, psychosocial risk factors such as social exclusion, behavioural risk factors such as poor nutrition and physiological risk factors such as stress
- *by* policy development, community action for social change, health education, health information, screening and surveillance
- *using* frameworks such as the Ottawa Charter for Health Promotion to guide you.

To keep developing your skills and expertise in the area of health promotion you can do the following:

- *Use the information in this book to develop your skills.* Put the ideas into practice and see which ones work for you and the community within which you work.

- *Keep reading about the areas covered in this book.* Each area is based on sound theory and practice. As you develop your background in the areas, you'll be more effective in developing your practice.

- *Talk with your colleagues.* Discuss your ideas, your successes and your challenges with anyone who is interested to learn with you.

- *Ask questions.* Successful people draw on the expertise of others.

- *Share your learning professionally by joining professional associations, attending conferences and presenting papers on your work.* So many people who do great work fail to recognise how many people would like to hear about their work and learn from it.

- *Work together, supporting and encouraging each other and promoting the health of the team.* A great many of the strategies described in this book need to be implemented within health organisations first. Developing the self-efficacy of everyone in the team is vital. Work together, support and encourage each other and promote the health of the team. The ripples of this work will be felt far beyond the confines of the organisation and you will be able to establish a team environment that will achieve so much more than that which individuals alone may achieve.

- *Continue working to keep the development of comprehensive primary health care on the agenda, and to ensure that the system moves towards critical health promotion practice.*

4 Health promotion practice

COMPREHENSIVE PRIMARY HEALTH CARE

SOCIO-ECOLOGICAL APPROACH

SELECTIVE PRIMARY HEALTH CARE

BEHAVIOURAL APPROACH

BIOMEDICAL APPROACH

| Healthy public policy to create environments and settings that support health and wellbeing | Community development action to support social and environmental change | Health education and health literacy to develop knowledge and skills for health and wellbeing action | Health information and social marketing to raise awareness about health and wellbeing priorities | Vaccination, screening, risk assessment and surveillance to monitor and reduce risk of disease conditions |

Health promotion community assessment, program planning, implementation and evaluation

INTRODUCTION

This chapter describes the health promotion practice cycle of community assessment, planning, implementation and evaluation. Models and theories underpinning the health promotion practice cycle inform all action areas of the *Framework of health promotion practice in a comprehensive primary health care context* which was introduced in Chapter 1. Using the health promotion practice cycle facilitates the development of a research base for health promotion action in a way that both strengthens the relevance of health promotion work and enables practitioners to be accountable for their practice. Strengthening partnerships between communities, practitioners, governments and researchers is recommended to increase the likelihood of successful outcomes from health promotion programs (Jackson & Greenhalgh, 2015).

Health promotion programs are a coherent series of activities, which together contribute to improving quality of life. A health promotion program is usually developed in response to an identified health and wellbeing priority (Hawe et al., 1990). This chapter begins with health promotion models for practice, followed by the role of research in informing practice. This is followed by the four main sections of the health promotion practice cycle (see Fig. 4.1). The first section provides a rationale for and steps taken in community assessment to identify community health and wellbeing assets and needs. The second section describes the process of program planning in response to the findings of the community assessment. The implementation of a health promotion program plan is addressed in the third section. The fourth section describes the methods used to evaluate the process, impact and outcome of a health promotion program. Before starting the chapter, take some time to review *Putting the Ottawa Charter into Practice* on p. 168.

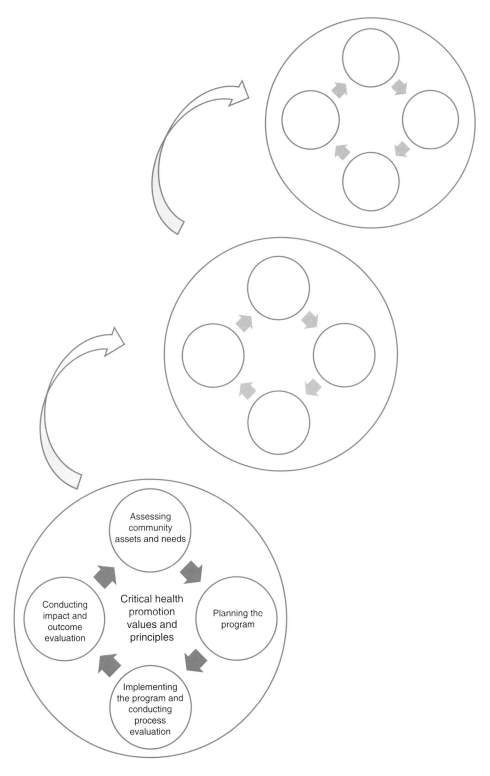

FIGURE 4.1 Health promotion practice cycle

PUTTING THE OTTAWA CHARTER INTO PRACTICE

The following questions, arranged in the Ottawa Charter action areas, are presented to guide health practitioners to reflect on and critically evaluate their professional role and practice and the health promotion philosophy of their organisation. Content of this chapter will assist practitioners to develop the necessary professional knowledge and skills to conduct community assessment and plan, implement and evaluate health promotion programs.

PUTTING THE OTTAWA CHARTER INTO PRACTICE

Build healthy public policy

- Can national, state and local policy priorities provide a rationale for a health promotion program?
- Are there agency protocols for funding community assessment, planning, implementation and evaluation?
- Are there existing international, national, state or local policies that address the health and wellbeing priorities of a community?
- What new policies, legislation, standards or codes of practice are required to address the health and wellbeing priorities of a community?

Create supportive environments

- Are there existing environmental structures or institutions that address the health and wellbeing priorities of a community? These may be in social, economic, built or natural environments.
- What new environmental structures or institutions are required to address the health and wellbeing priorities of a community?
- Are communities adequately supported so they are not set up to fail?

Strengthen community action

- Does the rationale for the program clearly state the importance of community engagement and capacity building?
- Is the process of engaging community members clearly documented?
- What methods are being used to engage people?
- Who is participating in the community assessment, planning, implementation and evaluation stages of the health promotion program?
- What roles do they have?
- What is their role in decision making?
- Who is not participating in the community assessment, planning, implementation and evaluation stages of the health promotion program?
- How could they be more engaged?
- Can the community showcase its skills to others?
- What community development strategies or actions are being used in the implementation of the health promotion program?

Continued

PUTTING THE OTTAWA CHARTER INTO PRACTICE Cont.

Develop personal skills

- Are community members supported to develop their skills in community assessment, planning, implementation and evaluation?

Reorient health services

- What role are health services playing in the community assessment, planning, implementation and evaluation of health promotion programs?
- What resources are health services contributing to health promotion programs?
- Do the health services have policies or strategic plans for working with communities on health promotion programs?
- Do the health services have health promotion responsibilities included in the job descriptions of health practitioners?
- To what degree do health services wish to have control or 'ownership' over health promotion programs? Are they willing to share or hand over governance to the community?
- Who are the influential people within a health service?
- Do the health services have a process of responding to the evaluation results of health promotion programs?

HEALTH PROMOTION MODELS

A comprehensive primary health care (CPHC) approach ensures that the process and outcome of health promotion action are acceptable to the community and mindful of social justice, while ensuring the efficiency and effectiveness of the organisation or agency undertaking the action. The fundamental proposition of health promotion action is that health and wellbeing priorities are influenced by multiple interrelated socio-ecological determinants. As such, health promotion efforts must be multidimensional and multisectoral.

Conceptual health promotion models provide structure and organisation to a health promotion program. There are no perfect models and all have their strengths and weaknesses. However, all models address the components of the health promotion practice cycle. There are many useful resources to help practitioners in the health promotion practice cycle.

Models used by practitioners to guide their health promotion practice include: *Ottawa Charter for Health Promotion* (WHO, 1986); *PRECEDE–PROCEED Model* (Green, n.d.); *Needs Assessment and Planning Model* (Hawe et al., 1990); *Program Management Guidelines for Health Promotion* (New South Wales Department of Health, 1994); and *Circle of Health, Health Promotion Framework* (Prince Edward Island Health and Community Services System, 2003). There is considerable variation in the level of technical detail provided across the models. For example, both the *PRECEDE–PROCEED Model* and *Needs Assessment and Planning Model* provide more comprehensive detail about undertaking community assessment and evaluation. The *Needs Assessment and Planning Model* and Program Management Guidelines for Health Promotion provide moderate to comprehensive detail on planning and the latter provides a moderate level of detail on implementation. There is very limited detail across the models about implementation and sustainability. Program Management

Guidelines for Health Promotion is the only model that explicitly incorporates sustainability as a structural component, and the *PRECEDE–PROCEED Model* identifies it as an important tenet.

With respect to theoretical foundations, the only model that articulates the theoretical foundations upon which the model is based is the *PRECEDE–PROCEED Model*. Both *PRECEDE–PROCEED* and *Circle of Health* models indirectly identify the relevant health paradigm. The only model that refers to values and principles is the *Circle of Health Model*. Even though a list of values and principles is provided, there is no detail about how these values and principles might be applied in practice. Recognition of these gaps in existing models led to the development of the *Red Lotus Health Promotion Model* (Gregg & O'Hara, 2007).

The *Red Lotus Health Promotion Model* was published in 2007 by Jane Taylor (nee Gregg) and Lily O'Hara, two of the authors of this book, in response to the need for a model of health promotion practice that explicitly included the values and principles of critical health promotion and their application (Gregg & O'Hara, 2007). Since then it has been used in teaching, research and practice in Australia, the UK, USA, United Arab Emirates and Qatar. The model has recently been revised and is now known as the *Red Lotus Critical Health Promotion Model*. The model uses the image of a lotus plant to depict the essential components of critical health promotion. The pod of the flower represents holistic health and wellbeing, with the multiple seeds in the pod reflecting the various aspects of health and wellbeing, including physical, cognitive, emotional, social, cultural and spiritual aspects across the spectrum from illness and disability through to flourishing. Some seeds may be more robust than others, and will inevitably change over time. Likewise, health and wellbeing is not a set or complete state, but a complex and ever-changing set of states.

The stamens surrounding the pod and the first layer of petals represent the determinants of health and wellbeing, using a socio-ecological approach. The stamens represent the aspects of individual people that contribute to the various aspects of health and wellbeing, including: biological factors (age, sex, genetics and physiological status); socio-economic factors (education, employment, ethnicity, income, and marital status); cognitive factors (knowledge, attitudes, values and beliefs); affective factors (emotions, feelings and moods); and people's behaviours (physical, mental, social, cultural and spiritual).

The first layer of petals represents the environmental determinants of health and wellbeing, including the social, cultural, economic, policy, natural and built environments, operating at multiple levels from the individual through to the family, group, community, population and global levels. The pod (health and wellbeing), stamens (individual-level determinants) and first layer of petals (environmental determinants) are organically interconnected and therefore multidirectional impacts are recognised. Changes to any of the individual or environmental determinants impact on health and wellbeing, but so, too, do changes in health and wellbeing influence or affect the determinants.

The other four petal layers of the lotus flower represent the health promotion practice cycle components of community assessment, planning, implementation and evaluation. Together, the whole lotus flower represents health and wellbeing, the determinants of health and wellbeing and the health promotion process required to enhance health and wellbeing. The pod cannot survive without the stamens and petals of the flower, and so enhanced health and wellbeing cannot be achieved without all of these components being considered.

In addition to flowers, the plant produces leaves which represent sustainability. The leaves are the permanent component of the plant and remind us to always consider processes that will enhance the sustainable outcomes of health promotion action. The leaves and the flowers of the lotus plant are connected by stems to the plant's roots. The roots and stems represent the values and principles of critical health promotion that must be present for the plant to produce leaves and flowers. All parts of the lotus plant impact on each other, and the whole of the plant is greater than the sum of its parts.

Values are regarded as the process or outcome that is valued, and principles are the action required to attain the value. The values and principles of the *Red Lotus Critical Health Promotion Model* are described in Table 4.1. They are contrasted with the values and principles of selective health promotion, which is the type of health promotion practice more consistent with selective primary health care. The *Red Lotus Critical Health Promotion Model* explicitly articulates the ethical and technical values and principles required for critical health promotion. In doing so, it encourages health practitioners to engage in critical reflection to determine the extent to which their current practice is reflective of these values and principles, and consider strategies that will enable them to move their health promotion practice towards a more critical approach.

HEALTH PROMOTION PRACTICE CYCLE

The health promotion practice cycle (see Fig. 4.1) is an ongoing iterative cycle of assessing community assets and needs, planning a health promotion program, implementing the program strategies, and evaluating the implementation process, short-term impacts and long-term outcomes of a program. This is followed by re-assessing, re-planning, re-implementing and re-evaluating, in a continuous cycle of reflection and action (Baum, 2016; Bauman & Nutbeam, 2014; Wadsworth, 1997). All health promotion models include these stages of the health promotion practice cycle; however, only the *Red Lotus Critical Health Promotion Model* explicitly identifies the critical health promotion values and principles that relate to each stage. The steps within each stage of the cycle are outlined in Table 4.2. A detailed description of each stage and the steps follows.

The stages of community assessment and evaluation are often framed as research processes, as they involve the collection of data to answer research questions about the community before a program, and then questions related to the process, impact and outcome of a health promotion program during and after the program. However, the whole health promotion practice cycle may be framed as a research process, as even the planning and implementation phases must involve critical reflection on practice-oriented questions. As such, before delving into each stage of the cycle, it is important to discuss issues related to health promotion as a research process.

RESEARCH AND PRACTICE

Systematically collecting and analysing information about communities is integral to the health promotion practice cycle. Evidence improves practice and limits wasting resources that are often scarce. When research is integral to practice, practice is strengthened in several ways. First, health promotion practice will be built around the assets and needs of the people for whom it is designed. It will be responsive to those assets and needs and based on recognition that priorities are dynamic rather than static and therefore change over time. Second, with grounding in community health and wellbeing priorities, health practitioners are less likely to implement programs that do not meet these priorities, thus

TABLE 4.1 Health promotion values and principles

Focus of Value and Principle	Red Lotus Critical Health Promotion Model		Selective Health Promotion Practice	
	Value	Related principle – action on the value in practice	Value	Related principle – action on the value in practice
Health paradigm	Holistic health paradigm	Seeing health as a complex concept that includes physical, mental, spiritual, social, and cultural aspects of wellbeing that relate to the whole person.	Biomedical-behavioural health paradigm	Seeing health as the absence of disease or injury, and the absence of 'unhealthy' behaviours, primarily related to the body and mind, excluding social and spiritual health and wellbeing.
Program approach	Salutogenic approach	Emphasising salutogenic factors that create and support health, wellbeing, sense of coherence, happiness and meaning in life.	Deficit approach	Emphasising risk factors for disease.
Scientific approach	Ecological science	Using the science of ecology, which recognises that: people exist in multiple ecosystems, from the individual, to the family, group, community and population levels; all parts within systems impact on each other; the whole of any system is greater than the sum of the parts.	Reductionist science	Using reductionist science in which understanding about the whole comes from simply understanding each part.
Who to work with	Focus determined by equity	In recognition that access to health promoting conditions of living is a human right, prioritising work with people and communities that are most marginalised, vulnerable, and disadvantaged based on considerations of equity.	Focus on whole groups or populations	Prioritising work with more visible groups or whole populations, or the less vulnerable and more accessible populations.
Professional role	Working with people as an ally	Working with people as a culturally competent ally and resource who is respectful of all aspects of diversity.	Working on people as an expert	Working on people as an outside expert who assumes they know what is best for them.

Assumptions about people	Assume people are doing the best for their wellbeing	Assuming that when left to their own devices, people will do the best for their wellbeing and that of their families and communities, given their circumstances and available resources.	Assume people are not doing the best for their wellbeing	Assuming that left to their own devices, people will naturally adopt "unhealthy" lifestyles".
Basis for practice	Comprehensive use of evidence and theory	Basing health promotion practice on evidence of community assets and needs, sound theoretical foundations, and evidence of effectiveness.	Limited or selective use of evidence and theory	Basing health promotion practice on selective use of evidence of need and/or effectiveness; not applying appropriate theory to practice.
Strategy approach	Portfolio of multiple strategies	Using a portfolio of strategies incorporating all action areas of the Ottawa Charter.	One or two strategies	Using predominantly one or two strategies, particularly legislation and regulation, and developing personal skills for behaviour change.
Engagement processes	Empowering engagement processes	Using participatory enabling processes that empower and meaningfully engage people most impacted by an issue in collaborative governance and decision making to gain increased control over their lives and the determinants of their health and wellbeing.	Disempowering engagement processes	Using non-participatory patriarchal processes that exclude people most impacted by an issue from collaborative governance and decision making by targeting those 'at risk' and that do not address the determinants health and wellbeing.
Personal autonomy	Respect personal autonomy	Ensuring all relevant parties consent to health promotion change processes and acknowledging and respecting that not all people will choose the same actions.	Restrict personal autonomy	Expecting all people to adopt the same actions, irrespective of their own preferences.
Beneficence	Maximum beneficence	Actively considering what the benefits of any health promotion change process may be to the full range of beneficiaries.	Limited beneficence	Considering what the benefits of any health promotion change process may be to a limited range of beneficiaries.
Non-maleficence	Non-maleficence is a priority consideration	Actively considering what the potential harms of any health promotion change process may be; who may be harmed by the change processes and in what way; taking steps to minimise or avoid this harm; communicating risks involved in a truthful and open manner.	Scope of maleficence not fully considered	Considering only a limited range of potential harms (due to a belief that health promotion processes will result in positive health outcomes).

preventing expensive mistakes. Third, when research is integral to practice, health promotion and other activities of health practitioners are routinely evaluated and the findings used to improve the quality of health promotion work. The principles underpinning *The WHO Strategy on Research for Health* (WHO, 2012) are that research is of high quality, designed to have the greatest impact, in a style of inclusiveness and collaboration.

A CPHC approach to research can be described by the following elements.

- Research is a dynamic cyclical process, inextricably intertwined with action. Its aim is to improve the conditions under which people live.
- The research process is guided by critical self-reflection on the part of the 'researcher' and the research participants. The values of researcher and research participants are acknowledged up front and are the subject of critical self-reflection as part of the research process.

TABLE 4.2 Stages in the health promotion practice cycle

Stage 1 Assessing community assets and needs
Identify the resources and activities required for community assessment.
Examine the characteristics of the community, including identifying its strengths and assets.
Gather primary and secondary data about health and wellbeing status from primary and secondary data sources.
Analyse the primary and secondary data collected.
Work with the community to identify the health and wellbeing priorities.
Investigate the individual and environmental level determinants of the health and wellbeing priorities.
Ensure a participatory decision-making process.
Clarify what the stakeholders are attempting to achieve.
Investigate what types of health promotion actions are most acceptable and feasible for specific populations and circumstances.
Review existing practice to assess whether the health promotion action is meeting a justified health and wellbeing priority.
Stage 2 Planning the health promotion program
Determine the program goal, objectives and sub-objectives relevant to the health and wellbeing issue, determinants and contributing determinants respectively.
Ensure the program goal, objectives and sub-objectives are specific, measurable, achievable, relevant, and time bound.
Select a portfolio of appropriate strategies to achieve the goal, objectives and sub-objectives.
Develop an action plan to implement the strategies using relevant theories or models.
Assign responsibility to specific stakeholders for each of the actions in the action plan.
Develop an evaluation plan to evaluate the implementation of strategy activities, and the short-term impact and long-term outcomes of the program.
Assign responsibility to specific stakeholders for each of the actions in the evaluation plan.
Ensure collaborative decision making in all aspects of planning.

TABLE 4.2 Stages in the health promotion practice cycle—cont'd

Stage 3 Implementing the health promotion program and conducting process evaluation
Implement the strategy activities as planned.
Prepare materials and resources and train staff.
Inform everyone involved with the program of the implementation requirements.
Collect process evaluation data for the implementation of strategy activities: • Are the actions being implemented as planned? If not, why not? • What is working well? What is not working well? Why? • Are the program materials and services good quality? • Who is being served by the program? Who is missing? Why? What can be done to increase the involvement of equity populations? • Are people happy with the program? What is the actual level of satisfaction? How can it be improved? • Are the resources available for the program? • Are there other unplanned opportunities that have arisen to enhance the reach and quality of the program?
Make changes to the program in light of the process evaluation.
Stage 4 Evaluating the program
Collect data for impact and outcome evaluation.
Analyse the data.
Write the evaluation report.
Distribute the evaluation report to all stakeholders.
Use the evaluation report to advocate for continuing the program or redirecting energies to a different health and wellbeing priority.

- The relationship between researcher and research participants is a partnership that itself acts to change the status quo by breaking down the traditionally 'top-down' approach of researchers. Thus, all people involved in the research process are best described as research partners.

Working on, for and with others in research

The health promotion practice cycle requires practitioners to collect various forms of data. It is important to distinguish between research arising from, being assigned to, or imposed on, the community (O'Leary, 2005). Health promotion research is ideally conducted in ways that are 'democratic, participatory, empowering and life-enhancing' (Stringer & Genat, 2004, p. 28). The centrality of community participation in health promotion, discussed further in Chapter 6, is embedded in the Ottawa Charter definition of health promotion as 'the process of enabling people to increase control over, and improve their health' (WHO, 1986). The emphasis must be on working with people as equal partners, involving them in the research process and acknowledging their expertise. This will ensure that the research conducted is relevant to their priorities and therefore useful. This approach to research involves working collaboratively with community members while drawing on a wide range of research methods. Planning committees comprising researchers, health practitioners and community members can work together to undertake community assessment, planning, implementation and evaluation of health promotion programs. Contributions of community members in defining the parameters of the research and reviewing priorities that arise, from their perspectives as community members, add much to the value of the research.

Some research methods have this participatory approach embedded in the research process. Of note here are participatory action research (PAR) and feminist research (Wadsworth, 1997). They are ideal approaches to working with community members, enabling them to reflect on their own experiences, plan how they can act to change their situation, act and then evaluate the impact of the changes in order to then re-plan, re-act and re-evaluate in a continuing cycle of change, development and learning. PAR also provides a framework for health practitioners to continually analyse and develop their own practice. That is, it provides a framework for good reflective practice (Baum, 2016).

Challenges to participatory research approaches

Developing participatory research in a way that is both rigorous and accepted by professional colleagues and funding bodies on the one hand, and meaningful and acceptable to community members participating in the process on the other, is a challenge. Involving community members as partners in the process means that the process may become unpredictable and uncontrollable. This may create difficulties for people if the framework in which they are working doesn't allow for flexibility, or if the community members want to take the process in a direction that is against the principles of health promotion and CPHC. This is by no means a simple issue. How do practitioners balance the need to be flexible in their approach, ensure community members are true partners in the process and maintain the rigour of research at the same time? It is necessary to grapple with these challenges.

Baum (2016) highlights the issue of power in PAR and whose worldviews dominate the research (see More to Explore at the end of this chapter). She argues that 'PAR is the only empirical method available to public health that will allow such wide-ranging assessments of complex realities and policy and political engagement' (Baum, 2016, p. 407). Discussion of the worldviews or philosophies that underpin all research is beyond the scope of this chapter; however, the principles of health promotion and CPHC outlined in Chapter 1 and the values discussed in Chapter 2 are a starting point for the conduct of any research in communities. Further, it is important to reflect on the discussion about culture and cultural safety and competence in Chapter 2.

Research with Indigenous communities

The principle of working in partnership with people is central to health promotion, but unfortunately is not always evident. Arabena's discussion (2010) of Indigenous knowledge across the world and research in Indigenous communities in Australia is instructive (Kendall et al., 2011; O'Donahoo & Ross, 2015). The way we conduct research has been traditionally based on 'Western' ways of doing research with 'culturally insensitive research designs and methodologies that fail to match the needs, customs, and standards of Aboriginal communities' (Kendall et al., 2011, p. 21). In New Zealand, research involving Māori or Pacific peoples is expected to be conducted or facilitated by people of the same ethnicity—in recognition of not researching 'on' but researching 'with' these population groups.

Research conducted within Indigenous communities, minority groups and other cultural groups requires specific knowledge of those groups that makes it imperative that they are involved in every aspect of the research. Engagement with communities needs to start before a research proposal is put forward and continued throughout. It is also imperative that health practitioners are aware of ethical guidelines that provide clear procedures for the initiation, protocols, participation and ownership of the research process.

Guidelines for ethical practice

Health promotion research should be conducted with all the considerations and safeguards expected of all forms of research. There are international and national rules governing how research is conducted based on the core ethical values of merit and integrity, justice, respect and beneficence. In Australia, the Australian Health Ethics Committee advises the National Health and Medical Research Council (NHMRC) on ethical issues relating to health and the development of guidelines for the conduct of medical research involving humans. *Guidelines for Ethical Research in Australian Indigenous Studies 2012* (Australian Institute of Aboriginal and Torres Strait Islander Studies, 2012) guides research in Australian Indigenous communities so that researchers follow a process of meaningful engagement and reciprocity between the researcher and the individuals and/or communities involved in the research. Jamieson and colleagues (2012) have published 'Ten principles relevant to health among Indigenous Australian populations'. The Health and Disability Ethics Committee (n.d.) provides guidance for New Zealand researchers. Human research ethics committees (HRECs) oversee research on behalf of many organisations. These committees are found in large organisations such as universities, education departments, health departments and large hospitals. It is not proposed that we deal comprehensively with ethical issues here. (Also see, for example, Bamberger et al., 2012, Chapter 9; Centers for Disease Control and Prevention, n.d.; Jamieson et al., 2012; Posavac, 2011, Chapter 5; Purtillo & Doherty, 2011 for a comprehensive discussion of codes of behaviour and ethics.)

Approval for community assessments and evaluations

There has been some debate about whether HREC approval is needed for health promotion practice, particularly community assessments and evaluations (Allen & Flack, 2015; Posavac, 2011). Some argue that much can be gained by seeking approval from HREC in any circumstance. Others argue that if the community is involved in identifying their own health and wellbeing priorities, and planning, implementing and evaluating appropriate health promotion initiatives to address these priorities, then seeking approval from an outside HREC is unnecessary. Allen and Flack (2015) argue that although the overall objective of research may be of public benefit and people may choose to participate in research for altruistic reasons, research activity may not necessarily have a direct individual benefit, and so great care must be taken. Awareness of power relationships is the most important consideration. Power imbalances may emerge in the research procedures in community assessments and evaluation. The values and principles of critical health promotion and CPHC provide a solid foundation for conducting community assessments and evaluation within the health promotion practice cycle. However, given Baum's (2016) discussion of power and PAR, and the issues raised about culturally insensitive research above, further discussion is needed concerning some of the ethical issues for health practitioners to consider.

Five categories of ethical issues have been identified:

1. *Treating people ethically*
2. *Recognising role conflicts*
3. *Using valid methods*

> 4. *Serving the needs of the program participants*
> 5. *Avoiding the negative effects of the research.*
>
> *(Posavac & Carey, 2003, p. 97)*

Treating people ethically

Health practitioners need to consider whether any harm will be done during the research process. Practitioners may need to take training in cultural awareness and there are four major principles to consider. First, treating people ethically means having an understanding of, and respect for, the culture and history of the community. Second, there needs to be clear and sustainable benefits to the community. Third, culturally sensitive methods need to be observed, and fourth, meaningful participation of the community in the entire research process is imperative (Kendall et al., 2011; O'Donahoo & Ross, 2015).

A core ethical value is respect and it is important to reflect on how this is demonstrated. Involving the community in the design and implementation of the research has been discussed. The quality of the data collection process is another and several aspects need to be considered including whether the people conducting the research have the necessary skills. For example, Allen and Flack (2015) argue that HRECs should not be asked to approve a survey written by someone with no expertise in survey design.

Obtaining informed consent prior to research is routine research practice. The emphasis here is on *informed*, which means that the information explaining the research and negotiating the participants' role must be done in a way that can be understood, therefore enabling communities to truly make an informed decision about whether to participate or not. O'Donahoo and Ross stated that 'permission without understanding is inherently exploitative' (2015, p. 5305). Further, confidentiality agreements may need to be considered too. It is often not necessary to identify the participants or the community, because usually it is their opinion that is needed, not a record of their name and contact details. However, if it is necessary, utmost care must be taken to protect these, and, if confidentiality is promised, it must be preserved (Posavac, 2011).

Recognising role conflicts

Ethical dilemmas sometimes arise from the conflicting interests of the stakeholders. A conflict of interest may occur if someone has a personal interest in a particular outcome (Allen & Flack, 2015). How the stakeholders could be affected by the findings is a significant issue to be considered before the research takes place.

- Why is the research being done?
- Who is conducting the research?
- Who will have access to the findings?
- How will the findings be used?

These are important questions which, when addressed, prevent conflict and compromised research procedures (Posavac, 2011). A negotiated Indigenous research agreement may be needed (Allen & Flack, 2015; Kendall et al., 2011). O'Donahoo and Ross (2015) suggest story-telling in Indigenous communities enables a two-way transaction in communication. This 'back and forth' process may need to happen many times. Translating Western ideas into Indigenous narratives about the research and enabling researchers to see the research within the community worldview ensures genuine engagement and understanding. They advise that knowing who can speak on behalf of the community is imperative. In a fragmented community this can be a challenge, but this is not a reason to bypass ethical practice guidelines.

Using valid methods

When potential harms have been considered and minimised, and benefits to the community are clear, it is important to focus on the validity of the program. Research design must fit the needs of those who will utilise the information. Conducting research that is not suitable for the purposes for which it was commissioned is unethical. Interpersonal skills need to be highly developed. Experienced data collectors and analysts need to be involved in research. If quantitative methods are to be used, then a standardised test appropriate to the setting will minimise the risk of invalid results (Posavac, 2011). If interviews form part of the process, then experienced and culturally appropriate interviewers are required to avoid cultural insensitivity or wasting the interviewee's time and research program funds through meaningless or inadequate interviewing. Good interviewing practice requires tremendous skill and sensitivity.

Serving the needs of the program participants

People will not benefit from the findings if they are not published (Posavac, 2011) and as we have said, working with participants in program development and evaluation maximises the chances of addressing the priorities of the participants. Collecting data that do not address the priorities of the participants, directly or indirectly, is unethical.

Avoiding the negative effects of the research

People can be hurt through a lack of due diligence leading to insensitive research and inaccurate findings. Disclosure of personal information carries risks for an individual, including embarrassment, loss of dignity, stigmatisation and discrimination in employment (Allen & Flack, 2015). The process and outcomes of research undertaken in Indigenous communities has largely been a negative experience for Indigenous community members (Kendall et al., 2011). O'Donahoo and Ross noted that 'Indigenous communities are heartily sick of being told they are poorer, sicker and less functional than mainstream Australia' (2015, p. 5307). Evidence-informed program design can minimise the negative effects of research.

Now that we have a sound ethical base for conducting health promotion research, we can move on to describing the stages in the health promotion practice cycle in more detail. We begin with Stage 1 Community assessment.

STAGE 1: COMMUNITY ASSESSMENT

Assessing community assets and needs is the first stage in the health promotion practice cycle (see Fig. 4.1 and Table 4.2) and the essential starting point for health promotion work. Community assessment can be defined as a process that results in:

> ... a comprehensive description of the (assets and) needs of a population that is defined, or defines itself, as a community, and the resources that exist within that community, carried out with the active involvement of the community itself, for the purpose of developing an action plan or other means of improving the quality of life in the community.
>
> *(Hawtin et al., 1994, p. 13)*

This definition highlights considerations central to meaningful community assessment (adapted from Hawe et al., 1990).

- Community assessment is a process of determining both the assets and needs of a community. While considerable attention tends to be focused on the needs of communities, and these certainly are important, a focus on needs alone tends to paint a 'deficit' picture of communities. This can be a negative, disempowering experience for communities and ignore the positive characteristics and resources of that community. Community assets can be a source of pride for the community and may hold a key to successfully addressing the needs that arise.

- Community assessment should be carried out with the active participation of community members. Community members have the right and ability to be meaningfully engaged in identifying what their assets and needs are. Good community assessment is a participatory process.

- Community assessments are carried out for the specific purpose of achieving change that improves the health and wellbeing and quality of life of those living as part of that community. A community assessment is not an end in itself, but a guide to action. Unless community assessments are acted on, they are a waste of time and resources. Community assessments that leave few resources for acting on what is found, or for which there is no real commitment to act on after their completion, are unethical. They do little to help those for whom the community assessment is purportedly being carried out, and are likely to result in significant community frustration.

In preparing to assess the assets and needs of any individual, group or community, it is vital to know why the assessment needs to be done. What needs to be known, and to what end? This will help determine how the assessment should be conducted. Adequate resources need to be available. As discussed, identifying needs, creating the expectation that something will be done about them, then not acting, is unlikely to develop confidence in those whose time has been wasted. Community assessment should reflect the socio-ecological perspective of health and wellbeing, and involve both formal and informal assessment of assets, needs and resources. It should be conducted in partnership between community members and practitioners.

Before expanding on the steps in a community assessment, we need to think about who or what the 'community' is and what is meant by community assets and needs. Community is defined in Chapter 2 and discussed further in Chapter 6. In the health promotion practice cycle, the essential initial questions are:

- Is the community local, state/territory or national?
- Is it a community of interest or a geographical community?
- How homogeneous or heterogeneous is the community?
- How will you engage as many people in the community as possible?

Community assets and needs

Assets

Kretzmann and McKnight (1995) have demonstrated that assessment of community assets, such as community members' skills, is essential in program planning. To encourage and build healthy communities, the unique capabilities that communities offer in developing, nurturing and caring for their citizens must be identified (Cavaye, n.d.; McKnight, 2010). This approach does not imply that communities do not need additional resources from the outside. Rather, that outside resources will be much more effectively used if the local community is fully mobilised and engaged, and if members can define the agendas for which additional resources must be obtained. The primary reason for incorporating this approach is that there is considerable evidence to suggest that community action is successful when local communities are committed to investing in themselves, including identifying and developing their own assets (McKnight & Kretzmann, 2005, p. 158).

Assets fall into three main categories: primary, secondary and potential building blocks (McKnight & Kretzmann, 2005). These assets are mapped alongside the needs of the community. Primary building blocks comprise assets in the community, largely under community control. These include the skills and connections within a community, as well as the community-controlled organisations such as citizens associations, business associations and religious organisations. Secondary building blocks are assets in the community but controlled by outsiders. These can be divided into three main categories: private and non-profit organisations; public institutions; and resources such as hospitals, social service agencies, schools, police, libraries and parks. Partnerships between individuals and agencies can be formed to run these facilities. Potential building blocks are resources outside the community controlled by outsiders. These include major public assets such as public capital improvement expenditures, which empowered communities may begin to redirect to community building purposes (McKnight & Kretzmann, 2005). In Bajayo's (2012) discussion of building resilience in the face of climate change, four sets of networked resources are proposed that individually and collectively build resilience in the face of natural disasters (see Chapter 3 on climate change and health system responses). The resources include economic development, social capital, information and communication, and community competence.

Needs

While comprehensive community assessment examines both the assets and needs of a community, the notion of needs has a central place in community assessment. This is especially so when there is a focus on social justice and working to achieve equity for those who are most marginalised. Arguably, any community assessment should start with an examination of what need is and a review of some of the issues surrounding the definition of something as a need. Need has been defined as 'the condition marked by the lack of something requisite' (Yallop, 2005). This definition highlights the fact that the very concept of need itself is value-based and socially constructed. Whether something is identified as a need will depend on the perspectives and values of those involved. In addition, the way in which health and wellbeing priorities are defined at a social and political level influences how individuals, groups and societies come to decide which issues are of concern to them and which things they need. Given the value-laden nature of need, it is important to be clear about which values are driving the needs-identification process.

There are several different ways in which needs can be classified. Bradshaw's (1972) typology of *felt need, expressed need, normative need* and *comparative need* is useful. Which health and wellbeing priorities are constructed as needs depends on the particular values in place in the society or group. The categories of felt and expressed need include need determined by community people themselves, while the category of normative need represents need determined by experts, and comparative need by past responses to similar priorities or differences between one community and another. With an emphasis on equal partnership between practitioners and community members in a CPHC approach to health promotion, all these types of need have something useful to contribute to an assessment of need and an over-reliance on one type of data has its limitations. All these needs described below tell practitioners different things.

Felt need

Felt need is most easily described as what people say they need (Bradshaw, 1972). For example, if a local community is surveyed regarding its highest priorities for health promotion action, people may say that they want more intensive-care beds, safer streets in which their children can play or less youth unemployment in the local area. Felt need is important because it involves asking people themselves what their needs are. However, on its own it may not give a complete picture of need for several reasons.

First, people may limit what they tell practitioners they need to what they think they can have. If they believe that meeting some of their needs is beyond their reach, they may not ask for them. Second, people may only voice needs that they believe practitioners are interested in. For example, if a practitioner asks someone about their health and wellbeing needs, that person may interpret the question as referring to his or her illness problems alone and may not think of health in its broad context.

A third reason why felt needs should not be the sole source of information is that powerful groups in the community can have a strong influence in determining how people see their needs. Community members' beliefs about what they need can be socially constructed by interest groups, opinion leaders and the mass media. Groups and communities may 'adopt' certain needs as their own because these have been sold to them through the mass media. In many instances, it is not the need alone but also one potential response to the need that is presented as the 'solution'.

Finally, the perspective of a small group of community members may not reflect the perspective of the whole community. Careful consideration needs to be made of whom a group of community informants represents—a section of the community, a small subsection or only themselves. A useful consideration when conducting a community assessment is whose voices are not represented. This will provide some insight into the most marginalised people in the community. Effort will need to be made to connect with these people using culturally appropriate and ethical processes.

The principles of equity, empowerment and sustainability mean that health and wellbeing are promoted when health promotion programs are based on people's own assessment of their felt needs. However, because of the forces that influence people's perceptions of felt need, they may not have had a real opportunity to decide for themselves. In health promotion, as in any other area of health, practitioners need to ensure that people can make informed decisions and that they have access to the information they need to make those decisions. Of course, this process may require more than giving people information; it may require them to examine the forces that influence their decisions. That is, this process of helping people clarify their felt needs may involve the process of conscientisation (Freire, 1974). In Chapter 3, Insight 3.4 is an example of a process of local conscientisation in Australia on issues related to gas and coal.

Another important point to note is that the felt need is often expressed in the form of a solution, which can be very limiting. It is worth asking what is the health and wellbeing priority rather than what is the solution to the priority. There may be many creative solutions to identified priorities. Furthermore, health promotion funding is currently made available for specific programs, often aimed at particular diseases or risk factors. Frequently, funding may be granted and the program begun without any prior systematic assessment of the community's felt needs. The program being funded may be a long way down the community's list of priorities, and people may not be motivated to participate in the activities. It is imposed on the community, and, at best, the community is simply told about why they should want it. This approach to funding presents some very real dangers, as it encourages practitioners and others to ignore a community's own assessment of its needs, or regard them as a simple 'add on' rather than an integral part of the program.

The project focused on linking community participation and therapeutic landscapes to develop social prescriptions for health (Aitken et al., 2015) (Insight 4.1) is a good example of community-based research that explored the felt needs of a community. Community members were asked to identify places in their community that affected their health positively or negatively. Participants could focus on healthy places, develop strategies to deal with unhealthy places and change their therapeutic landscape by adding health to place.

The identification of felt need is important, but not sufficient to identify health and wellbeing priorities. What if a group or community wants something but there is no evidence to demonstrate the need for it? In such a situation, more information may be needed. Does the group or community know that it is comparatively well off in the area concerned? This may change the priorities that the group sets. Conversely, is it the case that there is a lack of formal evidence in this area because of the shortcomings of information

---

INSIGHT 4.1 Linking community participation and therapeutic landscapes to develop social prescriptions for health

Building social capital in rural communities encompasses the notion of 'boundary crossing' where:

> *Boundary crossers understand the culture and language of community and health service domains and have the trust of both. Rural health professionals living within the communities they serve are ideally placed to harness community capacity so as to influence community-level determinants of health.*
>
> **(Kilpatrick et al., 2009, p. 284)**

As a rural pharmacist, I was interested in exploring the notion of community participation to improve rural health outcomes of the community in which I live and work. Part of my journey resulted in me enrolling in a PhD to become the researcher of the '*Improving the health of communities through participation*' research project. The research included asking community members to locate on a map the places that affected their health and wellbeing. These places became a therapeutic landscape for participants, which could have a positive or negative effect on health. Community members wanted a place that promoted healthy living, got retired people 'off the couch' and encouraged socialisation and intergenerational dialogue. Adding health to places involved developing three community gardens in Warracknabeal, Beulah and Hopetoun. Dietitians, physiotherapists and other allied and community health staff became involved in the program. Community participants reported greater socialisation, healthier eating habits and pride in the shared outcomes of the program.

One of the themes of this research is about capacity building for community stakeholders. The collaboration between the university and the health service has improved the academic focus of the health service staff, built research capacity within the organisation, and improved both health service and community sustainability. Even though I have lived and worked in one of these communities, as the researcher, I have learnt new skills, developed capacity and new relationships with university staff. I am treated as a peer by fellow academics and I have presented research findings at national conferences; outcomes that I would never have been able to achieve in the dispensary, behind a desk or 'on the couch'.

Source: Aitken et al., 2015.

collection, rather than that there is no objective need? These questions demonstrate the importance of collecting information on other types of need.

Expressed need

Expressed need is need that is demonstrated by people's use of services or demand for new or more services. That is, expressed need can be described as 'felt need turned into action' (Bradshaw, 1972). Examples of expressed need include waiting lists for services such as child care, housing or public dental services.

Expressed need has limitations, as people can only add their names to waiting lists for services that already exist or are about to come into existence. Indeed, waiting lists are limited to issues of service provision: for example, it is not possible to join a waiting list for a new public policy; however, the number of letters written to a politician on an issue may be regarded as another form of expressed need.

The constraints on people's choices here are even greater than in felt need, since the specific service they are demanding must already be there. Moreover, expressed need can easily be misinterpreted. For example, a waiting list at the local dentist might be interpreted as the need for more dental treatment services, when in fact it could reflect inadequate oral health promotion or lack of awareness of school dental therapy services. Another problem with expressed need is that in many situations people may add their names to all available waiting lists for a particular service, although in reality they would accept only one place (e.g. a nursing home placement). In such a situation, adding up the numbers of names on waiting lists is likely to give an inaccurate impression. In other situations, people may refrain from placing their names on waiting lists if they believe the waiting lists are already long and their chances of success low. In addition, people's beliefs about whether they have a right to particular services, or deserve to have access to them, will influence whether they act to formally express a need.

Normative need

Normative need is need determined by 'experts' on the basis of research and professional opinion. Examples of normative need include safe levels of air and water quality, recommended daily allowances of different food groups, and unsafe levels of lead ingestion. Normatively determined need is often regarded as objective and unbiased because it has been determined by experts. It often carries the assumption that it is value-free and beyond reproach, but this assumption needs to be called into question. Professional opinion often changes over time, leaving the public confused. Normative need may reflect some level of paternalism and it can provide conflicting information, depending on the values of the experts themselves (Bradshaw, 1972, p. 641).

One crucial issue that influences normative need and requires examination is that many professional groups act, often unconsciously, as gatekeepers in society. They may be unable or unwilling to acknowledge publicly that something is occurring at an unsafe level, such as lead levels in a mining town, if their judgement in this case has political implications. This then represents another possible limitation of normatively determined need.

Comparative need

Comparative need is determined by comparing the services or resources in one population or geographical area with those in another population or geographical area. Sometimes it is argued that a particular area requires a certain service because other areas with similar demographic characteristics have one. Comparative need can be useful in highlighting relative deficiencies in some communities. However, it can also be problematic because it is based on the assumption that the service provided in the place of comparison was the most appropriate response to the problem (Bradshaw, 1972), and that the needs of the two areas are the same.

Collecting community data using the socio-ecological determinants of health and wellbeing

Health practitioners need to make themselves aware of what information is already known about a community. (Before we look at this in more detail, a note about the term 'data'. Data is the plural of datum, and although data is used as a singular or plural in common language, it is generally used as a plural in scientific papers. We use it as a plural throughout the book.) There are a number of data sources and collation services to assist this process in the process of collecting community data. All sources of available information must be explored before committing resources to community assessments. Information about a community is only as good as the techniques used to collect it. Qualitative and quantitative methods used in the collection of community data are briefly discussed later. A lot of time and money can be wasted collecting data that are unuseable, or in planning and implementing activities based on data that do not reflect community priorities. Sources of data about a community fall into two main categories.

- *Secondary data sources* provide data from existing sources such as statistical and epidemiological data sources or peer-reviewed published literature. It is important to establish what is already known about the community before setting out to gather more information, and so the secondary sources of data should be explored first.

- *Primary data sources* provide new data directly from community members or by observation of the relationships between the system or subsystems within the community. Primary data can help to develop a deeper understanding of the secondary data, or to address gaps in the secondary data.

Secondary data sources

Secondary data are data that already exist and generally can be accessed relatively easily. These data contribute to the overall picture of a community and are essential to providing a strong rationale for a new program. Conducting a review of the peer-reviewed literature is usually the first task health practitioners take when looking for information about a community and its assets and needs. Furthermore, national databases such as the Australian Bureau of Statistics (ABS) or Statistics New Zealand (Stats NZ), national and regional 'burden of disease' reports, and local government databases that draw on databases such as .id (http://home.id.com.au/) with demographic information, are all rich sources of secondary data. These sources are often referred to as 'grey literature', and are equally as important for sourcing secondary data about communities as the 'black literature' published in peer-reviewed journals. This section deals first with the process of reviewing the black literature, followed by the numerous sources of grey literature.

Peer-reviewed literature

A literature review is defined as '… an extensive, exhaustive, systematic and critical examination of publications relevant to a chosen topic' (Seaman & Verhonick, 1982 in LoBiondo-Wood & Haber, 2002, p. 78). It has two main purposes: first, to critically evaluate published research material; and second, to place current information and activities in the context of previous research. Literature reviews are applied to all parts of the health promotion cycle, from identifying needs and assets, to analysing health and wellbeing priorities, and planning, implementing and evaluating programs. Conducting a literature review before commencing a program not only allows health practitioners to draw wisdom from the experts, but also prevents wasting time, or making the same mistakes that others have made. A later review of the literature may allow an extension of existing knowledge, identification of methods that could be used, or to guide modification of previously tried approaches in order to enhance their effectiveness locally. A literature review sets the current activity into the context of wider health promotion practice. Skills in accessing and reviewing literature are essential to informing different phases of a community assessment.

Searching the literature: There are different types of literature reviews such as systematic reviews, scoping or narrative reviews, and rapid reviews, each with strengths and weaknesses (Grant & Booth, 2009; Robinson & Lowe, 2015). For comprehensive guidance on the literature searching and reviewing process, consult a research methods text. University libraries also provide tutorials online (see More to Explore at the end of this chapter). However, basic principles of conducting a literature review apply. The following provides a brief overview of the main steps in the process and some practical guidelines.

- Primary research, reported in refereed journals, should be the key criteria used for selecting literature. Primary sources are first-hand accounts—research reports written by the researcher.

- Primary sources are preferred because anything interpreted by a second author has the potential to be biased by the views of the second author (LoBiondo-Wood & Haber, 2002, p. 83).

- A literature review requires good knowledge of data sources and skills in using them effectively. McKenzie and colleagues (2013, p. 94) provide a useful diagrammatic outline of a literature search strategy. Be wary of using the easily accessible, but completely non-validated writings and opinions contained in many internet addresses that turn up from a 'keyword' search.

There are many challenges for practitioners in accessing reliable evidence. Many organisations do not provide access to primary data through journal subscriptions or databases such as Proquest or CINAHL. There are some easily accessible websites that can be used to obtain reliable information. Google Scholar, the Cochrane Library and the Campbell Library are three good resources for students and health practitioners to start a literature review. Researchers sometimes post their articles on ResearchGate and similar websites that are free to access. Government websites sometimes provide primary data sources or reviews, and university libraries also provide access to databases and journals to individuals and organisations for a fee.

Secondary literature sources are at least once removed from the primary author. These could include summaries of research studies (e.g. an annotated bibliography). The Cochrane or Campbell libraries and databases of systematic reviews may be useful. Textbooks provide a foundation, particularly in historical, theoretical and conceptual areas, including definitions. However, they contain material assembled from other sources.

The process of searching the literature begins with a question and framing this question clearly helps with the next four steps of: searching the relevant bodies of literature; appraising that literature and managing the results; synthesising the literature; and writing an assessment. The process is iterative in that as you gain more understanding of the topic you will rethink, refine and rework your review (Harvard Graduate School of Education, n.d.). Following the development of the question, keywords are specified and 'included' or 'excluded' to begin a search strategy.

Critical evaluation of the literature: It is essential to critically evaluate published material in order to determine the quality of the research that is being reported and the trustworthiness of the information that is retrieved. The review must identify the strengths, weaknesses, conflicts and gaps in the literature. A literature review is not simply a matter of reading large amounts of literature and providing a narration. It should provide some critique to the reader as to the usefulness of the findings for the current purpose.

Use the following questions as a guide to reflect on each piece of literature.

- Is each piece relevant to the community/group/topic you are working with or does the paper report on a community/group very different from the one you are working with?
- Are the research processes and outcomes credible and sound?
- Are there flaws in the research design?
- Are reasonable conclusions drawn?
- Is the information vital to this review?

Be systematic in collecting the material (McKenzie et al., 2013). After deciding that an item is relevant and useful for the purpose, keep a copy of the article so it can be re-read, and quoted from if required. Be sure to have all the citation requirements at the time. How broad the review needs to be depends on its purpose. A review to inform data gathering for a major research process or higher degree will necessarily be very comprehensive. A short review for a small funding grant may be limited to literature that relates to the local context.

Two simple visual diagrams (Table 4.3 and Fig. 4.2), the literature review grid and the funnel, can be used to explain the techniques and phases in literature management to inform program planning. Concepts that are presented in diagrams or models provide valuable frameworks to assist when searching the literature and when structuring the review (Talbot & Verrinder, 2008).

Making a literature review grid: Making a grid in the reviewing process, before commencing writing, is a useful activity that will assist those who are less experienced with writing literature reviews to collate relevant material and to structure their review well (Talbot & Verrinder, 2008). Set up a grid/table in Microsoft Word or Excel. Some people

TABLE 4.3 Literature review grid

Journal details	Theme 1	Theme 2	Theme 3	Theme 4
Article 1 *Author* *Title summary* *Location*				
Article 2 *Author* *Title summary* *Location*				
Article 3 *Author* *Title summary* *Location*				

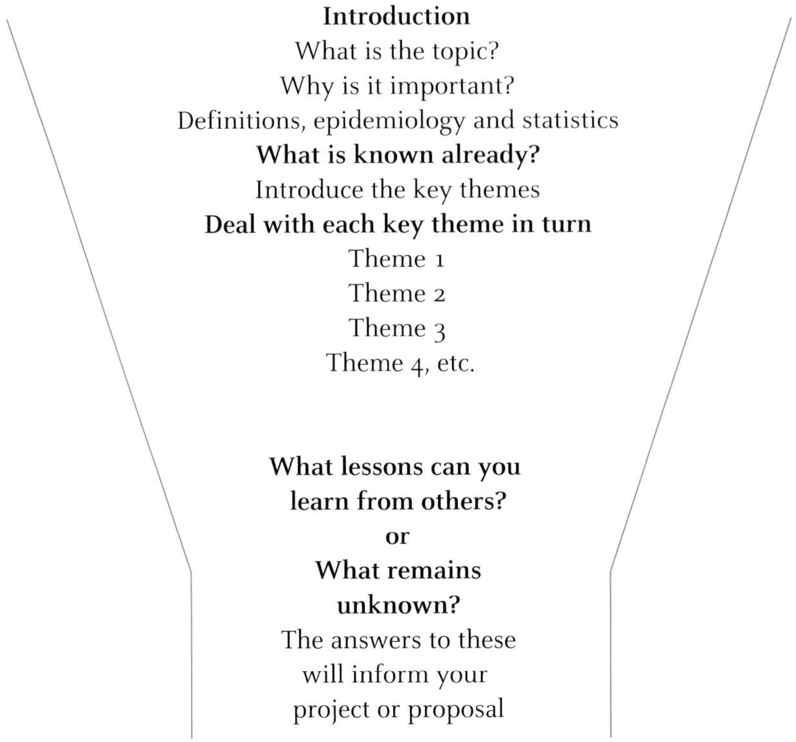

Introduction
What is the topic?
Why is it important?
Definitions, epidemiology and statistics
What is known already?
Introduce the key themes
Deal with each key theme in turn
Theme 1
Theme 2
Theme 3
Theme 4, etc.

**What lessons can you
learn from others?**
or
**What remains
unknown?**
The answers to these
will inform your
project or proposal

FIGURE 4.2 Literature review structural funnel

find it easier to have a hard copy of key articles, so they can highlight main points, but this can also be done within digital files like PDFs. Read all the materials the first time without marking them, to get an idea of what the key themes are. In this way, new keywords can be generated and specific subtopics identified and explored.

In the second reading, highlight aspects of the paper, according to the key themes that are emerging, using the series of questions mentioned in the previous section to evaluate each piece. During this review process, collate the grid—add new themes into new columns as they arise. Use a new row for each article. In the cell, write very brief prompts to enable easy identification of the section of the paper when writing the review (see Table 4.3). (Different-coloured highlighters can also be used to highlight different theme(s) in each paper—one colour per column.) As new themes emerge, the literature searching is broadened to explore its significance in the original topic (Talbot & Verrinder, 2008).

When the literature reading, reviewing process and grid construction are complete, the grid is used to help structure the writing of the literature review so it tells a logical 'story' to the reader, theme by theme.

A good review should answer the following questions.

- What is known about the topic?

- Why is it an important topic?

- What is not known about the topic?
- Why is it important that the knowledge gap is filled?
- What activities or processes might fill the existing knowledge gap?

The process is the same, irrespective of the size of the review. It is useful to conceptualise a literature review as a funnel, which takes the reader from the broad general topic or problem at the start and narrows through the exploration of key themes to the specific focus of the research or program that emerges at the end of the review.

This conceptual diagram (see Fig. 4.2) is useful and draws directly on the grid that was constructed during the reading phase. Commence with an introduction that sets out the purpose of the review and provides a rationale as to why it is a worthy topic. Introduce any key terms and definitions that are necessary for the reader. Outline any limitations in the breadth of the topic being explored or the search parameters. Next, provide a summary of current knowledge of the problem and introduce the key themes that the review will address (i.e. list off the column headings from the grid, in an order that will tell a logical 'story'). The grid provides a 'map' for the review. The key point of advice when using the grid is that the grid rows are assembled horizontally as literature is read and analysed, but when using it to construct the written review, use the vertical columns, one theme at a time, integrating all the points and papers that are made in the cells in that column. This prevents the common problem of simply summarising individual papers sequentially.

Depending on the size of the review, a separate section is composed for each of the themes (or columns). Use a series of headings as 'signposts' to ensure that everything that is included in the section directly relates to that theme (the headings can be taken out at the end). Each theme becomes a 'mini-essay' in itself and so needs a strong introduction. This is followed by a discussion of the literature relating to that theme. Include the following in the discussion for each theme: the critique of what was useful, relevant, reliable about the research; what other research concurs or contradicts the findings; and the gaps in the knowledge related to the theme. After each theme is dealt with, the conclusion should highlight the purpose of the review. For instance, if it has a research purpose, the conclusion should highlight the topic that requires further exploration. If the purpose of the review was to inform health promotion planning or practice, the conclusion should highlight key action areas or wisdom from the field.

The literature review is usually the first step in compiling information about a community's assets and needs. Once this is completed, the health practitioner needs to identify sources of information from the grey literature, including any epidemiological or local profiles that have been compiled about a community, and information about specific determinants at the individual and environmental levels relevant to the community.

Epidemiological profile

Epidemiology has been defined as dealing 'with the incidence, distribution, and control of disease in a population' (Merriam Webster Dictionary, n.d.). However, this definition is more consistent with a biomedical model of health. Holistic approaches to epidemiology frame it as the study of the incidence and geographic, demographic and temporal distribution of states of health and wellbeing and their determinants. Hence, traditional epidemiological data focus on levels of death (mortality) and disease (morbidity) and their distribution in the community according to such criteria as gender, age and place of residence. The holistic application of epidemiology also includes data about levels of physical, mental, spiritual and social health and wellbeing. Epidemiological data come from a number of sources including:

- registries of births and deaths
- health surveys and studies; for example, those conducted by the Australian Institute of Health and Welfare (AIHW)
- social surveys and studies
- hospital discharge records
- reports of notifiable infectious diseases.

By providing information at a population level, epidemiology provides a useful tool to confirm or question the hunches of health practitioners and community members regarding health and wellbeing priorities. This can be valuable because assumptions about priorities in a community may not always be correct. The reports produced by the AIHW (2018), Organisation for Economic Co-operation and Development (OECD) (2019) or Stats NZ (Statistics New Zealand) (www.stats.govt.nz) for example, are of particular value in providing and analysing up-to-date epidemiological data. Also, local public health or health promotion units may prepare epidemiological data relevant to their own areas. Much of these data are available on the internet, especially in the validated reports of government agencies in areas such as women's health, domestic violence, injury surveillance, and mental health and wellbeing.

It is important to note that epidemiological data are not equally available for all health and wellbeing priorities. Some health and wellbeing priorities have well-developed databases (e.g. cardiovascular disease) while others do not. Until relatively recently, the seriousness of Aboriginal and Torres Strait Islander health in Australia was ignored because data were not collected. Relying on pre-existing epidemiological data risks focusing further attention on conditions that are already well identified, at the expense of those that may be serious but that have been ignored in the past.

Morbidity and mortality data are useful when planning health promotion programs; however, used in isolation they are not sufficient to enable us to see all of the determinants of health and illness. Epidemiological data are of limited use in situations where no simple cause-and-effect relationship exists or where delayed onset of symptoms occurs. This may particularly be the case, for example, with environmental health issues where a relatively long timeframe is required before evidence of a problem emerges, by which time a number of people will have already experienced illness or even death. Epide-miology data usually express morbidity and mortality, not the extent of wellness of a community.

Local community profile

Community profiles are usually available on local government municipality websites. Most municipalities have a great deal of information about the community derived from national data repositories and other sources that are valid and updated at regular intervals. Every agency or service that has responsibility to a community will need to have access to a relatively up-to-date profile of that community. This is necessary to have a sense of what needs there may be and what demographic and social issues are likely to be shaping the lives of people in the community. Health practitioners may be part of the team that sets about preparing or updating a community profile.

It is worthwhile to examine what sort of information will be needed to include in a community profile and some of the general principles involved in preparing it. Data gathering in the community can be guided by a series of categories, which can be used to document community assets and needs. Taken together, the information in these categories will provide a picture of the community. However, communities are dynamic and changing and so information will need to be added along the way. A community profile is not something that can be completed and then filed away. Explore all possible sources of second-ary data first, but you may be required to collect additional information. It is important to note that community profile data obtained from governmental sources may not match the specific community that is being assessed. Further data may need to be collected, or the results of the existing profile should be used with caution when applying it to the community being assessed.

In addition to epidemiological and local community profiles, data about other individual and environmental-level factors impacting on a community need to be gathered in order to provide the most detailed picture of the community possible. Data about the individual people can include a range of social and economic factors.

Social and economic data about the people within a community help to construct a richer, more detailed picture of that community. Data may be gathered from national census data and broken down into regions, municipalities and suburbs. Data such as proportions of people in each age group, country of origin, cultural groups, religion, income, education, employment, housing status and use of public transport are examples of the information that is useful in helping to construct a picture of the community. State and local governments and community organisations may also have data about the community. For example, Community Indicators Victoria (CIV) measures wellbeing in the state of Victoria (Community Indicators Consortium, 2017). CIV provides a comprehensive framework of community wellbeing measured by local-level data. The wellbeing indica-tor data can be accessed through Wellbeing Reports, Live Reports or Data Maps. These reports are an example of the combination of secondary data from the ABS and Victorian State Government department sources and primary data from surveys conducted for this site. CIV enables municipalities to gauge the strengths and challenges facing their communities.

In addition to data about people, it is important to gather data about the various environments operating within the community, including the policy environment, physical (built and natural) environments, and social and cultural environments.

Policy environment

Policy documents often provide material from a combination of sources, particularly epidemiological data, social and economic indicators, and the views of professionals. They are developed with varying degrees of community consultation, depending on political will and timeframes. They are often used in rapid reviews and provide an overview or summary rather than systematically searching and critically analysing documents. It is important to note that policy documents are often reflective more of political priorities and processes than of the priorities of the community. The politically determined nature of these documents must be acknowledged. They need to be compared with local evidence of health and wellbeing priorities rather than be assumed to reflect the local picture. With recognition of these issues in mind, such documents can be useful sources of information and should be used wherever possible as one component of identifying needs. They are certainly useful for identifying funding priorities. It is worthwhile finding out about the process by which these documents were developed. Were they simply summarised from state and national documents, or were regional community assessments carried out? They may have been prepared without consulting the community members in the region. Their value may therefore be limited.

Built and natural environments

The physical environment in which people live strongly influences the way in which they can interact with each other. It also may be the source of some health problems for the community. A town that includes a number of dirty industries and is situated in a valley may face serious environmental pollution; a community may have little recreational space within its boundaries; or a suburb may be designed around the needs of cars, often resulting in lack of access to services for those who do not own cars. Evidence to support the importance of connection with nature is burgeoning (Cleary et al., 2017; Folke et al., 2016) and the potential for adverse environmental and ecosystem impacts on public health is increasing. An obvious example is the adverse socio-ecological impacts associated with extractive industries, which 'range from environmental degradation to income inequality to structural violence and beyond' (People's Health Movement et al., 2014, p. 229). Another example, and to a lesser extent, is the provision of shade through the urban tree canopy which Cook and colleagues (2015, p. 7) argue is 'critical to resilience, health, social equity, urban amenity and child-friendly cities in a warming world. Despite these benefits, tree cover remains uneven across metropolitan cities with those most vulnerable experiencing shade and cooling-deficits'. Community assessment processes can raise the issues for public concern and scrutiny, and prompt local action. Health impact assessments outlined in Chapters 3 and 9 are often used.

Social and cultural environments

The social environment of a community includes the social capital (the glue that binds people—see Chapter 2), social justice (see Chapter 2), social structures (organisations) operating within a community, the communication mechanisms used within the community, and the distribution of power and leadership within a community. The cultural environment includes the range of cultural groups and their respective cultural practices. It also includes the history of a community.

Organisations: Several organisations may operate and have influence in a community. Their presence and the role they play in the community could provide very useful information. Organisations can be classified under a number of categories, including local and state government bodies, industrial and commercial organisations, religious bodies, non-profit agencies and voluntary organisations. It is worthwhile finding out about the roles played by each of the organisations in the community and their relationships or partnerships. For example, is there a company that is the main employer? Is there a religious organisation that involves itself in a lot of community work?

Communication: Bajayo (2012) reports that communication is the most important resource for community resilience and further, that local and trusted communications systems best enable resilience. Knowing which mass communication methods are used in the community helps health practitioners understand the community in greater detail. For example, what radio and television stations are received in the area, and which stations seem to be listened to or viewed by which groups of people? Which newspapers are available locally? Is there a local newspaper? Several other effective communication options may also be operating. For example, are there community noticeboards that are well used? Do certain groups use blogs or Twitter? Are there community email networks or Facebook pages?

Power and leadership: Power and leadership can be both formal and informal, and an understanding of both is needed when health practitioners work with a community. Information of value here includes details about leaders of local political parties, local government and community groups as well as key influential people within those organisations. It may also include information about people who seem to have a strong voice in influencing public debate or a particular organisation but who may not necessarily hold a current position of formal authority. All of these types of secondary data are important to gather in order to paint as detailed a picture of the community as possible, and to identify gaps where additional primary data may need to be gathered.

Primary data sources

As per the definition provided earlier, primary data provide new data directly from community members or by observation of the relationships between the system or subsystems within the community. Primary data can help to develop a deeper understanding of the secondary data, or to address gaps in the secondary data. However, it is vital that data gathering is purposeful and ethical.

A great deal of time and money has been spent and an enormous amount of information has been gathered from community members by researchers doing 'data raids'; that is, gathering primary data without a clearly defined purpose in mind, and then making no use of the findings. Such processes are clearly unethical. Successful program outcomes and sustainability depend on community participation from the beginning. Participants in a potential program need to engage with the process and understand the outcomes. Community members may have many under-utilised and under-valued skills.

It is useful to use a conceptual framework such as the *Red Lotus Critical Health Promotion Model* to assist in the collection of primary data. There are qualitative and quantitative options for collecting primary data. It is important to have a basic understanding of each before conducting research to collect primary data in a community.

Qualitative research approach

A qualitative research approach is useful for exploring the 'how?' and 'why?' questions in the community, rather than the 'how many?' questions, which can often be answered from national and local census data and do not usually provide sufficient detail to be a basis for planning a community health promotion program. The aim of a qualitative research approach is to encapsulate the understandings, interpretations and experiences of community members in their everyday lives and environments (Denzin & Lincoln, 2011). A qualitative approach often involves face-to-face methods. There are a number of advantages and disadvantages of using a qualitative approach in community assessments. Some of the advantages include:

- People have a greater chance of defining and describing what is important to their health and wellbeing and why.
- It gives the researcher the opportunity to follow up on cues and explore priorities in detail.
- People are not forced to choose one way or the other—they are able to take a middle ground, or to put up options that have not been previously determined.
- People can begin to contribute to solutions and strategies.

Some of the disadvantages include:

- It is time-consuming and requires a skilled interviewer.
- Some people are unable or unwilling to share personal or private information with others.
- Anonymity cannot always be guaranteed.

- The process may generate more questions than answers, or problems that cannot be managed by a proposed program, and therefore generate further community frustration.

- Vocal participants can dominate.

It will not be practical to talk to all of the chosen community, so the aim is to canvass a broad range of opinion from all of the subgroups represented. Consider a data-gathering approach that will enable best access to as many people as possible, taking account of age, gender, ethnic or language background, employment status and area of residence. Informal networks as well as mass advertising may be the best way of recruiting participants from the various subgroups. Choose an acceptable and convenient location for the interviews or meetings. Prepare a broad interview protocol in advance, which will take only about half an hour. Keep the questions specific to the general theme of health, but be flexible enough to follow strong responses from participants. Use a planning model or theoretical framework (such as the Ottawa Charter) to develop the question framework. Pilot test the questions and then refine them. Have a research assistant or colleague 'scribe' the responses or record the session (with participants' permission). Allow plenty of time to prepare the seating and facilities. Focus groups and public forums need skilled facilitators to ensure that all potential participants have the chance to be heard. Journal and record overall impressions and reflections after each session. Involve local community people as researchers, and ensure you provide them with the appropriate training and support.

Preliminary consultations: The first data-gathering process may be informal and its purpose is to determine the need for, and breadth of, a community assessment. The community may inform health practitioners of issues of concern to them, which may trigger informal information gathering to clarify the felt need. Conversations with other people such as concerned community members, police, teachers, medical practitioners, community workers, local government council staff and others may occur. These groups may contribute a great deal to the assessment of health and wellbeing priorities. In particular, other health practitioners may themselves have listened to community members or may have conducted formal community assessments in the past. Furthermore, several different practitioners may discuss a priority and each brings to it a slightly different perspective, based on individual experience and professional background. Similarly, they may each notice slightly different priorities in the same community. This can all be useful in gaining an understanding of the scope of health and wellbeing priorities facing the community.

Community forum: A community forum is a public meeting to which residents are invited to express their opinions about community priorities. It is important to have a semi-structured plan for the meeting, and to have strategies in place to enable participation from all people who attend, not just the most vocal.

Focus groups: A focus group is a group interview or discussion with a particular focus. The group is also focused because it has people or characteristics in common. These can be either face-to-face or via various online means such as Google Hangouts or Zoom. The group is encouraged to discuss issues of concern to them with a facilitator guiding the discussion to ensure all participants have an opportunity to express their views.

Nominal group process: This process is highly structured where five to seven representatives of a community (usually a subgroup) are asked to qualify and quantify specific priorities. Responses of the group are recorded for all participants to see without further discussion. The group is then asked to rank or order the responses by importance (McKenzie et al., 2013).

Interviews: Face-to-face or telephone interviews are conducted with members of the community. Participants may volunteer to take part or they may be identified because they have some particular relevance to the future wellbeing of the community, its services and its people. Interviews may be conducted with subsections of the community, those who are affected by a particular issue, significant others, key informants or opinion leaders.

In the qualitative data-gathering options mentioned here, it is advisable to use a broad schedule of open questions and themes to guide discussion that prompts full responses, rather than narrow, closed questions that prompt monosyllabic responses (yes or no) and give no guidance for planning future strategies with the community. Consider using the WHO definition of health discussed in Chapter 1.

- What factors make it easier or more difficult for you to achieve good physical wellbeing in your community?
- What determinants make it easier or more difficult for you to achieve good emotional and mental wellbeing in your community?
- What factors make it easier or more difficult for you to achieve good social wellbeing in your community?

These three questions explored thoroughly and sensitively with a range of people in a community may be all that are needed to gain sufficient primary data to inform a health promotion program to build on their assets and address their health and wellbeing priorities.

Observation: Observation of the environment or people is another way of collecting data. These methods require the same attention to ethical standards as any other data collection method. Observations can be direct or indirect, obtrusive or unobtrusive. Individual or community behaviour can be observed. 'Windshield tours or walk-throughs' and photovoice can also be used to make assessments of the environment such as the types and condition of housing, recreational facilities, roads and the natural environment. Photovoice is a method of data collection where community members are provided with training and cameras to capture images of their community's strengths and needs as they see them. The aim is to promote dialogue between community members, practitioners and policymakers about issues the community members have identified using images (Community Toolbox, n.d.; Minkler & Wallerstein, 2008; Wang, 1999).

Analysing qualitative data: Qualitative data are managed systematically using a four-step procedure.

1. Organising the data into a useable form, which may include collating notes and/or transcribing interviews.
2. Shaping the data, which means identifying key themes and categories. The interview schedule will be useful for this, but some data may fall outside what was anticipated by the questions.
3. Summarising the data by identifying the extremes of views or the range of opinion. All responses must be represented, but it is not appropriate to attempt to quantify the results.
4. Explaining what is meant by the data, consistent with the responses you have received.

In many approaches to qualitative research, researchers are advised to interrogate the data by exploring the transcripts line-by-line or paragraph-by-paragraph in a process of constant comparison with previously analysed text to draw out both similarities and disparities. The data are then explored further to establish whether or not there are relationships, patterns or interconnections between the concepts. Grbich (2007, p. 32) describes the process of managing the data as 'block and file' or 'conceptual mapping or a combination of both'. Creswell (2003) describes a similar process of identifying specific segments of information and labelling these to create categories. A process of reducing redundancy among the categories then occurs and a model is created that incorporates the most important categories. Computer software programs such as NVivo can be used to manage qualitative data. These programs are particularly useful in organising large sets of data.

This is a complex process requiring research expertise that is best obtained through practitioners gaining appropriate qualifications in research procedures or working with people who have expertise. Research skills are often limited in health promotion (Chambers et al., 2015). Wood and Leighton (2010, cited in Farmer et al., 2012) suggest that 'third organisations' in particular—that is, social enterprise organisations—are poorly equipped to conduct evaluation (which requires the same skill as community assessments), because there is a lack of skill, resources and time.

Quantitative research approach

A quantitative research approach is useful for exploring the 'how many?' and 'amongst whom' questions about a community. In epidemiology terms, these are referred to as the prevalence, incidence and distribution of issues. Examining distribution includes exploring how issues may differ across geographic areas, between different demographic groups, and over time. There are numerous methods used to collect quantitative data about communities, with the most common being the community survey.

Survey: Few communities are small enough for it to be possible to ask everyone to define their needs and assets. Therefore, often, a community survey will be conducted with a sample of people. Determining which people and how many to ask in order to obtain an appropriate sample is a key component of planning a survey, and requires the involvement of people with expertise in survey development.

Surveys are particularly useful to study 'How often?' or 'How many?' questions about assets and needs. A well-designed survey will enable the researcher to generate a large amount of data at the least cost. It is important to plan the survey process carefully to collect data that informs future planning. The terms survey and questionnaire are often used interchangeably; however, they are not the same thing. The survey is the overall method—to survey means to look over or across. Surveys can involve people surveys, environmental surveys, policy surveys, etc. The instrument used to collect data from people is most commonly a questionnaire. People may participate in a survey by completing a questionnaire. The questionnaire is often referred to as the survey instrument.

Questionnaire design: Designing a questionnaire requires a high level of planning and skill. Using a previously validated questionnaire whenever possible is therefore recommended. For instance, the SF-36™ Short Form Health Survey (Ware, 2000) is a 36-item questionnaire that provides a validated and very quick indicator of health status. It was developed to provide a general health survey that is 'comprehensive and psychometrically sound, yet short enough to be for practical use in large scale studies' (Stephenson, 1996). It covers themes such as physical, social and emotional functioning, role limitations due to health problems, vitality and general health perceptions. As a means of validating the instrument for use in Australia, standard norms for the Australian population have been derived from ABS census data.

If the questionnaire has not been previously validated, it is imperative to pilot test it to ensure the questions can be readily understood, that there is a logical sequence and questions do not lead the respondent into a certain response. As we have said, HRECs should not be asked to approve a questionnaire written by someone with no expertise in survey instrument design (Allen & Flack, 2015). Questionnaires can be distributed by mail, telephone, online tools or in person.

A multistep or Delphi technique may be used instead of a one-off questionnaire. In this approach participants are asked to make more than one contribution. The aim is to build consensus through a series of questionnaires. Broad questions are developed for the first questionnaire. The responses are analysed and the same participants are asked more specific questions in a second questionnaire, which are then analysed. This refinement of questions continues each round until consensus about priority issues is reached (McKenzie et al., 2013).

Analysing quantitative data: Quantitative data can be presented as frequencies of categorical data (such as what proportion of participants agree or strongly agree with a particular statement), or means and standard deviations of continuous data, such as the score on the SF-36^{TM}. These calculations can be made with readily accessible programs such as Microsoft Excel. Higher-level statistical analysis may be conducted to determine relationships between different factors. It may be necessary to recruit someone with higher-level skills in this area to assist with data analysis.

Reporting the findings to the community

Reporting the findings is an essential part of any community assessment, particularly to the people involved to ensure that the information obtained accurately reflects what people said. It will then enable community members to be involved in the priority-setting process discussed in the next section of this chapter. Responses should be presented in a succinct manner, with key findings in an Executive Summary. The report should be made available through a range of venues/forums, so that all people who took part in the data gathering have an opportunity to know of and discuss the results, and to take part in priority setting. Use the media options that will provide the best access, according to the characteristics of the community. Present the information in a format that makes the findings clear and which can be easily understood by all who participated—use tables, graphs, colours, quotes and plain language. Infographics are a common way to communicate research findings to a range of audiences. Unless appropriate probabilistic sampling techniques are used to recruit participants, the researcher must be cautious about making generalisations that apply to the whole community.

Health practitioners' relationships with community

To conclude this stage, it is worthwhile examining the relationship between health practitioners and their communities. Sometimes practitioners suggest that, because they are a part of their community, there is little need to canvass community needs—what they themselves see as problems is an accurate reflection of community needs. However, although health practitioners may be members of a community, they cannot represent all groups in it, and in fact no one can. Because of their professional education and socialisation, health practitioners bring a particular perspective to health and wellbeing priorities. Certainly, this perspective is a valuable one that contributes much to the debate about health and wellbeing and health promotion. Nevertheless, it is only one perspective and cannot be substituted for the opinions of other community members. Therefore, while professional opinion offers a great deal, it cannot be assumed to reflect the views of the whole community or remove the need for listening to the community or checking external assessments of priorities.

Undertaking a comprehensive community assessment will enable the health practitioner to collect data from a broad range of primary and secondary sources about the community's assets and needs. This is the foundation required for moving to the next stage of planning health promotion action.

STAGE 2: PLANNING THE HEALTH PROMOTION PROGRAM

The purpose of planning health promotion action is to devise a program that addresses the health and wellbeing priorities of a community identified in Stage 1 of the health promotion practice cycle (Fig. 4.1), within the available resources.

Separating priorities from solutions

Before designing the health promotion program, the community's health and wellbeing priorities need to be separated from any prematurely proposed solutions. In presenting and analysing the findings of a community assessment, it is possible that the priorities will be expressed in terms of solutions to the priorities, rather than the priorities themselves. Often when this occurs, the assumption is that the solutions presented are the only mechanisms for addressing the priorities. The reason for this may stem from the way people interpret questions about their health and wellbeing assets and needs, which may lead them to think about a solution rather than the priority itself. You may need to 'peel the onion' to get to the deeper layer of understanding: ask what is the priority that leads them to this one solution?

It is very important to develop a vision of the priority as separate from any potential solutions, and so broaden the scope for addressing the priority by coming up with a range of possible solutions. This process is one in which community members and practitioners can think creatively together. It provides an excellent opportunity for consciousness-raising to occur. As people discuss the priorities in their community they may, layer-by-layer, be able to work their way through to alternative conceptualisations of them. This may broaden quite markedly the choices available in addressing those priorities.

Setting priorities for action

It is rarely the case that a community assessment identifies only one priority. Sometimes a number of priorities may be able to be dealt with together if they all share a similar root cause and you have recognised this in your analysis, but this will not always be the case. It will, therefore, be necessary to set some priorities, as it is rare to have the time or other resources to be able to deal with all the priorities at once.

How do you set priorities for action? Some people suggest that you deal with the easiest or most 'winnable' priorities first (e.g. Minkler, 1991), but there are some problems with this approach. The easiest priorities to deal with may not be the ones that make the biggest difference in people's lives. The most difficult ones may well have the biggest impact if they are acted on successfully. Priority setting, done in partnership with community members and other organisations, is likely to be the most successful approach because of the community support for, and action on, any decisions made. Health practitioners need to be aware of complementary programs that already exist in the community, to avoid duplication, and at the same time they may 'piggy-back' strategies for added impact. Of course, there may be times when the health priorities are urgent and time for community involvement may be limited. Even then, maximum possible involvement by community members should be built into the decision making.

Priorities set by national health agencies or organisations can be taken up if they are identified as local health and wellbeing priorities. The advantage here is that if they are national priorities, it is more likely that funding will be available to support health promotion programs and health practitioners will be encouraged to take action in this area. Similarly, some areas may be included in the charter of the agency for which health practitioners work, and so these may need to be addressed first. Furthermore, some priorities may be able to be dealt with first because the necessary expertise is available in the team with which you are working or because you have ready access to it. While it would be a mistake to build an agency's work around the interests of the staff rather than the priorities of the community, acknowledging and working with the expertise of the staff and other available expertise is a valuable use of resources.

There are several questions worth asking about each identified priority in order to help to set priorities for action. The questions to consider could include the following.

- Prevalence: Is the priority widely experienced? How many people are affected?

- Severity: Does the priority cause major or minor problems? Is this a critical priority that should be addressed before other priorities? What will the consequences be if this priority is not addressed?

- Selectivity: Does the priority affect one group within the community more than another?

- Amenability to health promotion action: Are there known successful programs addressing this priority? How can this priority best be addressed? Is it likely to be affected by health promotion action? What programs are presently available to address the priority? Does the priority coincide with the organisation's mission statement or policies? If not, why not? Can the organisation's policies be influenced? What assets (funds, staff, connections, infrastructure, etc.) are available to address the priority? Which community members and other partners are most appropriate to work on these health and wellbeing priorities?

The answers to these questions will lead to the selection of one or more health and wellbeing priorities to address. For each priority, a comprehensive analysis must then be undertaken.

Health and wellbeing priority determinants analysis

A health and wellbeing priority determinants analysis involves the identification of the range of socio-ecological health and wellbeing determinants that contribute to the health and wellbeing priority. One of the common frameworks used to categorise the determinants of a priority that are amendable to change involves identifying the predisposing, enabling and reinforcing determinants or factors (Green, 2005).

- *Predisposing factors*: a person's or population's knowledge, attitudes, beliefs, values and perceptions that facilitate (predispose towards) or hinder (predispose against) the capacity for change to people or environmental conditions.

- *Enabling factors*: people's skills and resources and environmental conditions that facilitate (enable) or hinder (disable) the capacity for change. Facilities or community resources may be ample or inadequate; laws may be supportive or restrictive. Enabling factors thus include all the factors that make a change to people or environmental conditions possible.

- *Reinforcing factors:* the feedback received from others, the rewards, the punishments that result from a change to people or environmental conditions.

Knowing whether the factors are predisposing, enabling or reinforcing will guide the type of program that is ultimately developed. For example, will the program need to increase a community's knowledge (predisposing factor) on a particular topic? Do policies (enabling factors) need to be developed in an organisation or municipality? Are there community elders or other members who need to be engaged in the process of change (reinforcing factors)?

Fig. 4.3 provides an example of a health and wellbeing determinants analysis for the priority issue of exclusive breastfeeding until six months of age. The immediate determinants, and the contributing determinants—the factors that contribute to the immediate determinants—are identified across individual and environmental factors (see, for example, Rollins et al., 2016). Within this analysis, we can categorise factors as predisposing, enabling and reinforcing. For example, some of the factors in the analysis can be categorised as follows:

- Predisposing: mother's intention to exclusively breastfeed, knowledge about the benefits, knowledge about good attachment, perception of adequate milk supply, confidence in feeding in public, knowledge of right to breastfeed in public
- Enabling: self-efficacy to breastfeed, antenatal information about normal sleeping and feeding patterns, access to lactation consultants, workplace policies for maternity leave and breastfeeding, limited exposure to advertising and promotion of infant formula through the media
- Reinforcing: infant issues well managed resulting in infant thriving, knowledge in the community about mothers' rights to breastfeed in public.

The health and wellbeing priority issue analysis also identifies the priority populations for whom the health and wellbeing issue is a high priority, based on considerations of equity. In the breastfeeding example, the priority equity populations are Aboriginal and Torres Strait Islander women (Ogbo et al., 2016), women under 25 years of age (Baxter et al., 2009; Hauck et al., 2011; Meedya et al., 2010; Ogbo et al., 2016; Quinlivan et al., 2015), women living in rural areas (Hauck et al., 2011), women experiencing domestic violence (Ogbo et al., 2016).

Developing the health promotion program plan

The health promotion program plan includes goals, objectives, sub-objectives, strategies, activities and evaluation. (Use of the terms 'goals' and 'aims' varies across disciplines. In this book we use the term 'goals' for consistency.) The skills to develop all of these components for a health promotion program are an essential part of any health practitioner's 'toolkit'. Good goals, objectives and sub-objectives clearly define what changes the health promotion program aims to achieve. This provides the foundation on which the entire program is built. A solid foundation is essential to the development of appropriate strategies and activities that will be enacted in order to achieve the goals and objectives, and for developing the evaluation plan that will enable the health practitioner to evaluate if the program actually achieved what it set out to achieve. Fig. 4.4 (program logic) illustrates the relationship between goals, objectives, sub-objectives, strategies and evaluation. Program logic is underpinned by a theory of change. Fig. 4.5 provides a worked example of the development of a program goal, objectives and sub-objectives for the health priority of breastfeeding.

Goals

Goals express the changes in the health and wellbeing priority that the community wants to achieve. Sometimes these can be long term, depending on the nature of the priority. In the breastfeeding example, the priority issue is exclusive breastfeeding until six months

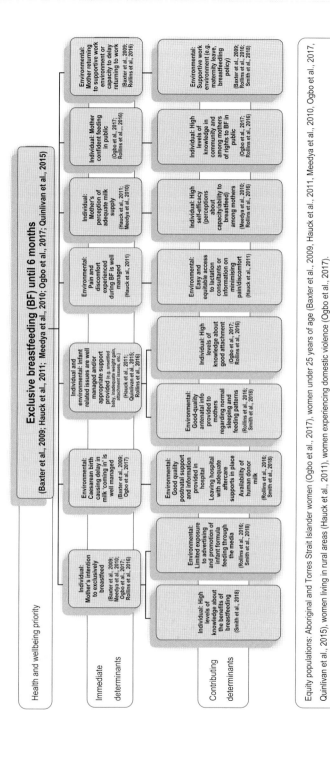

Equity populations: Aboriginal and Torres Strait Islander women (Ogbo et al., 2017), women under 25 years of age (Baxter et al., 2009, Hauck et al., 2011, Meedya et al., 2010, Ogbo et al., 2017, Quinlivan et al., 2015), women living in rural areas (Hauck et al., 2011), women experiencing domestic violence (Ogbo et al., 2017).

FIGURE 4.3 Health and wellbeing priority determinants analysis

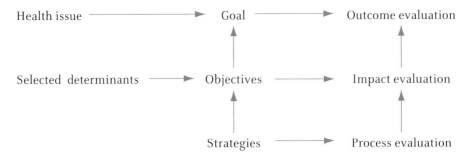

FIGURE 4.4 Health promotion program logic

of age. The goal developed to address this priority issue is to increase the rates of women exclusively breastfeeding for six months to 50% by 2025 (Smith et al., 2018).

Objectives and sub-objectives

Objectives state what must occur for the goal to be achieved. They address the determinants of the health and wellbeing priority identified in the analysis. Depending on the nature of the priority, they can also be expressed as learning objectives, action/behavioural objectives and environmental objectives. Objectives identify the type and degree of changes to the immediate determinants that are necessary to achieve the goal. Sub-objectives identify the type and degree of changes to the contributing determinants that are necessary to achieve the objectives. Writing goals, objectives and sub-objectives takes considerable time, research and practice to make them SMART, which means they should be:

Specific: clearly state who is the focus, where the program will occur, and using terms that are able to be operationally defined

Measurable: indicate what will change and the degree of change expected

Achievable: ensure the degree of change is realistic and able to be achieved in the timeframe; refer to what other programs have managed to achieve as a reference

Relevant: ensure that the goal is directly relevant to the health and wellbeing priority and the objectives are directly relevant to the determinants

Timescale: state when the change is to be achieved.

In the breastfeeding example, one of the individual-level determinants that contributes to exclusive breastfeeding is the mother's intention to exclusively breastfeed, which is influenced by her knowledge about the benefits of exclusive breastfeeding, and limited environmental exposure to advertising and media portraying infant formula as normal and easier than breastfeeding. The objective is therefore to increase to 60% the number of women who intend to exclusively breastfeed for six months by 2025. The sub-objectives to address the contributing determinants are to increase to 75% the number of women who can identify the major benefits of exclusive breastfeeding by 2020, and to decrease by 40% the number of advertisements for infant formula and media that portray formula feeding as normal and easier than breastfeeding by 2020. The program plan must identify what women it is referring to, where the program will be focused (e.g. local, regional, statewide or national), and the operational definitions of the constructs of exclusive breastfeeding, intention, knowledge and number of advertisements and media.

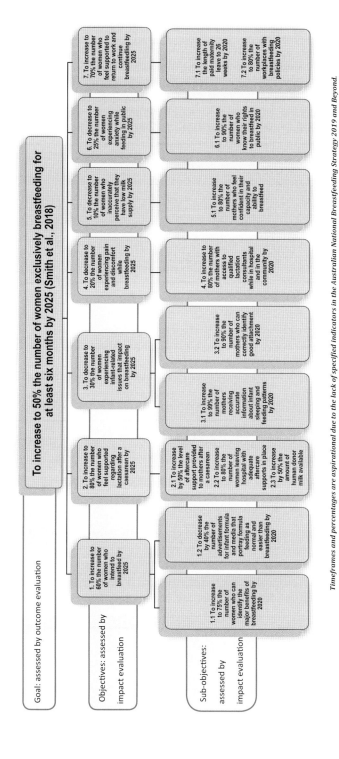

Timeframes and percentages are aspirational due to the lack of specified indicators in the Australian National Breastfeeding Strategy 2019 and Beyond.

FIGURE 4.5 Goal objectives and sub-objectives

It is important to note that one organisation's goal can be another organisation's objective. For example, the national government's goal may be to reduce the incidence of suicide in young people and one of the objectives is to increase knowledge of the signs and symptoms of depression. There are many things that contribute to youth suicide, and in your town you may have identified a higher than normal incidence of depression and poor social support for marginalised youth. Rather than focusing your health promotion program goal on reducing suicide rates, your goal might be focused on reducing the incidence of depression in youth in your town. The program objective may be focused on increasing the social support networks for marginalised youth.

Strategies and activities

Once the program goal, objectives and sub-objectives have been established, a complementary mix of strategies to bring about the planned changes can be developed. This combination of strategies is referred to as a strategy portfolio. Strategies should be based on theories or models appropriate to the nature of the strategy. These will be explored further in the subsequent chapter on health promotion strategies. Health practitioners may be familiar with behaviour change theories, such as the social cognitive theory or the health belief model, but these are only applicable to developing personal skills. It is essential to seek out theories and models that can be used to build healthy public policy, create supportive environments, strengthen community action and reorient health services. In addition, a review of the literature is required to learn from the experience of others about what has worked in other similar programs. In this way, a portfolio of complementary theory-based and evidence-informed strategies and activities can be developed.

A useful framework for developing the strategy portfolio is the Ottawa Charter for Health Promotion (WHO, 1986). Achieving the goals, objectives and sub-objectives related to most health and wellbeing priorities will require building healthy public policy, creating supportive environments and strengthening community action. Some priorities will also require developing people's personal skills and/or reorienting the health system towards a greater emphasis on health promotion. Activities may need to take place on different levels to address the health and wellbeing priority in the short term and longer term. For example, working for public policy change may take some time, but in the meantime people may need resources to strengthen the community capacity to address the priority. Each of these areas of health promotion action is underpinned by various theoretical frameworks and will be discussed in the following chapters.

In the youth suicide example above, where the goal is focused on reducing the incidence of depression in youth in your town, and one of the objectives is focused on increasing the social support networks for marginalised youth, you may decide that strengthening community action and creating supportive environments are the major strategies you will use to achieve this goal and objective. To strengthen community action, you may initiate an activity to develop a youth health Facebook page. Another activity may include engaging marginalised groups to develop this health page. To create a supportive social environment, your activities may include identifying potential youth facilitators from the marginalised group for the development of peer support programs in your town. All of these goals, objectives, strategies and activities contribute to addressing the nationally identified priority of reducing youth suicide rates, but at different levels to suit local conditions. Documenting the explicit logic of the program at the local level is just as important as at the national level.

Resources

An assessment of the resources available to implement the planned strategies and activities is required in the planning stage. Depending on the context of the health practitioner and the community, additional funding may be required to implement the program. Funding bodies usually provide very clear guidelines and it is important to read them carefully. Finding examples of successful applications from the funding body may be useful. Successful applications are the result of systematic program planning and careful budgeting. Part of the assessment is necessarily concerned with the organisational capabilities and resources for the development and implementation of the program. Limitations of resources, policies and abilities, and time constraints are investigated as part of the community assessment process. Resources for finding funding for community activities can be found at the end of this chapter. Funding proposals are generally expected to include the following sections.

Program summary

The program summary outlines very *succinctly* what will be done, why it will be done, how it will be done and who will be doing it; that is, the people for whom the program is designed. It outlines the health and wellbeing priority and the goal, objectives, sub-objectives, strategies, activities, evaluation and partners. This section is probably the most important part of the application. Busy reviewers will read the rest of the proposal if the summary provides a clear, organised overview.

Background

The background describes what the priority is and how that was determined. Evidence from the primary and secondary data sources is described.

Determinants of health and wellbeing

This describes the determinants of health and wellbeing for this particular priority.

Program goal, objectives and sub-objectives

This is a clear outline of the expected changes that will occur in the short and long term as a result of the program.

Implementation plan

The implementation plan outlines the program strategies and key activities, who will be involved, what resources will be needed and a tentative timetable.

Evaluation plan

The evaluation plan describes the process, impact and outcome evaluation. The plan should assess how effectively the program goal, objectives and sub-objectives have been met, and how process-related elements will be evaluated (refer back to the program logic diagram in Fig. 4.3). The section below on evaluation describes each of these in greater detail.

Program budget

The financial resources required to implement and evaluate the program are described in detail. Some funding agencies require applicants to also detail in-kind support that may be provided by the applicant's own agencies and other collaborating organisations. This is the support that is not financial, but may include the allocation of human resources, space, time, communication technologies or any other type of support that contributes to the program. Evidence of in-kind support from collaborating organisations is usually viewed very favourably by funding agencies.

STAGE 3: IMPLEMENTING THE HEALTH PROMOTION PROGRAM

Once the planning stage is complete, and resources are available, the health promotion program can begin. Implementation requires activation of the strategies and activities according to the plan, and keeping good documentation about what is being done. It is also important in the implementation stage to be aware of other opportunities that may arise related to the program, and to document any changes to the plan and the reasons why such changes may have occurred. Process evaluation (described in the next section) is undertaken in the implementation phase.

STAGE 4: EVALUATING THE HEALTH PROMOTION PROGRAM

Health promotion programs need to be fully evaluated. The theoretical frameworks used in community assessment, planning and implementation stages are also applied to health promotion program evaluation. Some of the important elements of evaluation applied to daily practice are described here and the importance of making evaluation itself a participatory, potentially empowering, experience for both health practitioners and community members is discussed in the following section.

What is evaluation?

Evaluation has been described as 'the process by which we judge the value or worth of something' (Suchman, 1967 in Hawe et al., 1990, p. 10). Evaluation is used to determine the strengths and weaknesses of an activity, program or system-wide plan. Evaluations can provide information about 'what works, for whom, and under what circumstances' (Baum et al., 2014, p. i134). Evaluation may be as specific as determining the effectiveness of a particular learning aid or activity, or as general as gauging the effectiveness of a community-driven social activity. Evaluation allows us to identify inconsistencies that may exist between program goals or objectives and implementation processes.

Why evaluate?

Evaluation contributes to knowledge in a number of ways including: gaining a better understanding of the impact of health promotion action with individuals, communities or populations; improving an individual program; informing policy development; and being accountable to the funding body. Evaluation will almost always be a requirement of an organisation that funds the program and, quite reasonably, they want to know that their investment is making an improvement in the health of the particular population. Guba and Lincoln (1989) argue that evaluation is the process of sharing accountability, not assigning accountability. On one hand, health practitioners have a responsibility to the funding body to work in accordance with any reasonable demands made of them, while on the other hand, they have a responsibility to the individuals and communities they are working with.

Dual responsibility has implications for each health practitioner's practice and the evaluation of the work of an agency. Whether working as a sole practitioner, in a team within a larger institution or as part of a small agency or centre, a health practitioner will need to find out if their work addresses the health and wellbeing priorities of those to whom they are accountable. If health bureaucracies and employers uphold a CPHC approach, they are supportive of this primary responsibility and help health practitioners to respond to the priorities of the communities within which they work. Unfortunately, health bureaucracies in high-income countries are not often oriented to a CPHC approach (see Chapter 1), and health practitioners may often find themselves experiencing some difficulty as they attempt to grapple with their dual accountabilities to central planning agencies and communities. Evaluating against the values and principles of critical health promotion and the principles of CPHC on the one hand, and the sometimes-competing requirements of bureaucratic expectations on the other, may present some challenges. Some of the different and competing perspectives that may underpin a health practitioner's decision about evaluation of a program include the following (Sarvela & McDermott, 2003):

Community's perspective

- To learn about the value of planned change
- To increase community participation in a program
- To promote positive public relations
- To be accountable to the community

Health practitioner's perspective

- To be clear whether program activities occurred as planned
- To determine whether the program achieved its objectives, and if not, why not
- To identify program elements that could be changed
- To inform planning of a new program or developing a comparable one
- To contribute to professional knowledge
- To identify areas for further research, or unmet community needs

Organisation's perspective

- To decide if resources were well spent
- To be accountable, to meet accreditation requirements
- To inform future planning and allocation of resources
- To secure future funding by fulfilling funding body's requirements

Funding body's perspective

- To demonstrate program effects for political purposes
- To provide evidence for more program support
- To contribute to the evidence base

Evaluating practice can be a part of every working day. It can also be part of a more formal process in which health practitioners, either individually or as part of the team with which they are working, take time out every so often to formally review the activities with which they have been involved and the priorities they have been working towards. Building informal and formal evaluation into one's practice will add greatly to the relevance and the power of health promotion work.

It is vital that health practitioners build knowledge and skills in both formal and informal evaluation, including critical reflection. This process involves developing a 'culture of evaluation' (Wadsworth, 1997, p. 57) and is an essential part of health promotion practice. Questions such as 'What went well?', 'What would I do differently next time?' and 'What else would I like to trial next time?' are questions that can be asked as a matter of course at the end of each activity. Such questions can easily be asked by every health practitioner on a regular basis throughout their working day as well as at various stages throughout health promotion programs. Colin and Garrow (1996) describe this process as thinking, listening, looking, understanding and acting as you go along.

Who is the evaluation for?

Evaluation has been described as a 'complex process of measurement and judgment which includes gathering and organising and interpreting information' (Bedworth & Bedworth, 1992, p. 407). Judgements and interpretations can be based on different views of the world, by people or organisations holding contrasting values to those of the participants. The challenge is not to remove values from the evaluation process, but to ensure that the process reflects the values of the community as well as those of the health and/or funding agencies (Coombe in Minkler, 2012, Chapter 19) (see Insight 4.1). Community members or program participants are not the only people interested in the outcomes of health promotion evaluation. Funding bodies, managers and other practitioners may be keen to see a health promotion program evaluated, and their needs may be very different to those of community members participating in the program. So, despite the impression we are often given that evaluation is an objective process that will inform us of the 'best' way to proceed, it is clearly a process of judgement—and this judgement can never be value-free. We may describe evaluation by using such terms as 'measurement', 'appraisal', 'assessment' or 'calculation', but when we use terms such as these it is clear that the objects of interest are compared with some sort of standard or benchmark. Such baselines may be driven by competing values, such as cost control or prior political or organisational decisions to change services. Perceptions of successful outcomes can be time dependent, and influenced by political aspirations or perceptions (Farmer et al., 2012).

Evaluation is a value-driven process and in a CPHC approach it is the values of CPHC that drive the evaluation. That is, the needs of the people for whom the activity is carried out are foremost, as are issues of community control, social justice and equity.

Approaches to evaluation research

Evaluating any activity needs to be built around methods appropriate to health promotion action. A level of flexibility sufficient to respond to the needs of the people for whom it is being implemented needs to be maintained. Both qualitative and quantitative methods may be used, depending on the evaluation question. Each approach has strengths and limitations although it seems that the primacy of the quantitative approach remains, particularly with many funding agencies. Certainly, quantitative approaches to evaluation can contribute significantly to evaluation processes when they are used appropriately and in balance with other approaches. However, they are often unable to provide the answers to questions regarded as important in health promotion, particularly to inform program refinement or redesign.

Planning for evaluation

An evaluation plan is integral to the health promotion practice cycle. Developing an evaluation plan ensures transparency, robustness, and clarity of purpose, which enable a program to be communicated to others (Farmer et al., 2012). Guiding principles include: having a clear process; being useful, relevant and practical; and using multiple and appropriate data-collection methods. Evaluation findings need to be plausible; that is, they need to reflect the experience of all stakeholders, which means paying attention to power structures and politics. Leaving evaluation planning until after the program has been planned (or worse, after it has been implemented) means the impact or outcome of a program is difficult to demonstrate.

There are many perspectives that have to be incorporated at the planning stage. Health promotion programs are often complex with multiple components and expectations (Bauman & Nutbeam, 2014; Smith & Petticrew, 2010). Evaluations cannot be all things to all people and so evaluations conducted for different reasons can be conducted separately. Thinking through the implications of all these perspectives at the planning stage will mean that much of the information that is required by the different perspectives can be built into the implementation phase, making even formal evaluation for the managers or those funding a program easier than it might be if evaluation is regarded as an 'add-on' activity.

There are a number of steps that guide planning an evaluation:

- Identifying the purpose of the evaluation
- Formulating evaluation research questions related to the goals, objectives, sub-objectives, strategies and activities of the program
- Determining the most appropriate design for the evaluation including where and when the evaluation will take place
- Determining the most appropriate data-collection and analysis methods
- Considering the range of ethical issues related to evaluation research
- Clarifying the roles and responsibility of those involved in the evaluation
- Outlining how the results will be disseminated
- Costing the evaluation.

Evaluation research ethics

The four principles of ethical practice outlined in this chapter are integral to evaluation research: merit and integrity, justice, beneficence, and respect.

Merit and integrity

Applying the ethical principle of merit and integrity means that the evaluator must be competent and experienced, the evaluation study must be well designed and carefully planned, and the evaluation process, outcomes and benefits must be clear to all involved.

Justice

Enacting the ethical principle of justice means that the evaluation must be fair and inclusive, and no section of the population is excluded unfairly. This principle also means that it is unethical to expose one group of people to the risks of the evaluation solely for the benefit of another group, and provides special protections for vulnerable persons including children, pregnant women, prisoners, people with intellectual disability, people who are illiterate or have limited education and people with limited access to services.

Beneficence

The ethical principle of beneficence means that the evaluator is responsible for the physical, mental, social and spiritual wellbeing of participants, and all participants should receive some benefit from the evaluation. It also means that the evaluation should do no harm to people participating in the evaluation, including harm to social standing or social relationships, psychological harm to mental or emotional wellbeing, financial harm, legal harm through exposure to legal proceedings, or physical harm to person or property. Harm may result from the data-collection process, or from a breach of privacy or confidentiality, which are described in the next section on respect.

Respect

Applying the ethical principle of respect in evaluation means treating people with dignity, respecting people's rights to privacy and confidentiality, and ensuring fully informed and voluntary consent to participate in the evaluation study. Protecting privacy and ensuring confidentiality are key components of respecting the safety and dignity of evaluation participants. Privacy and confidentiality are similar concepts, and the terms are often used interchangeably, but they are different concepts and both need to be considered in any evaluation process.

Privacy relates to having control over the extent, timing and circumstances of sharing oneself with others. In other words, it relates to the methods used to gather information from participants. Evaluation methods that might pose concerns related to privacy include observational studies, focus groups, snowball sampling, intrusive or inappropriate questions in a questionnaire or interview, and knowledge about participation in a study on sensitive, stigmatising or illegal topics.

Confidentiality relates to the treatment of information that a participant has disclosed in a relationship of trust and with the expectation that it will not be divulged to others. It refers to the obligations of researchers and institutions to appropriately protect the information disclosed to them. Evaluation participants must be able to decide what measure of control over their personal information they are willing to relinquish to researchers. Protecting confidentiality does not mean that participants in an evaluation are not able to be identified or their information protected from disclosure. It means that the participant gets to decide that for themselves. Some participants want to be identified and quoted. Some agree to have their photographs, audio or video recordings published or otherwise made available to the public. The key consideration here is what participants provide informed consent for.

Ensuring confidentiality in the data-collection process is easiest if data are collected anonymously. However, if identity is required for follow-up purposes, then the evaluator should remove direct identifiers from the data set as soon as possible, use pseudonyms when reporting results, and/or only report aggregate results. After the data are collected, confidentiality must also be ensured through data protection. Decisions regarding where the data will be stored and for how long, what procedures will be in place to protect the data from inappropriate access, and who will have full access to the data all need to be carefully considered. Strategies for reducing breaches of confidentiality include encrypting the data, storing data on computers without an internet connection, ensuring computer and data files are password protected with different passwords, and data are stored in locked cabinets.

The final requirement of the ethical principle of respect is ensuring fully informed and voluntary consent to participate in the evaluation study. People must be provided with sufficient and understandable information about the evaluation to enable a fully informed decision about their participation. Information must be in the participants' own language and at an appropriate comprehension level. The process of informed consent begins with recruitment and continues throughout the evaluation.

Evaluation challenges for health promotion

Health promotion work is often very difficult to evaluate because it can be long term, developmental and complex, and attributing the cause of changes to specific activities is often impossible. This is a serious challenge when funders interpret it as a problem of the work itself rather than the realities of evaluation research. Changes in systems and communities are non-linear and often unpredictable, and evaluation may not assess the wider ripple effects of a health promotion program.

Another challenge is that detailed evaluation of the effectiveness of programs is often beyond the scope of small organisations and more in the realm of special evaluation projects conducted by skilled research teams. Research shows that health promotion programs have not been well evaluated in Australia (Chambers et al., 2015; Jolley et al., 2007). Specific challenges in evaluating community-level health promotion programs include:

1. Methodological (choosing the appropriate and measurable unit of analysis)
2. Differentiating program effects from other trends
3. Identifying very small effects from community-level programs
4. The time it takes for any level of community penetration effect
5. The limitations of linking theory to the complexity of actions and levels of influence (Pommier, 2010 in Farmer et al., 2012, p. 146).

Evaluation of a health promotion program can also be influenced by influencers, fashion, dissemination routes and 'tipping points' (Farmer et al., 2012, p. 134). With increasing evaluation requirements placed on health practitioners, there is a great danger that short-term, simple (and potentially less useful) health promotion activities will be implemented because they are easier to evaluate and outcomes can be reported in a short timeframe, rather than more innovative, longer-term programs, which have the potential to make a much bigger difference to the socio-ecological determinants of health, but are more difficult to evaluate (Baum, 1999, p. 38). As a result, health practitioners may be so pressured to provide evaluation evidence that health promotion programs are developed to match the evaluation methods and short-term timeframes, rather than the other way around. 'Too often the evaluation tail wags the program dog as health practitioners choose objectives amenable to evaluation' (Freudenberg, 1984, p. 46). This may also have the effect of discouraging health practitioners from taking up innovative health promotion work because it may be difficult to evaluate. Underhill and colleagues (2016) provide insight into the learnings from the Healthy Together Mildura evaluation, and the difference made by applying systems thinking to their previous work. They support real-time feedback and adaptation, and evaluating with a focus on the whole rather than individual parts.

Evaluation in 'high-risk' and 'low-risk' programs

Health promotion is an investment package, balancing innovative but high-risk strategies (because definitive statements about outcome may not be possible) with more straightforward low-risk strategies on which evidence of effect is provided in the research literature (Hawe & Shiell, 1995). This portfolio approach is needed if health promotion is to address the range of socio-ecological determinants. For example, working to increase health equity and improve the health chances of poor or Indigenous people are the central goals of health promotion in Australia and New Zealand. Such goals require long-term commitment and resources. However, if outcome criteria revolve around whether or not a program is easily measurable, specific and achievable within a short funding cycle, a great deal of evaluation may occur, but it may do little in the long term to improve health.

INSIGHT 4.2 GoWell

The Glasgow Community Health and Wellbeing Research and Learning Program—GoWell—is a partnership between the Glasgow Centre for Population Health, the University of Glasgow's Department of Urban Studies and the Medical Research Council and Chief Scientist Office (MRC/CSO) Social and Public Health Sciences Unit. GoWell is sponsored by the Glasgow Housing Association, the Scottish Government, NHS Health Scotland and NHS Greater Glasgow and Clyde.

GoWell investigates the impacts of investment in neighbourhood regeneration initiatives on the health and wellbeing of individuals, families and communities. Regeneration initiatives include:

- housing improvements
- transformational regeneration
- resident relocation
- the creation of mixed tenure communities
- changes in housing type (demolition of high-rise blocks and replacement with lower-rise flats and houses)
- community engagement and empowerment.

Launched in 2005, GoWell measures health and wellbeing before, during and after the implementation of these regeneration initiatives. The evaluation research includes a longitudinal community survey, qualitative research, ecological analysis and an economic evaluation. The evaluation findings are fed back into the planning and implementation process.

A range of outcomes has been reported across six themes:

- Communities
- Neighbourhoods
- Health and wellbeing
- Empowerment
- Housing
- Mixed tenure.

Source: https://www.gowellonline.com/

Furthermore, evaluating programs beyond a reasonable level acts as a drain on the very limited resources available for health promotion. For those reasons, evaluation activities need to be critically reviewed and carefully considered so that inappropriate evaluation does not become part of the problem. The GoWell longitudinal research project in Glasgow, Scotland (Insight 4.2), and the Victorian Healthy Supermarket Trials (Insight 4.3), are examples of evaluations conducted by skilled researchers in collaboration with communities, with the aim of placing evaluation in a broad theoretical framework that links health determinants and program outcomes.

Cautions with evaluation

Failing to accurately indicate where the problems lie with a program can largely be avoided with thorough planning. After all, it is a significant waste of resources if health practitioners cannot be sure why a program works so well (or why it doesn't). If a program is very successful, success should be shared with others, to save valuable resources and time, or to prevent them from making costly mistakes. There are two common pitfalls with evaluation.

INSIGHT 4.3 Victorian healthy supermarket trials

Low nutrient food consumption is now one of the biggest contributors to the burden of disease in Australia. The primary drivers of this are food environments that encourage eating of low-nutrient high-energy foods and beverages. With supermarkets accounting for the majority of food spending in Australia, marketing techniques involving manipulation of promotion, product, price and placement in the supermarket environment have the potential to improve the nutrient quality of consumer food purchases at a population level.

The award-winning trials in supermarkets in Bendigo (regional Victoria) assessed the real-world feasibility and impact of activities designed to create supermarket environments that encourage purchases of nutrient-rich foods. The program was initiated by the retailer, who wanted to support the community's health and wellbeing. A partnership between Champions IGA, City of Greater Bendigo, Deakin University and VicHealth was formed to test a range of low-cost, scalable changes to supermarket store environments that aimed to increase purchasing of nutrient-rich foods and while maintaining profit for the retailer. Activities were selected by the research partners, based on evidence from the academic literature, feasibility of implementation and the interests of the retailer. The activities included: shelf tags for all products achieving a 4.5- or 5-star rating in the Australian Health Star Rating nutrition labelling scheme; and custom-developed signage in all trolleys and baskets promoting consumption of nutrient-rich foods. Sales data were collected and activity monitoring was undertaken in three stores implementing the program and four control stores during the baseline periods, the 6–8-week program periods and the washout period.

The health promotion program led to significant positive effects on the nutrient quality of consumer food purchases, with no detrimental effect on retailer profit observed. The relationships formed during the program and the positive feedback from customers led to a willingness among all partners to extend and expand the collaboration, with more trials planned for the future.

Source: Dr Adrian Cameron, Senior Research Fellow Global Obesity Centre (GLOBE), WHO Collaborating Centre for Obesity Prevention, School of Health & Social Development, Faculty of Health, Deakin University, and Amy Brown, Research & Evaluation Officer, Active and Healthy Communities, City of Greater Bendigo.

1. Not sufficiently resourcing evaluation. It is better to do a thorough job of one form of evaluation, than to do a hasty, scant job of too many forms. Inadequate resourcing, in terms of time, personnel and funds, can mean either that the valuable aspects of a good program failed to be demonstrated, or you are unable to recognise where there may be issues of concern in a program.

2. Ignoring the results of the evaluation because of evaluation faults. A poorly planned evaluation may not identify the logical link between goal, objectives and strategies. Therefore, no matter how effective the activities or strategies are, the evaluation will never demonstrate achievement of an overly ambitious goal. Likewise, evaluation will fail to demonstrate that any form of activity has been effective if the program framework is based on an inadequate community assessment (Hawe et al., 1990).

Types of evaluation

There are various types of evaluation, and the choice of evaluation type depends on the purpose of the evaluation. Taking a systems approach to evaluation by integrating a range of evaluation types should paint a relatively comprehensive picture of the health promotion action (Bauman & Nutbeam, 2014). Fig. 4.3 (program logic) earlier in the chapter shows the relationship between health and wellbeing priorities, their determinants and contributing determinants, the goals, objectives and sub-objectives of the program, and the types of evaluation linked to each. In addition to impact and outcome evaluation, there are a number of other types of evaluation for the health practitioner to consider.

Organisational evaluation

This evaluation occurs at the organisational level and assesses management practices; for example, quality assurance processes such as regular review of planning processes, accounting for the day-to-day use of funds or staff development processes. Evaluating the work of an agency or team is a vital process to prevent it wandering from its original goals or away from addressing the health and wellbeing priorities of the community. Informal evaluation can be incorporated into the normal work of the agency or team; for example, through discussion and reflection at weekly staff meetings. It will be necessary, however, for the agency or team to take time out to evaluate itself more formally and to involve the community in this process. This can be done by setting time aside specifically for evaluation and strategic planning. Although much of this can occur as a regular internal process, such as yearly evaluation and planning days, it can also be done by involving the agency or team in formal evaluation processes that include external evaluators. In these situations, however, care must be taken to ensure that the process is a supportive and useful one for the practitioners and community members concerned.

Process evaluation

Process evaluation is about evaluating the way in which health promotion strategies and activities are being implemented. Because of the centrality of *process* in the CPHC approach to health promotion, examination of the strategies and actions is particularly important. Furthermore, health promotion actions are often multifactorial and delivered in systems that are unpredictable so it is important to examine the progress, or the quality and quantity, of what was actually implemented in a program to understand what did or did not work and why. Hawe and colleagues (1990) recommend asking:

- Is the program or activity reaching the people for whom it was designed?
- What do the participants, staff and organisational partners think of the program or activity?
- Is the program or activity being implemented as planned?
- Are all aspects of the program of good quality?

The particular process elements important in a CPHC approach will also include the extent to which the direction of the program has changed in response to the needs of the participants, and evaluating the relationships between the organisational partnerships.

Evaluating how power was shared between health practitioners and participants—that is, what kind of participation occurred—may also be part of process evaluation. Process evaluation needs to show how populations facing the greatest inequality were engaged in a culturally and socially appropriate way.

Impact evaluation

In impact evaluation, the immediate effects of the program are assessed. The questions relate to whether the objectives and sub-objectives of the program have been achieved. The evaluation therefore relates to changes in the immediate and contributing determinants of the health and wellbeing priority. In impact and outcome evaluation (discussed in the next section), quasi-experimental and non-experimental evaluation designs are often used as opposed to experimental designs. There are advantages and disadvantages of each evaluation design. Experimental designs use statistical methods, and randomisation of participants into control and program groups. The sample size is necessarily large to obtain statistical significance. There are strict protocols around the conduct of the research; the design therefore can be replicated. Experimental designs have traditionally been highly regarded but they are time-consuming and costly, and randomisation may discriminate against subgroups of the population. They are not necessarily the best design for participatory health promotion programs. In quasi-experimental designs, comparison groups are used, rather than randomly assigned control groups. These evaluation designs can be rigorous and implemented relatively easily but they can also be costly. Pre-test/post-test designs are used in both quasi-experimental and non-experimental designs. Non-experimental designs do not use any comparison groups. They can be useful to obtain baseline data or data obtained at the end of a program. They are useful when the purpose is to understand the implementation process and are the least expensive option.

Outcome evaluation

Outcome evaluation assesses the long-term effects of the program. The questions relate to whether the goals of the program have been achieved. The evaluation therefore relates to changes in the health and wellbeing priority, and so it is often the type of evaluation conducted beyond the organisational level. Health departments usually measure health and wellbeing indicators. Evaluation designs for outcome evaluation are discussed in the previous section on impact evaluation.

Goal-free evaluation

Evaluation carried out by comparing results with goals and objectives is not a complete evaluation of a program's outcomes because it does not provide an opportunity to note any outcomes that do not relate directly to the goals and objectives. These outcomes may either add greater benefit to the activity or undermine some of its other benefits. In either case, these unpredicted consequences are an important part of the program, and reliance solely on evaluation against goals and objectives would have caused them to be missed. For these reasons, some evaluation not directly linked to the goals and objectives is useful. This type of open-ended inquiry can be described as 'goal-free evaluation' (Wadsworth, 1997, p. 39). Wadsworth (1997) highlights the importance of conducting this type of evaluation before impact and outcome evaluation. This is because the process of measurement against goals and objectives is by definition constrained to the short- and long-term changes desired, and does not encourage creativity. Undertaking impact and outcome evaluations first may make it very difficult for people to think broadly and creatively. However, conducting open-ended inquiry first will not make it difficult to undertake impact and outcome evaluation, and in fact may help health practitioners evaluate goals and objectives themselves. Wadsworth (1997, pp. 48–49) suggests that the philosophical values that guide the development of an organisation may provide better guidance for an evaluation than the specific goals and objectives. This is because goals and objectives may not reflect the value base and long-term goals of the organisation, and the extent to which this has been implemented may in fact be the most important thing to evaluate.

The quality and appropriateness of the goals and objectives is critically important. The complexities of capturing what is happening in a community program also highlights the importance of writing SMART objectives which describe the quantitative impacts of a program, as well as the more qualitative social impacts. Relying solely on goals and objectives that may not have been drawn up under optimum conditions severely limits the potential value of any evaluation. Further, sometimes the length of time it takes to realise outcomes, the cost of conducting robust evaluation and the changes in policies, structures and the community and unforeseen impacts make assessment of the process elements all the more important.

Economic evaluation

This type of evaluation is based on a cost–benefit analysis. Value for money is assessed and is assigned to the funding body. In this evaluation the resources consumed, such as time and money, are assessed as being efficient relative to the population served and outcomes achieved. For example, social return on investment (SROI) has been used internationally to evaluate the impact of programs, organisations, businesses or policies (Millar & Hall, 2013). The methodology assists to identify the benefits generated in the social, economic and physical environment and place a value on this impact. This value can then be compared to the investment required to generate the benefits. These evaluations are relatively complex and resource intensive (Farmer et al., 2012) but the same questions are asked, and similar processes occur, as for any other evaluation.

Evaluating community participation and empowerment

One of the key features of working with a CPHC approach is that the evaluation process actively involves the people for whom the program is running, building on their active involvement in the community assessment, planning and implementation of health promotion action. It is for this reason that participatory evaluation fits most comfortably with a CPHC approach—because it is built on the active involvement of community members in the evaluation process. There are four overarching dimensions of community participation that need to be examined in participatory evaluation (Baum, 2016; Coombe in Minkler, 2012, Chapter 19; Jolley et al., 2008; Wadsworth, 1997):

- the extent and scope of community participation
- the processes of working together
- the capacity and support for practitioners and community participants
- the impacts of participation.

Wadsworth points out that while non-participatory research may come up with useful outcomes, 'a non-participatory, non-democratic process of evaluation cannot ensure a user-appropriate outcome' (Wadsworth, 1997, p. 16). In addition to what is done to promote health, how it is done is very important and can have a positive or negative impact on the people as discussed previously. It is recognition of this, along with recognition of the expertise community members have about local factors that concern them, that is behind support for participatory evaluation. Drawing conclusions about a health promotion activity in a way that is disempowering will be of limited value for community members (Coombe in Minkler, 2012, Chapter 19).

In Chapter 6, the discussion centres on using community development approaches to support citizens increasing their abilities to control decisions that affect their community. A number of principles presented in that chapter can be used as the basis for formulating an evaluation plan. For example:

- the six principles of community development processes can be used to formulate objectives, and as the basis for impact evaluation discussions or in a community survey

- the DARE criteria for reflecting on community empowerment through goal setting are a useful evaluation benchmark
- the two principles of community development outcomes can be used to formulate a program goal, and as the basis for outcome evaluation.

As one of the essential characteristics of community development, community members would decide on the evaluation criteria or what they see as measures of success.

Community participation and empowerment are also indicators of individual and community wellbeing. Rifkin and colleagues (1988) suggested a means of evaluating the quality of community participation. The community identifies the various concepts or domains that they consider would be indicators of participation in their community. Rifkin and colleagues suggest these domains could be:

- the level of involvement in community assessments
- the degree to which community is heard and their opinions are valued in decision outcomes
- whether there is a reference group with a majority of community members, guiding the program
- whether existing organisations are included in new community processes; or
- whether program money is used to employ, increase the capacity of and improve the health of community members.

The domains can be imagined, for example, as a five-item Likert scale with a higher score being allocated to the most desirable or successful end of the scale. To improve the visual clarity and impact of the scoring process, the findings can be represented diagrammatically in the form of a spider's web. Each domain forms an arm of the web. Lines are drawn between the average scores for each domain. The domains can be used for evaluation in different ways:

- members of a community or reference group can score each domain and the results can be compared between members
- reference group and management can score the domains and compare perspectives as a basis for discussion
- the scores from each group can be compared over time as a basis for tracking improvements in the effectiveness of participation
- the extent of participation and the different perceptions of the stakeholders about the degree of the participation can be mapped over time by overlaying the webs.

Laverack (2007) has drawn on the work of Rifkin and colleagues (1988) in his work describing community empowerment. He identifies that the spider's web configuration can be created using readily available spreadsheet packages, such as Chart Wizard (see Fig. 4.6 as an example).

Evaluating partnerships

Health promotion is everyone's business. Community health and wellbeing priorities are complex and require the perspectives and resources of many, particularly when we are applying systems thinking. Forming organisational partnerships to work towards common goals becomes essential and whether partnerships are working well can be evaluated. The extent of collaboration, whether there is genuine collaboration or whether there is a dominant person or organisation, are central questions. Other elements for consideration in

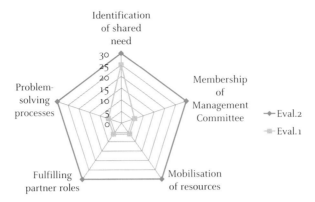

FIGURE 4.6 Spider web configuration

evaluating partnerships might be whether there is a common vision, whether trust is valued and given time to develop and whether the partners think the relationship is productive and enjoyable (Jolley et al., 2008). The outcomes of a successful partnership could be evaluated by considering whether there are more equitable, effective and accessible services or whether the population is experiencing an improvement in health status, wellbeing and quality of life (Jolley et al., 2008). Partnership logic models guides are available (see, for example, the Centers for Disease Control and Prevention (2011), the National Collaborating Centre for Methods and Tools (n.d.) and the VicHealth Partnership Tool (VicHealth, 2011)).

Evaluation reports

Having done the evaluation, it is then necessary to write the evaluation report. This helps health practitioners, organisations and funding bodies make decisions about the changes that need to be made to the program (if any). The evaluation report brings the community health and wellbeing priorities to the attention of others and promotes greater understanding. Individual, community or policy changes may take place as a result of disseminating the evaluation report. All stakeholders need to have access to the information, particularly those who designed the program or for whom the program was designed. In order that the evaluation report meets the needs of the widest possible audience, health practitioners must consider who the report is for and the most appropriate format. Different audiences have different expectations and you may need to develop more than one report. Research reports for funding agencies may have a template to follow. If not, there are numerous resources available to help you with different styles of report writing. In preparing the report you will need to think about the most appropriate length, language and visual presentation of results. In a written report, the executive summary is extremely important. It is often the only component of the report that the majority of the people will read; therefore it must summarise each section of the report. It is useful to think about the executive summary as a document in its own right. You will need to report on what has been done, why it was done, how it was done, what the outcomes were and how it contributes to best practice.

Finally you will need to consider how the report should be disseminated. You could conduct face-to-face presentations, provide printed materials, make a video, a series of social media posts, or develop a web page.

CONCLUSION

This chapter has described the health promotion practice cycle of community assessment, program planning, implementation and evaluation. Research evidence and skills form the basis of the ongoing cyclical process, which must be underpinned by the values and principles of critical health promotion. Models and theories underpinning the health promotion practice cycle inform all action areas of the *Framework of health promotion practice in a comprehensive primary health care context.* Community assessment incorporates assessment of both assets and needs and results in the identification of health and wellbeing priorities. Community assessment may be both a formal and an informal process, but it is only the first step to improving the health and wellbeing of community members; it is never an end in itself. Planning involves developing the goal, objectives, strategies, activities and evaluation plan, together with identifying the required resources to deliver the plan. Implementation involves implementing the strategies and activities and documenting the process. Evaluation involves putting the evaluation plan into place and is an integral component of good health promotion practice. All stages of the health promotion practice cycle should be transparent, and detailed documentation of processes and dissemination of evaluation findings are important to maintaining the credibility of health promotion.

MORE TO EXPLORE

PARTICIPATORY ACTION RESEARCH
- Power and glory: Applying participatory action research in public health (Baum, 2016)

COMMUNITY ASSESSMENT, PLANNING, IMPLEMENTATION AND EVALUATION TOOLS
- Community Health Assessment and Group Evaluation (CHANGE) action guide: building a foundation of knowledge to prioritise community needs (Centers for Disease Control and Prevention, 2010)
- Conducting a community needs assessment (Our Community, n.d.)
- Planning and Evaluation Wizard (PEW) (Flinders University, 2019)
- The Health Equity Assessment Tool: A user's guide (Signal et al., 2008)
- Community Sustainability Engagement Evaluation Toolbox (Evaluation Toolbox, n.d.)

LITERATURE REVIEWS AND SECONDARY DATA SOURCES
- A typology of reviews: an analysis of 14 review types and associated methodologies. Review Article (Grant & Booth, 2009)
- The literature review: a research journey (Harvard Graduate School of Education, n.d.)
- PHIDU (Public Health Information Development Unit), Torrens University Australia (Torrens University Australia, n.d.)

PLANNING MODELS IN HEALTH PROMOTION
- The PRECEDE–PROCEED Model of health program planning and evaluation (Green, n.d.)

- Planning, implementing, and evaluating health promotion programs: a primer (McKenzie et al., 2013)
- Health promotion planning: planning and strategies (Tones & Green, 2010)

EVALUATION (SEE REFERENCE LIST)

- Bamberger et al. (2012)
- Bauman and Nutbeam (2014)
- Evaluation Toolbox (n.d.)
- Hawe et al. (1990)
- Patton (2011)
- Posavac (2011)
- Tones and Green (2010)
- Wadsworth (2010)

ETHICS IN RESEARCH AND EVALUATION

- National Statement on Ethical Conduct in Human Research, Preamble, Ethical background: National Health and Medical Research Council (2007, updated 2018a)
- National Statement on Ethical Conduct in Human Research, Section 1: Values and principles of ethical conduct (National Health and Medical Research Council, 2007, updated 2018b)

RESOURCES FOR FINDING FUNDING FOR COMMUNITY ACTIVITIES

Funding is available from local, state and national government and philanthropic sources. A number of resources are available to assist health practitioners to find funding, including the following.

- Our Community Pty Ltd (https://www.ourcommunity.com.au/community/) is a useful website that includes a publishing house and several knowledge and service hubs. It contains some good resources that can help community groups, individuals and businesses to find funding and write effective applications. Each organisation tends to use its own application proforma; small grants offered by local government and local service clubs are a good place to start.
- Philanthropy Australia (https://www.philanthropy.org.au/) provides a primary resource to identify the priorities of trusts and foundations and provide information about corporate funding available in Australia. Health organisations and public libraries often subscribe to this service. The application process and reporting expectations are often less daunting than public health agencies and services.

IUHPE Core Competencies for Health Promotion

The IUHPE Core Competencies for Health Promotion (International Union for Health Promotion and Education, 2016) comprises nine domains of action. Each domain has a series of core competency statements and a detailed outline of the knowledge and skills that contribute to competency in that domain.

The content of this chapter relates especially to the achievement of competency in the health promotion domains outlined below.

1. Enable change	*1.2 Use health promotion approaches which support empowerment, participation, partnership and equity to create environments and settings which promote health*
	Determinants of health and health inequities
	Theory and practice of collaborative working including facilitation, negotiation, conflict resolution, mediation and teamwork
	1.4 Facilitate the development of personal skills that will maintain and improve health
	Health promotion models
	1.5 Work in collaboration with key stakeholders to reorient health and other services to promote health and reduce health inequities
	Knowledge of strategy and policy development and how legislation impacts on health
	Partnership building and collaborative working
2. Advocate for health	*2.5 Facilitate communities and groups to articulate their needs and advocate for the resources and capacities required for health promotion action*
	Methods of stakeholder engagement
	Knowledge of strategy and policy development
3. Mediate through partnership	*3.1 Engage partners from different sectors to actively contribute to health promotion action*
	Systems, structures and functions of different sectors, organisations and agencies
	3.2 Facilitate effective partnership working which reflects health promotion values and principles
	Principles of effective intersectoral partnership working
	Networking
4. Communication	*4.1 Use effective communication skills including written, verbal, non-verbal, listening skills and information technology*
	Communication skills including written, verbal, non-verbal, listening skills and information technology
	Working with individuals and groups
	Use of electronic media and information technology
	4.4 Use interpersonal communication and groupwork skills to facilitate individuals, groups, communities and organisations to improve health and reduce health inequities
	Ability to work with individuals, groups, communities and organisations in diverse settings

5. Leadership	*5.1 Work with stakeholders to agree a shared vision and strategic direction for health promotion action* Principles of effective intersectoral partnership working
	5.5 Contribute to mobilising and managing resources for health promotion action Principles of effective human and financial resource management and mobilisation
6. Assessment	*6.1 Use participatory methods to engage stakeholders in the assessment process* Ability to work with stakeholders from community groups/organisations
	6.2 Use a variety of assessment methods including quantitative and qualitative research methods Range of assessment methods/processes using both qualitative and quantitative methods
	6.3 Collect, review and appraise relevant data, information and literature to inform health promotion action How to obtain, review and interpret data or information Qualitative research methods including participatory and action research Quantitative research methods including statistical analysis Critical appraisal skills
	6.5 Identify the health needs, existing assets and resources relevant to health promotion action Evidence base for health promotion action and priority setting
	6.6 Use culturally and ethically appropriate assessment approaches Understanding social and cultural diversity
	6.7 Identify priorities for health promotion action in partnership with stakeholders based on best available evidence and ethical values How to obtain, review and interpret data or information
7. Planning	*7.1 Mobilise, support and engage the participation of stakeholders in planning health promotion action* Use and effectiveness of current health promotion planning models and theories

	7.2 Use current models and systematic approaches for planning health promotion action
	Principles of project/program management
	Principles of resource management and risk management
	7.3 Develop a feasible action plan within resource constraints and with reference to existing needs and assets
	Use of health promotion planning models
	7.4 Develop and communicate appropriate, realistic and measurable goals and objectives for health promotion action
	Analysis and application of information about needs and assets
	Use of project/program planning and management tools
8. Implementation	*8.1 Use ethical, empowering, culturally appropriate and participatory processes to implement health promotion action*
	Use of participatory implementation processes
	8.2 Develop, pilot and use appropriate resources and materials
	Theory and practice of program implementation
	8.3 Manage the resources needed for effective implementation of planned action
	Use of project/program management tools
	Collaborative working
	8.4 Facilitate program sustainability and stakeholder ownership through ongoing consultation and collaboration
	Use of participatory implementation processes
	8.5 Monitor the quality of the implementation process in relation to agreed goals and objectives for health promotion action
	Quality assurance, monitoring and process evaluation
9. Evaluation and research	*9.1 Identify and use appropriate health promotion evaluation tools and research methods*
	Knowledge of different models of evaluation and research
	Critical appraisal and review of literature
	Write research reports and communicate research findings effectively and appropriately
	9.2 Integrate evaluation into the planning and implementation of all health promotion action
	Formative and summative evaluation approaches
	Qualitative and quantitative research methods

	9.3 Use evaluation findings to refine and improve health promotion action
	Data interpretation and statistical analysis
	Evidence base for health promotion

In addition, IUHPE (International Union for Health Promotion and Education, n.d.) specifies knowledge, skills and performance criteria essential for health promotion practitioners to act professionally and ethically, including having knowledge of ethical and legal issues, behaving in an ethical and respectful manner and working in ways that review and improve practice. Full details are available at: http://www.iuhpe.org/index.php/en/the-accreditation-system.

Reflective Questions

1. You have been assigned the task of leading a community assessment to identify the assets and needs of your local geographical community. Develop a plan for undertaking this task including the range of assets and needs you will need to collect data about, the sources for the different types of secondary and primary data needed, and your approach to working with the local community and stakeholders.

2. Using Fig. 4.5 'Goals, objectives and sub-objectives', develop an outcome and impact evaluation plan to evaluate the goal and related objectives and sub-objectives.

3. Reflect on the *Red Critical Health Promotion Model* values and principles in Table 4.1. Identify which values and principles are *most* relevant to each stage of the health promotion practice cycle. Discuss the extent to which these values and principles are evident in health promotion initiatives that you are aware of.

REFERENCES

Aitken, J. C., Dickson-Swift, V., & Kenny, A. (2015). Linking community engagement and therapeutic landscapes to develop new social prescriptions for health and well-being. Bendigo: La Trobe Rural Health School Higher Degree Research Festival, 27 November 2015.

Allen, J., & Flack, F. (2015). Evaluation in health promotion: thoughts from inside a human research ethics committee. Health Promotion Journal of Australia, 26(3), 182–185. doi:10.1071/HE15062.

Arabena, K. (2010). All knowledge is Indigenous. In V. Brown, J. Harria, & J. Russell (Eds.), Tackling wicked problems: through the transdisciplinary imagination. London: Earthscan.

Australian Institute for Health and Welfare (AIHW). (2018). Australia's health 2018. Retrieved from https://www.aihw.gov.au/reports/australias-health/australias-health-2018/contents/table-of-contents.

Australian Institute of Aboriginal and Torres Strait Islander Studies. (2012). Guidelines for ethical research in Australian Indigenous Studies 2012. Retrieved from https://aiatsis.gov.au/sites/default/files/docs/research-and-guides/ethics/gerais.pdf.

Bajayo, R. (2012). Building community resilience to climate change through public health planning. Health Promotion Journal of Australia, 23(1), 30–36. doi:10.1071/HE12030.

Bamberger, M., Rugh, J., & Mabry, L. (2012). RealWorld evaluation: working under budget, time, data, and political constraints (2nd ed.). Thousand Oaks, CA: Sage.

Baum, F. (1999). The role of social capital in health promotion: Australian perspectives. Paper presented at the Proceedings of the 11th National Health Promotion Conference, Perth.

Baum, F. (2016). Power and glory: applying participatory action research in public health. Gaceta Sanitaria, 30(6), 405–407. doi:10.1016/j.gaceta.2016.05.014.

Baum, F., Lawless, A., Delany, T., et al. (2014). Evaluation of health in all policies: concept, theory and application. Health Promotion International, 29(suppl1), i130–i142. doi:10.1093/heapro/dau032.

Bauman, A., & Nutbeam, D. (2014). Evaluation in a nutshell. Sydney: McGraw-Hill Education Australia.

Baxter, J., Cooklin, A. R., & Smith, J. (2009). Which mothers wean their babies prematurely from full breastfeeding? An Australian cohort study. Acta Paediatrica, 98(8), 1274–1277. doi: 10.1111/j.1651-2227.2009.01335.x.

Bedworth, A., & Bedworth, D. (1992). The profession and practice of health education. Dubuque IA: WC Brown.

Bradshaw, J. (1972). The concept of social need. New Society, 30(March), 640–643.

Cavaye, J. (n.d.). Community capacity building toolkit for rural and regional communities. Retrieved from http://inform.regionalaustralia.org.au/process/regional-development-processes/item/community-capacity-building-toolkit

Centers for Disease Control and Prevention. (2010). Community Health Assessment and Group Evaluation (CHANGE) Action Guide: Building a Foundation of Knowledge to Prioritize Community Needs. Retrieved from http://www.cdc.gov/nccdphp/dch/programs/healthycommunitiesprogram/tools/change/pdf/changeactionguide.pdf.

Centers for Disease Control and Prevention. (2011). Evaluation technical assistance document: division of nutrition, physical activity, and obesity (DNPAO) partnership evaluation guidebook and resources. Retrieved from https://www.cdc.gov/obesity/downloads/PartnershipEvaluation.pdf.

Centers for Disease Control and Prevention. (n.d.). Public health ethics. Retrieved from https://www.cdc.gov/od/science/integrity/phethics/index.htm.

Chambers, A. H., Murphy, K., & Kolbe, A. (2015). Designs and methods used in published Australian health promotion evaluations 1992–2011. Australian and New Zealand Journal of Public Health, 39(3), 222–226. doi:10.1111/1753-6405.12359.

Cleary, A., Fielding, K. S., Bell, et al. (2017). Exploring potential mechanisms involved in the relationship between eudaimonic wellbeing and nature connection. Landscape and Urban Planning, 158, 119–128. doi:10.1016/j.landurbplan.2016.10.003.

Colin, P., & Garrow, A. (1996). Thinking, listening, looking, understanding and acting as you go along. Alice Springs: Council of Remote Area Nurses of Australia.

Community Indicators Consortium. (2017). Community indicators Victoria. Retrieved from https://communityindicators.net/indicator-projects/community-indicators-victoria/.

Community Toolbox. (n.d.). Implementing photovoice in your community (Chapter 3, Section 20). Retrieved from https://ctb.ku.edu/en/table-of-contents/assessment/assessing-community-needs-and-resources/photovoice/main.

Cook, N., Hughes, R., Taylor, E., et al. (2015). Shading liveable cities: exploring the ecological, financial and regulatory dimensions of the urban tree canopy. Working Paper. Retrieved from http://ro.uow.edu.au/cgi/viewcontent.cgi?article=4168&context=sspapers.

Creswell, J. W. (2003). Research design: qualitative, quantitative, and mixed method approaches (2nd ed.). Thousand Oaks CA: Sage.

Denzin, N. K., & Lincoln, Y. S. (Eds.). (2011). The SAGE handbook of qualitative research (4th ed.). Thousand Oaks CA: Sage.

Evaluation Toolbox. (n.d.). Community sustainability engagement evaluation toolbox. Retrieved from http://evaluationtoolbox.net.au/.

Farmer, J., Hill, C., & Munoz, S.-A. (2012). Community co-production: social enterprise in remote and rural communities. Cheltenham, UK: Edward Elgar.

Flinders University. (2019). Planning and Evaluation Wizard (PEW). Retrieved from https://www.flinders.edu.au/southgate-institute-health-society-equity/planning-evaluation-wizard.

Folke, C., Biggs, R., Norström, A., et al. (2016). Social-ecological resilience and biosphere-based sustainability science. Ecology and Society, 21(3):1. doi:10.5751/ES-08748-210341.

Freire, P. (1974). Education for critical consciousness. London: Sheed & Ward.

Freudenberg, N. (1984). Training health educators for social change. International Quarterly of Community Health Education, 5(1), 37–52.

Grant, M. J., & Booth, A. (2009). A typology of reviews: an analysis of 14 review types and associated methodologies. Health Information & Libraries Journal, 26(2), 91–108. doi:10.1111/j.1471-1842.2009.00848.x.

Grbich, C. (2007). Qualitative data analysis: an introduction. London: Sage.

Green, L. (2005). Health program planning: an educational and ecological approach (4th ed.). New York NY: McGraw-Hill.

Green, L. (n.d.). The PRECEDE–PROCEED Model of health program planning and evaluation. Retrieved from http://www.lgreen.net/precede.htm.

Gregg, J., & O'Hara, L. (2007). The red lotus health promotion model: a new model for holistic, ecological, salutogenic health promotion practice. Health Promotion Journal of Australia, 18(1), 12–19. doi:10.1071/HE07012.

Guba, E. G., & Lincoln, Y. S. (1989). Fourth generation evaluation. Newbury Park CA: Sage.

Harvard Graduate School of Education. (n.d.). The literature review: a research journey. Retrieved from https://guides.library.harvard.edu/literaturereview.

Hauck, Y., Fenwick, J., Dhaliwal, S., & Butt, J. (2011). A Western Australian survey of breastfeeding initiation, prevalence and early cessation patterns. Maternal and Child Health Journal, 15(2), 260–268. doi:10.1007/s10995-009-0554-2.

Hawe, P., Degeling, D. E., & Hall, J. (1990). Evaluating health promotion: a health worker's guide. Sydney: MacLennan and Petty.

Hawe, P., & Shiell, A. (1995). Preserving innovation under increasing accountability pressures: the health promotion investment portfolio approach. Health Promotion Journal of Australia: Official Journal of Australian Association of Health Promotion Professionals, 5(2), 4–9.

Hawtin, M., Hughes, G., & Percy-Smith, J. (1994). Community profiling: auditing social needs. Buckingham: Open University Press.

Health and Disability Ethics Committee. (n.d.). Latest updates. Retrieved from https://ethics.health.govt.nz/

International Union for Health Promotion and Education. (2016). Core competencies and professional standards for health promotion 2016. Retrieved from https://www.iuhpe.org/images/JC-Accreditation/Core_Competencies_Standards_linkE.pdf.

International Union for Health Promotion and Education. (n.d.). The IUHPE health promotion accreditation system. Retrieved from http://www.iuhpe.org/index.php/en/the-accreditation-system.

Jackson, C. L., & Greenhalgh, T. (2015). Co-creation: a new approach to optimising research impact? Medical Journal of Australia, 203(7), 283–284. doi:10.5694/mja15.00219.

Jamieson, L. M., Paradies, Y. C., Eades, S., et al. (2012). Ten principles relevant to health research among Indigenous Australian populations. Medical Journal of Australia, 197(1), 16–18. doi:10.5694/mja11.11642.

Jolley, G., Lawless, A. P., Baum, F. E., et al. (2007). Building an evidence base for community health: a review of the quality of program evaluations. Australian Health Review, 31(4), 603. doi:10.1071/AH070603.

Jolley, G., Lawless, A., & Hurley, C. (2008). Framework and tools for planning and evaluating community participation, collaborative partnerships and equity in health promotion. Health Promotion Journal of Australia, 19(2), 152–157. doi:10.1071/HE08152.

Kendall, E., Sunderland, N., Barnett, L., et al. (2011). Beyond the rhetoric of participatory research in Indigenous communities: advances in Australia over the last decade. Qualitative Health Research, 21(12), 1719–1728. doi:10.1177/1049732311418124.

Kilpatrick, S., Cheers, B., Gilles, M., & Taylor, J. (2009). Boundary crossers, communities, and health: exploring the role of rural health professionals. Health and Place, 15(1), 284–290. doi:10.1016/j.healthplace.2008.05.008.

Kretzmann, J., & McKnight, J. (1995). Assets-based community development. Retrieved from https://onlinelibrary.wiley.com/doi/abs/10.1002/ncr.4100850405.

Laverack, G. (2007). Health promotion practice building empowered communities. Maidenhead: Open University Press.

LoBiondo-Wood, G., & Haber, J. (2002). Nursing research: methods, critical appraisal, and utilization (5th ed.). St Louis MO: Mosby.

McKenzie, J. F., Neiger, B. L., & Thackeray, R. (2013). Planning, implementing, and evaluating health promotion programs: a primer (6th ed.). Boston MA: Pearson.

McKnight, J. (2010). Asset mapping in communities. In A. Morgan, M. Davies, & E. Ziglio (Eds.), Health assets in a global context: theory, methods, action (pp. 59–76). New York NY: Springer.

McKnight, J., & Kretzmann, J. P. (2005). Mapping community capacity. In M. Minkler (Ed.), Community organizing and community building for health (2nd ed.). New Brunswick: Rutgers University Press.

Meedya, S., Fahy, K., & Kable, A. (2010). Factors that positively influence breastfeeding duration to 6 months: a literature review. Women and Birth, 23(4), 135–145. doi:10.1016/j.wombi.2010.02.002.

Merriam Webster Dictionary. (n.d.) Epidemiology. Retrieved from https://www.merriam-webster.com/dictionary/epidemiology.

Millar, R., & Hall, K. (2013). Social Return on Investment (SROI) and performance measurement: the opportunities and barriers for social enterprises in health and social care. Public Management Review, 15(6), 923–941. doi:10.1080/14719037.2012.698857.

Minkler, M. (1991). Improving health through community organization. In K. Glanz, F. M. Lewis, & B. K. Rimer (Eds.), Health behavior and health education: theory, research and practice. San Francisco CA: Jossey-Bass.

Minkler, M. (2012). Community organizing and community building for health and welfare (3rd ed., Vol. 9780813553146). New York NY: Rutgers University Press.

Minkler, M., & Wallerstein, N. (Eds.). (2008). Community-based participatory research for health from process to outcomes (2nd ed.). San Francisco, CA: Jossey-Bass.

National Collaborating Centre for Methods and Tools. (n.d.). Partnership evaluation: the partnership self-assessment tool. Retrieved from https://www.nccmt.ca/knowledge-repositories/search/10.

National Health and Medical Research Council. (2007, updated 2018a). National statement on ethical conduct in human research, preamble, ethical background. Retrieved from https://www.nhmrc.gov.au/about-us/publications/national-statement-ethical-conduct-human-research-2007-updated-2018#toc__15.

National Health and Medical Research Council. (2007, updated 2018b). National statement on ethical conduct in human research, section 1: values and principles of ethical conduct. Retrieved from https://www.nhmrc.gov.au/about-us/publications/national-statement-ethical-conduct-human-research-2007-updated-2018#toc__95.

New South Wales Department of Health. (1994). Program management guidelines for health promotion. Sydney: New South Wales Department of Health.

O'Donahoo, F. J., & Ross, K. E. (2015). Principles relevant to health research among Indigenous communities. International Journal of Environmental Research and Public Health, 12(5), 5304–5309. doi:10.3390/ijerph120505304.

O'Leary, Z. (2005). Researching real-world problems: a guide to methods of inquiry. London: Sage.

Ogbo, F. A., Eastwood, J., Page, A., et al. (2016). Prevalence and determinants of cessation of exclusive breastfeeding in the early postnatal period in Sydney, Australia. International Breastfeeding Journal, 12(1), 16. doi:10.1186/s13006-017-0110-4.

Organisation for Economic Co-operation and Development (OECD). (2019). OECD health statistics 2019. Retrieved from http://www.oecd.org/els/health-systems/health-data.htm.

Our Community. (n.d.). Conducting a community needs assessment. Retrieved from https://www.ourcommunity.com.au/management/view_help_sheet.do?articleid=10.

Patton, M. Q. (2011). Developmental evaluation: applying complexity concepts to enhance innovation and use. New York NY: Guilford Press.

People's Health Movement, Medact, Medico International, Third World Network, Health Action International, & Asociación Latinoamericana de Medicina Social. (2014). Global health watch 4: an alternative world health report. London: Zed Books.

Posavac, E. J. (2011). Program evaluation: methods and case studies (8th ed.). Boston MA: Prentice Hall.

Posavac, E. J., & Carey, R. G. (2003). Program evaluation methods and case studies (6th ed.). Englewood Cliffs NJ: Prentice Hall.

Prince Edward Island Health and Community Services System. (2003). Circle of health: Prince Edward Island's health promotion framework. Canada: The Quaich Inc.

Purtillo, R., & Doherty, R. (2011). Ethical dimensions in the health professions (5th ed.). St Louis MO: Elsevier Saunders.

Quinlivan, J., Kua, S., Gibson, R., et al. (2015). Can we identify women who initiate and then prematurely cease breastfeeding? An Australian multicentre cohort study. International Breastfeeding Journal, 10(1), 16. doi:10.1186/s13006-015-0040-y.

Rifkin, S., Muller, F., & Bichmann, W. (1988). Primary health care: on measuring participation. Social Science & Medicine, 26(9), 931–940. doi:10.1016/0277-9536(88)90413-3.

Robinson, P., & Lowe, J. (2015). Literature reviews vs systematic reviews. Australian and New Zealand Journal of Public Health, 39(2), 103. doi:10.1111/1753-6405.12393.

Rollins, N. C., Bhandari, N., Hajeebhoy, N., et al. (2016). Why invest, and what it will take to improve breastfeeding practices? The Lancet, 387(10017), 491–504. doi:10.1016/S0140-6736(15)01044-2.

Sarvela, & McDermott. (2003). Health promotion short course facilitators guide: Module 1. Melbourne: State Government of Victoria, Department of Human Services.

Signal, L., Martin, J., Cram, F., & Robson, B. (2008). The Health Equity Assessment Tool: A user's guide. Retrieved from https://www.flinders.edu.au/southgate-institute-health-society-equity/planning-evaluation-wizard.

Smith, R. D., Cattaneo, A., Iellamo, A., et al. (2018). Review of effective strategies to promote breastfeeding. Retrieved from https://www.saxinstitute.org.au/publications/review-effective-strategies-promote-breastfeeding/.

Smith, R. D., & Petticrew, M. (2010). Public health evaluation in the twenty-first century: time to see the wood as well as the trees. Journal of Public Health, 32(1), 2–7. doi:10.1093/pubmed/fdp122.

Stephenson, C. (1996). SF-36 interim norms for Australian data. Retrieved from https://www.aihw.gov.au/getmedia/13a09319-2ec0-4030-aa54-ac43478573e1/SF-36%20Interim%20norms%20for%20Australian%20data.pdf.aspx?inline=true.

Stringer, E., & Genat, W. (2004). Action research in health. New Jersey: Pearson, Merrill Prentice Hall.

Talbot, L., & Verrinder, G. (2008). Turn a stack of papers into a literature review: useful tools for beginners. Focus on Health Professional Education: A Multi-disciplinary Journal, 10(1), 51–58.

Tones, K., & Green, J. (2010). Health promotion planning: planning and strategies. Thousand Oaks CA: Sage.

Torrens University Australia. (n.d.). PHIDU (Public Health Information Development Unit), Torrens University Australia. Retrieved from http://phidu.torrens.edu.au/#JtKQqgqtoeBzCAiH.97

Underhill, G., Sloane, A., McCracken, J., et al. (2016). Healthy together Mildura. Evaluation paper 2012–2016. Retrieved from http://healthytogethermildura.com.au/wp-content/uploads/2013/10/HTM-Evaluation-Paper_270616_Final.pdf.

VicHealth. (2011). The partnerships analysis tool. Retrieved from https://www.vichealth.vic.gov.au/search/the-partnerships-analysis-tool

Wadsworth, Y. (1997). Everyday evaluation on the run (2nd ed.). Sydney: Allen & Unwin.

Wadsworth, Y. (2010). Building in research and evaluation human inquiry for living systems. Sydney: Allen & Unwin.

Wang, C. C. (1999). Photovoice: a participatory action research strategy applied to women's health. Journal of Women's Health, 8(2), 185. doi:10.1089/jwh.1999.8.185.

Ware, J. E. (2000). SF-36 health survey update. Retrieved from https://journals.lww.com/spinejournal/Fulltext/2000/12150/SF_36_Health_Survey_Update.8.aspx

World Health Organization (WHO). (1986). The Ottawa Charter for Health Promotion. Retrieved from https://www.who.int/healthpromotion/conferences/previous/ottawa/en/.

World Health Organization (WHO). (2012). The WHO strategy on research for health. Retrieved from https://www.who.int/phi/WHO_Strategy_on_research_for_health.pdf.

Yallop, C. (Ed.) (2005). Macquarie dictionary (4th ed.). Sydney: Macquarie Library.

5 Healthy public policy to create environments and settings that support health and wellbeing

COMPREHENSIVE PRIMARY HEALTH CARE

SOCIO-ECOLOGICAL APPROACH			
		SELECTIVE PRIMARY HEALTH CARE	
	BEHAVIOURAL APPROACH		BIOMEDICAL APPROACH
Healthy public policy to create environments and settings that support health and wellbeing	*Community development action to support social and environmental change*	*Health education and health literacy to develop knowledge and skills for health and wellbeing action*	*Health information and social marketing to raise awareness about health and wellbeing priorities*	*Vaccination, screening, risk assessment and surveillance to monitor and reduce risk of disease conditions*

Health promotion community assessment, program planning, implementation and evaluation

INTRODUCTION

Developing healthy public policy is key to creating environments and settings that support health and wellbeing, and one of the five Ottawa Charter for Health Promotion action areas (WHO, 1986). Healthy public policy describes the decisions enshrined in the legislation, policy, strategic plans or rules of operation of a sector of government or an organisation, made on behalf of the relevant population or group to protect or enhance their health and wellbeing. Public policy includes national policy, state policy, local government policy, regulatory activities including executive orders, local laws, ordinances, organisational position statements, regulations and formal and informal rules. As noted by Alaszewski and Brown, 'policy making involves defining desirable ends, especially improvements in society, as well as evaluating and deciding the best means to achieve such ends' (2012, p. 26). This chapter explores stages in the development of policy generally and healthy public policy in particular that is designed to protect and improve health and wellbeing at global, local and organisational levels, and the factors that influence policy developments.

Chapter 1 outlined a framework for health promotion practice. At one end of this framework is healthy public policy, highlighting policy activities that create supportive environments and settings for health and wellbeing. Healthy public policy can enhance health and wellbeing in ways that cannot be achieved through other health promotion strategies because of the capacity that policy has to move responsibility for health and wellbeing away from the individual and onto the shoulders of those who have the power to control the environment or setting.

Healthy public policy can achieve long-term impact on the socio-ecological determinants of health and wellbeing. Recent developments in the Health in All Policies (HiAP) approach are recognition of the broad range of social and ecological factors that determine health or illness, and the value of policy in shaping population health and wellbeing status.

PUTTING THE OTTAWA CHARTER INTO PRACTICE

The following questions, arranged in the Ottawa Charter action areas, are presented to guide health practitioners to reflect on and critically evaluate their professional role and practice and the health promotion philosophy of their organisation. Content of this chapter will assist health practitioners to develop the necessary professional knowledge and skills to work in different settings for health promotion, and advocate for and develop healthy public policy.

Build healthy public policy

- Are there organisational or discipline-specific policies that can be used as a lever for health and wellbeing enhancement in the setting you work in?
- What are the organisational constraints that would impact on your capacity to develop policies to address the socio-ecological determinants of health and wellbeing affecting local community members?
- What changes to policies, guidelines or rules are needed to ensure fairness of access to resources for health and wellbeing for all?
- How is local government healthy public policy protecting and enhancing the health and wellbeing of the population?

Create supportive environments

- Are community members being provided with opportunities to know what is happening in their community? Is the process for engaging with community embedded in the strategic plans and strategies of the organisation?
- Is advocacy for policy change being conducted in partnership with community members?
- How is local government involved in making it easier for people to be healthy and well?

Strengthen community action

- Is there benefit clearly evident and desired by community members?
- Are community members advocating for policy change which will ensure health and wellbeing gains for future generations?
- Is there effective community engagement for the development of new local government policies and strategies? How could engagement be improved further?

Develop personal skills

- Does the agency have a policy or commitment in their strategic plan to support capacity building for community members?
- Is capacity-building training provided that will enable development of transferable skills?
- Is funding used to facilitate the development of transferable and useful skills?

Continued

PUTTING THE OTTAWA CHARTER INTO PRACTICE Cont.

Reorient health services

- Is the health and wellbeing agency able to take a long-term view about social change?
- Are agencies in the community flexible enough to deal with a stronger and more skilled community?
- To what extent are health and wellbeing considered in the strategic plans of core agencies in your community?
- Is health promotion part of the core business of local government?

Healthy public policy may be developed at the international, national and local levels, with all three levels working in concert with one another. Working to build healthy public policy and create supportive environments for health and wellbeing often takes place in settings that have characteristics in common, such as schools, healthcare agencies and entire residential areas. Using the settings approach, work for structural change usually occurs through partnerships between those with an interest in that setting, including those who have the capacity to initiate policy changes or new policy. Community members and professionals from all sectors work with government to improve people's health and wellbeing in geographic areas, communities and organisations. Before starting the chapter, take some time to review *Putting the Ottawa Charter into Practice* on p. 233.

BUILDING HEALTHY PUBLIC POLICY

Building healthy public policy is one of the five action areas of the Ottawa Charter for Health Promotion (WHO, 1986) and the foundation strategy in any health promotion strategy portfolio. It is important, however, to distinguish between health policy and healthy public policy as the two are often confused. Health policies are a process where the visions or aspirations of a government or authority with power are translated into actions designed to improve the health of a population or group (Alaszewski & Brown, 2012). Health policy sets requirements for health service provision and funding allocations, and aspirational targets for various health improvements. Initially, health policy was developed to ensure the proper functioning of and funding for hospitals.

The development of public health policy is a more recent phenomenon that commenced with epidemiological evidence demonstrating the role that environmental factors and so-called 'lifestyle choices' can have in protecting the health and wellbeing of the population. Healthy public policy has a focus on creating the supportive environment around people rather than regulating their individual behaviour (Alaszewski & Brown, 2012). For example, the importance of landscape planning and applying 'healthy by design' principles is recognised as key to healthy public policy.

Irrespective of the differences in focus, all policies have certain characteristics in common.

1. *Policies belong to an entity such as an organisation, a department or a political party.*

2.   *Policy conveys a commitment to some form of action and achievement of a certain outcome.*

3.   *Policy denotes a certain status; it has the backing of a group of influential people.*

(Alaszewski & Brown, 2012)

'Health' policies can be *about* health or *for* health. Policies that are developed within the health sector have four distinct ways of affecting people. Several authors; for example, Salisbury and Heinz (1970) and Palmer and Short (2000), have used Lowi's (1964) typology as the basis for discussion. These policy types are not mutually exclusive.

1.   Distributive policies lead to the provision of services or benefits to a particular segment of the population; for example, family allowances or baby bonuses provided by governments.

2.   Regulatory policies are specific statements that have a narrow impact. They guide or control action. They usually take the form of legislation, such as the Acts concerned with smoking, food, water and environmental quality standards, or local government by-laws or regulations, such as building codes, design regulations or land development strategies.

3.   Self-regulatory policies are sought by organisations or groups to maintain control of their actions. Professionals are bound by codes of practice. Contemporary relevance of self-regulatory policies may be upgraded through peer review and use of quality assurance processes in an organisation.

4.   Redistributive policies are the most contested; they are attempts by governments to change the distribution of income, wealth, property or rights between groups in the population. The national pharmaceutical subsidies (Pharmaceutical Benefits Scheme [PBS]) and nationalised healthcare services such as Medicare in Australia are good examples of redistributive healthy public policies. Both are designed to improve access to healthcare for the whole population. Access to medicines and services is based on need rather than the ability to pay. This form of redistributive policy is often dependent on the political philosophy of the governing authority at the time they are introduced, but after implementation they are politically very difficult to reduce or remove, because the population comes to view them as 'rights'.

Healthy public policy

Healthy public policy sets guidelines and requirements for changes to the environment or setting to make it easier for people to be healthier. Healthy public policy may evoke complex and high-level action that does not seem relevant to 'hands-on' health practitioners. It may sound like something that a national government would put in place to outline how health funds are to be spent, and this is correct; but it can mean much more, which is why we need to analyse the elements of the term in more detail. 'Healthy' in this context relates to health enhancement and health protection, supporting people's wellbeing. 'Public' refers to all of the groups or communities that health practitioners may work with, or who may be affected by the policy. 'Policy' can mean any set of decisions expressed in a national, state or local government policy, a strategic plan, mission statement or organisational philosophy, agreed regulations, organisational guidelines or rules or statements that can be taken by or applied to all members of that group, community, organisation or population. When analysed in this way, 'healthy public policy' is a very broad term that encompasses a range of efforts designed to protect and enhance the health and wellbeing of the population.

It is useful to recognise that while a national road toll initiative, which has a number of regulations about vehicle and road design and construction as well as safe driving, is healthy public policy, so too is the decision made within an organisation to erect a shade shelter over an outside dining area and to encourage use of the sunscreen that is provided.

By its name, 'healthy public policy' may seem grand, and not something that a health practitioner, community nurse or land use planner would be directly involved in. However, these professionals are often key policy actors, and their professional expertise is highly valuable in ensuring the settings in which they work are health enhancing. Healthy public policy is designed to make it easier for people to be healthy and well; however, this area may be one of the most challenging areas of health promotion in which to work.

Healthy public policy at a national level is often redistributive policy. Health practitioners working within comprehensive primary health care are likely to support national redistributive policies because of their commitment to social justice. Their work might include being an advocate for a particular group of people and lobbying government to ensure that redistributive policies are considered. It is therefore important not only to understand how policies affect people but how they are developed.

Healthy public policy activities discussed in this chapter are those involving the application of regulatory and financial frameworks across a community or population that create opportunities for healthy living (Lin et al., 2014). These regulatory processes or healthy public policies can be aimed at building and landscape design or social or environmental change at the local/community level, or change within an organisation or a group of organisations, or regulations relating to individual actions that are a risk to health and wellbeing. In the framework for health promotion action outlined in Chapter 1, these activities are associated with the socio-ecological approach; they can bring about change across a society, environment or setting. In this chapter, we use the term 'healthy public policy' to include all the activities described here.

Role of healthy public policy

Healthy public policy is central to the promotion of health and wellbeing because, without the support of healthy public policy, other health promotion actions are likely to be of limited value. Healthy public policy has the largest and most sustainable impact of all health promotion strategies because policy has the capacity to redistribute resources more fairly, and it can structurally change the environment or setting. Policy usually remains in place even when a political party or organisational leader has changed. Policy is the most important factor in maintaining and improving a situation over time and can provide both an impediment to change, and a powerful argument to resist change.

The Ottawa Charter for Health Promotion (WHO, 1986), with its emphasis on building healthy public policy as the foundation component of health promotion action, marked the formal recognition of the powerful role that all public policy plays in influencing health and wellbeing, and the role of settings and environments in shaping opportunities for health. People's social, cultural, economic, natural and built environments impact significantly on their opportunities for health and wellbeing. All public policies, mandated or regulated activities, not just those labelled as 'health' policies, have health consequences. The role of healthy public policy is to create lasting positive health and wellbeing influences across a community or population.

Social policies deal with such issues as welfare and access to health services and education, access to housing, social support and transport, while economic policies affect employment, inflation, income distribution, unemployment and taxation policies. Policies that impact the natural and built physical environments include urban and land use planning, building codes, air quality, sun protection, environmental protection and water quality. All these policies contribute to safeguarding the environments in which people live. The notion of public policies having a substantial impact on health protection and enhancement makes good sense, and the need for all types of policies to be responsive to the risks and requirements of the population is apparent. Two recent examples of the growing recognition of the importance of population health protection through building healthy public policy are the increasing concern for the link between health and wellbeing and the state of the environment, set out in Chapter 3, and concern about the lasting impact of economic globalisation and neoliberalism, especially in increasing inequities and their consequent impact on quality of life, discussed in the first two chapters (Labonté & Schrecker, 2006; Lin et al., 2014; Mooney, 2012; Tesoriero, 2010). A policy that protects or enhances the health and wellbeing of a population or group can be used as the basis for very persuasive arguments for a change in a local area, group or setting and/or for funding to support a change. For example, the National Aboriginal and Torres Strait Islander Health Plan 2013–2023 (NATSIHP) sets out policy direction for the Aboriginal and Torres Strait Islander populations for a 10-year period (Australian Government Department of Health, 2013).

Values underpinning policy

New policies reflect the values of those who develop them, and thus may increase inequalities across a nation, or make healthcare services more difficult to access. Similarly, new policy may create environments and settings that enhance health and wellbeing or increase social support for vulnerable community members. Policy values depend on the political philosophy of the party (or person) in power (Alaszewski & Brown, 2012). Policies may also reflect underlying values of an organisation in its mission statements, aims and objectives, and organisational values should be reflected in its policies.

In earlier chapters, we discussed the values of equity, equality, social justice and sustainability underpinning CPHC. The development of healthy public policy, even within an organisation or local setting, requires political will to consider a change that may challenge the status quo. Making a commitment to equity and human rights would ensure members of a society or community received the health and wellbeing benefits of social or environmental change, but there may be additional financial costs associated with change that cannot be directly controlled. Most nations have a range of social and welfare services that have resulted from new policies introduced over time, including unemployment benefits, pension payments for vulnerable groups and older people, sickness benefits and payments for children and students. Governments with a social welfare philosophy will be more inclined to broaden welfare state provisions. It is always politically difficult to remove or reduce a welfare payment or to make it harder to access, such as increasing the retirement age, or imposing eligibility criteria on benefits. Healthy public policy will always be influenced by values and attitudes which can be influenced by a range of external factors, including political expediency and financial considerations.

HEALTH IN ALL POLICIES

'Health in All Policies' (HiAP) (WHO, 2010a), introduced in Chapter 1 as an approach to creating healthy public policy, has been endorsed by the WHO through a number of global health promotion charters and declarations (WHO, 2010a; WHO, 2011b; WHO 2013a; WHO, 2016b). Following recommendations from the World Conference on the Social Determinants of Health, convened by the WHO and Commission on Social Determinants of Health (2008), there has been increased advocacy in health promotion for countries, states and regions to adopt a HiAP approach whereby policymakers are required to consider the health and wellbeing impacts of any new policy under development or refinement. The approach recognises that responsibility for many of the socio-ecological determinants of health and wellbeing fall outside of the health sector; for example, housing, transport and education. It also recognises that many population health and wellbeing gains are dependent on other sectors and all levels of government considering how they contribute to health and wellbeing through their policy agendas. Most recently HiAP has been endorsed as a tool for achievement of the SDGs, particularly Goal 3 Health and wellbeing (Government of South Australia & WHO, 2017).

The Government of South Australia and the WHO have had a longstanding collaborative partnership on HiAP since Professor Ilona Kickbusch was South Australia's Thinker in Residence in 2007. The partners produced the *Adelaide Statement on Health in All Policies* in 2008, and since that time they have developed, implemented and evaluated a HiAP approach to address the social determinants of health. The three recommendations arising from the Conference on the Social Determinants of Health were to:

1. *improve daily living conditions*
2. *tackle the inequitable distribution of power, money and resources*
3. *measure and understand the problem and assess the impact of action.*

(WHO & Commission on Social Determinants of Health, 2008, pp. 202–206)

These recommendations were used to guide development of the six strategic directions in the South Australian Strategic Plan (Cappo, 2009) demonstrating a strong link between international public health philosophy and government policy. The South Australian HiAP initiative is an approach to working across government sectors in collaborative processes designed to improve population health and wellbeing.

> *The South Australian Health in All Policies model seeks to build strong intersectoral relationships across government and facilitate policy work of mutual benefit to the health sector and the partnering sector. By incorporating a focus on population health into the policy development process of different agencies, the government is able to better address the social determinants of health in a systematic manner.*
>
> **(Health in All Policies Unit, 2010, p. 8)**

There has been considerable investment in training policy advisers across many government departments and industry sectors, academics and international learners to develop a 'community of practice'. Various stakeholder sectors identify and adopt approaches that support better quality of life (Delany et al., 2016; WHO, 2011a). The implementation model has two key elements.

1. Central policy control by the South Australian Government, guided by the South Australian Strategic Plan and specific population health targets. Collaborative partnerships between departments and sectors are mandated.

2. A health lens analysis process, where prospective policies and projects are analysed by the Health in All Policies Unit of the government and other partner agencies, to ensure they will make a positive contribution to population health enhancement.

Public policy and health and wellbeing outcomes are measured against the strategic priorities of the SA Strategic Plan as well as public policy outcomes set by the relevant departments (SA Health, 2019b). In 2018, the South Australian Department for Health and Wellbeing was designated a WHO Collaborating Centre for Advancing Health in All Policies to work with the WHO to:

- *increase capabilities for action on the determinants of health and health equity through HiAP approaches*
- *contribute to the knowledge base on the critical success factors for collaborative practices to enhance systems for health*
- *support WHO in strengthening the alignment between the determinants of health and the SDGs to drive collaborative action on the achievement of the Sustainable Development Agenda*
- *support WHO to strengthen research to policy translation on the determinants of health to increase evidence-based strategies for prevention and population health.*

(SA Health, 2019c)

This is a highly structured and systematic approach to implementing HiAP that is at the forefront of HiAP initiatives internationally. There is a great deal to read and learn from the publications that are guiding and documenting the processes, and the training manual and educational programs, available from the SA Health website (SA Health, 2019a).

More broadly in Australia, the philosophy of HiAP is being endorsed and taken up by state governments, health promotion agencies and some geographic localities, although to date it is not being mandated in the same way as in South Australia, and there is not the same level of analysis. A focus on particular settings as the location for health promotion effort provides opportunities for the use of policy and integrated strategies to address the socio-ecological determinants of health and wellbeing, and improve equity of access to social services and resources.

The Victorian Government is also moving to a HiAP agenda by using the legislated requirement for local government areas to prepare and implement a 4-yearly integrated and strategic municipal public health and wellbeing plan to guide health promotion action across the municipality. The rationale is that delivering the greatest impact on health and wellbeing outcomes for communities requires better alignment of existing services and activities across agencies and across a geographic area (Department of Health and Human Services, 2016).

In New Zealand, the Canterbury Health in All Policies Partnership (CHIAPP), initiated by the Canterbury District Health Board, is an agreement between Community and Public Health District Health Board, Christchurch City Council and Environment Canterbury to ensure they work together to embed health and wellbeing in policy across the three organisations (Community & Public Health, 2020). A recent example of the HiAP approach was its application in 2015 to renew the Greater Christchurch Urban Development Strategy Update (Greater Christchurch Partnerships, n.d.) which is included as a case example in the WHO Progressing the SDGs through HiAP resource (2017). The Canterbury District Health Board has provided leadership for the *Integrated Planning Guide—For a healthy, sustainable and resilient future*, updated in 2019 (Community and Public Health, 2019). The guide is founded on a HiAP approach and used as a tool to support a collaborative approach for health and wellbeing-related policy development and renewal locally.

HiAP is the next stage of building healthy public policy; it has an aim of 'joined up' policymaking that 'addresses complex health and wellbeing challenges through an integrated and dynamic policy response across portfolio boundaries' and 'allows government to address the social determinants of health in a more systematic manner' (Health in All Policies Unit, 2010, p. 10). There will be significant developments in this area as governments come to terms with the need to make long-term investments in critical health promotion and CPHC, and acknowledge that the only way to achieve desired health and wellbeing and improved equity is through collaboration across policy areas and departments.

PUBLIC POLICYMAKING PROCESS

Public policymaking is a 'dynamic social and political process' (Milio, 1988, p. 3), but the process has also been described as messy and circuitous (Lin et al., 2014). Public policymaking is not a smooth linear progression because it must synthesise 'power relationships, demographic trends, institutional agendas, community ideologies [and] economic resources' (Brown, 1992, p. 104). Evidence-based research also informs policy development (Alaszewski & Brown, 2012).

There are three key groups of people involved in the policymaking process: the public, including formal interest groups, industry and professional representatives and stakeholders; political and bureaucratic policymakers; and the mass media (Lin & Gibson, 2003; Milio, 1988). Some interest groups involving themselves in the policymaking process have a great deal more power than others because of their political or financial position and their ability to influence the views represented in the mass media. If an organisational or local community policy is being developed, the three groups of 'policy actors' described above will be similar: stakeholders (those with something at stake if there is no policy); management or power-brokers (who often have something to lose if there is a new or policy change); and the people affected by the policy (with whom a communication process may or may not be transparent and inclusive) (Alaszewski & Brown, 2012).

Public comment on proposed healthy public policy is always valuable. There is now greater acknowledgement of the importance of community participation in decision making, including policy development. Community engagement is core to CPHC and this has built on growing disquiet about decision makers' willingness to act in the community's best interest, and an increasing desire to influence decisions made by governments. Controversy about environmental protection has been an example of this (Tesoriero, 2010). In addition, there is recognition that implementation of strategies enshrined in a policy will be more positively accepted if community members have taken part in its formulation. Nevertheless, it is usually the politicians, bureaucrats and powerful interest groups who set the agenda and decide the framework and philosophy of a policy. It is essential to avoid the situation where members of the public have to try to change the policy after the framework has been set because they have been excluded from the policy development process (Alaszewski & Brown, 2012; Lin & Gibson, 2003).

Policy cycle

Several authors have described the public policymaking process using a variety of similar models. Jenkins (1978 cited in Palfrey, 2000, p. 35) described a seven-stage model, with feedback loops, and Palmer and Short (2000) described five stages. Lin and colleagues (2014, p. 140) presented an eight-stage process and represented it as a cyclical process (Fig. 5.1). This model focuses on policies that are formally developed, rather than those that develop incrementally or may never reach the public agenda. However, the stages

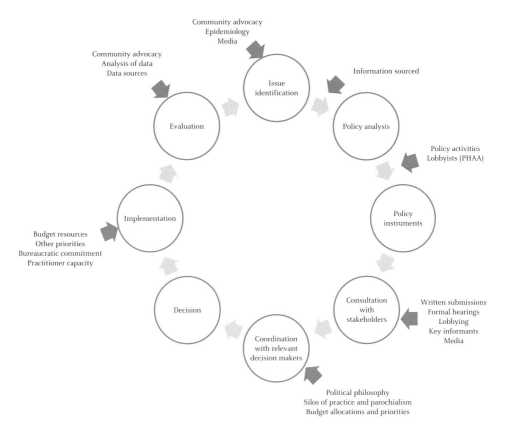

FIGURE 5.1 The policymaking process
Source: Adapted from Lin et al., 2007.

and potential external influences at each stage will be similar, even at the community level. Presenting the process as a cycle is useful because policymaking is not clear-cut; there is always potential to go back and review, and for external parties to have influence that changes the process along the way.

Influencing the policymaking process

Those who are affected or have potential to be affected by a policy, or who have a vital interest in it, may be able to influence the policymaking process at any stage in its life. These are the 'policy actors'. Influence is more likely to occur during policy formation and policy evaluation/review. In addition, because of the cyclical nature of the process, policy actors can be part of the process (represented by the darker arrows in Fig. 5.1) that puts priorities back onto the policy agenda (Alaszewski & Brown, 2012). With regard to issues that gradually rise to prominence in community awareness, community members can advocate for getting the matter onto the public agenda and reviewed critically, perhaps for the first time, to commence the policymaking process.

Influencing public policies through social advocacy and lobbying are discussed in more detail later in this chapter. It is important to note, however, that affecting public policy in this way is often a slow process and it may take several years of concerted effort by a number of people or groups to change the major direction of a policy (Alaszewski & Brown, 2012; Lin et al., 2014). In addition, it is not always clear which groups are seeking to alter a policy, or who may be involved during the policy development processes. It is a very 'political' process, where the stakes are significant.

Regulatory policies such as international laws that address issues of pollution of the oceans, or national laws such as quarantine, or local laws such as residential planning or garbage disposal, are developed for the 'common good'. However, these healthy public policies are sometimes controversial because they are perceived to infringe upon the rights of some individuals.

Health practitioners working in any setting have a core function as policy actors to advocate for policy that enhances health and wellbeing and embodies CPHC values for a sustainable future. Ideally, the need for a new policy, local law or organisational decision should be identified by the community and the policy developed with community and expert knowledge combined with the experience of policymakers. This collective wisdom will make it socially acceptable to most people, and ethically and scientifically sound.

Levels of policy—global to local

If the socio-ecological determinants of health and wellbeing are to be addressed, then new policies relating to a broad range of sectors are necessary. It is well established that health and wellbeing are created by conditions outside the health system. Policy and regulatory activities involve the application of legislative and financial frameworks that create or enhance opportunities for healthy living. Policy and regulatory activities are developed at international, national and local levels and may work alongside other policies and regulations. Addressing poverty, for example, will require international and national policy across the world if significant progress is to be made (Mooney, 2012). The Declaration of Human Rights, Agenda 21, Healthy Cities, and the WHO Framework Convention on Tobacco Control are examples of regulatory activities developed at the international level and adopted at national and local levels that aim to create supportive environments for health and wellbeing.

Organisational policies which set regulations across a certain sector, a local geographic area, or that are internal to an organisation create supportive environments and opportunities for health and wellbeing in smaller settings. Supportive environments are created in settings such as local councils, workplaces, schools, universities, prisons and recreational clubs. VicHealth, the Victorian Health Promotion Foundation, for example, provides leadership and funding for organisations to create supportive environments for health and wellbeing. In these settings, health promotion principles are integrated into the policies or service directions of the organisation. At any level, healthy public policy usually requires advocacy by groups to gain political commitment, social acceptance and systems or management support for the change.

HEALTHY PUBLIC POLICY AT ALL LEVELS: TOBACCO CONTROL CASE EXAMPLE

Developing healthy public policies that can be implemented at all levels has the greatest impact on creating supportive environments for health and wellbeing. Successive policy development on the use of tobacco, given the personal and social costs of tobacco consumption, is a good example. Here, an overview of tobacco control policy at international level through to national, state and local-level frameworks in Australia and New Zealand is used as an illustration.

National and state policies have also enabled some innovative strategies to improve health. Many of these have used social marketing techniques, with powerful messages displaying health warnings in large print on cigarette packets, and advertisements in various media with images such as measuring and displaying the tar and nicotine content of cigarettes, and graphic images depicting the risks associated with tobacco use, such as gangrenous toes and a diseased lung (Chapman & Wakefield, 2001, cited in Baum, 2008; Scollo et al., 2015; Wakefield et al., 2015).

International-level tobacco control—WHO

WHO's Framework Convention on Tobacco Control (FCTC) came into force on 27 February 2005 (WHO, 2005) and continues to have a significant effect on tobacco-related ill-health of the population worldwide. The WHO FCTC is the first legal instrument designed to reduce tobacco-related deaths and disease worldwide. The 181 parties that have currently ratified the treaty and which cover more than 90% of the global population, are bound by their endorsement and expected to legislate according to its provisions (WHO, n.d.-d). The Convention has provisions that set out international minimum standards on tobacco-related issues, such as tobacco advertising, promotion and sponsorship, tax and price measures, packaging and labelling, education and communication, demand reduction measures, illicit trade and protection from second-hand smoke. These provisions are designed to guide governments, which are free to legislate at higher thresholds if desired (WHO, 2005). Australia was actively involved in the development of the WHO FCTC and ratified it in October 2004, preceded by New Zealand in January 2004. A conference of the parties to the Convention meets regularly to discuss new approaches to reducing the risk from tobacco and tobacco-like products and provide guidelines to signatory countries.

Periodically, new protocols are added to the framework that can provide guidance for the development of broader legislation within countries (WHO, 2013b). Most recently in October 2018 the *Global Strategy to Accelerate Tobacco Control: Advancing Sustainable Development through the Implementation of the WHO FCTC 2019–2025* (WHO, n.d.-a) was developed. This strategic framework, referred to as GS2025, will guide implementation of the WHO FCTC and aims to:

- *empower parties to work multisectorally, with the health and non-health sectors and other stakeholders engaged in the fight against tobacco at the global, regional and country levels*

- *help parties prioritise their actions to fulfil their obligations under the Convention*

- *elevate the profile and visibility of tobacco control issues, including the Convention itself, internationally and domestically*

- *manage increased demands and limited resources while ensuring effectiveness of the work of the Convention Secretariat.*

(WHO, n.d.-a)

The GS2025 (WHO, n.d.-a) has a vision for a world free of tobacco and a range of strategic goals, objectives and indicators to achieve this vision, as well as making a significant contribution to the achievement of SDG Goal 3 Good Health and Well-being target 3.A—to strengthen implementation of the WHO FCTC (United Nations, n.d.).

Trade policy impacts

Trade policy variations between nations can inadvertently facilitate illicit trade in tobacco products that both bypass the taxation system to make cheaper tobacco products available, and increase population risks of tobacco-related harm because the quality of the products is not safeguarded. Countries such as Australia and New Zealand that have high taxes on cigarettes and small-volume local tobacco production are especially vulnerable to illicit trade in unprocessed tobacco (colloquially known as chop chop) (Geis et al., 2003; Scollo et al., 2015). Article 15 of the WHO FCTC (WHO, 2005) relates to eliminating trade in illicit tobacco products and the protocol adopted in 2014 provides the framework for securing the supply-chain for tobacco products internationally (WHO, 2013b). However, 'free trade' agreements between nations that have the aim of reducing trade barriers (such as import duties) between partner nations, have the potential to undermine adherence to international protocols such as the FCTC, and thus can have a negative effect on health policy within nations. For example, a collaborative team (Hirono et al., 2015) undertook an assessment of the draft Trans-Pacific Partnership Agreement, and their finding was that the agreement, if adopted as planned, would potentially undermine Australian policy that regulates tobacco advertising. Similarly, regulations that control alcohol advertising, the use of alcohol warning labels for pregnant women, and labelling of foods could also be undermined, and the price of some pharmaceuticals, currently managed under the Pharmaceutical Benefits Scheme, would increase. These measures have the potential to affect the least powerful, most vulnerable members of society to the greatest extent. After his election in 2016, US President Donald Trump signed an executive order removing the USA from the proposed Trans-Pacific Partnership (TPP) free trade agreement, which resulted in the agreement not being ratified and therefore never coming into effect. This was seen as a significant loss for many exporters of primary produce. The remaining partners, including Australia and New Zealand, negotiated a new trade agreement called the Comprehensive and Progressive Agreement for Trans-Pacific Partnership, which incorporates most of the provisions of the TPP. The new agreement was ratified and entered into force in 2018.

National-level tobacco control—Australia and New Zealand

The Australian and New Zealand governments have taken responsibility for a mixture of regulatory activities in tobacco control over many years. Both countries have imposed an excise tax on tobacco products since the early 1900s, although at that time, the tax would probably have been a revenue-raising activity rather than for the purposes of improving health and wellbeing. After the Second World War, when three-quarters of adult males were smokers, the New Zealand Health Department began using posters linking smoking with cancer, to try to reduce smoking rates.

In the early 1990s, the National Health Policy on Tobacco (Australian Government, 1991) and the *Smoke-free Environments Act 1990* (and subsequent amendments) through the Department of Health in New Zealand resulted in national tobacco strategies incorporating a series of incremental changes designed to curb smoking. Strategies included bans on cigarette advertising and smoking in designated public places and eventual bans on tobacco sponsorship for sporting events. Public support for the changes was strong and significant reductions in smoking were achieved in both nations, although reductions in Māori smoking rates were far less significant at that time (New Zealand Smokefree Coalition, 2015). The process of incremental changes continues, with both countries developing specific population strategies which continue to reaffirm the WHO's FCTC and further extend the national agendas to reduce the social and physical harm of tobacco.

In Australia, this process of incremental change is encompassed in the National Tobacco Strategy, 2012–2018 (Intergovernmental Committee on Drugs, 2012) that was developed by the Intergovernmental Committee on Drugs Standing Committee on Tobacco as a sub-strategy under the National Drug Strategy 2010–2015, and endorsed by the Commonwealth, state and territory Health Ministers. The goal of the strategy is to improve the health of all Australians by reducing the prevalence of smoking and its associated health, social and economic costs, and the inequalities it causes. It also details objectives and targets for tobacco control until 2018 and sets out nine priority areas for action as follows.

1. *Protect public health policy, including tobacco control policies, from tobacco industry interference.*

2. *Strengthen mass media campaigns to: motivate smokers to quit and recent quitters to remain quit; discourage uptake of smoking; and reshape social norms about smoking.*

3. *Continue to reduce the affordability of tobacco products.*

4. *Bolster and build on existing programs and partnerships to reduce smoking rates among Aboriginal and Torres Strait Islander people.*

5. *Strengthen efforts to reduce smoking among people in populations with a high prevalence of smoking.*

6. *Eliminate remaining advertising, promotion and sponsorship of tobacco products.*

7. *Consider further regulation of the contents, product disclosure and supply of tobacco products and alternative nicotine delivery systems.*

8. *Reduce exceptions to smoke-free workplaces, public places and other settings.*

9. *Provide greater access to a range of evidence-based cessation services and supports to help smokers to quit.*

(Intergovernmental Committee on Drugs, 2012, p. iii)

New Zealand also has a comprehensive tobacco control program under which strategies have been adopted, especially in response to national survey data, including the 2009 New Zealand Tobacco Use Survey and the Māori Smoking and Tobacco Use 2011 profile (National Smokefree Working Group, 2015). A key initiative of the New Zealand Government in 2011 was the establishment of a goal to be smoke-free by 2025, referred to as *Smokefree Aotearoa 2025* (Ministry of Health, 2020).

Strategies designed to achieve tobacco control goals and priorities in Australia and New Zealand include abolishing any remaining forms of tobacco promotion, reducing the visibility of tobacco products, reducing the affordability of tobacco, eliminating exposure to environmental tobacco smoke, providing advice to consumers about the dangers of tobacco smoking, and 'developing a regulatory system for tobacco products' to reduce the harm of tobacco-delivered nicotine and the trade in illegal tobacco products (Intergovernmental Committee on Drugs, 2012; National Smokefree Working Group, 2015). The plain or standard packaging of tobacco products is a good example of tobacco control policy action.

The Australian Government, in its response to the National Preventative Health Taskforce, announced in 2010 that it would introduce a policy that mandates plain packaging of tobacco products. The Australian Parliament passed the relevant Act in 2012 in a move that was applauded internationally as a new benchmark in tobacco control legislation. The legislation has been appealed by tobacco manufacturers on a number of grounds, but Australia's move has also strengthened the resolve of several other governments to introduce similar policies. The New Zealand Government announced agreement in principle to introduce plain packaging in 2012 after it had undertaken essential consultation with relevant stakeholders (Greenhalgh & Bayly, 2017). The New Zealand Government introduced standardised tobacco packaging in 2018, which closely aligns with regulations introduced in Australia.

While federal governments have taken responsibility for a range of coordinated nationwide strategies, service delivery primarily rests with the states and territories or regions. The state of Victoria, for example, has been an international leader in tobacco control programs and it is used here to illustrate the policy implementation process at different levels of government. In New Zealand, similar strategies are coordinated through the New Zealand Smokefree Coalition.

State-level tobacco control—Victoria

Victorian tobacco action is guided by the principles set out in the international FCTC and the National Tobacco Strategy (2012–2018) in parallel with state initiatives including the Victorian Health and Wellbeing Plan (2019–2023). The Quit Victoria Strategic Plan (2016–2019) sets out five priority areas.

1. Create a tobacco-free environment. Strategies include:
   - protecting people from exposure to tobacco smoke in public places and shared private spaces
   - removing opportunities for exposure to tobacco advertising
   - increasing social norms about the unhealthy effects of smoking.

2. Prevent new nicotine addictions. Strategies include:
   - reducing the uptake of smoking, aiming for no new smokers
   - reducing the uptake and use of alternative nicotine delivery systems (e-cigarettes).

3. Help smokers become tobacco-free. Strategies include:
   - a broad range of education and support mechanisms through Quit
   - providing people with the information and tools to become and remain tobacco-free.

4. Enhance and tailor efforts for priority populations. Strategies include specific efforts designed for high-risk groups including:
   - people from low socio-economic status groups
   - Aboriginal people
   - people with mental illness and prisoners.

5. Quit Victoria to lead and facilitate Victoria's efforts to end the tobacco toll including:
   - undertaking research and data management
   - providing policy advice and information for relevant organisations.

The strategy sets out a range of activities to further reduce tobacco-related health risks, especially in highly vulnerable groups. It has a clear focus on the social determinants of health and provides evidence that tobacco use increases social and health inequalities. While there are whole-of-population strategies, such as banning smoking in cars carrying children under 18 years and banning point-of-sale displays and advertising, there are also strategies that focus on groups with high smoking rates, such as the strategy to provide improved access to smoking cessation programs for Aboriginal people and prison populations.

Regulatory activities to create supportive environments for health have been part of Victoria's landscape for some time. The purpose of the *Tobacco Act 1987*, for example, was to prohibit certain sales or promotion of tobacco products and to establish the Victorian Health Promotion Foundation (VicHealth, n.d.-b). Since then many statutory regulations have emerged to regulate sales, advertising, labelling and pricing of tobacco in Victoria. Recent developments in tobacco control in Victoria include smoke-free dining, including outdoors, and bans on point-of-sale tobacco advertising and display restrictions, and smoking restrictions in bars, clubs and gaming venues, and smoking bans in school grounds. The Quit Strategic Plan 2016–2019 outlines various new policy advocacy priorities, including restrictions on alternative nicotine delivery systems.

The Victorian State Government provides information and support to local governments, which are seen as key sites for implementation of the strategies, including implementing and enforcing relevant local laws (Scollo et al., 2015; Wakefield et al., 2015). This strategic advice is designed to assist local governments in conducting their education and enforcement responsibilities under the *Tobacco Act 1987*. It provides local councils with information, resources and training for environmental health practitioners who are legally responsible for enforcing the Act.

Organisational-level tobacco control

VicHealth, Australia

The Victorian Health Promotion Foundation (VicHealth) was established in 1987 using a portion of the tax from tobacco sales. In Victoria, VicHealth works to promote and support smoking cessation and prevent people from taking up smoking, advocates for stronger anti-smoking policy, especially relating to creating smoke-free environments, and supports new research in the area. These actions have more than halved smoking rates in Victoria from 34% to less than 15%. VicHealth provides substantial funding to Quit Victoria and the VicHealth Centre for Tobacco Control as well as conducting its own tobacco control activities, such as working with sports, arts and local government sectors. For example, community members are engaged through sporting associations to develop smoke-free policies within sporting associations and local clubs, and the Arts for Health Program supports agencies to develop policies and procedures to create smoke-free environments in art settings (VicHealth, n.d.-b).

Hapai Te Hauora, Aotearoa

Hapai Te Hauora Tapui (Hapai) is a community-based public health organisation funded by the New Zealand Ministry for Health. Hapai is responsible for providing strategic direction and solutions to address health inequities regionally and nationally across four priority service areas including the *Hapai National Tobacco Control Advocacy Service*. Hapai facilitates engagement between numerous stakeholders and communities to progress the *Smokefree Aotearoa 2025* agenda through a range of public health and advocacy activities that contribute to four objectives:

1. *To reduce smoking initiation*
2. *To increase quitting*
3. *To reduce the social, economic and health harms of tobacco*
4. *To reduce inequalities.*

Hapai publishes a fortnightly newsletter on health promotion activity, research and events related to tobacco control from the local through to international levels.

Local government strategies

Local laws enforced by a local council have a role in enforcement of smoke-free legislation and making local laws around new smoke-free locations such as schools and hospitals. In 2019, under the Activities Local Law 2019, the City of Melbourne local government introduced 11 smoke-free areas in and around the city, including the Bourke Street Mall, where it is a finable offence to smoke (City of Melbourne, n.d.). Palmer and colleagues (2013) make the case that further local laws requiring licensing of tobacco retailers, in a similar way to licensing restrictions for the sale of other hazardous substances such as pharmaceuticals, may further reduce smoking by restricting the availability of tobacco products.

HEALTH PROMOTING SETTINGS

Throughout the world, various settings in which people live, work and play are the focus of health promotion programs to facilitate the improvement of people's health and wellbeing. The WHO defines settings as 'the places and social contexts in which people engage in daily activities, and in which environmental, organisational and personal factors interact to affect health and wellbeing' (n.d.-c). Different forms of settings can be used as the focus for tailored health promotion action including building healthy public policy. Settings can be defined geographically (e.g. cities, villages, municipalities, islands) or organisationally (e.g. schools, workplaces, hospitals, universities, prisons, sporting clubs, ageing facilities). They can also be defined more fluidly, producing hybrids of the geographic and organisational forms (e.g. community gardens, markets). Additionally, they can take the form either of a physical space where people come together on occasions for shared interaction (e.g. a mass gathering) or of a virtual space where they communicate electronically (e.g. a socially oriented website or service).

Health promoting settings use integrated and multidisciplinary approaches to enhance the protective factors and reduce the range of risks to health and wellbeing across an entire system or setting. For example, a local government may support a whole-of-community approach to increasing active transport or specific policies may apply to school settings to improve children's nutrition, such as a breakfast program or policy related to food provided in school canteens/tuckshops. At a different policy level, hospitals may involve their staff members in increasing client awareness about prevention of cross-contamination and universities may initiate peer education programs to support mental wellbeing. Policies that apply to a specific setting or organisation can have a big impact on people's lives, and health practitioners can contribute to the development of these policies.

The health promoting settings approach is built on the Ottawa Charter for Health Promotion (WHO, 1986), including the principles of equity, empowerment, community participation and partnerships, and was reinforced in the subsequent Sundsvall Statement on Supportive Environments for Health (WHO, 1991). In 1997, the Jakarta Declaration also emphasised the value of settings for implementing comprehensive strategies and providing an infrastructure for health promotion action. A range of settings-based movements, networks, frameworks and guides are available to health practitioners to support health promotion action in different settings. The WHO Western Pacific Region, which includes New Zealand and Australia, supports a range of health promoting settings initiatives under its Program on Healthy Settings and Environments (WHO, n.d.-e).

Health promoting cities

The healthy cities movement is the best-known health promoting settings approach. The movement is focused on using core principles to build collaboration for health across social, economic and environmental sectors. The WHO Healthy Cities project is a global movement with the aim of promoting healthy public policies and comprehensive local strategies to enhance health and wellbeing and sustainable development. The WHO project was launched in Europe in 1988 and there are now more than 1400 cities and towns in more than 30 countries that have adopted this policy approach to creating supportive environments at the local level. The primary goal of the current phase of the Healthy Cities Network is to put health and wellbeing high on the social, economic and political agenda of city governance. It works by engaging local governments in supporting community wellbeing through processes of political commitment, institutional change, capacity building, partnership-based planning and innovative projects. There is a special emphasis on addressing the social and environmental determinants of health and wellbeing, health inequalities and urban poverty, and the needs of vulnerable groups (WHO, n.d.-c). Healthy Cities aims to:

- create a health-supportive environment
- achieve a good quality of life
- provide basic sanitation and hygiene needs
- supply access to healthcare.

Successful implementation of this approach requires explicit local government political commitment, leadership and institutional change, and innovative actions addressing all aspects of health and living conditions (WHO, n.d.-c).

More recently, there has been increased emphasis on the idea of healthy urbanisation due to the global population becoming increasingly urbanised with the expectation that 60% of the world's population will live in an urban setting by 2030. Uncontrolled urbanisation puts the health and wellbeing of the most vulnerable new residents most at risk. The WHO Regional Framework for Urban Health in the Western Pacific 2016–2020 proposes a whole-of-system approach to good urban governance that supports health and wellbeing that contributes to the attainment of health-related SDG2 zero hunger, SDG3 good health and wellbeing, SDG6 clean water and sanitation, SDG7 affordable and clean energy, SDG11 sustainable cities and communities, and SDG13 climate action (WHO, 2016a).

The vision for the urban health framework is 'Healthy and resilient cities and urban communities' (p. 12) which is underpinned by the principles of good governance, rule of law, equity and universal health coverage (WHO, 2016a). The framework outlines the following five domains of action to achieve this vision:

1. *Urban health governance and coordination infrastructure*
2. *Urban health program planning, management and quality improvement*
3. *Urban health information and surveillance systems*
4. *Urban health workforce and network capacities*
5. *Urban health system roles and functions.*

(WHO, 2016a, p. 13)

Health promoting municipalities

While there is a WHO Healthy Municipalities and Communities movement (WHO, n.d.-c), it is centred in the Americas. In Australia and New Zealand, the focus for healthy municipalities is being driven by state and regional priority setting and policy initiatives and local government decision making. The HiAP approach discussed earlier is gaining traction as the basis for integrated and collaborative health and wellbeing planning across municipalities. It enables a shared understanding of population characteristics and the impact of the socio-ecological determinants of health and wellbeing in the local area. Collaboration through planning, policymaking and service delivery produces improved economic and social outcomes (Department of Health and Human Services, 2016; SA Health, 2019b). The 'Go Goldfields' project centred in Maryborough, Victoria, is a collaborative project across the Central Goldfields Shire that brings together community members, agencies and government departments to make improvements for children, young people and families. The stewardship team has set a 'collective impact' agenda that is guided by agreed values and beliefs. The group is auspiced by the shire council and brings together resources from the different departments and agencies. Go Goldfields has been able to attract additional external funding and is achieving stronger collaboration between community members and agencies than has been possible in the past (Go Goldfields, n.d.).

Role of local government in healthy public policy

Although healthy public policy developed at the international and national levels has a great influence on the way our daily lives are structured, a remarkably large number of policy decisions that shape the context of our lives occur at the local level, particularly through local government. Responsibility for such issues as land use, urban design and development, placement of industry, housing standards, availability of recreational areas and location of shopping areas is all exercised at the local level. Local laws control the sale of cigarettes and enforcing smoke-free settings, safety of food premises, levels of noise and other nuisances. Developing healthy public policy at the local level is not without its challenges. The same tensions between policy for economic development and healthy public policy exist at the local level (Lin et al., 2014), albeit to a lesser degree, as they do on a national and international scale.

Local councils are challenged by demands of changing population profiles, sometimes without support or encouragement from community or higher levels of government. Urban and industrial expansion are highly regarded by society generally. Using local population health data and commissioned local research about priorities and preferences can provide significant leverage for introducing healthy public policy in the local government setting. Many local governments are adding to widely available data sources through local community planning processes to gain a detailed picture of the characteristics of their communities. Health practitioners have a role in presenting the information and the implications of change in accessible forms, supporting community members to be involved in community planning, and lobbying local councils to take their concerns about healthy public policy seriously.

Local government has a unique capacity to bridge the gap between separate 'silos' of local action and wider social action. In local government, there is increasing recognition that healthy public policy to address local health issues and support community-wide health promotion approaches is possible if there is the political will and enough funding. For example, municipal planning guidelines relating to land use, residential design, parking and transport infrastructure are having a significant role in creating environments that can support people to be more physically active. Some of the approaches that make a link between urban design and enhanced health and wellbeing follow.

1. *Designing public areas around people, not cars*

   o Shifting transport to active forms such as walking and cycling by creating accessible infrastructure and public transport that improves opportunities for people to engage in physical activity.

   o Enhancing the walkability of geographic areas which can be measured using Walk Score ratings on a scale from 0–100 based on walking routes to destinations such as grocery stores, schools, parks, restaurants and retail. Walk Score is a private company that maintains the maps and scores. Walk Score ratings are being used to market the attractiveness of certain areas, especially because of the potential public health benefits (Walk Score, n.d.).

   o Walking and cycle-friendly streets can encompass a range of policies and design principles such as penalties for 'car-dooring' cyclists, separating cycle lanes from vehicle traffic, and reducing urban road traffic speeds (Gilderbloom et al., 2015; Riggs & Gilderbloom, 2016). Design approaches include: linking up cycle and walking paths to schools, commercial and recreational centres; cycle-friendly roundabout design; and making crossing signals accessible to cyclists. Other local government and organisational approaches can include bike-share schemes, convenient cycle parking and workplace change and shower facilities (Armstrong et al., 2015).

   o Integrating transport and land use planning is a process of strategically planning to facilitate all forms of transport to meet the needs of each sector of the community from, for example, commercial and manufacturing sectors through to the residential population. Integrating planning to meet all user needs is an incremental process that begins with acceptance that more freeways and more parking will not solve problems in the long term; 'the best transport plan is a great landscape plan' (Public Salon, 2012).

   o Reducing land consumption is important because facilitating car use takes a great deal of land area for roads and parking spaces. This results in loss of viable agricultural land and a sprawling city where people must commute for long distances for work, retail and social connection.

   o Increasing housing density makes owning a car less essential and promotes social connectedness. Local government policies can support limiting the urban growth boundary and increasing residential density through its housing policy.

   o Single-occupancy cars are a major contributor to greenhouse gas emissions. Promoting and rewarding car-sharing, making streets narrower and traffic slower and imposing taxes on congested areas will eventually reduce the number of cars. Some expert commentators consider traffic congestion to be the greatest threat to the future of our cities (Armstrong et al., 2015).

2. *Urban design principles with a priority on health and wellbeing*

   o Principles of urban design encompass a broad range of factors in the built environment that can impact on health and wellbeing, including those mentioned earlier. For example, they may be considered in the landscape plan for a new residential and commercial area, or as guidelines for incremental changes in 'renewal' projects in existing urban areas.

    ◦   Principles can encompass the concept of 20-minute neighbourhoods, where most of people's daily needs can be met within a 20-minute walking distance.

    ◦   Pedestrian movement is a key priority; therefore making places where it is appealing to be active, that support access to local, nutritious food and fresh water, and that encourage opportunities for people to connect, need to be integrated into local laws for new residential spaces. (See the Building Healthy Places Toolkit for a detailed overview, Urban Land Institute, n.d.).

3. *Greening cities*

    ◦   Green cities is a global movement to make urban landscapes more sustainable, with priorities around reducing greenhouse emissions, reducing energy and resource consumption and promoting biodiversity.

    ◦   Greening cities and neighbourhoods is also a movement to reintroduce greenery into the landscape of urban areas, through tree planting, encouraging biodiversity especially in plantings in local neighbourhoods, streetscapes and vertical gardens, and encouraging community participation in nurturing the natural environment, including facilitating and providing support for urban agriculture and community gardens. Other strategies include rainwater harvesting and beekeeping.

4. *Promoting social and mental wellbeing*

    ◦   Since the presence of cars and related infrastructure has dominated public space in many cities, urban design policymakers and planners have realised that the intrusions and losses are impacting on the physical and emotional wellbeing of urban residents.

    ◦   Public open spaces were originally created for social purposes and urban planners are again recognising the importance of public places in people's life and learning. As urban populations become more diverse, public places provide opportunities for people to observe, meet, mix with and learn about others. It is in the public places of cities, the squares and streets accessible to all the city's inhabitants, that all can see and hear each other.

    ◦   A growing body of literature in contemporary social research is telling us that healthy, well-functioning communities need face-to-face meeting, interaction and communication among their members; something that electronic 'social media' cannot replace, which requires high-quality physical space.

    ◦   Urban planners are increasingly planning to ensure the interface between built structures such as roads and buildings provides places that are attractive to be in, using seemingly simple measures such as street furniture, wider footpaths, traffic calming, better lighting and shade or shelter (Lennard, 1995, Chapter 5).

    ◦   There are numerous causal pathways between loneliness and social isolation and poor mental wellbeing, including the sense of social failure loneliness fosters, the physiological effects of stress (such as increased adrenaline and cortisol production) and increase in risk-taking behaviour associated with boredom and inactivity, especially substance abuse (Price, 2016).

    ◦   Local government has the capacity to enshrine building codes that foster the positive social and psychological benefits of attractive public places into their urban design frameworks, thereby ensuring that future developments are also guided by these principles.

Municipal public health and wellbeing planning

Municipalities are complex settings, but they are also ideal for taking integrated and collaborative action to address local health and wellbeing priorities, protect public health and address the socio-ecological determinants of health and wellbeing; they are therefore ideal settings for a HiAP approach. Local government health planning activities differ between states or regions depending on legislative frameworks. The priorities also differ between municipalities, reflecting local demographics, priorities and funding capacity. Most municipalities deliver some direct health services, which may include immunisation, maternal and child health services, and home and community care. Other services with health benefits are also provided, including waste services, food and dining safety, water and swimming pool safety and pet animal safety. Many of these are governed by statutory requirements. Some local governments in Australia also deliver health promotion programs to enhance community health and wellbeing, such as nutrition awareness and cooking skills development programs. Councils have a traditional role in providing and maintaining sports and recreation facilities, bicycle paths, walking tracks and traffic-calming measures that all create supportive environments for people to go about their daily lives.

Local governments undertake a range of statutory planning activities that set out a municipal approach to promoting and protecting the health and wellbeing of their population. For example, in Victoria councils are required to develop a municipal public health and wellbeing plan (MPHWP) every 4 years to align with the state level health and wellbeing plan, currently the Victorian Public Health and Wellbeing plan 2019–2023 (State Government of Victoria, 2019). For example, the City of Melbourne Municipal Public Health and Wellbeing Plan is integrated into the Council Plan (2017–21) (City of Melbourne, 2017a). Current health and wellbeing priorities include: Active living, Healthier living, Preventing crime, Violence and industry, Planning for people, and Social inclusion (City of Melbourne, 2017b). In other states, strategies may be integrated with other municipal planning documents. From a local government perspective, health services and health promotion actions should not be seen in isolation; effective health policy and programs at the local level must be integrated with the direct services provided by community and mental health, medical services and services for specific groups in the population.

The socio-ecological determinants of health and wellbeing are commonly used as a framework for such plans and strategies. Recent Australian research exploring barriers and enablers for local governments incorporating health and wellbeing into their policy process (Lilly et al., 2019) is presented in Insight 5.1.

Health promoting schools

Schools play a central role in the lives of children all around the globe and their potential as health promoting settings is enormous (Langford et al., 2015). Health promoting schools is a WHO initiative that creates strong links between the school and wider community (WHO, n.d.-f).

> *A health promoting school is where all members of the school community work together to provide students with integrated and positive experiences and structures which promote and protect their health. This includes both the formal and informal curriculum in health, the creation of a safe and healthy school environment, the provision of appropriate health services and the involvement of the family and wider community in efforts to promote health.*
>
> *(WHO, 1999, p. 3, cited in WHO, n.d.-c)*

INSIGHT 5.1 Integrating health and wellbeing into local government (municipality) policies

There are three tiers of government in Australia, with constituted federal and state/territory governments and a non-constituted local government under the powers of each state or territory in which they reside. The role and responsibility for hospitals and healthcare mainly rests with the state/territory government. However, local governments have long been recognised for their community development role of working across sectors, their proximity to the communities which they support (Rantala et al., 2014), and responsibility (albeit varied) for the social, built and economic environments related to their local populations (WHO, 2012). For these reasons, there is a longstanding argument that they may be the best tier of government to address the wellbeing of populations by incorporating the socio-ecological determinants of health and wellbeing into a range of policy areas (de Leeuw & Clavier, 2011).

Recent Australian research found that 90% of local government survey respondents reported that health and wellbeing was 'always' or 'most of the time' considered in at least one policy outside of the traditional health agenda, such as transport, housing or economic development. The research sought to identify the enablers and barriers for local governments in Australia to integrate health and wellbeing into local policy, giving recognition to the complexity of the policy process as its foundation (Lilly et al., 2019). The survey identified the following key factors that contribute to either enabling the integration of health and wellbeing into policy or are likely to challenge the policy process.

Factors likely to enable local governments to integrate health and wellbeing in policy include:

- Understanding of a socio-ecological perspective of health
- Priority of health and wellbeing as a policy issue
- Leadership within local government
- Strong organisational obligation to the community
- Cooperation across a broad range of departments within local government
- Shared personal obligations and values of decision makers
- Perception that investing in health and wellbeing is of cost-benefit.

Factors likely to challenge local governments to integrate health and wellbeing in policy include:

- Lack of cooperation across sectors outside of local government
- Lack of broader political support from federal and state/territory government
- Lack of policy entrepreneurs to identify 'windows of opportunity'
- Lack of measurable indicators for health and wellbeing
- Limited financial and staff resources
- Lack of lobbying efforts within local government.

Source: Written by Kara Lilly, Associate Lecturer in Public Health, University of the Sunshine Coast, Australia, www.usc.edu.au

The health promoting schools approach contributes to the development of in the school environment, including healthy public policies, school ethos and culture and enhanced parental participation (Stewart-Brown, 2006). Improving access to nutritious food for vulnerable children has been the focus of a number of health promoting schools initiatives along with creating a supportive environment for physical activity (Langford et al., 2015). Government-supported health promotion practitioners and school health nurses are valuable members of the school community because they are able to identify children who are vulnerable in a variety of ways, including through poor nutrition, family violence and emotional distress, and become a conduit between other professional services, family members and school administration to ensure the best outcome for the children.

Evidence shows that the approach is effective in improving the physical and mental health and educational outcomes of children. Evaluation of the health promoting schools initiative has identified that insecure funding to implement initiatives is the greatest challenge to its success. As with many other programs and initiatives that rely on volunteerism, energy wanes after a period of time, and this is especially so in the primary school setting because children's (and parents') time there is transient (Deschesnes et al., 2003). A systematic review reported limited evidence of the full impact of the health promoting schools framework on children's educational attainment. However, the authors did conclude that using the health promoting schools framework has a positive impact on some elements of children's health; for example, increasing fruit and vegetable intake and physical activity, and decreasing bullying and smoking incidence (Langford et al., 2015). Many countries have advocated over many years for the adoption of a health promoting schools approach by schools in partnership with their communities. For example, in New Zealand, the Ministry of Health endorses the use of the heath promoting schools approach and in 2010 introduced a guiding national framework and website to support adoption by schools (Ministry of Health, n.d.). In Western Australia (WA), the WA Health Promoting Schools Association (Inc.) now 30 years old, supports school communities to develop and implement a range of health promotion initiatives to enhance the health and wellbeing of children; for example, food and nutrition, mental health, physical activity, and health and safety (WA Health Promoting Schools Association (Inc), n.d.).

Health promoting workplaces

Health promoting workplaces have become increasingly important as people spend more time than ever before in the workplace. A health promoting workplace is defined by the WHO as '... one in which workers and managers collaborate to use a continual improvement process to protect and promote the health, safety and wellbeing of all workers and the sustainability of the workplace ...' (2010b, p. 6). The WHO Jakarta Declaration acknowledged the importance of workplace health for sustainable social and economic development, and called on health practitioners to act in partnership with employers to protect and enhance the health of their workforce (WHO, 1997). Core areas include the primary prevention of all forms of risk to health through workplace hazards, occupational health and safety, and an integrated response to the specific health and wellbeing priorities of the workplace community. Workplace policies that enable workers to increase control over hours worked, supervision and autonomy can increase wellbeing and productivity, and workplace education programs are an important means of reducing bullying and harassment, or having it managed appropriately.

The WHO has prepared the Healthy Workplace Framework and Model to guide organisations to implement the approach into their setting (Burton, 2010; WHO, n.d.-b). The model includes four focus areas: physical and psychosocial work environments, personal health resources and community involvement. The model also includes the process of assessing assets and needs, planning, implementation of strategies and evaluation, underpinned by core principles of leadership and worker involvement (WHO, 2010b). Many larger organisations have health and wellbeing strategies that set out a range of health promotion, screening and support services for mental and physical wellbeing and family assistance that are available to their staff with the help of organisational management.

Staff members with health promotion competencies are particularly valuable in these settings because they can bridge the knowledge gap in a workforce where health and wellbeing are not core business. Health practitioners play a vital role in supporting the development of healthy public policy within the organisation. The ways in which health practitioners can advocate for healthy organisational policy will vary depending on the institution, the ways in which the policy will influence the wellbeing of the public, and the health practitioner's relationship with the organisation. When a health practitioner seeks to incorporate healthy public policy into an organisation, they may be required to use their skills in social or policy advocacy set out below, or media advocacy, set out in Chapter 8. Creating an employer–employee partnership in policy development responds to the felt and expressed needs of the employees, which is an empowering process. Priorities are identified and health goals and strategies for the organisation as a whole are mutually agreed upon (WHO, n.d.-b).

Key characteristics of a health promoting workplace include:

- clearly expressed principles or values (such as in a mission statement) that directly inform the organisation's policies and strategies, such as equity, empowerment, participation and access
- support for organisational capacity to implement these principles through activities such as leadership, and through professional, technical and political skills, culture, resources, networks and partnerships
- a range of programs and services geared to promoting physical and mental wellbeing that are made accessible to all staff
- facilities whose design, location and function contribute to the health and wellbeing of service users and employees that enable them to take health promotion actions, and which also are an amenity to the local community.

Health promoting sporting organisations

Sporting clubs are the social hub for many smaller communities, especially those in rural settings. They have provided strong links between community members even when other services have been lost from the communities and local population numbers have declined. However, despite the strong social capital, many of the activities have also been characterised by unhealthy role modelling in excess alcohol consumption and hierarchical bullying. The Good Sports program is a national program in Australia funded by the Alcohol and Drug Foundation that works together with local sporting clubs to build healthier sporting clubs to provide a safe and inclusive setting for all people, including players of all ages and abilities and other community members. The program supports clubs to progressively introduce a set of practices and policies that create a culture of responsible drinking within the club. The program includes direct assistance with a health promotion project officer and other resources to build the capacity of each club to make the physical and cultural changes that are needed, and this helps to ensure the sustainability of the new procedures and culture in the long term (Alcohol and Drug Foundation, n.d.).

Health promoting hospitals

The health promoting hospitals program was established by WHO in 1988 and relates to integrating health promotion activities into existing practices in healthcare settings, to increase health literacy of staff and clients, and gradually move the focus of the health sector to health promotion, rather than illness care (WHO, n.d.-c). WHO envisages health promoting hospitals as those that incorporate processes to improve the health of staff and patients (Carlson & Warne, 2007). Some success has been reported in hospitals in the United Kingdom, Australia, New Zealand and the United States where 'collaborative leadership styles' have been encouraged (Carlson & Warne, 2007, p. 508). A strong association has also been found between a healthy nursing workforce and improving patient health (Carlson & Warne, 2007, p. 509). In these health promoting hospitals, nurses have become empowered, which has resulted in better teamwork, greater levels of nurses' work satisfaction, and decreases in staff illness, absenteeism, turnover and patient mortality rates.

For nurses, the main barriers to promoting health are organisational and educational (Carlson & Warne, 2007; Mooney et al., 2011). Organisational barriers include inadequate opportunities to develop health promotion knowledge and skills in the nursing curriculum and the hospital culture of providing illness care rather than healthcare, resulting in a lack of time for promoting health due to workload pressures and inadequate resources. Nurses with postgraduate qualifications in health promotion are better equipped to advocate for health promotion (Carlson & Warne, 2007) but this is not possible for everyone. The IUHPE competency statements included at the end of every chapter provide a useful framework for including core health promotion competencies in the education curriculum for all health practitioners and professional development.

A current focus of the WHO Healthy Hospitals approach is reducing the climate change impacts generated by the significant emissions and waste from hospitals and health services. The Global Green and Healthy Hospitals framework sets out 10 key points in the design and functioning of healthy hospitals that will reduce climate change impacts. These are as follows (adapted from Global Green and Healthy Hospitals, 2015):

- leadership: prioritise environmental health in strategic objectives and purchasing decisions
- chemicals: advocate to substitute harmful chemicals with safer alternatives; have strict protocols for dose management
- waste: reduce, treat, safely transport and dispose of healthcare waste
- energy: implement energy-efficiency programs within the organisation and advocate for use of renewable energy consumption
- water: reduce hospital water consumption and supply potable water, rather than bottled water
- transportation: improve transportation strategies for patients and staff, including measures to foster use of public transport
- food: purchase and serve sustainably grown, local healthy food
- pharmaceuticals: safely manage and dispose of pharmaceuticals
- buildings: support green and healthy hospital design and construction
- purchasing: buy safer and more sustainable products and materials—reducing disposables and waste where possible.

Health promoting universities and colleges

The health promoting universities and colleges concept aims to promote the health of staff, students and the wider community by incorporating health and wellbeing into institutional core business (Suárez Reyes et al., 2019). The Health Promoting Universities initiative emerged as part of the WHO's settings approach in the 1990s and the University of Central Lancaster was a very early adopter (Came & Tudor, 2020). Although the movement has been in existence for some time, there has been less guidance on how universities incorporate health promotion action within their own setting. This has been attributed to a range of different theoretical approaches being used and highlights the potential benefits of a more unified approach (Dooris et al., 2014). The role and responsibilities of universities in embedding health promotion into university policies and programs is an emerging discussion in both Australia and New Zealand (Came & Tudor, 2020; Taylor et al., 2019).

The Okanagan Charter for Health Promoting Universities and Colleges was an outcome of a conference in Kelowna, British Columbia, Canada, in 2015 in recognition of the unique role that higher education plays 'in all aspects of the development of individuals, communities, societies and cultures—locally and globally' (International Conference on Health Promoting Universities & Colleges, 2015). The aim of the Charter is to provide a unified framework that sets out the principles and processes to build the health promoting universities' movement and to advance action on the HiAP initiative internationally. The Charter has two calls to action for higher education institutions.

1. Embed health into all aspects of campus culture, across the administration, operations and academic mandates.

2. Lead health promotion action and collaboration locally and globally.

Each of these calls to action has several strategies to guide implementation in each location (International Conference on Health Promoting Universities & Colleges, 2015). A recent study that explored how the Okanagan Charter was being implemented across 54 universities in 25 countries found that while there was variation in the way it was being implemented, universities were adhering to the implementation of the framework components (Suárez Reyes et al., 2019). A case example of how the framework has been used at the University of the Sunshine Coast, Queensland, Australia, is provided in Insight 5.2.

ADVOCATING FOR HEALTHY PUBLIC POLICY

Policy influencers

Health professionals

Influencing policy is an important and legitimate role of the entire health professional workforce and those with an agenda based in support for community wellbeing and equity principles. Health practitioners are strategically positioned to influence policy that impacts on health and wellbeing in community agencies and settings as well as on broader state, regional, territory or national agendas. They can bring together information about the social, economic and environmental determinants affecting the health and wellbeing of people in their local communities, with knowledge of the wider structural mechanisms influencing health and wellbeing and use it to influence change through policy. They are articulate, passionate about social justice concerns, and frequently have access to parliamentarians or public health or rural health policy advocacy groups. Healthy public policy relating to an issue or risk to health and wellbeing can provide a powerful and ongoing tool to ensure a health promoting environment or to enable equitable access to community resources for the most vulnerable people. The most sustainable way to enhance equity through local policy change is to include it in the strategic plan, mission or values or local laws of the local government or organisation. When written into their policy, decision-makers have to be true to their word!

INSIGHT 5.2 Healthy University Initiative, University of the Sunshine Coast, Australia

The *Healthy University Initiative* at the University of the Sunshine Coast (USC), Australia, acknowledges the responsibility and commitment of the university to contribute to the health and wellbeing of the USC community through the creation of healthy working and learning environments.

The process began in 2004 when the health promotion faculty in the Public Health Discipline initiated a strategy for USC to become a Health Promoting University. The first steps involved undergraduate public health students undertaking a series of studies for the community assets and needs assessment phase. A community profile was developed, followed by a qualitative study of student, staff and faculty opinions about the environmental factors that affect their health and wellbeing. A large survey was then undertaken to determine the health and wellbeing status, health and wellbeing-related behaviours and interactions with health- and wellbeing-related environments among students, staff and faculty. Based on the results of these studies, the health promotion faculty in the Public Health Discipline successfully advocated for the creation of a staff position with the Student Services and Engagement department dedicated to facilitating the development of a university-wide plan consistent with the Health Promoting Universities framework. As a result, the *Healthy University Initiative* was established.

Health and wellbeing activities at USC are now organised according to the principles of the Okanagan Charter for Health Promoting Universities and Colleges (International Conference on Health Promoting Universities & Colleges, 2015):

- Support personal development.
- Create supportive campus environments.
- Provide equitable access to campus health services.
- Strengthen community action.
- Advance health promotion research, teaching and training.
- Integrate health, wellbeing and sustainability.
- Create healthy campus policies.
- Develop partnerships for health promotion.

The *Healthy University Initiative* is a fundamental component of the university's strategic plan commitment to 'protecting the health, safety and wellbeing of all our people'. The next phase of the initiative seeks to strengthen the coordination of health and wellbeing activities across the university; align systems and processes to consider impacts on health and wellbeing; build student and staff capacity and awareness; and balance the needs and resources of our people with organisational and educational outcomes.

Written by David Duncan, Lily O'Hara and Jane Taylor. For further information about current initiatives, see: https://www.usc.edu.au/current-students/student-support/health-and-wellbeing/healthy-usc/healthy-university-initiative

Community members

Health practitioners can be powerful advocates working in partnership with, or on behalf of, community members. It is important to ensure the capacity of community members is built so they too have skills that are transferable to new settings and different health and wellbeing priorities. Community members may be able to influence the policymaking process about a priority of concern at any stage, but they are more likely to have influence during the policy formation and policy evaluation phases (Lin et al., 2014). For priorities that have never been formally adopted into policy, but which have arisen incrementally, community members may be active in the important process of getting the priority onto the public agenda and critically appraised by policymakers for the first time. Public policy is cyclical in nature so community members and interest groups can be active in putting issues back onto the policy agenda. Fig. 5.1 sets out this process.

Citizens' juries

Citizens' juries are an increasingly common way that community input can have a significant influence on new policy. Local government is one sector using or considering the process with development of a new strategic plan, or when seeking feedback on a specific policy area or proposal (Bolitho, 2013). The process involves establishing conditions that can enable deep conversation with a small number of people, rather than broad but shallow consultation. This can include online forums as well as face-to-face activities. It can be described as 'deliberative democracy' where the chosen group is provided with detailed background information and they spend significant time together deciding on the best response to the chosen priority. For example, in 2016 the City of Melbourne council engaged a citizens' jury as one strategy to refresh the *Future Melbourne 2026 Plan* (City of Melbourne, 2016b). The citizens' jury comprised 50 invited local business owners, workers and residents from the municipality who came together over six weeks online and for three half-day workshops to deliberate and ensure the relevance of the plan for the next 10 years.

Advocacy and lobbying

Advocacy and lobbying are recognised in the Ottawa Charter for Health Promotion as key competencies for building healthy public policy. Health practitioners have two key roles in social or health advocacy: acting as advocates and lobbyists themselves, and encouraging and supporting other community members to take up advocacy and lobbying. Developing competencies in this area, as well as assisting others to do so, is a vital part of health promotion work. To have maximum influence on policy formulation or policy directions, health practitioners and interest groups work in collaboration across sectors with peak industry bodies such as the National Rural Health Alliance, the Public Health Associations in Australia and New Zealand and the Rural Health Alliance Aotearoa New Zealand. Community members seeking to change policy at any level would be well advised to articulate their priorities through the wider networks or lobby groups and peak advisory bodies, including with what are traditionally regarded as non-health sectors, in order to maximise the joint actions necessary to promote health, rather than acting in isolation. This could include colleagues in industry, transport, agriculture, education and local government working in collaborative relationships. Advocacy through effective use of the media is also a key component of this process. Notable success in initiating or changing policy has been achieved by issue-based lobby groups working in this way (Lin & Gibson, 2003).

Advocacy

Defining advocacy

Advocacy occurs when a person in authority or an agency with negotiating power represents the interests, views or needs of a person, group or community, to change a situation to improve their lives, which may not be possible if the people were to make their own case for change (Stewart, 1999). Advocacy activities centre on seeking to change an issue rather than raising the profile of the individual or group who raises the issue. The definition of health advocacy was refined by Moore and colleagues as:

> the act of supporting or arguing in favour of a cause, policy or idea. It is undertaken to influence public opinion and societal attitudes or to bring about changes in government, community or institutional policies. It may include the strategic use of mass media for advancing a social or public policy initiative.
>
> *(Moore, et al., 2015, p. 1)*

Advocacy may be used in community situations when there are unequal power relations and the least powerful have been unable to get their message across or to change their situation using usual communication mechanisms, or when community values about proposed changes are not strong. A health practitioner, for example, may advocate on behalf of young people to have a late-night safe transport space or bus service implemented to reduce the risks of assault. A health promotion organisation may advocate for incorporating environmental and equity considerations into the Australian Physical Activity Guidelines.

People can do advocacy work as individuals, to represent the views or principles of their organisation, or as part of an organisation that includes advocacy and lobbying work in its activities. This may include direct approaches and the strategic use of mass media to advance positive views about the issue.

Moore and colleagues (2015) recommend 'Kotter Plus—a 10-step plan for Policy Advocacy' to ensure that advocacy is successful in achieving the desired outcome.

Step 1: Establishing a sense of urgency

Step 2: Creating the guiding coalition

Step 3: Developing and maintaining influential relationships

Step 4: Developing a change vision

Step 5: Communicating the vision for buy-in

Step 6: Empowering broad-based action

Step 7: Being opportunistic

Step 8: Generating short-term wins

Step 9: Never letting up

Step 10: Incorporating changes into the culture

A number of key organisations advocate for community members and consumers in the health system (Lin et al., 2014). Some exist specifically for community and consumer advocacy work; for example, the Consumers Health Forum of Australia and the Health Issues Centre. Others are professional organisations that include community and consumer advocacy as part of their role; for example, the Australian Health Promotion Association, National Rural Health Alliances and Public Health Associations of Australia and New Zealand. Most local governments and state or regional government departments provide a range of opportunities for members of the public and organisations to make comment or formal submissions on proposed new policies or strategies.

Community members and health practitioners can involve themselves in advocacy with all of these organisations. Check the websites of public health, health promotion and consumer advocacy organisations and local government (council) to see the scope and extent of the lobbying and advocacy they undertake on important health and wellbeing priorities, and the opportunities for community input into priority setting and strategy development.

Advocacy is the key to getting political commitment for a priority. Advocacy can directly influence policy direction when it is being formulated or revised at local governance level, or within an organisation or agency. Advocacy is an overtly political activity, and to be effective, advocates work across a range of sectors to bring a groundswell of engagement with a new perspective or approach (Alaszewski & Brown, 2012; Lin et al., 2014; Stewart, 1999). Advocacy can cause economic and political instability because it challenges the status quo. Longstanding agreements, informal arrangements and allegiances may be challenged (see Lin & Gibson, 2003, Part 3).

Tesoriero (2010) cautions against assuming that a health practitioner is automatically better able to represent the views of community members, and that community members will naturally need to be advocated for in their efforts to bring about change or to raise a priority in public debate. Advocacy is potentially further disempowering for community members who are already in a vulnerable position. Sometimes it is better for people to represent their own interests, rather than to feel they always need someone else to do it for them (Buse et al., 2012). Advocacy work should be accompanied by an analysis of power relations between community members and advocates (Buse et al., 2012). Power relations are dealt with in more detail in Chapter 2 and later in this chapter.

Purpose of advocacy

There are four key purposes in advocating with or on behalf of a community.

1. Mobilise resources—advocacy usually argues for a different distribution of funds to what is currently in place.

2. Change opinions—advocacy may involve persuading those in decision-making positions to see an alternative perspective, in new policy development or policy revision.

3. Catalyse change—sometimes individuals or agencies may be willing to change their perspective or approach, but need guidance to commence or to implement new policies that are appropriate to another worldview.

4. Cause actions—advocates can act as mentors to guide implementation of different strategies.

Skills for effective advocacy

Advocacy involves using skills to put a priority into public and policy debate, thereby encouraging those who can influence policy to report it in such a way that the change is supported by the wider population (Egger et al., 2005; Egger at al., 2013). Effective advocacy relates to collectively articulating the message about a priority very clearly and repeating it as often as is necessary to change values, opinions or actions. Refer to the stages in the cycle of policy development in Fig. 5.1 (Lin et al., 2014, p. 140) as you consider the following policy advocacy strategies.

1. *Be clear about what the group wants.* What is the aim or goal? What is it they want to change? What do they want the agency they are approaching to do about the priority? The group, community or organisation seeking change needs to be very clear and precise in this statement before it is taken into a wider domain and make sure it represents the unified views of the group.

2. *Establish common themes.* What are the key messages about why this change needs to be made? Articulate the rationale clearly, linking it with other

philosophical or political approaches. That is, use principles of social justice or existing policy as an argument supporting the change that is being advocated for. Think about issuing messages and arguments that will appeal to a broad range of people, rather than a narrower point of view.

3. *Never stray away from the message.* It is easy to be impassioned by the urgency of the change or the strong values held by the group, and this can bring advocates into arguments that result in the key points being lost. Reiteration of the key message, rather than counterargument, is a wiser strategy.

4. *Use all opportunities to get the message across.* The aim is to generate news coverage that is sympathetic to the point of view of the policy advocates and thus to reframe public debate on this societal issue.

5. *Become political in a range of forums that already operate at different levels in the community.* For instance, consider approaches to community-based organisations and support groups that already exist, formal community organisations such as committees of management or business networks and all levels of government (local councillors, state and federal government members), and approach other advocacy or peak body groups for support, such as the national Public Health Association, or environmental action groups (Dugdale, 2008).

6. *Use a range of media, especially targeting those your audience will access.* Publicise the message in a variety of ways in your community. These various approaches reinforce the importance of having a clearly stated message and reasons why the change is essential. Whatever publicity option is available will entail restating the key points in more, or less, detail. More guidance for media strategies is provided in Chapter 8.

7. *Develop media contacts.* Keep a careful note of the approaches that are made, who is contacted and what responses are received. Be prepared to 'cultivate' those media contacts that provide rapid and positive responses.

8. *Own the statistics and 'quantify' your arguments.* People in positions of influence will be more readily swayed if your arguments in favour of change can be backed up with evidence. Use statistical evidence that will substantiate your argument. Making contact with researchers in the area can be advantageous (see Lin & Gibson, 2003, Part 3). Use new and existing evidence to gain media attention and clearly convey the public health importance of a priority. Have the statistics ready to use and be prepared to provide a printed summary to back up publicity. Always provide valid sources for the evidence. There is nothing to be gained by not being able to back up the claims that are made—it provides an avenue for criticism.

9. *Repetition is essential.* Be prepared to repeat the message any time an audience can be created. The message will only be 'news' the first time around, so don't expect a media outlet to keep publishing the same item— they are there to report the news and the advocate's role is to make the item newsworthy. Seek new forums for the message to be heard.

10. *Find a suitable internal spokesperson.* Identify a person who can be the public image of the priority, a person who becomes associated with the cause. This person must be prepared to be accessible and have their name associated with the cause. This person also needs to have a positive public image, because

remember, this is a very political process and some serve an agenda in opposition by discrediting the messenger, not the message.

11. *Use icons with credibility.* Sometimes interest groups employ persons with a public profile for another reason—to advocate for their cause (such as sportspeople advocating quit smoking programs). Be sure that the values and behaviours of the 'icon' are, and will remain, congruent with the priority they are advocating.

12. *Be persistent.* The work of advocacy requires determination and a 'thick skin'. These are the characteristics associated with all forms of political processes and social change. A refusal at one approach may mean that an alternative approach is tried, or a different person is contacted.

13. *Make it OK to talk about.* There are a number of priorities that have previously been 'taboo' or not widely spoken of in public; for example, sexual behaviours. Advocates wishing to change policy have been fundamental in changing social values and putting topics onto the public agenda.

14. *Find corporate allies.* Corporate sponsorship of a priority allows it to enter a whole new domain of influence. Sponsorship provides advocates with additional purchasing power and public profile. However, sponsorship does not come without its costs. Ensure that the values of the corporations are in line with that of the advocated agenda. Remember also that a corporation will expect some return on their investment, so be sure the demands can be met before the contract is signed.

Social media for advocacy

Social media advocacy and community engagement activities add impact to other advocacy efforts. Social media is increasingly being used by people of all ages, and it has the potential to reach people faster than all other forms of media and advocacy. Social media as a form of advocacy or community engagement should be seen as one of a suite of advocacy tools, rather than as a stand-alone strategy. It is not always possible to know in advance what form of advocacy will resonate with different audiences on differing topics, so it is better to use a range of approaches. The advantages of social media are that it is low- or no-cost, it has almost instantaneous dispersal and has the potential for the message to be spread widely without further action. The disadvantages are the potential unreliability of responses, and the permission that anonymity gives people to express unethical or antisocial values that are in contrast to those of the organisation that is undertaking the advocacy. There is a range of views about how unethical social media posts should be managed; some organisations moderate the responses, and remove them when necessary, while others consider social media users to be the best moderators and will take those making unethical posts to task, thus adding to the richness of discussion.

As with other forms of advocacy, it is important to have a digital media strategy—understand the social media and which groups are likely to use the different forums. It is possible to commission paid advertisements with some social media such as Facebook, and this can be a good investment to focus attention on specific priorities. Preparation of the questions and posts is an advantage to keep this form of advocacy in parallel with the other forms that have been chosen. In order to achieve maximum impact and gain full and rich information from social media advocacy, it is also an advantage to be responsive to the posts and to pose new questions and provide additional information to keep the discussion 'live'.

Social media is increasingly used by many parliamentarians to communicate with the public. Organisations and individuals can use social media and email to express views, as members of parliament use this to gauge public responses about a topical issue. Twitter is now widely used by parliamentarians to 'test' their point of view or to gauge opinion about an issue. For example, when Julia Gillard was Prime Minister of Australia (2010–2013), she participated in OurSay in 2012 (https://home.oursay.org/). OurSay then teamed up with Crikey to ask questions of the federal independents. As they said, 'remember, democracy is not a spectator sport'. This initiative set the scene for broader use of social media by politicians to reframe the debate on social issues and to gauge public opinion about a topical issue. Using social media is now an important component of the health practitioner's toolkit, because it is widely used to build health literacy, engagement with a priority, and awareness of a new development or changed policy. Conducting competitions using social media can also be a valuable way of building engagement with a new initiative or among a new audience group; for example, asking people to post an image on Instagram of them using a new cycle path, walking to school and so on.

Lobbying

Defining lobbying

Lobbying is the process or the activities involved in advocating on behalf of a group or a priority. The term 'lobbying' usually describes advocacy to parliamentarians or to media sources. The term originated from the habit of policy advocates standing in the lobby of parliament in order to approach members as they entered or exited the parliamentary chambers. Lobbyists may be professionals in this role, including specialist media services paid by organisations seeking policy change, who want their issue advocated directly to a minister or who are seeking to raise public awareness about an issue or perspective, particularly during the policy development phase (Alaszewski & Brown, 2012).

Lobbying members of parliament

Appealing to members of parliament to act on priorities that impact on the health and wellbeing of the community can be a useful way of having certain views represented and (hopefully) taken account of when decisions are being made at the political level. Members of parliament have limited access to staff who can research priorities for them, so they rely on constituents and lobbyists for information.

There are several possibilities for health practitioners to engage in lobbying. First, it is worthwhile when communicating with members of parliament to emphasise the impact of the concern for the local people, as parliamentarians are elected by local people in the expectation that they will represent those people's interests. Second, members of parliament responsible for particular portfolios relevant to the priority at hand can be lobbied. For example, the government ministers for health may be approached regarding concerns about a health priority. Ministers responsible for other relevant portfolios can also be approached. The transport, agriculture, sport, education and environment ministers are just some of those whom it may be appropriate to approach regarding different health and wellbeing priorities. Third, the party leaders can be approached if you believe the priority has more serious or urgent consequences. They are best reached via their electoral offices, as their offices at Parliament House are often unattended (Alaszewski & Brown, 2012). Contacting a member of parliament by letter or email rather than by telephone is more likely to be successful because a written request is more difficult to ignore, and you have a chance to put the arguments forward clearly and in more detail. Encouraging other people to lobby members of parliament, or organisational/management authorities, and to keep at it by regularly contacting them, will increase the chances of success, and this is much easier than previously, with the use of internet-based communications including social media.

However, nothing beats face-to-face contact if it is possible. Ask for an appointment time, and go well prepared, with documentation to reinforce the main points you wish to make. Explain why the priority should matter to them, but attempt to understand and acknowledge their perspective. Consider using stories from the field to illustrate and add impact to the argument. Legislators and managers like to be treated with respect. Always be polite and be sure to thank them for their time. You may need their support on another priority in the future.

Departments of health, regional planning and other government sectors canvass public opinion on various issues, such as inviting public comment on a strategic direction or draft policy, or inviting involvement in an activity or application for funding, by placing advertisements in all the major metropolitan newspapers, usually on a Saturday, or by advertising online. National research organisations, such as the National Health and Medical Research Council in Australia, and philanthropic trusts, also invite applicants for funding in the same manner and, in addition, a number of agencies collate lists of potential funding sources. It is therefore valuable to examine the major newspapers and peak body or organisational web pages regularly, and subscribe to relevant email lists in order to identify calls for public comment, which provide a valuable opportunity to influence government policy on priorities affecting health and wellbeing, and planning for the future (Lin et al., 2014).

Unfortunately, many health practitioners do not take the opportunities to respond to these calls because they assume that others in more powerful or public positions will take on this role on their behalf, or they liken it to engaging in 'politics'. Regrettably, this may mean that the final reports of government do not accurately reflect a broad range of professional and public opinion. This does not mean that a clinical nurse, for example, needs to become a political 'activist', but working with colleagues to prepare a submission on a proposed policy, strategy or change, or contacting a professional organisation about practices that endanger health and wellbeing, are clearly within the role of advocacy.

It may be a good idea to arrange for a group of people with local wisdom or specific knowledge about the priority to get together to discuss these draft documents, and perhaps to put together a group response. This is a useful strategy if the people who may be affected by the proposal are unlikely to respond individually because they feel they do not have enough time, confidence or skills.

In situations where a government may need to explore a priority in some depth, or may decide to review a policy, a parliamentary committee may be established to investigate the priority and make recommendations to parliament. When a parliamentary committee conducts an inquiry, submissions are called for in the press, and from organisations with a key responsibility for implementing that policy. Regional hearings may be held, where all members of the public are invited to respond. The hearings are usually open to the public, although it is possible to request to speak to the committee in private if necessary.

Using mass media

As a key influence in placing priorities on the policy agenda, the mass media is a powerful tool to get a large number of people involved in working for healthy public policy (Egger et al., 1993; Lin et al., 2014). Using the media in this way is known as 'media advocacy', which is discussed further in Chapter 8. Consider the growing impact of professional lobby organisations, such as GetUp and OurSay, which use email and social media as their means of public engagement to gain enormous support on some emerging social issues.

In addition, lobbyists can use social media such as Facebook and Twitter and produce media resources such as 'infomercials' and YouTube videos as a means of persuasion about social values or specific issues (Neiger et al., 2013).

Responding to calls for public comment, writing letters to the editor and preparing media releases can all put forward an alternative view and help to reshape the public perception of an issue. There is widespread acknowledgement that politicians increasingly rely on the mass media for much of their information about public issues, so the value of using the mass media to lobby for change should not be underestimated (Neiger et al., 2012, p. 13). Media skills are recognised as a core competency in health promotion practice and they are especially useful because of the potential they bring to influence policy.

Community representation on committees

If public policy will guide strategies relevant to a community, its members or consumers need to be adequately represented in formulating the policy. Health practitioners have an important role in lobbying for community representation on, and ensuring effective participation in, policy development. It is an important way in which policy remains in touch with community perspectives, and this activity in itself constitutes policy activism by the practitioner.

Some people may wonder why community representatives are necessary if health practitioners are committed to presenting a community perspective. There will be times when the perspective of community members may differ from that of health practitioners, and health practitioners should not assume that they are always able to represent the community perspective in an unbiased way while also representing their professional interests (Consumers Health Forum of Australia, n.d.). Furthermore, accepting community members as partners with health practitioners means according them partnership status, not simply speaking on their behalf (Labonté, 1997). In situations in which community representatives are present, health practitioners can assist where appropriate by adding their voice to those presenting the perspective of community members.

Representing consumer interests, whether as the community representative or as a health practitioner concerned with representing the consumer perspective, is not always a comfortable position to be in. The perspective of community members can be threatening to many professionals and organisations if they believe that it is their job to make decisions on behalf of the community and that they know what is best. This is especially so if the consumers or community members do not agree with these professionals' opinions. Recognising that the community perspective may challenge professionals' views may help community representatives deal with any negative feedback they receive during the process. Supporting members of the community in this position, or finding support for yourself if you are in this position, is vital if the community perspective is to be maintained on the policy or other committee for a length of time that enables things to be achieved. Consumers may also be directed to the Australian Charter of Healthcare Rights (Australian Commission on Safety and Quality in Health Care, n.d.) where there are relevant guidelines about the quality of care they can reasonably expect within the Australian healthcare system. Knowing your health rights can be a very useful starting point for evaluation, reflection and arguing for change.

The Health Issues Centre runs a training program and provides a number of other resources including an email bulletin, a journal and research for Consumer Leadership (Health Issues Centre: A Voice for Everyday People, n.d.). The Consumers Health Forum of Australia also provides many resources for health consumer advocacy and community participation (Consumers Health Forum of Australia, n.d.). Similar resources are available from many state and federal government departments. It is worthwhile ensuring that agencies utilise resources such as these and make them available to any community members or budding community representatives, so as to help them increase their impact as consumer/community representatives and build their capacity for active and useful participation.

INTERSECTORAL COLLABORATION AND PARTNERSHIPS

Intersectoral collaboration

Governments recognise the value of collaborative approaches to addressing the socio-ecological determinants of health and wellbeing by enshrining collaboration as a condition for developing and implementing healthy public policy. This process is described as 'intersectoral collaboration', which occurs between sectors and organisations involved in promoting and/or creating health and wellbeing in a particular setting. For example, health, housing, finance and social development sectors may collaborate in a strategy to address inequalities in Aboriginal health status (Australian Government Department of Health, 2013). Collaboration is a process through which parties that have different perspectives about a health and wellbeing priority, or who can address different aspects of it, can create solutions together (Chircop et al., 2015). Collaboration aims to reduce the barriers between sectors and create solutions across sectors that go beyond one partner's vision of what is possible. Intersectoral action is defined by the WHO as:

> working together across sectors to improve health and influence its deter-minants. The objective is to achieve greater awareness of the health and health equity consequences of policy decisions and organizational practice in different sectors and thereby move in the direction of healthy public policy and practice across sectors.
>
> *(WHO, 2011a)*

The intersectoral collaborative approach is recognised in international, national and local health- and wellbeing-related policies. The ability to achieve intersectoral collaboration in policy formulation will depend on the political, social and economic context (Buse et al., 2012). An example of the potential for intersectoral collaboration is the examination of tobacco policy presented earlier. On a national scale, an ideal outcome of intersectoral collaboration would be to have a *Health in All Policies* approach where there is systematic consideration of health and wellbeing priorities in the policy processes of all sectors, and to identify and adopt health promotion action that supports better quality of life (Delany et al., 2016; WHO, 2011a).

The WHO (2011a, pp. 2–6) developed a 10-step process for intersectoral collaboration in health.

1. Conduct self-assessment to assess the sector's capacity and readiness for collaboration, and if necessary improve the capacity of relevant staff by enhancing their policy knowledge.

2. Achieve a better understanding of other sectors, their policies, goals, language, values and priorities, and how these align or differ.

3. Gain a good understanding of the area of concern and what factors would improve quality of life.

4. Choose the level of engagement. Should it be across the entire sector, related to one common issue, or more localised about one potential program or strategy?

5. Develop a strategy to engage the collaboration partners, setting out the terms of reference that would be agreed.

6. Use a common framework, such as a socio-ecological determinants of health and wellbeing conceptual diagram, so other sectors can see where they fit within the whole.

7. Strengthen governance structures, political will and accountability by documenting expectations, outcomes and accountability measures.

8. Enhance community engagement to achieve real dialogue and wide opportunities for consultation, using a range of approaches.

9. Choose other processes that promote collaboration including transparency, reciprocal respect and participation, and adhering to human rights obligations.

10. Monitor and evaluate the processes and use the findings to inform and improve further policy developments.

Intersectoral collaboration is the basis of the settings approach to health promotion where sectors that have a role in settings such as schools, workplaces, health service facilities, and cultural and recreational venues, come together to work on a health and wellbeing priority of mutual concern. The approach draws on what works best in each setting and uses the skills and strengths of the collaborating agencies. Collaborative action can take many forms; for example, policy development, health promotion, community development, advocacy, and service delivery models, such as shared management. Collaborations may be between organisations from areas of interest, such as education, child care or agriculture; large organisational structures such as local, state or national government; and community-based structures such as neighbourhood centres, service clubs and other non-government agencies.

Intersectoral action is likely to be effective in health promotion for a number of reasons.

- It enables broad multi-focused approaches to address the determinants of health and wellbeing that would not be possible by smaller agencies working in isolation.

- The availability of support services is not the business of any one sector.

- If the collaboration allows those most affected to take part in decision making and action about a priority, then the information used and strategies developed are acceptable to the group and more sustainable over time.

- It promotes efficient use of resources without duplication.

- The process multiplies the impact because of its breadth of health promotion actions and this extends the capacity to influence policies elsewhere.

- It gives credibility and legitimacy to the issues and those involved in the processes that are further strengthened over time.

- During the process, partners will develop new skills and capabilities that enhance their commitment to the outcome and are transferable to other settings.

Intersectoral action is less likely to be effective when:

- Power relations between sectors remain unequal.

- It is a 'top-down' approach, set up by formal agreements between managers or bureaucrats, and the collaboration may be underpinned by hierarchical power relations; signatories to an agreement may not perceive a partnership of care.

In addition to formally negotiated collaborative partnerships outlined by the WHO and used in national or state policy development, at a local level collaborative action can use a wide range of strategies such as an agreement between managers, joint approach to a common priority, collaboration of practitioners in a specific case, and a change in local policy or legislation (e.g. developing a new municipal public health and wellbeing plan).

State and regional governments in Australia and district health boards in New Zealand encourage intersectoral collaboration between health and human service providers across local geographic areas to improve access to services, reduce morbidity associated with chronic illnesses and deliver integrated health promotion services. Examples include the Primary Care Partnerships strategy (PCP) (Department of Health and Human Services, n.d.-b) and Health Alliances in New Zealand where nine networks of primary health care providers and district health boards are collaborating to implement the government's Better, Sooner, More Convenient Health Care in the Community initiatives (Ministry of Health, 2011). The Healthy Together Victoria initiative (Department of Health and Human Services, n.d.-a) is a partnership approach supported between federal, state and local governments taking a systems-wide approach to creating health environments for healthy eating and physical activity at home, in childcare centres, schools, workplaces, shops and sporting facilities. Multiple health promotion strategies, policies and initiatives are implemented in places where people spend their time. However, the risk to sustainability of such initiatives is ongoing political commitment at each level.

There are advantages for community members when collaborative and interdisciplinary approaches are used to address a health and wellbeing priority. They benefit from the collective wisdom and combined funding, rather than having separate 'silos' of professional roles, within single disciplines of practice, dealing with one facet of a priority (Delany et al., 2016). There are also advantages for health practitioners in working collaboratively; they share their expertise and agency resources, provide interpersonal and inter-agency support in tackling the most difficult challenges, and achieve greater financial efficiencies, so they can have more impact for the dollars spent. Sustainable improvement in health and wellbeing can be achieved when the full range of sectors work together to address the socio-ecological determinants of health and wellbeing through health promotion action (WHO, 1986). Guidelines for putting intersectoral collaboration into professional practice are presented in Insight 5.3.

Partnerships

The term 'partnership' is usually used to describe the most effective working relationships between groups of agencies or between agencies and community groups dealing with a health and wellbeing priority. 'Partnership' is an indicator of the quality of the relationships between two or more agencies. While an intersectoral collaboration may also be a successful partnership, not all collaborations result in effective partnerships. Agencies or groups participating in collaboration may not be there as equal partners. As suggested by Arnstein's Ladder of Citizen Participation, presented in Chapter 6 (Fig. 6.1), there are a number of forms of participation, but partnerships are the most mutually beneficial and desirable. The process of establishing and maintaining effective partnerships is as important as the outcome. In the partnerships approach, there should be recognition that agencies and community groups all have wisdom to contribute. Partner agencies and community representatives are directly involved in decision making and implementation, and there is negotiation and agreement between partner agencies and groups. VicHealth, in Victoria, has developed a Partnerships Analysis Tool for representatives of agencies planning to work in collaboration. It provides guidelines for agencies to develop a clear understanding

INSIGHT 5.3 Guidelines for putting intersectoral collaboration into practice

1. The collaboration has a purpose. The collaboration may arise out of a formal or informal community assessment process. The key priority to be addressed becomes the purpose for bringing stakeholders together. Some of the agencies or groups represented may already be working on the priority.
2. All relevant stakeholders are involved. Thinking broadly considers all those who may have a role to play in the approach to the issue. In the early stages of development, a 'reference group' could be formed, representing the stakeholder agencies or groups. The reference group could then identify strategic approaches, and other relevant sectors to be approached. As the action evolves, different sectors may need to be co-opted.
3. Stakeholders' interests and concerns are considered. By definition the nature of the collaboration will need to be described in detail to make sure that no stakeholder is later confused about expectations.
4. Each sector or organisation outlines its level of support for a proposed action. Small and large organisations will be able to commit different levels of contribution, including financial, staff or in-kind contribution. In the same way, different agencies will be inclined to commit at different levels according to how closely the priority being addressed aligns with the core business or strategic plan of their agency.
5. Effective action must engage all major stakeholders. Stakeholders should be invited to collaborate because they have a defined role to play, not because they 'should' be invited. Each agency partner has a role that is congruent with their core business. Even when an agency refuses to join the collaboration, their views should be considered. It may mean that they are more willing to participate later.
6. Organisations need to recognise their interdependence in achieving a common end.

For more information about effective collaborative partnerships, refer to the Vic Health Partnerships Analysis Tool and other guidelines at the Victorian Government Health website at: http://www2.health.vic.gov.au.

of how different forms of collaboration may work for them, to use as a means of evaluating the quality of collaborative partnerships they have formed, and to focus on ways to strengthen new and existing partnerships (VicHealth, 2011).

Achieving partnerships begins with consideration of two important concepts discussed in Chapters 2 and 6—power and participation. Participation involves sharing power, rather than one organisation achieving power over the others. Power is often vested in those who hold the financial purse-strings or who are seen to have the 'expert' knowledge, such as health practitioners (Tesoriero, 2010). It is often a new and complex role for the health practitioner to relinquish control by working in partnership with other agencies and/or community members. Working to overcome powerlessness is the essential first step in mobilising community action to make structural social, political and economic change. It brings immediate benefits to the individual because they gain a sense of control, hope and purpose (Syme, 1998). An empowering process is to work collaboratively with individuals and communities to form partnerships based on mutual respect, where decision making is shared. This assists people to move from an inward-looking focus on day-to-day crisis management to a focus on broader social and environmental priorities that affect their future health and wellbeing through active participation in forming and implementing healthy public policy.

Within the context of the discussion about enhancing the quality of community partnerships, the approach health practitioners take towards community members they are employed to work with can impact on how and what health and wellbeing changes are achieved. A health practitioner's approach will influence how controlling or supportive they are of community members and the significance of community members' contribution to local healthy public policy and action. Health practitioners' elitism has the potential to stifle or discourage the development of policies and skills that will allow people to work more effectively for what they need in the future. Across the spectrum of health promotion action, from community action or policy guidelines to health education, the work of health promotion is to enable, mediate and advocate on behalf of community members. Participation is essential if the community is to achieve equitable access to health and wellbeing opportunities, and to become empowered as part of the process by being able to take an active part in decisions that affect them.

CONCLUSION

The WHO encourages development of healthy public policy at global, national and local levels as this strategy will have the most impact on the socio-ecological determinants of health and wellbeing in settings and environments that support collaborative approaches to create health and wellbeing. Supportive environments and settings provide people with an opportunity to live a healthy and full life.

This chapter has reviewed some of the ways in which we can work for healthier communities, especially through being active in forming and using healthy public policy. There is potential to have more significant and lasting improvements on population health and wellbeing when governments adopt the Health in All Policies approach. Working collaboratively across sectors and communities, the health promotion effort is directed at changing the environment rather than the individual. Policy change is assisted by lobbying, advocacy and working in partnership with communities, and health practitioners have key roles in facilitating policy action. Health practitioners—whether they are specialists in health promotion, they work in local, state or national government or in a clinical field—have an ongoing role as policy actors. It is in this policy action area more than in any other area of health promotion practice that developments are occurring, as health practitioners develop more innovative ways to work with colleagues, communities and client groups. Changes in a setting or environment that are enshrined in policy have the potential to be sustained over time. In the long term, the health and wellbeing advantage will become a 'normal' part of life, even after program funding has finished, or there has been a change of administration or government.

MORE TO EXPLORE

- VicHealth—Preventing tobacco use (VicHealth, n.d.-a)
- WHO Collaborating Centre for Advancing Health in All Policies (SA Health, 2019c)
- Progressing the sustainable development goals through health in all policies: case studies from around the world (Government of South Australia & WHO, 2017)
- VicHealth partnership tool (VicHealth, 2011)
- The Future Melbourne 2026 citizens' jury (City of Melbourne, 2016a)

IUHPE Core Competencies for Health Promotion

The IUHPE Core Competencies for Health Promotion comprises nine domains of action. Each domain has a series of core competency statements and a detailed outline of the knowledge and skills that contribute to competency in that domain.

The content of this chapter relates especially to the achievement of competency in the health promotion domains outlined below.

1. Enable change	*1.1 Work collaboratively across sectors to influence the development of public policies which impact positively on health and reduce health inequities* Theory and practice of collaborative working including facilitation, negotiation, conflict resolution, mediation and teamwork
	1.2 Use health promotion approaches which support empowerment, participation, partnership and equity to create environments and settings which promote health Knowledge of strategy and policy development and how legislation impacts on health
	1.5 Work in collaboration with key stakeholders to reorient health and other services to promote health and reduce health inequities Health promotion settings approach
2. Advocate for health	*2.1 Use advocacy strategies and techniques which reflect health promotion principles* Advocacy strategies and techniques
	2.2 Engage with and influence key stakeholders to develop and sustain health promotion action Knowledge of strategy and policy development
	2.3 Raise awareness of and influence public opinion on health issues Knowledge of strategy and policy development
	2.4 Advocate for the development of policies, guidelines and procedures across all sectors which impact positively on health and reduce health inequities Use of advocacy techniques
	2.5 Facilitate communities and groups to articulate their needs and advocate for the resources and capacities required for health promotion action Working with a range of stakeholders Knowledge of strategy and policy development
3. Mediate through partnership	*3.1 Engage partners from different sectors to actively contribute to health promotion action* Systems, structures and functions of different sectors, organisations and agencies

	3.2 Facilitate effective partnership working which reflects health promotion values and principles Principles of effective intersectoral partnership working
4. Communication	*4.2 Use electronic and other media to receive and disseminate health promotion information* Theory and practice of effective communication including interpersonal communication and group work Applications of information technology for social networking media and mass media
5. Leadership	*5.1 Work with stakeholders to agree a shared vision and strategic direction for health promotion action* Theory and practice of collaborative working including facilitation, negotiation, conflict resolution, mediation, decision making, teamwork, stakeholder engagement and networking
	5.3 Network with and motivate stakeholders in leading change to improve health and reduce inequities Principles of effective intersectoral partnership working Collaborative working skills
	5.5 Contribute to mobilising and managing resources for health promotion action Emerging challenges in health and health promotion
7. Planning	*7.1 Mobilise, support and engage the participation of stakeholders in planning health promotion action* Ability to work with: groups and communities targeted by the health promotion action; stakeholders and partners
	7.2 Use current models and systematic approaches for planning health promotion action Use and effectiveness of current health promotion planning models and theories
8. Implementation	*8.4 Facilitate program sustainability and stakeholder ownership through ongoing consultation and collaboration* Quality assurance, monitoring and process evaluation
9. Evaluation and research	*9.4 Use research and evidence-based strategies to inform practice* Data interpretation and statistical analysis Evidence base for health promotion

In addition, IUHPE specifies knowledge, skills and performance criteria essential for health promotion practitioners to act professionally and ethically, including having knowledge of ethical and legal issues, behaving in an ethical and respectful manner and working in ways that review and improve practice. Full details are available at: http://www.iuhpe.org/index.php/en/the-accreditation-system

Reflective Questions

1. Identify a new healthy public policy under development in your local area. Now review the policymaking process set out in Fig. 5.1. For each stage of the policymaking process, identify the three groups of policy actors: stakeholders (those with something at stake if there is no policy); management or power brokers (who often have something to lose if there is a new policy change); and the people affected by the policy. Discuss the difference in perspectives on a health and wellbeing issue between the policy actor groups.

2. What healthy public policies do you think contributed to the following public health achievements during the last century: reduction in motor vehicle-related deaths; reduction in fatal occupational injuries and deaths; reduction in deaths from coronary heart disease; decreased maternal mortality in childbirth in developing nations; reductions in tooth decay in children in your country; and prevention of smoking-related deaths?

3. Think of a setting that you are familiar with. It might be a school, hospital, university or any workplace. Using the guidelines for putting intersectoral collaboration into professional practice presented in Insight 5.3, develop an intersectoral collaboration plan to improve health and wellbeing in this setting.

REFERENCES

Alaszewski, A., & Brown, P. (2012). Making health policy: a critical introduction. Cambridge: Polity.

Alcohol and Drug Foundation. (n.d.). Good sports. Retrieved from https://adf.org.au/programs/good-sports/.

Armstrong, B., Davison, G., Malan, J. D. et al. (2015). Delivering sustainable urban mobility. Retrieved from https://acola.org/sustainable-urban-mobility-saf08/.

Australian Commission on Safety and Quality in Health Care. (n.d.). Australian charter of healthcare rights. Retrieved from https://www.safetyandquality.gov.au/sites/default/files/migrated/Charter-PDf.pdf.

Australian Government. (1991). National health policy on tobacco. Canberra: AGPS.

Australian Government Department of Health. (2013). National Aboriginal and Torres Strait Islander health plan 2013–2023. Retrieved from https://www1.health.gov.au/internet/main/publishing.nsf/Content/natsih-plan?Open=&utm_source=health.gov.au&utm_medium=redirect&utm_campaign=digital_transformation&utm_content=natsihp.

Baum, F. (2008). The new public health (3rd ed.). South Melbourne: Oxford University Press.

Bolitho, A. (2013). The role and future of citizen committees in Australian local government. Retrieved from https://www.uts.edu.au/sites/default/files/ACELG_Citizen_Committees_Report_.pdf.

Brown, A. (1992). Groupwork community care practice handbooks. Aldershot, England: Ashgate.

Burton, J. (2010). WHO healthy workplace framework and model: Background and supporting literature and practice. Retrieved from https://www.who.int/publications-detail/who-healthy-workplace-framework-and-model.

Buse, K., Mays, N., & Walt, G. (2012). Making health policy: understanding public health (2nd ed.). Maidenhead, England: McGraw-Hill Education/Open University Press.

Came, H. A., & Tudor, K. (2020). The whole and inclusive university: a critical review of health promoting universities from Aotearoa New Zealand. Health Promotion International, 35, 102–110.

Cappo, D. (2009). People and community at the heart of systems and bureaucracy: South Australia's social inclusion initiative. Retrieved from https://apo.org.au/node/2343

Carlson, G. D., & Warne, T. (2007). Do healthier nurses make better health promotors? A review of the literature. Nurse Education Today, 27(5), 506–513. doi:10.1016/j.nedt.2006.08.012.

Chircop, A., Bassett, R., & Taylor, E. (2015). Evidence on how to practice intersectoral collaboration for health equity: a scoping review. Critical Public Health, 25(2), 178–191. doi:10.1080/09581596.2014.887831.

City of Melbourne. (2016a). Citizens' jury ready to help shape our city's future. Retrieved from https://www.melbourne.vic.gov.au/news-and-media/Pages/future-melbourne-2026-citizens-jury-ready-to-help-shape-our-citys-future.aspx.

City of Melbourne. (2016b). Future Melbourne 2026. Retrieved from https://s3.ap-southeast-2.amazonaws.com/hdp.au.prod.app.com-participate.files/6814/7027/1508/Future_Melbourne_2026_Plan.pdf.

City of Melbourne. (2017a). Council plan 2017–21. Retrieved from https://www.melbourne.vic.gov.au/about-council/vision-goals/pages/council-plan.aspx.

City of Melbourne. (2017b). Municipal public health and wellbeing plan. Retrieved from https://www.melbourne.vic.gov.au/about-council/vision-goals/Pages/municipal-public-health-and-wellbeing-plan.aspx.

City of Melbourne. (n.d.). Smoking and tobacco. Retrieved from https://www.melbourne.vic.gov.au/community/health-support-services/health-services/pages/smoking-and-tobacco.aspx.

Community & Public Health (CPH). (2019). Integrated Planning Guide for a healthy, sustainable and resilient future. Health in All Policies Team, CPH. Retrieved from ttps://www.cph.co.nz/wp-content/uploads/IntegratedPlanningGuideV3.pdf

Community & Public Health (CPH). (2020). Health in All Policies approach at Community and Public Health. Retrieved from https://www.cph.co.nz/your-health/health-in-all-policies/

Consumers Health Forum of Australia. (n.d.). Consumers Health Forum of Australia. Retrieved from https://www.chf.org.au/.

de Leeuw, E., & Clavier, C. (2011). Healthy public in all policies. Health Promotion International, 26(Suppl_2), ii237–ii244. doi:10.1093/heapro/dar071.

Delany, T., Lawless, A., Baum, F., et al. (2016). Health in all policies in South Australia: what has supported early implementation? Health Promotion International, 31(4), 888–898. doi:10.1093/heapro/dav084.

Department of Health and Human Services. (2016). Delivering place-based primary prevention in Victorian communities. Retrieved from https://iepcp.org.au/wp-content/uploads/2017/04/Discussion-Paper-delivering-place-based-prevention-Sept-2016.pdf.

Department of Health and Human Services. (n.d.-a). Preventive health. Retrieved from https://www2.health.vic.gov.au/public-health/preventive-health.

Department of Health and Human Services. (n.d.-b). Primary care partnerships. Retrieved from https://www2.health.vic.gov.au/primary-and-community-health/primary-care/primary-care-partnerships.

Deschesnes, M., Martin, C., & Hill, A. J. (2003). Comprehensive approaches to school health promotion: how to achieve broader implementation? Health Promotion International, 18(4), 387–396. doi:10.1093/heapro/dag410.

Dooris, M., Wills, J., & Newton, J. (2014). Theorizing healthy settings: a critical discussion with reference to Healthy Universities. Scandinavian Journal of Public Health, 42(15_suppl), 7–16. doi:10.1177/1403494814544495.

Dugdale, P. M. (2008). Doing health policy in Australia. Sydney: Allen & Unwin.

Egger, G., Donovan, R., & Spark, R. (2005). Health promotion, strategies and methods (2nd ed.). Sydney: McGraw-Hill.

Egger, G., Donovan, R., & Spark, R. (2013). Health promotion strategies and methods (3rd ed.). Sydney: McGraw-Hill.

Egger, G., Spark, R., & Donovan, R. (1993). Health and the media: principles and practices for health promotion. Sydney: McGraw-Hill.

Geis, G., Cartwright, S., & Houston, J. (2003). Public wealth, public health, and private stealth: examining the black market in cigarettes in Australia. Australian Journal of Social Issues, 38(3), 349–364. doi:10.1002/j.1839-4655.2003.tb01150.x.

Gilderbloom, J. I., Riggs, W. W., & Meares, W. L. (2015). Does walkability matter? An examination of walkability's impact on housing values, foreclosures and crime. Cities, 42(a), 13–24. doi:10.1016/j.cities.2014.08.001.

Global Green and Healthy Hospitals. (2015). GGHH agenda and its sustainability goals. Retrieved from http://www.greenhospitals.net/sustainability-goals/.

Go Goldfields. (n.d.). About us. Retrieved from https://gogoldfields.org/about-us/.

Government of South Australia, & World Health Organization (WHO). (2017). Progressing the Sustainable Development Goals through Health in All Policies: case studies from around the world. Retrieved from https://www.sahealth.sa.gov.au/wps/wcm/connect/ 4760078042fd0137a2cff68cd21c605e/17061.3+HiAP+Who+Case+Study+Book -ONLINE.PDF?MOD=AJPERES&CACHEID=ROOTWORKSPACE-4760078042fd 0137a2cff68cd21c605e-mN5ICGv

Greater Christchurch Partnerships. (n.d.). Urban development strategy. Retrieved from https:// greaterchristchurch.org.nz/projects/strategy/.

Greenhalgh, E., & Bayly, M. (2017). Trends in the prevalence of smoking. Tobacco in Australia: facts and issues. Retrieved from https://www.tobaccoinaustralia.org.au/chapter-1-prevalence.

Health in All Policies Unit. (2010). Implementing health in all policies: Adelaide 2010. Retrieved from https://www.sahealth.sa.gov.au/wps/wcm/connect/0ab5f18043aee450b600feed1a914d95/ implementinghiapadel-sahealth-100622.pdf?MOD=AJPERES&CACHE=NONE&CONTENTCAC HE=NONE

Health Issues Centre: A Voice for Everyday People. (n.d.). Health Issues Centre: a voice for everyday people. Retrieved from https://hic.org.au/.

Hirono, K., Haigh, F., Gleeson D., et al. (2015). Negotiating healthy trade in Australia: health impact assessment of the proposed Trans-Pacific Partnership Agreement. Retrieved from http://www.hiaconnect.edu.au/wp-content/uploads/2015/03/TPP_HIA.pdf.

Intergovernmental Committee on Drugs. (2012). National tobacco strategy 2012–2018. Retrieved from https://www.health.gov.au/resources/publications/national-tobacco-strategy-2012-2018.

International Conference on Health Promoting Universities & Colleges. (2015). Okanagan charter: an international charter for health promoting universities & colleges. Retrieved from https:// open.library.ubc.ca/collections/53926/items/1.0132754.

Labonté, R. (1997). Power, participation and partnerships for health promotion. Retrieved from https://www.vichealth.vic.gov.au/media-and-resources/publications/power-participation-and-pa rtnerships-for-health-promotion.

Labonté, R., & Schrecker, T. (2006). Globalization and social determinants of health: analytic and strategic review paper. On behalf of the Globalization Knowledge Network. Retrieved from https://www.researchgate.net/profile/Ronald_Labonte/publication/228780092_Globalization _and_social_determinants_of_health_Analytic_and_strategic_review_paper/links/ 02bfe51012578333f3000000/Globalization-and-social-determinants-of-health-Analytic -and-strategic-review-paper.pdf?origin=publication_detail.

Langford, R., Bonell, C., Jones, H., et al., (2015). The World Health Organization's health promoting schools framework: a Cochrane systematic review and meta-analysis. BMC Public Health, 15(1), 130. doi:https://doi.org/10.1186/s12889-015-1360-y.

Lennard, S. H. C. (1995). Livable cities observed: a source book of images and ideas for city officials, community leaders, architects, planners and all other committed to making their cities livable. Carmel, CA: Gondolier Press.

Lilly, K., Hallet, J., Robinson, S., & Selvey, L. A. (2019, Aug 29). Insights into local health and wellbeing policy process in Australia. Health Promotion International. doi:10.1093/heapro/ daz082.

Lin, V., & Gibson, B. (2003). Evidence-based health policy: problems & possibilities. Melbourne: Oxford University Press.

Lin, V., Smith, J., & Fawkes, S. (2007). Public health practice in Australia: the organised effort. Crows Nest, N.S.W.: Allen & Unwin.

Lin, V., Smith, J., & Fawkes, S. (2014). Public health practice in Australia: the organised effort (2nd ed.). Sydney: Allen & Unwin.

Lowi, T. J. (1964). American business, public policy, case-studies, and political theory. World Politics, 16(4), 677–715. doi:10.2307/2009452.

Milio, N. (1988). Making policy: a mozaic of Australian community health policy development. Canberra: Department of Community Services and Health, AGPS.

Ministry of Health. (2011). Better, sooner, more convenient health care in the community. Retrieved from https://www.health.govt.nz/system/files/documents/publications/better-sooner-more-convenient-health-care_0.pdf.

Ministry of Health. (2020). Smokefree Aotearoa 2025. Retrieved from https://www.health.govt.nz/our-work/preventative-health-wellness/tobacco-control/smokefree-aotearoa-2025#achievingsf2025.

Ministry of Health. (n.d.). Health promoting schools. Retrieved from https://www.health.govt.nz/our-work/life-stages/child-health/health-promoting-schools.

Mooney, B., Timmins, F., Byrne, G., & Corroon, A. M. (2011). Nursing students' attitudes to health promotion to: implications for teaching practice. Nurse Education Today, 31(8), 841–848. doi:10.1016/j.nedt.2010.12.004.

Mooney, G. (2012). Health of nations: towards a new political economy. London: Zed Books.

Moore, M., Yeatman, H., & Pollard, C. (2015). Evaluating success in public health advocacy strategies. Retrieved from https://www.phaa.net.au/documents/item/620.

National Smokefree Working Group. (2015). Smokefree Aotearoa 2025 action plan 2015–2018. Retrieved from https://www.smokefreenurses.org.nz/site/nursesaotearoa/nsfwg-action-plan-2015-2018.pdf.

Neiger, B. L., Thackeray, R., Burton, S. H., et al. (2013). Evaluating social media's capacity to develop engaged audiences in Health Promotion settings: use of Twitter metrics as a case study. Health Promotion Practice, 14(2), 157–162. doi:10.1177/1524839912469378.

Neiger, B. L., Thackeray, R., Van Wagenen, S. A., et al. (2012). Use of social media in Health Promotion: purposes, key performance indicators, and evaluation metrics. Health Promotion Practice, 13(2), 159–164. doi:10.1177/1524839911433467.

New Zealand Smokefree Coalition. (2015). Smokefree Aotearoa 2025 action plan for 2015–2018. Retrieved from https://www.smokefreenurses.org.nz/site/nursesaotearoa/nsfwg-action-plan-2015-2018.pdf

Palfrey, C. (2000). Key concepts in healthcare policy and planning: an introductory text. Basingstoke, Hampshire: Macmillan Press.

Palmer, G. R., & Short, S. D. (2000). Health care and public policy: an Australian analysis (3rd ed.). South Melbourne: Macmillan Education Australia.

Palmer, K., Bullen, C., & Paynter, J. (2013). What role can local authorities play in tobacco 'end-game' policies in New Zealand? Policy Quarterly, 9(3).

Price, S. (2016). Loneliness, urban design, and form-based codes. Public Square: A CNU Journal. Retrieved from https://www.cnu.org/publicsquare/loneliness-urban-design-and-form-based-codes.

Public Salon. (2012, 5 July 2012). Brent Toderian speaks at the Vancouver Urban Forum [YouTube]. Retrieved from https://www.youtube.com/watch?v=eRk93Wgdv1g

Rantala, R., Bortz, M., & Armada, F. (2014). Intersectoral action: local governments promoting health. Health Promotion International, 29(suppl_1), i92–i102. doi:10.1093/heapro/dau047.

Riggs, W., & Gilderbloom, J. (2016). Two-way street conversion: evidence of increased livability in Louisville. Journal of Planning Education and Research, 36(1), 105. doi:10.1177/0739456X15593147.

SA Health. (2019a). Health in all policies. Retrieved from https://www.sahealth.sa.gov.au/wps/wcm/connect/public+content/sa+health+internet/about+us/about+sa+health/health+in+all+policies

SA Health. (2019b). The South Australian model of health in all policies. Retrieved from https://
www.sahealth.sa.gov.au/wps/wcm/connect/public+content/sa+health+internet/about+us/
about+sa+health/health+in+all+policies/the+south+australian+model+of+health+in+all
+policies.

SA Health. (2019c). WHO Collaborating Centre for advancing health in all policies. Retrieved
from https://www.sahealth.sa.gov.au/wps/wcm/connect/public+content/sa+health+internet/
about+us/about+sa+health/health+in+all+policies/who+collaborating+centre+for
+advancing+health+in+all+policies.

Salisbury, R., & Heinz, J. (1970). A theory of policy analysis and some preliminary applications.
In K. Sharkansky (Ed.), Policy analysis and political science. Chicago: Markham.

Scollo, M., Bayly, M., & Wakefield, M. (2015). Availability of illicit tobacco in small retail outlets
before and after the implementation of Australian plain packaging legislation. Tobacco
Control, 24(e1), e45. doi:10.1136/tobaccocontrol-2013-051353.

State Government of Victoria. (2019). Victorian public health and wellbeing plan 2019–2023.
Retrieved from https://www2.health.vic.gov.au/about/publications/policiesandguidelines/
victorian-public-health-wellbeing-plan-2019-2023.

Stewart-Brown, S. (2006). What is the evidence on school health promotion in improving health
or preventing disease and, specifically, what is the effectiveness of the health promoting
schools approach? Health Evidence Network (HEN). Retrieved from http://www.euro.who
.int/__data/assets/pdf_file/0007/74653/E88185.pdf.

Stewart, R. G. (1999). Public policy: strategy and accountability. Melbourne: Macmillan Education.

Suárez Reyes, M., Serrano, M. M., & Van den Broucke, S. (2019). How do universities implement
the Health Promoting University concept? Health Promotion International, 34(5), 1014–1024.

Syme, S. L. (1998). Social and economic disparities in health: thoughts about intervention.
Milbank Quarterly, 76(3), 493–505. doi:10.1111/1468-0009.00100.

Taylor, P., Saheb, R., & Howse, E. (2019). Creating healthier graduates, campuses and
communities: why Australia needs to invest in health promoting universities. Health
Promotion Journal of Australia, 30, 285–289. doi:10.1002/hpja.175.

Tesoriero, F. (2010). Community development: community-based alternatives in an age of
globalisation (4th ed.). Sydney: Pearson Australia.

United Nations. (n.d.). About the sustainable development goals. Retrieved from https://
www.un.org/sustainabledevelopment/sustainable-development-goals/.

Urban Land Institute. (n.d.). Building healthy places toolkit: strategies for enhancing health in the
built environment. Retrieved from https://bhptoolkit.uli.org/#banner.

VicHealth. (2011). The partnerships analysis tool. Retrieved from https://www.vichealth.vic.gov.au/
search/the-partnerships-analysis-tool.

VicHealth. (n.d.-a). Our work: preventing tobacco use. Retrieved from https://www.vichealth
.vic.gov.au/our-work/preventing-tobacco-use.

VicHealth. (n.d.-b). Preventing tobacco use. Retrieved from https://www.vichealth.vic.gov.au/
our-work/preventing-tobacco-use.

WA Health Promoting Schools Association (Inc). (n.d.). WA Health Promoting Schools
Association (Inc). Retrieved from http://wahpsa.org.au/.

Wakefield, M., Coomber, K., Zacher, M., et al. (2015). Australian adult smokers' responses to plain
packaging with larger graphic health warnings 1 year after implementation: results from a
national cross-sectional tracking survey. Tobacco Control, 24(Suppl 2), ii17. doi:10.1136/
tobaccocontrol-2014-052050.

Walk Score. (n.d.). Retrieved from https://www.walkscore.com/

World Health Organization (WHO). (1986). The Ottawa Charter for Health Promotion. Retrieved
from https://www.who.int/healthpromotion/conferences/previous/ottawa/en/

World Health Organization (WHO). (1991). Sundsvall statement on supportive environments
for health. Retrieved from https://www.who.int/healthpromotion/conferences/previous/
sundsvall/en/.

World Health Organization (WHO). (1997). Jakarta declaration on leading health promotion into the 21st century. Retrieved from https://www.who.int/healthpromotion/conferences/previous/jakarta/declaration/en/.

World Health Organization (WHO). (2005). WHO framework convention on tobacco control. Retrieved from https://www.who.int/fctc/text_download/en/.

World Health Organization (WHO). (2010a). Adelaide statement on health in all policies. Retrieved from https://www.who.int/social_determinants/hiap_statement_who_sa_final.pdf.

World Health Organization (WHO). (2010b). Healthy workplaces: a model for action, for employers, workers, policy-makers and practitioners. Retrieved from https://www.who.int/occupational_health/publications/healthy_workplaces_model.pdf?ua=1.

World Health Organization (WHO). (2011a). Discussion paper: Intersectoral action on health: a path for policy-makers to implement effective and sustainable intersectoral action on health. Retrieved from https://www.who.int/nmh/publications/ncds_policy_makers_to_implement_intersectoral_action.pdf

World Health Organization (WHO). (2011b). Rio political declaration on social determinants of health. Paper presented at the World Conference on Social Determinants of Health, Rio De Janeiro, Brazil. Retrieved from http://www.who.int/sdhconference/declaration/Rio_political_declaration.pdf.

World Health Organization (WHO). (2012). Addressing the social determinants of health: the urban dimension and the role of local government. Retrieved from http://www.euro.who.int/en/publications/abstracts/addressing-the-social-determinants-of-health-the-urban-dimension-and-the-role-of-local-government.

World Health Organization (WHO). (2013a). Helsinki statement on health in all policies. Retrieved from http://www.who.int/healthpromotion/conferences/8gchp/8gchp_helsinki_statement.pdf?ua=.

World Health Organization (WHO). (2013b). Protocol to eliminate illicit trade in tobacco products. Retrieved from https://www.who.int/fctc/publications/en/.

World Health Organization (WHO). (2016a). Regional framework for urban health in the Western Pacific 2016–2020: healthy and resilient cities. Retrieved from https://iris.wpro.who.int/bitstream/handle/10665.1/13047/9789290617525_eng.pdf.

World Health Organization (WHO). (2016b). Shanghai Declaration on promoting health in the 2030 agenda for sustainable development. Retrieved from https://www.who.int/healthpromotion/conferences/9gchp/shanghai-declaration.pdf?ua=1.

World Health Organization (WHO). (n.d.-a). Global strategy to accelerate tobacco control: advancing sustainable development through the implementation of the WHO FCTC 2019–2025. Retrieved from https://www.who.int/fctc/cop/g-s-2025/en/.

World Health Organization (WHO). (n.d.-b). Healthy workplaces: a WHO global model for action. Retrieved from https://www.who.int/occupational_health/healthy_workplaces/en/.

World Health Organization (WHO). (n.d.-c). Introduction to healthy settings. Retrieved from http://www.who.int/healthy_settings/about/en/.

World Health Organization (WHO). (n.d.-d). Parties to the WHO framework convention on tobacco control. Retrieved from https://www.who.int/fctc/cop/en/

World Health Organization (WHO). (n.d.-e). Regional activities. Retrieved from https://www.who.int/healthy_settings/regional/en/.

World Health Organization (WHO). (n.d.-f). What is a health promoting school? Retrieved from https://www.who.int/school_youth_health/gshi/hps/en/.

World Health Organization (WHO) & Commission on Social Determinants of Health. (2008). Closing the gap in a generation: health equity through action on the social determinants of health. Final Report of the Commission on Social Determinants of Health. Retrieved from https://www.who.int/social_determinants/thecommission/finalreport/en/.

6 Community development action for social and environmental change

COMPREHENSIVE PRIMARY HEALTH CARE

SOCIO-ECOLOGICAL APPROACH

SELECTIVE PRIMARY HEALTH CARE

BEHAVIOURAL APPROACH

BIOMEDICAL APPROACH

Healthy public policy to create environments and settings that support health and wellbeing

Community development action to support social and environmental change

Health education and health literacy to develop knowledge and skills for health and wellbeing action

Health information and social marketing to raise awareness about health and wellbeing priorities

Vaccination, screening, risk assessment and surveillance to monitor and reduce risk of disease conditions

Health promotion community assessment, program planning, implementation and evaluation

INTRODUCTION

In Chapter 1, the framework for health promotion practice was introduced. In the previous chapter we explored building healthy public policy to create environments and settings that support health and wellbeing. In this chapter we address the complementary strategy of community development for social and environmental change. Community development has been prominent in health promotion practice since the Declaration of Alma-Ata highlighted it as an important strategy for promoting health. Before that, many health practitioners were unfamiliar with the concept of community development, despite community development philosophy and methods being used in other fields, and by health practitioners in low-income countries, for many years. (See Craig et al., 2011; DeFilippis & Saegert, 2013; Minkler, 2012 for detailed overviews of the historical development and evolution of community development approaches.)

Community development action for social and environmental change is an essential component of the socio-ecological approach to health promotion, as it relates to making changes in the settings of people's lives that improve their health and wellbeing. Changes are made by people in their own locality to address local determinants of health or wellbeing. Community members may be engaged in new communication and power relationships. Changes are likely to be sustained over time if community members are directly involved in identifying the issues and their determinants, and then planning, implementing and evaluating health promotion programs to address their priorities. Sustainability is more likely when community members are able to gain new skills and there are advancements in health and social equity. The role of the health practitioner in community development practice is to facilitate the desired changes through their work as advocate, mediator and enabler, working with the particular community.

In the previous chapter, the advantages of using intersectoral collaboration across organisations to assist with policy advocacy, policy development and implementation was

PUTTING THE OTTAWA CHARTER INTO PRACTICE

The following questions, arranged in the Ottawa Charter action areas, are presented to guide health promotion practitioners to reflect on and critically evaluate their professional role and practice and the health promotion philosophy of their organisation. Content of this chapter will assist practitioners to develop the necessary professional knowledge and skills to work effectively with communities.

PUTTING THE OTTAWA CHARTER INTO PRACTICE FOR COMMUNITY DEVELOPMENT ACTION FOR SOCIAL AND ENVIRONMENTAL CHANGE

Build healthy public policy

- Are there policies that disadvantage people in the community who are already vulnerable or disadvantaged?
- Would a change in policy make it easier for some to be healthy?
- Is policy working to the advantage of those who are already in positions of authority or power?
- Are you able to act as an advocate for change that can be enshrined in agency or government policy?
- Are appropriate human ethics procedures being followed—are the rights of community members being protected?
- Does the proposal and its procedures make false promises to community members—are they expecting more than can be delivered?

Create supportive environments

- Is a health promotion practice framework being used as a guide for gathering data that reflect a holistic view of health?
- Are you hearing the voices of all sections of the community?
- Are the processes of community assessment excluding some, because of language, locality or other forms of barriers?
- How are you treating people who are 'different'?
- Is the cultural safety of community members being safeguarded and respected at every stage?
- Are you enabling all to learn from the process of assessment?
- Can you ensure that community members will not become scapegoats if decisions do not work out as planned?

Strengthen community action

- Who defined the health and wellbeing priorities?
- Are all community members being consulted?
- Is their participation more than tokenism?
- Can the community strengthen their claims by using research and epidemiological data?

Continued

PUTTING THE OTTAWA CHARTER INTO PRACTICE Cont.

- Are all community members able to understand the assessment findings, and do they all know where to find them?
- Is the community itself leading the decision making?

Develop personal skills

- Are there opportunities to gain new skills?
- Can you act as a mentor?
- Can you facilitate skills in accessing other relevant information?
- Are the communication methods appropriate to build respect and health literacy?

Reorient health services

- Are funds being allocated ethically, given the health and wellbeing priorities identified in the community assessment?
- Is a new iteration of the health promotion practice cycle based on the outcomes of a previous cycle?
- How can health promotion be put on the agenda more often?
- Is there an agency agreement or a policy statement that enables support for the most vulnerable community members?
- Is there a focus on providing an environment of support, rather than individual behaviour change?

emphasised. In this chapter, the focus of health promotion practice is on working to develop effective partnerships with community and relevant organisations or individuals who can enable the community to reach its goals.

Due to the breadth of potential practice in the area, community development practice can be difficult to describe; there is no one correct way to practise community development. In an effort to provide clarity and guidance to practitioners new to the field, the bulk of the chapter is presented in three main sections:

1. community development *philosophy*, where the two main concepts fundamental to community development—community participation and empowerment—are discussed
2. community development *practice* including community development models, processes and outcomes
3. community development practice *roles, skills and attributes.*

The chapter then examines the role of social enterprise and social entrepreneurship in community development, challenges for community development, and the evaluation of community development. Before starting the chapter, take some time to review *Putting the Ottawa Charter into Practice* on p. 283.

PHILOSOPHY OF COMMUNITY DEVELOPMENT

In community development practice the environment or setting, rather than the individual, is the focus of change. Health practitioners using a community development approach are responsive to the health and wellbeing priorities of the community in which they are working. Their tasks are to advocate for the community, mediate relations with people and organisations who may have control over resources and decision making, and help the community to find ways that enable them to reach their goals (WHO, 1986). Working with communities to improve community wellbeing can be achieved using 'bottom-up' or 'top-down' approaches, or a mixture of both. The change process can be introduced by community members (bottom-up) or from institutions, such as through a new policy or strategic direction from government, or by a social enterprise initiative led by an individual or group (top-down).

Bottom-up community development approaches are those in which communities are central in the identification of priorities and decision making about their own future; change is driven from the grass roots of the community (Walter & Hyde in Minkler, 2012). A community may come together because of a wider social issue of concern, such as racism or social isolation being experienced by a subgroup in the community, or poor maintenance of their public housing. In other bottom-up approaches, communities may be supported to develop a local community plan as a means of identifying local strengths and future priorities. People may develop a local response designed to build community connections, such as organising regular shared meals, building a community garden, undertaking group advocacy or a range of different activities.

In top-down community development approaches, organisations with the power to direct policy, control finances, decide on priorities or set up a social enterprise initiate changes that have been identified by evidence 'about' the community. This is sometimes in the form of non-negotiable development that is provided 'for' the community. For example, an urban renewal program may be funded by a federal, state or regional government because of statistical data reporting the high incidence of poverty, risk and violence, and other socio-ecological determinants of illness. Similarly, a social enterprise organisation may be established by a group of hospitality professionals to build work-readiness for vulnerable young people. In top-down community development approaches, health practitioners or social entrepreneurs with expertise and knowledge about a population develop a health promotion program aimed at improving the lives of vulnerable groups, without necessarily including members of those groups in the process. Additional efforts are essential to develop a partnership that successfully engages vulnerable community members and to ensure the program is implemented in ways that meet the needs of all parties.

A combined approach may have perceived benefits; federal funding and local action can be a 'win–win' (see Kearns and Mason, 2015, and the other research evaluation outcomes of the GoWell urban renewal program in Glasgow, Scotland, at the time of the Commonwealth Games in 2014), but very often a federal policy perspective based on individualist values tends to be at odds with local community empowerment initiatives (DeFilippis & Saegert, 2013).

There is a long history of success in improving the wellbeing of poor, disempowered and vulnerable groups through health promotion programs based on working in partnership with members of those groups. They include programs focused on adult literacy, skills development, better nutrition and clean water supply. Micro-enterprise credit schemes around the world are also an example of community development that creates personal independence and social capital (Minkler, 2012). More recently, diverse social enterprise or social entrepreneurship initiatives are demonstrating enormous success in making lifelong changes, building self-esteem and developing skills for some of the most vulnerable community members.

Working with community has the potential to address some of the structural issues, specifically at the local level, that lead to poor health. As mentioned in Chapters 1 and 2, the conditions in which people are born, live, work and age have a powerful influence on their health and wellbeing. Social factors create the life experiences and opportunities that make it easier or more difficult for people to achieve optimal health. Equity of access to social, environmental and health resources, and ensuring cultural safety are important factors in determining enhanced health outcomes.

In addressing structural issues, community development action for social and environmental change is obviously political, since it means working for change to create social justice. While any form of health promotion practice can be political, by using the approaches described here, the political nature of community development practice is more explicit.

Community development defined

Community development has been defined as a process of 'working with people as they define their own goals, mobilise resources, and develop action plans for addressing problems they collectively have identified' (Minkler, 1991, p. 261). The terms 'community development' and 'community organisation' are both defined variously and often overlap in their definitions (Craig et al., 2011). The term 'community development' is most often used in Australia and New Zealand, but in the United States (USA) and Canada the term 'community organisation' is more common. As Minkler's definition identifies, community development and community organisation processes are directed at overcoming a problem or issue of concern.

'Community building' is another term commonly used in this field of practice. Community building has a wider focus on bringing about social change and increasing equity, rather than addressing one specific problem, such as substance use or racism. Community building brings a deeper analysis of politics and power relations. It has a focus on 'building capacities, not fixing problems' (Minkler, 2012, p. 10). An example may be social action to build stronger social connections between people, which will often have aspects of economic development as part of overall community building. Labonté (in Minkler, 2012) emphasises that community building involves a change in power relations between community and others that moves towards greater equity.

Note that Minkler's definition of community building focuses on building capacities, not fixing problems. From Chapter 1 you will recall that critical health promotion values a salutogenic approach, which means building on strengths and assets, and not just on problems. As such, the term community building is more consistent with critical health promotion than the term community development, with its focus on problems. However, due to the widespread use of the term 'community development' in the health promotion field, we will continue to use this term throughout this chapter. It is important to remember that health promotion practice in general, and community development specifically, should not just be deficit-oriented, but must take a salutogenic approach.

In Chapter 2 we noted that the term 'community' has different meanings. Definitions of community commonly encompass elements of geography, culture and social stratification (DeFilippis & Saegert, 2013; Naidoo & Wills, 2010). These three factors are viewed as bringing together people into a positive and desirable common entity, although DeFilippis and Saegert (2013) caution against developing an idealised view of 'community'. In community development, emphasis has traditionally been placed on community as a social system, bound by geographical location or common interest, recognising that each of these community types will have webs of ties and interaction between families, associates and organisations; these ties are not always geared towards healthy social purposes. 'Social' or 'virtual' communities are important as they can have the same capacities to build social capital as communities that meet face-to-face (Minkler, 2012). The notion of a 'sense of community' was also discussed in Chapter 2. It has connotations of an ideal state of solidarity and connectedness in which everyone affected by the life of the community participates positively in community life. This 'sense of community' can be an important component of people feeling as though they belong to a certain community, and it also has implications for the process of community development (Lawson & Kearns, 2014).

Two further points are worth making here. First, care must be taken not to oversimplify the consequences of humans being a part of, or living in, communities; communities can be unsafe, disempowering and they can work towards unhealthy outcomes. Second, it cannot be assumed that having a sense of community is an ideal or desirable state for everyone, in that some people may not choose to be a part of that community as their ideal. These issues are of particular importance in considering community development, as aspects of community disempowerment and social alienation may become evident during the community development process (Lawson & Kearns, 2014). Indeed, health practitioners using community development processes may have to regularly consider the implications of disempowerment and alienation in their work. Tesoriero (2010, p. 99) suggests that community is a subjective experience that means different things to different people; that communities evolve over time with ongoing dialogue, consciousness-raising and action. Some characteristics of the 'ideal' community include:

- sharing equal responsibility for and commitment to maintaining its spirit
- a highly effective working group
- a consensual decision-making body
- celebrates a wide range of gifts, talents and individual differences
- is inclusive
- facilitates healing
- is reflective, contemplative and introspective.

Community participation

Community participation can be described broadly as people taking part in some action or activity with others. Preston and colleagues (2009) define community participation as 'people from a community of place or of interest participating together in advisory groups, fundraising, attending consultations, planning, or in other activities' (p. 2).

Participation is difficult to describe because the purposes that bring different interested parties together will be diverse and, in addition, the course and outcomes of the coming together will be just as varied. The process of participation constantly changes, so there can be no predetermined set of steps to guide health practitioners. Arnstein (1971) suggested that there are at least eight types of participation (Fig. 6.1), ranging from forms of manipulation and co-option through to shared decision-making power. Despite being published some time ago, the 'Ladder of Citizen Participation' still provides a useful framework for reflecting on levels of community participation. Arnstein described two forms of community participation as 'non-participation', because they involve either including people in a community process in order to gain their support ('manipulation') or because they are seen as opportunities to change people's behaviour rather than give them any involvement in decision-making ('therapy'). 'Informing', 'consultation' and 'placation' are described as forms of tokenism because, while people may be heard, there is no guarantee that their ideas will be acted upon, because they have no power. It is only at the levels on the ladder of

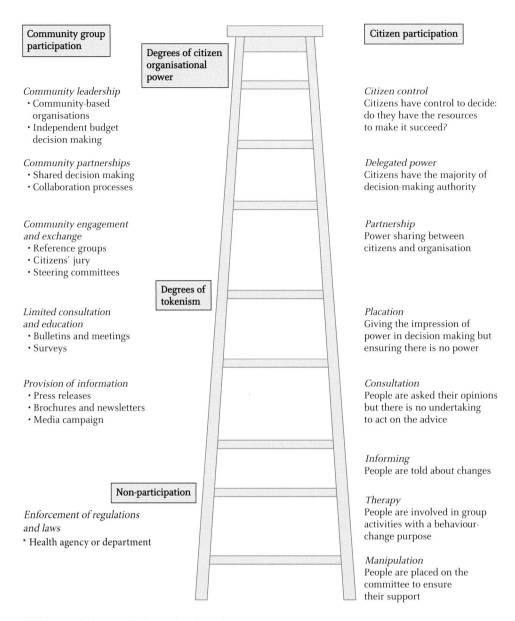

FIGURE 6.1 Ladder of Citizen Participation: approaches to participation

Source: Adapted from Arnstein (1971).

'partnership' and above that people have decision-making power. There is 'delegated power' when citizens have most of the decision-making power, while with 'citizen control' citizens have total control (Arnstein, 1971, p. 73).

Morgan and Lifshay (in Minkler, 2012) document how Arnstein's Ladder of Citizen Participation can be further adapted to reflect the levels of participation in decision making that community groups can have. The ladder diagram in Fig. 6.1 is useful to highlight how individuals and community groups can be empowered or disempowered in the ways information is provided to them or shared with them, the capacity they have as individuals or groups to take part in decision making, and ultimately whether they have control of the resources and how they are used.

Using Arnstein's ladder as an analytical tool, it is possible to see that a great many instances of participation are actually non-participation or tokenism and few cases of participation actually result in shared power or power being handed over to community members. However, it is this power sharing that we are aiming for in health promotion practice within a comprehensive primary health care context. In many instances, power sharing will result only from the decentralisation of decision making.

Another widely used model of community participation is the International Association for Public Participation (IAP2) Public Participation Spectrum. This framework includes five levels of community participation according to the potential, or lack of opportunity, for impact on decision making. The spectrum includes provision of information (inform), obtaining public feedback (consult), community consultation that achieves full understanding (involve), partnering with community to identify options and preferred outcomes (collaborate), and placing the final decision making in the hands of community (empower). Each level involves different approaches and communication methods. Both models help to remind us that informing community members about a decision made elsewhere is not the same thing as active engagement in decision making, and does not give people any sense of control or empowerment.

Clearly, community members cannot be partners in every health-related decision, but providing opportunities to hear their views will still be valuable (see Mooney, 2012, for a discussion of this issue with reference to population health in Cuba, Kerala and Venezuela). What is important is to be honest and transparent about the true level of participation, and not to claim that lower levels of participation are actually shared decision making. Critical health promotion requires the health practitioner to always be working towards real shared collaboration and decision making wherever possible.

The benefits of community participation in decision making are relevant to individuals, the community, the health promotion program and government agencies. For the individual, benefits include enhanced self-esteem, new skills, a sense of power over the forces that determine their own lives, and connectedness with the community, which has physical, mental and social health and wellbeing benefits. For the community, benefits include a more educated public, more cohesive community, identification and mobilisation of untapped community resources, use of citizens' knowledge, and enhanced capacity to act as change agents and advocates. For the health promotion program, benefits of high-level community participation include improved decision making by program proponents, increased accountability, and a better and more relevant community-wide (or system-wide) program. At a government level, the benefits of community participation include the development of policy responsive to the community, wider endorsement of policy, intersectoral action on complex issues and demonstration of government commitment.

Community empowerment

Community participation is important during the processes of 'doing' community development work and one of the outcomes of effective community development can be community empowerment. Health practitioners using a community development approach need to be particularly concerned with the needs of those who have little power. It is easy to assume that a community development project is empowering for community members, but a detailed analysis can reveal a different story, where the community participation may really just be a form of tokenism (Lawson & Kearns, 2014). Empowerment therefore needs to be analysed from the perspective of each party in the community development process.

Knowledge and health literacy are important preliminary skills in community development processes that may lead to empowerment (Lawson & Kearns, 2014). Health literacy is discussed in more detail in Chapter 7. If people are not skilled in articulating their needs, or believe they are unlikely to have them met, then they are not likely to express them. Finding out what they believe they need may be a slow process, but it is an important part of community development practice. Unless the work begins with getting a full understanding of the people's situation and perspective, it is unlikely to succeed. People will not be empowered to act on issues they do not see as relevant to them.

Through the processes of meaningful participation, people can gain a sense of confidence in their ability to work for change in the world around them. Participation enables people to develop a wide range of skills in areas such as working effectively with a group or within a workplace team, organisational and negotiation skills, submission writing, interview techniques, working with the mass media, and using social media for business expansion. The confidence and improved skills developed through these processes increase the people's ability to work effectively for change on future issues; that is, the conditions are right for people to become empowered.

Rifkin (1986, p. 246) suggested three rhetorical or reflective questions to ask about participation to determine the extent to which participation is likely to strengthen or deny people's empowerment. They are 'Why participation?', 'Who participates?' and 'How do they participate?'

Why participation?

Health practitioners undertaking health promotion practice in a comprehensive primary health care context must encourage participation from community members to bring their own perspective, expertise and wisdom to issues in their community. This wisdom may contribute a great deal more to the quality of decisions than if decisions are made by health practitioners alone. Exclusion is disempowering for those who are most vulnerable. These skills and the networks people establish with others in the community, and their sense of being able to negotiate the system and achieve something, are valuable, and sometimes they are more valuable than any outcome of the group's activity. Where community members have led the process and decision making, the outcomes are more likely to be sustained (Anderson et al., 2007; Eckermann et al., 2010; Kearns & Mason, 2015; Labonté & Laverack, 2008).

Who participates?

The short answer to this question is 'as many people as possible'. However, it is of particular importance to make sure that everyone has the opportunity to participate, not just the most articulate or well-resourced people within a community. Equitable access to full participation is important if people are to achieve empowerment. This may mean that it is particularly important to ensure that people most impacted by health and wellbeing priorities have authentic opportunities for participation in decision making (Lawson & Kearns, 2014). Specific approaches to get to the 'hard to reach' people of a community may be necessary, including using refined skills of communication and expending more effort and time to overcome some of the barriers people may experience. Examination of engagement processes to see exactly who is involved and who is not, provides an opportunity to reflect on whether the avenues for participation are enabling all people to participate fully (Lawson & Kearns, 2014).

How do they participate?

Dwyer (1989, pp. 60–61) outlined methods of participation in common use that all enable degrees of empowerment. They were client feedback and evaluation, voluntarism, consultation and public discussion, representative structures, and advocacy and public debate. These methods are reflected in the IAP2 community engagement framework discussed earlier. They remain the primary mechanisms for participation, although health practitioners have also been working at the local level to adapt the methods to suit particular situations, providing opportunities for community members or consumers to participate more fully in issues of concern to them. Some of the more active forms of participation, including using social media platforms such as GetUp, are less popular with government. As such, there are challenges to achieving meaningful community participation for health practitioners working in government organisations at any level (Aulich, 2009). Health practitioners therefore must develop innovative ways of ensuring that community members have meaningful opportunities to participate.

Potential risks of community participation

There are several reasons why health practitioners using community development approaches may encourage participation by members of the community; however, not all of the reasons may actually benefit those being encouraged to participate. Clarifying why community participation is sought is important, and an analysis of whose needs are being met by the process can illustrate the level of tokenism by partner agencies and disengagement or cynicism by community members (Lawson & Kearns, 2014). Health practitioners using community development approaches therefore have a fine line to walk in providing opportunities for participation by community members, to make those opportunities meaningful and appropriate, and having the capacity to oversee implementation of the priorities of the community with which they have partnered. It can be an extensive and exhausting process when it may seem easier to just get on and do it without community participation. However, this is not consistent with the values and principles of critical health promotion.

In some instances, community participation may be used more to control people than to encourage empowerment. Decisions about what types of participation are relevant in a particular situation are not necessarily straightforward, but are important. If there are no opportunities for people to participate in decisions that affect them, they are likely to feel disenfranchised and powerless, especially if they are not given the respect of being informed about a change or decision that has been made. People may be encouraged to participate because of the likely health or wellbeing benefits of the participation itself, rather than a belief in the value of what they may contribute. If, however, too much participation is expected or people are required to participate in order to obtain access to healthcare or other services, they are equally likely to feel powerless and the participation may feel like manipulation. Participation may also be used to 'buy' people's acceptance of a pre-planned change. There is evidence that people are less likely to resist a change if they have contributed to its development. Thus, in some instances, people may be encouraged to participate, not because their ideas are highly regarded and will be implemented, but because it is hoped that their involvement will prevent them from complaining about the final decision or result. It may also give the impression that the 'cost' of health-related services is compulsory participation in the development of those services.

Such an approach can be tantamount to victim or community blaming for disadvantaged communities.

Manipulating people, through co-opting them to take a predetermined action, or working in a way that does not encourage true community control, is a thoughtless and unscrupulous use of power likely to create distrust among community members. This is *not* community development.

COMMUNITY DEVELOPMENT PRACTICE

Community development practice can be undertaken in almost any setting, and includes a range of approaches. The health practitioner engaged in community development must choose the approach that best suits the needs and realities of the community they are working with.

> *Each community development group has to find its own unique path to success. There is no one model or recipe. People often want specific formulas, recipes, and models for community development that they can replicate, ... but that approach doesn't work very well because each situation is unique. Guiding principles about how things work in a community are much more useful than a recipe.*
>
> *(Green et al., 2009, pp. 17–18)*

There are a number of models for community development practice to assist the health practitioner undertaking this work. The tasks involved in community development can be diverse, depending on the existing strengths, vulnerabilities and culture of the community. Irrespective of the setting or approach to community empowerment, there are two themes to keep in mind when working with the community. These are: 1. that the processes involved in doing community development work are as important as the outcomes—there are no shortcuts; and 2. that the community identifies its assets and needs and sets the goals. To some extent this second theme is a product of the first one, but it is an important reflection point to keep in mind.

The following sections provide an overview of community development practice. In it we present:

- two models for community development practice
- six processes of community development practice
- two outcomes of effective community development practice.

Community development models

Theoretical models can be useful in providing a visual representation of the interrelationship of aspects that are key to a practice area. There are many models to guide community development practice, and in this section, we present two of these. The community development model presented in Fig. 6.2 was developed from the philosophy of asset-based

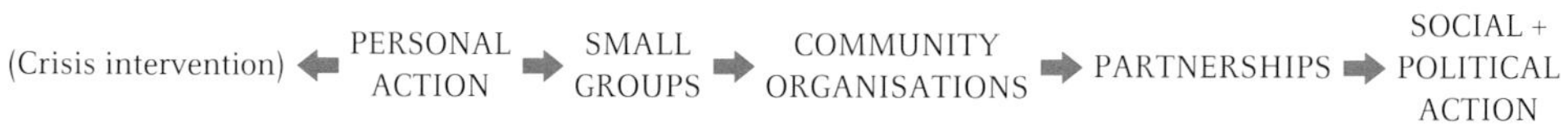

(Crisis intervention) ⬅ PERSONAL ACTION ➡ SMALL GROUPS ➡ COMMUNITY ORGANISATIONS ➡ PARTNERSHIPS ➡ SOCIAL + POLITICAL ACTION

FIGURE 6.2 The West Virginia Community Development Model
Source: West Virginia Community Development Hub (n.d.).

community development (ABCD) by the West Virginia Community Development Hub (n.d.). The Asset-Based Community Development Institute (2020) uses a strong evidence base to develop a range of unique approaches to community engagement and community strengthening, based on a philosophy that focuses on community assets, rather than their deficits or needs (Kretzmann & McKnight, 1993). Assessment of community assets is discussed in more detail in Chapter 4. A search for 'community development models' will return a range of designs with interrelated concepts, reflecting the complexity of community development practice. An exploration of the ABCD site will be valuable for any health practitioner using a community development approach because of the enormous range of evidence-based practical advice and tools freely available and downloadable. Other authors in the field of community development also developed models, including Tesoriero (2010, p. 106) drawing on his earlier work with Jim Ife. This model is valuable because it presents the interrelationship between ecology and social justice that is key to gaining a full understanding of sustainability in community development practice.

The model presented in Fig. 6.2 is included here because it provides a clear link to the important elements of community development practice, which are presented in some detail in this chapter. Health practitioners using a community development approach can envisage the different roles that they will undertake in building the capacity of communities and working to enable them to be stronger.

In the late 1980s community development practitioners and theorists in Australia (Jackson et al., 1989) and Canada (Labonté, 1990) independently developed very similar five-point models to conceptualise the various 'ways of working' to transform disempowered individuals, groups and communities based on the principles of equity and social justice. The model presented in Fig. 6.3 is a more recent modification of the two earlier versions (Labonté & Laverack, 2008). Jackson and colleagues (1989, p. 67) argued that:

> ... the choice of practice mode should be made in response to the needs and realities of the communities with whom one works, and that techniques from social action and locality development models, and from one-to-one case work, can be adapted to achieve community development goals.

The five points in the model identify the levels of empowerment that will be experienced by the person or group when community development guides professional practice.

Personal action

In crisis situations, health practitioners in personal action community development practice mode assist individuals, groups and families with everyday survival issues, because suffering is paralysing and incapacitating. Sometimes people are not in the position to think any more broadly than their day-to-day survival needs and, thus, it would be unethical not to address these as a first priority. However, with a community development approach, health practitioners need to nurture people's abilities to take control over decisions because 'all forms of social and political activism that change the conditions of people's lives inevitably start with the actions of discrete individuals' (Labonté & Laverack, 2008, p. 57). Maintaining a focus on strengths and assets enables the health practitioner to describe and build the strengths of individuals and communities. The role of the health practitioner may involve supporting an individual with a 'good' idea, an idea that may benefit them or the wider community, such as improved access to useful services and resources (Labonté & Laverack, 2008), or a new set of skills.

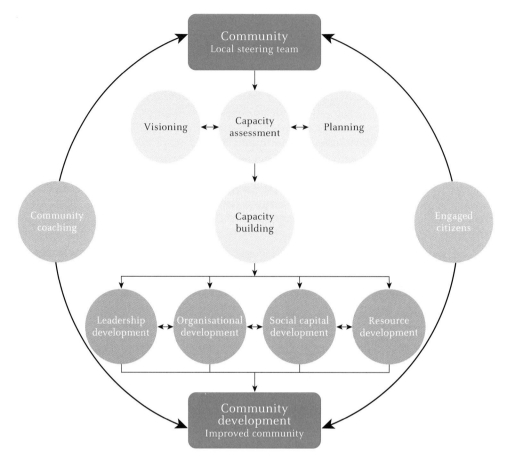

FIGURE 6.3 The community development empowerment continuum
Source: Labonté and Laverack (2008).

Small groups

In this community development practice mode, the health practitioner works to link vulnerable people into new or existing social networks, support groups or a community service network based on recognition that socially integrated people have a greater sense of empowerment and wellbeing. Social isolation and disempowerment is reduced through group discussion with others in similar situations, formation of self-help activities and facilitation of programs that enhance community integration. Social media can provide the ideal way for people to share their successes and gain a sense of belonging. The health practitioner supports activities that enable people to 'shift their safety net from dependence in unequal power relationships of practitioner/client to a more equal base amongst peers' (Jackson et al., 1989, p. 69). It may enable people to join others with similar 'good' ideas, although the focus of the groups tends to remain 'inward-looking' with a priority on solving their immediate needs. The groups may come together around a specific health priority, service issue or development of a range of skills (Labonté & Laverack, 2008). Working with small groups requires high-level communication and facilitation skills, which will be discussed in the next section and Chapter 7.

Community organisations

Forming community organisations is an important community development practice. Community organisations mark the transition of community members' capacity and strength to 'look outwards' and take part in community-wide and social issues that directly affect their lives in order to bring about wider change, including influencing policy at the local level, rather than as a means for their personal survival. In the early stages, it is important to support community members to choose a winnable issue or campaign, or to take small achievable steps in a personal journey. The role of the health practitioner is to have a 'repertoire of strategies' that 'foster confidence that joint action will achieve the desired change' (Jackson et al., 1989, p. 70). Community organisations build the capacity for participants to analyse their situation and the factors that are barriers to their empowerment (Labonté & Laverack, 2008). Various means of community advocacy are presented in Chapter 5, all of which can be empowering, and result in the development of skills transferable to other issues and campaigns.

Partnerships

A key role for health practitioners using the community development approach is building partnerships. Stakeholders coming together around an issue does not necessarily mean that effective participation is achieved (Labonté, 1997, Chapter 4); however, without participation there can be no partnerships. Labonté (1997, p. 45) argues that true partnership is the most desirable form of participation, since lesser forms of participation are merely tokenism. However, it is neither desirable nor possible to achieve true citizen control of decision making about health, because budget funds, with conditions about the way they can be spent, are always allocated by an external, more powerful agency. Community groups can partner with the organisations and agencies that will best enable them to meet their own interests. Partners should be chosen when they have a problem they cannot solve alone, with groups that have compatible agendas and which have the resources the group lacks (Labonté & Laverack, 2008). Collaborative partnerships mean community groups involved in the partnerships have the ability to negotiate their own style and conditions of relationship with agencies. The partners can agree on measures of success and working together they can achieve mutually satisfactory outcomes. As noted by Labonté, 'the goal of community development is not self-sufficiency; it is the ability of the group to negotiate its own terms of relationship with those institutions (agencies) that support it' (in Minkler, 2012, p. 104). Community members are encouraged to view this form of local participation as a means of building their confidence and skills before getting involved in wider social issues, networks and enterprises.

Community participation is often regarded in a rather romantic manner, but achieving partnership through effective participation can be a complex process—'the idea of citizen participation is a little like eating spinach: no one is against it in principle because it is good for you' (Arnstein, 1971, p. 71). Landcare in Victoria is an example of the partnership approach in Australia. It is a state-sponsored community participation program; that is, state government resources (and funds from private enterprise) are invested in volunteer organisations. The volunteers provide essential public goods. The organisation has had a strong long-term commitment to the participatory processes described above and to building community resilience. In Landcare, a large cross-section of the rural population has participated in the program, which has resulted in an increased awareness of land degradation and fauna decline, and increased skills in land management (Landcare, 2016).

Social and political action

In this community development practice mode, the health practitioner is facilitating the work of social activists who are engaged in far-reaching strategies to address inequalities in the distribution of power. Community members working in this way have already built significant skills in health literacy, knowledge of policy process and media awareness. The strength of this combined action is sufficient to change higher-level policy and/or power over political and economic decisions that enshrine disempowerment. People taking social and political action have the strength and capacity to 'see an important part of their lives to be ongoing commitment to social change' (Jackson et al., 1989, p. 71). Action based on the combined knowledge of the community and experts is most likely to be successful. For example, if a community is working for increased public housing in its area, evidence of a low rate of public housing or a high rate of people on low incomes (expert knowledge) will provide valuable support for increased housing, and will be a stronger argument than if residents' demand for more housing was the only rationale; a similar scenario can apply for a range of topics including unemployment for young people and people living with disability. Successful community-based movements brought about by local concerned citizens, social entrepreneurs or radical activists have ensured legal rights for vulnerable groups, established commercially successful enterprises and brought about changes in legislation (Farmer et al., 2012; Kernot, 2010). Outcomes might range from a change in the decision to dam a pristine river and lake, developing a new local government by-law, changes to refugee policy and treatment, or enabling greater access to employment options for people living in poverty or with a disability. Practical application of the community development empowerment modes is illustrated in Insight 6.1.

Processes and outcomes of community development practice

Earlier sections of this chapter have emphasised how important it is for the health and wellbeing of individuals and communities that they are enabled to make decisions about issues that affect their lives, property, environment and community. Core concepts of social justice and empowerment need to become the personal philosophy of health practitioners engaged in community development practice; the lens through which the quality of their activities is judged. The challenge for practitioners is to incorporate these concepts into each of their activities.

The following section provides more detail about working in community development. It distinguishes between the processes (or 'ways of working') in community development, and the long-term community development outcomes—what will happen as a result of working in these ways. The processes and outcomes of community development practice used as the basis for this section have been adapted from Butler and Cass (1993, p. 10). They provide practitioners with a systematic 'toolkit' of approaches to working with communities; they are guides for 'how you can do' community development. These processes and outcomes can be a very useful framework for self-reflection, organising a program logic for funding and reporting, and for community-based evaluation. In a program logic framework, the six processes could be used as the framework for expressing program/project objectives. See Chapter 4 for further guidance with this point.

Processes of community development practice

1. Control of decision making (valuing the wisdom of the community)

Alinsky (1972, p. 105) provided theoretical and personal leadership in community development strategies from his work with residents in ghettos in American industrial cities such

INSIGHT 6.1 Applying the community development practice modes to mental illness

Consider how the community development practice modes could be applied to supporting community members suffering a mental illness.

Personal action

In a mental illness crisis, therapeutic communication between client and practitioners is essential. Personal action may focus on building personal awareness such as through the use of Narrative Therapy.

Small groups

Small groups, such as a workplace team, may undertake Mental Health First Aid training (Mental Health First Aid Australia, 2019) as a means of providing a local network of support for vulnerable community members, and to increase knowledge about signs that early involvement from family or professionals may be necessary. This builds the capacity and unity of the group. Support groups may also be established and facilitated to support clients with a mental illness.

Community organisations

Community organisations and social enterprise groups are usually facilitated by a health agency or social enterprise initially, with the aim of increasing capacity for employment and building self-efficacy. A community garden developed with people who have experienced severe mental illness is an example, or a social enterprise in hospitality or a similar service area (see the Paul Ramsay Foundation (n.d.) as one example). Rural & Remote Mental Health (n.d.) is a social enterprise organisation that delivers mental health services and programs to people living and working in these areas. The three communities that are the focus of the service are Indigenous Australians, agricultural and farming communities, and mining communities, which all suffer high rates of mental illness.

Partnerships

Partnerships may develop between mainstream agencies. The outcomes will be increased community awareness of the barriers experienced by the participants, perhaps a commercial product or service, and increased sustainability of the service. An example of this form of success is PepperGreen Farm Catering (n.d.) in Bendigo, Victoria.

Social and political action

It is common to see a range of actions through the media, including the use of sportspeople, endurance activities, and petitions to raise community awareness of the impacts of racism. Similarly, people who have experienced mental illness are providing direct input into local strategy development and implementation, such as a Community Access and Inclusion Plan for local government.

as Chicago. Alinsky is often credited with laying the foundation of community-based action, and perhaps with coining the phrase 'Think globally, act locally'. His philosophy continues to resonate with local communities and political leaders, although in recent years there has been a strong move to the political right in the political philosophy guiding high-income nations, with a resultant focus on individual responsibility for health care, and community responsibility for 'building resilience'. DeFilippis and Saegert (2013, Chapter 44) provide an insightful analysis of the tensions in community development between a free-market economy (in the USA) and the community development redistributive philosophy aimed at equity and fairness. This is one key reason that a community development project proposal may not be supported, or may ultimately fail to make a difference.

In *Rules for Radicals*, Alinsky (1972) argued one of the challenges in working with disempowered communities is that 'if people feel they don't have the power to change a bad situation, then they do not think about it'. Alinsky advocated confrontational methods to empowerment which are not supported by most community development theorists (Minkler, 2012).

Community control of decision making allows a community to illustrate that it is the expert in its own affairs; that people 'on the ground' know best what they need and how this should be achieved.

> It is local community members who have this knowledge, wisdom and expertise, and the role of the community worker is to listen and learn from the community, not to tell the community about its problems and its needs.
> *(Holland & Blackburn, 1998, cited in Tesoriero, 2010, p. 121)*

There is nothing particularly complex about working in this way. The greatest attributes a health practitioner engaged in community development practice can bring are communication skills and patience. The greatest challenge to planners, policymakers and health practitioners is to relinquish the traditions of outside 'experts' making decisions on behalf of communities (Tesoriero, 2010, p. 120). Community control of decision making occurs on two fronts:

1. Decision making within the affected community, to ensure that decisions reflect the aspirations of the whole community
2. Decision making between the community and relevant agencies of authority, (including social enterprise management teams), to make sure the issue comes onto the authority's agenda for discussion, and that the community voice is heard.

Communities, whether they are a community of interest or members of a geographic community, can be in control of decision making when they are assisted to identify the issues and structures that prevent them from meeting their needs. After a community identifies its strengths and vulnerabilities, it must then decide what actions and changes it can make to become healthier. The emphasis here is on community identification, rather than expert 'diagnosis'. The processes of identifying community assets and needs and solution generation in communities is often called a community assessment or a needs assessment (Goetting & Green, 2010). The process is set out in detail in Chapter 4. For a health practitioner working with community development approaches to be effective in facilitating community control of decision making, they must get to know the community members, listen to, 'hear' and learn from the local people and validate with community members that the information provided is correctly interpreted. Effective communication between community and decision makers demands honesty, clarity and responsiveness by those running the participation process (Preston et al., 2009). A number of factors may get in the way of community members being 'heard', such as a professional being unable or unwilling to set aside their 'specialist' knowledge of how things should be, or the kinds of information provided by a community may not fit within the expected paradigms of what constitutes 'evidence' of need. An issue that has been a particular barrier to Aboriginal and Torres Strait Islanders and other minority community groups in Australia, and other nations taking control of decisions that affect their communities, has been that local knowledge and local solutions derive from different forms of 'knowledge', or 'worldviews'; ways of understanding the world. Another barrier to communities being heard is their inability to influence the wider public agenda, to influence social values and policy or legal decisions. It takes a great deal of effort, influence on structures of power and good fortune to raise an issue in the public profile sufficient to move it from a local concern onto the wider public agenda. Similarly, ensuring the cultural safety of participants and community groups requires real effort and an ongoing commitment; it cannot be tokenistic (Minkler, 2012). Many of the strategies of advocacy set out in Chapter 5, the guidelines for ensuring cultural safety presented in Chapter 2, and ethical guidelines in Chapter 4 are relevant to increasing community control of decision making.

2. Development of community competence (building a sense of empowerment)

The concept of community competence is strongly linked to community empowerment. A competent community is one that is able to recognise and address its problems. People and communities can feel powerless because their problems are complex and solutions often require knowledge and skills that they lack. Some feel powerless because they are left to deal with problems that they did not cause, such as unemployment or environmental degradation. They have been socialised to believe that authorities act in the best interests of the population and there is little they can do to challenge the decisions of authority. In some cases, a lack of action is also motivated by the fear that voicing or acting on concerns will worsen the risk or will have negative implications (Minkler, 2012). Minkler (2012, pp. 12–13) also emphasises the importance of advocating for social change through challenges to dominant political ideology in parallel to community empowerment in order to bring about lasting change to power relationships. Without social change, community empowerment may just be the rhetoric of government to pass responsibilities and costs to community members.

Being aware of the existing community resources is the first part of building competence. Community resources can be the knowledge and skills of community members, tangible things such as buildings and spaces, or they can include non-tangible resources such as the skills someone will share, the collaboration of others with more skills and resources or positive values such as trust and reciprocity; that is, the 'glue' of social capital (Putnam, 1993). It is important for the health practitioner engaged in community development practice to gain an understanding of these resources and existing social processes (such as communication patterns; social, commercial and economic networks; key informants and decision-making traditions) so the way they work in the community values and makes use of the assets, and does not exclude some people from participation, or act as a barrier that discourages people from getting involved.

Community development practice, especially in the early stages, frequently involves 'critical consciousness-raising, or critical conscientisation' (Freire, 1974), where the community members are assisted to recognise that existing values, structures and ways of viewing the world are keeping them feeling oppressed or powerless. Increased awareness of structural disempowerment can be the basis of collective social action. Feelings of powerlessness, felt for instance by many unemployed people, can be reinforced by social structures such as all forms of media, the health and education systems and religious institutions. Such seemingly simple issues as the use of jargon, or wearing certain clothing, or terms of communication or greeting, can be oppressive and exclusionary (Freire, 1974; Minkler, 2012; Tesoriero, 2010). See also Chapter 7 for further discussion of this concept.

Communities can gain collective strength by learning from the development journeys and the wisdom of experience of other communities in similar situations. A groundswell of opinion or reaction to an issue can create a culture of unity in the need for action. The large number and diversity of social enterprises that have developed in the hospitality industry is a good example of the groundswell of change that can occur (see, for example, Stephanie Alexander's Kitchen Garden Foundation (https://www.kitchengardenfoundation.org.au) and STREAT (https://www.streat.com.au)). Many social enterprises are resourced and expanded by internet-based crowdfunding campaigns. Crowdfunding is a way for businesses, organisations and individuals with a new idea or project to raise money to progress their activity or development. Building the collective culture of empowerment can make the issue public and political. It enables members of the community to portray and publicise their life experiences in the context of existing inequitable policy frameworks, or give wider recognition to an issue; it can be a means of advocating for policy change.

Health practitioners engaged in community development practice may consider applying the DARE criteria (Rubin & Rubin, 1992, p. 77) as a means of ensuring that decision-making continues to reflect the needs and concerns of the communities they work with.

- Who **D**etermines the goal?
- Who **A**cts to achieve the goal?
- Who **R**eceives the benefits from the actions?
- Who **E**valuates the actions?

3. Involvement in action (choosing a 'winnable' local issue)

If community members are expected to be active in local decision making, they need to believe that the action is worthwhile and likely to bring about change. Choosing the issues to focus on is important (Sterling, 2012). Minkler (1991, p. 272) suggested that if an issue is appropriate for a community development approach, the community must feel strongly about it, and it must be 'winnable, simple and specific'. She argued that this is particularly the case early in the community development process. Once people have started to develop a sense of their ability to effect change, they may be less easily swamped by resistance from others, or by lack of success on a particular issue. In the early stages, however, failure or resistance may lead the group to give up, so starting with winnable issues while people develop some skills can be productive. Other more difficult issues can then be addressed, with people building on the skills they have already developed through these experiences. Sterling (2012) provides a detailed overview of the personal benefits gained by vendors of *The Big Issue*, a social enterprise that produces a fortnightly magazine, sold on the streets by homeless and vulnerable community members, where the vendor retains half of the revenue.

At the start of a community development process, it may be the case that an outside 'expert' facilitator is employed to get the activity started; this is also when the commitment and skills of a social entrepreneur are key to the effectiveness of the project. The main aim of getting community members involved in the action is that they will become self-reliant in managing the issue or in solving the problem; the processes and outcomes are sustainable (Minkler, 2012; Sterling, 2012).

Spending the time, and using persistence, patience and creativity are all a part of being successful in bringing community members together. This is not a process that can be given scant attention or be done hastily. Getting to know community members, and being known and accepted in the community is important. Face-to-face contact helps, as does endorsement by community leaders and stakeholders. When working with Indigenous communities, the endorsement of community elders is essential (O'Donahoo & Ross, 2015).

The community development process must develop in such a way that when the initial resources are reduced to a bare minimum, or are removed altogether, the community strengths and capacity enable the activity to continue in a form the community is satisfied with, and the skills can be transferrable to a different setting (Minkler, 2012).

4. Development of community culture (working together successfully)

Development of a community culture, developing a collective voice or approach, or collaborating for a mutual outcome gives wider and more powerful recognition of an issue that a number of individuals may have believed affected only themselves. It allows them to move towards action for change (Tesoriero, 2010). Communities, whether they be people living in the same geographic area, or people with something in common, when they are acting together are far more effective in bringing about desired and sustained change than when trying to act alone, or they are pulling in different directions.

An essential element in building a culture of strength and unity in the community (or building on it if it already exists) is establishing mutually respectful dialogue between all parties involved in any activity. Respectful interaction relates particularly to agencies and personnel in authority, who are in positions of power because of their authority; for this reason they are at particular risk of perpetuating feelings of powerlessness or incompetence in members of the communities they work with. Effective communication with a community demands honesty, clarity and responsiveness (Munoz & Steinerowski in Farmer et al., 2012). Labonté (1997) refers to processes of working together successfully as community participation 'software', in an analogy with computer software. Software approaches spend energy on establishing group norms of behaviour and information sharing, exercises to build listening and respect, and creation of 'non-zero-sum power-with' (Labonté, 1997, p. 49).

In short, there are not specific activities involved in creating an empowered community culture, but it involves ways of working described in this chapter. The core comprehensive primary health care values that we have presented earlier, including equity, participation and social justice, can provide tools for health practitioners engaged in community development practice to illustrate where injustices are occurring. In this way, an issue can be framed as structurally inequitable, rather than being viewed as a personal complaint.

Development of an empowered community culture happens gradually from within the community, but health practitioners can be powerful catalysts in enhancing the culture when they link personal experiences of individuals to the wider political dimensions (Farmer et al., 2012). When one issue is resolved successfully, the empowered community will have no difficulty in finding another issue to address (Alinsky, 1972; DeFilippis & Saegert, 2013).

5. Learning (fostering skills that are transferable)

Community members who become engaged in the processes and decisions that concern them need to be open to the learning and dynamic changes that this entails. Communities of all descriptions constantly change and evolve, and as they become empowered to act on their own behalf, the process of change demands new skills and creates new opportunities for learning. While people learn as individuals, their additional knowledge is added to the community 'toolkit' of resources, to be used on other occasions in different settings. People may learn to complete a funding application, work with media agencies (for instance, to write a media release), read budgets and financial statements, analyse a piece of legislation, or chair a meeting. The community program may be based on skills development and this may lead to secure employment as well as professional skills and qualifications.

Gaining employment brings the greatest health benefit apart from secure housing (Cleland et al., 2016). People learn in a great number of ways; they may enter a training program, take part in action to challenge authority or inequitable systems, or learn new skills through mentorship and role modelling (Linnan et al. in Minkler, 2012, Chapter 13). People may feel they don't have the professional skills of those in formal organisations; however, the sheer weight of numbers coupled with enthusiasm and determination can be sufficient to raise the profile of an issue across the social spectrum, change social values over time, to bring about acceptance for their agenda, and support the sustainability of new initiatives for community members.

6. Organisational development (collaborating for mutual benefit)

The key process in community development—reflected in the definition presented at the start of the chapter—is that citizens increase their abilities to control decisions that affect themselves and their community. Whatever the reason that has brought community members to identify together, and no matter how disempowered they have felt, the challenge is to enable their progress along the continuum towards greater community/collective control. The wisdom and experiences of these people is the starting point on which all other processes are built. Tesoriero (2010, p. 128) has a salutary message for those health practitioners who want to impart their own expertise, or speed the community processes along:

> Barging in as the person with the expertise, intent on 'intervening' and bringing about change from a position of 'superior' knowledge and skills, is to guarantee failure, and will simply perpetuate structures and discourses of disadvantage and disempowerment.

For a start, the health practitioner engaged in community development practice must earn the trust and support of the community, who are likely to be distrustful on the basis of their prior experiences with 'professionals'. To be an advocate for a disempowered community may mean the health practitioner is seen as the enemy of the mainstream (Alinsky, 1972; Skerratt & Steiner, 2013). It can be a solitary, isolated role initially, until there is wider acceptance from the community. Some social enterprises collaborate widely across an industry sector, such as hospitality or disability support, and this is one way that opposition to a program is reduced and wider acceptance is built (Kernot, 2010; Sterling, 2012).

It is also easy when working with communities for the 'outside expert' to transfer control over community decisions to the 'elites' within the community; it is effectively a power transfer, rather than power sharing. These people may be the most vocal, articulate, active or politically or economically powerful community members (Skerratt & Steiner, 2013). Shared collaborative and consultative processes in the routine activities of the community are needed from the beginning, and are sometimes complex to establish because of the prior experiences and entrenched values of community members. Constant attention to democratic and participatory principles is required. The health practitioner engaged in community development practice models these processes in the way they work with the community. The community needs to make early decisions about how information is to be collated, distributed and acted on so that all members can be informed and be as active as they wish to be (Labonté, 1997; Minkler, 2012, Chapter 7).

The health practitioner engaged in community development practice, therefore, is not independent of the community, but joins the community team. The skills that they bring become part of the 'toolkit' of skills the community can call upon when needed. The more that people collaborate and share their skills and resources, the greater their future capacity to solve community problems through political action.

The six processes of community development practice presented above are more likely to be successful and to be sustained when communities work in partnership or collaboration with government and non-government agencies or private social enterprise that have similar philosophies or areas of interest, or are sympathetic to their cause. Working in ways that encompass these processes does not mean that a practitioner or agency loses power, or that there needs to be a power struggle. They describe a basis for shared decision making and negotiation to reach mutually satisfactory outcomes.

Outcomes of community development practice

While the processes of developing and strengthening a community that have been described so far are admirable, people tend to come together and give their energy voluntarily when they are trying to achieve a specific outcome or change; they have a reason for working together, a mutually agreed goal in mind. Although the processes of community development practice are extremely important, placing more importance on them than on the desired outcomes has some limitations. There is a real danger of this being paternalistic towards community members, for it effectively implies that, even though they worked long and hard and failed to achieve the goal they set themselves, the process was nonetheless still good for them. Community members themselves may not define this as success, but rather may be angered by the suggestion that the goal was unimportant (although they may acknowledge that they learnt from the process). Certainly, the processes of involvement may be very important for community members, but they may regard it as such only if they are successful in achieving the goal they set out to achieve. Lawson and Kearns (2014) also highlight the need for careful analysis of processes to ensure the community with whom a community development process is being implemented, are actually being empowered; what is the evidence it is 'good' for the community as well as being good for the funding agency and their public image?

The following community outcomes recognise the importance of having reasons for coming together. These outcomes provide people with the satisfaction and energy to tackle a new issue concerning their community. When developing a health promotion program that uses a community development approach (e.g. in a funding application or program logic), be sure to include both of these outcomes in the wording of the project goal. Further guidance on writing program goals is provided in Chapter 4.

1.   Concrete benefit

The key factor that makes all the processes of community development desirable and worthwhile is the issue that brings the community together in the first place. Careful selection of the issue to be addressed in a health promotion program using a community development approach is important. If the issue is a priority, it will attract the most community involvement. In practice, the idea of starting with winnable issues may not be possible as it may well be a difficult, even almost un-winnable, issue that brings a community to the point of wanting to act. In that case, the idea of starting with winnable issues is unrealistic. This is more likely to be so where the community development action begins spontaneously, as a result of people responding to an issue crucial to their lives, where change will bring a concrete benefit. The most important outcomes of community development are the tangible and lasting changes that occur as a result of the efforts of the community. The key concept that sums up the observable outcomes of community development activities is sustainability; for example, if there are improvements to housing or less pollution in the environment, a change to policy or if there are new skills and employment (Farmer et al., 2012; Minkler, 2012; Sterling, 2012). Gold fever (Insight 6.2) is an example of such outcomes.

INSIGHT 6.2 Gold fever—involvement in action

Wedders was a small country town where quite a bit of alluvial gold had been found in the distant past. Over time, it had settled into being a farming community. A mining company decided that it would like to search for any remaining gold around the town. They were 'strip' miners, bulldozing the trees, taking off the surface earth a bit at a time and running over the ground with metal detectors. The community was very much against this sort of 'development' because of the noise, the dust, the loss of amenity of the surrounding bushland and the loss of some nearby pistachio orchards. The miners applied for a planning permit, the local council refused it and the miners appealed to the civil administrative tribunal in the state capital. The community organised itself. The local council, the Community Health Centre, the returned soldiers, the Lions Club, the Gardening Club, the Mothers' Club, the Progress Association, the Tourist Development Association, the local businesses and the local real estate agent banded together to argue their case. The various groups vigorously debated the points and acquainted themselves with the relevant laws and regulations.

At the tribunal, they were up against highly paid lawyers hired by the miners. The community divided itself into teams to argue the main points: the dust and noise, the loss of amenity, the loss of productive orchards and the extent of miners' rights over citizens' rights. There was a telling moment when a long-term resident of the town openly wept when she described how she felt about the loss of the bushland that surrounded her little house on the edge of town. The lawyers pressed their case. Finally, commonsense prevailed and the tribunal ruled in favour of the community.

Source: Written by Dr Adrian Verrinder.

Goal setting in community development: It is difficult to bring ideal global visions of capable communities deciding their own courses of action down to practical, day-to-day achievable goals. A goal expresses what is desired by the community as an outcome of their activities. In community development, the goal will express both of the core elements of a tangible difference and an expression of new power relationships. It is also important to express a vision broader than meeting local objectives if real empowerment of the community is to be achieved and sustained.

2. New power relationships

Sustainable changes in communities will arise when members have acquired new skills and recognised their existing talents during the process, and they have made lasting structural changes in the community. Being involved in a community development project can change the social landscape of the community so that new and more equitable power relations are formed (Skerratt & Steiner, 2013). People reflect on, and acknowledge the value of, the process elements (Tesoriero, 2010). For instance, through the processes of community development, former adversaries may now be able to work together and relationships with government agencies may be less confrontational and more respectful than previously. There may be new business or commercial arrangements that have the capacity to transform the lives of people or the local economy (Steiner & Atterton, 2014).

Power relationships will change within the community and in the relationships between a community and wider society. For instance, there may be denser and stronger networks of association in the community creating the potential for settings that enhance health and wellbeing and build social capital (Talbot & Walker, 2007) and greater resilience to resist further challenges, including external policy and economic factors (Steiner & Atterton, 2014).

Health practitioners engaged in community development practice are agents of change for community-led ideas. The diffusion of innovation theory provides us with a way of understanding how new ideas are taken up (or not); that is, how change takes place in a community (Rogers, 2003). 'Diffusion' is defined as the process by which an innovation is communicated through certain channels over time among members of a social system. An 'innovation' is defined as an idea, practice or object perceived as new by an individual or other unit of adoption (Rogers, 2003). Communication channels serve as the link between those who know of the innovation and those who have not yet adopted it (Seabert, 2013). The process works in five steps: 1. innovation-gaining knowledge about the innovation; 2. communication challenges in becoming persuaded about the innovation; 3. decision step of adopting or rejecting the innovation; 4. implementation step of putting the innovation to use; and 5. confirmation step of either adopting the innovation or reversing the decision (Kanekar, 2008, p. 5). Different factors can influence the speed and success with which new ideas are adopted. These include the *relative advantage* or whether their idea is seen as better than what is currently in place; *compatibility* or the degree to which the innovation fits with existing values and needs, and people's past experience; *complexity*, the perception of the degree of difficulty the innovation is to achieve; *trialability*, the degree to which the innovation can be trialled and modifications made; and, *observability*, whether the results of the innovation can be observed by others, with visible changes more likely to promote adoption (Rogers, 2003). Social marketing strategies, including the use of social media, can enhance the effectiveness of the diffusion factors (Archibald & Clark, 2014). These are explored further in Chapter 8.

There are several kinds of adopters or consumers of the innovation, identified according to their willingness to adopt the innovation: innovators, change agents, transformers, mainstreamers, unwilling laggards, reactionaries; there are also iconoclasts, spiritual recluses and curmudgeons (AtKisson, 1999; Rogers, 2003; Seabert, 2013). Innovators are the progenitors of new ideas; they may be considered 'fringe', eccentric or unpredictable by the rest of the community and so may not be trusted. Change agents are the 'ideas brokers' for the innovator. Transformers or early adopters in the mainstream are open to new ideas and want to promote change. Mainstreamers can be persuaded that the innovation is a good idea and will change when they see the majority changing, but unwilling laggards (who are the late majority and who constitute about the same number as the mainstreamers) are the sceptics who need to be convinced of the benefits before they adopt a change. Reactionaries have a vested interest in keeping things as they are. Iconoclasts highlight problems but do not generate ideas; they are often silent partners of innovators. Spiritual recluses may proffer the philosophical underpinning and influence the atmosphere for change, while curmudgeons see change efforts as useless (AtKisson, 1999; Rogers, 2003).

Health practitioners engaged in community development practice are agents of change for community-led ideas. As such, they should work closely with the early adopters as this is the group with most influence in the adoption process (Seabert, 2013). Understanding the change role of different community members will facilitate adoption of a new idea leading to effective community decision making and long-term social change.

In theory, the success or otherwise of innovation depends on how it is seen by various groups—whether the innovation is seen as compatible with the established culture, for example, or the perceived relative advantage of the innovation. The simplicity and flexibility of innovation, together with its reversibility and the perceived risk of its adoption, will affect the extent to which innovation is taken up by the community. Finally, the observability of results will influence whether others take up the change (Rogers, 2003). Theoretical frameworks such as diffusion of innovation can just as readily be applied to the dissemination of new practice guidelines and other changes to clinical practice that are encompassed in evidence-based practice for health practitioners (Sanson-Fisher, 2004). An in-depth study of these factors and other theories may provide useful information for agents of change. The important thing is to know the community and what is likely to influence its response.

COMMUNITY DEVELOPMENT PRACTICE ROLES, SKILLS AND ATTRIBUTES

Start with what they know
Build on what they have
But of the best leaders
When their task is accomplished
Their work is done
The people all remark
'We have done it ourselves'

(Lao Tzu, founder of Taoism)

The approach described by the poem above is emblematic of a health practitioner using a community development approach. However, the breadth of community development practice is changing and it is now necessary to consider the realm of community development initiated by social enterprises and entrepreneurs, as well as when the community development process begins without the assistance of employed health practitioners (Farmer et al., 2012; Sterling, 2012). People outside the community may recognise an unmet need that will enhance the wellbeing of a community, and have the capacity to bring about change to a setting or access to services. Local people and community leaders are often committed to using that process and may work in their own areas or groups, attempting to build consensus and initiate collective action to address people's needs.

Community development practice roles

Health practitioners have an important role to play in supporting the people involved in community development, whether the community development process began through the efforts of external entrepreneurs, local leaders, as a policy initiative, or was instigated by health or community practitioners themselves. There are two main reasons for this. First, the philosophy of comprehensive primary health care and the action areas of the Ottawa Charter for Health Promotion guide health practitioners to take up community development strategies to promote the health of the people they are working with, and this may mean that their work is contrary to mainstream political philosophy. Second, health practitioners are well placed to engage in community development practice because they come into contact with members of marginalised groups. Special relationships of trust can develop in the context of the 'crisis' situations in which they often meet. Their close involvement with people in crisis situations means that they see quite clearly the health implications of poverty and disempowerment (Sterling, 2012). However, health practitioners may still need to break free from some community perceptions that they should be dealing directly with ill-health through clinical services only. If health practitioners join in the life of the community, make the most of opportunities to listen to the community, and develop relationships with community members, they will identify opportunities for community development that will support people to regain their self-sufficiency.

Integrated community development work requires health practitioners to be generalists. It is not appropriate to be confined to some roles more than others. There are some skills that are constantly required, others less so. The roles identified below are interdependent. They fit well with the roles of advocate, enabler and mediator which the Ottawa Charter for Health Promotion highlighted as important for health practitioners.

1. Catalyst: assisting the community to make the changes

Working in the role of a *catalyst*, the health practitioner engaged in community development practice is an instrument of change by assisting others to develop personal initiatives and to take action with others. Even though the role of the health practitioner is to support others, in the initial stages of change the practitioner may be more actively involved in providing initial support and bringing community members together, thus setting the agenda for action, perhaps by providing guidance on the first step to reduce inequalities. Spontaneously formed action groups may come together already prepared to take action, but need guidance about methods or approaches.

2. Facilitator: providing resources

Facilitating the process of turning decisions into actions by providing administrative or technical skills for small groups may also be required of a health practitioner engaged in community development practice. Practitioners can support the community by providing necessary resources for their program or assisting community members to make contacts or access resources they need. These might include access to personal resources to assist with presentation, photocopying and word-processing facilities, arranging a meeting with key stakeholders, and the use of meeting rooms. Negotiating to find accessible, neutral meeting places that are comfortable for group members will be an important component of this process, as some communities of interest commence from an extremely disadvantaged or vulnerable situation.

3. Educational: assisting with skills development

In the educational role, the health practitioner engaged in community development practice facilitates learning to increase the capacity of people through enhanced knowledge and problem-solving skills. Learning may come from a range of different sources, including peers in the community. People may need assistance with developing skills in such things as applications and interviews, communicating with the media, applying for funds, or writing letters to members of parliament, public services or local companies involved in a particular issue. Health practitioners can be active in assisting people to learn how to carry out these tasks effectively in order to build personal capacity, to get a message across and build capacity that is transferable to other settings for the future (Linnan et al. in Minkler, 2012).

4. Technical skills: planning action

If health practitioners have a better knowledge of bureaucratic processes, channels of enquiry and approaches to take, they are able to provide valuable information that will help the community group to plan and undertake an effective health promotion program. This can save much worry and uncertainty, and conserve valuable time and energy that might have been wasted if the group had acted inappropriately owing to lack of knowledge.

Assisting with applications for funding for some projects and other forms of advocacy may be necessary also.

Practitioners may have better skills than community members in researching information, better access to databases holding useful information and access to professional networks. They can assist communities in developing their research skills where appropriate and can themselves conduct research through information systems to which members of the public may not have easy access. Participatory evaluation (discussed in Chapter 4) relies on effective partnerships between community members and program evaluators to provide information and insights that may not otherwise be available, and to ensure the community perspective of 'success' is the focus of the evaluation (Coombe in Minkler, 2012, Chapter 19).

5.   Representation: supporting localism

The representational role in this context is as advocate or champion. While not all communities are locality-based, many of them are. Health practitioners and others with specific skills and assets they are willing to share can support community development action directly through the provision of new programs or by supporting the community to advocate for greater power in decision making, or improved access to employment, services and facilities. For example, encouraging the establishment of local credit cooperatives will help keep local money in the local area and will make more money available for financial support of local endeavours. Local employment initiatives also present valuable opportunities to support local economic development (Farmer et al., 2012; Sterling, 2012).

6.   Link making: supporting community members

A health practitioner engaged in community development practice may also be required to be a linking person between individuals, groups and organisations, or between the community and private or social enterprise or a government or semi-government agency. This may mean knowing where to go to link the different areas of expertise, bringing the parties together and being a translator for groups with different 'languages'. Technical skills may be required; for example, in research, or as a part of a social enterprise initiative.

Getting funds to start a project is often a big hurdle and what is often required is outlined in Chapter 4. Sometimes philanthropic organisations, individual benefactors or crowdfunding can provide the seed funding that enables the project to get under way. There are specific organisations that bring together information about philanthropic organisations that provide financial support for community initiatives and their specific funding priorities, including Philanthropy Australia (http://www.philanthropy.org.au). Local governments often allocate large one-off funding for capital projects such as building sporting facilities, community hubs and entertainment complexes. Rural communities with declining populations and struggling rural businesses may set a priority to attract visitors. It is useful to think of large community projects as a series of subprojects. It may be easier to attract smaller bundles of funding. Keep in mind also that most funding agencies are very positive about allocating funds where there is already some funding promised from another source. Crowdfunding is another option to consider.

Unless support is provided when necessary, community members involved in the process can end up 'burnt out', unable to continue and feeling disempowered. Community development is hard work and can be exhausting, physically and emotionally, for those involved. Community development work may also be a tiring process for the health practitioner, and so it is valuable for those using this approach to support each other. This can be particularly so when progress seems slow, and when community development is not endorsed enthusiastically by some decision-makers.

Community development practice skills and attributes

To perform these community development practice roles, there are some fundamental skills and attributes that health practitioners need. Communication skills, consensus building, collaboration and conflict management skills are constantly required.

1. Cultural competency

Working in multicultural communities will provide different challenges for the health practitioner engaged in community development practice. In Chapter 2 we discussed the concept of cultural safety where cultural awareness and intercultural sensitivity are essential to achieving cultural safety. The language, customs, attitudes, beliefs and preferred ways of doing things of different cultures need to be respected and reflected in the community development practice. Munford and Walsh-Tapiata (2006) provide an excellent example of this process in New Zealand. This example of change began at the grassroots level to create Te Kōhanga Reo ('Language Nest' or early childhood language centres). In this innovation, 'the dreams of kaumātua (older women) and women, who made a commitment' to reintroduce Māori children to their language was supported by formal policies and funding to develop this across New Zealand. 'The success of Te Kōhanga Reo has led to the development of schools for all age groups and university education where Māori language is the main medium of communication' (Munford & Walsh-Tapiata, 2006, p. 428). A more recent analysis of this approach supports its authenticity and re-emphasises the importance of understanding different worldviews and ensuring the cultural safety of disempowered community members of cultural minority groups.

2. Communicating effectively

Authentic, effective communication is probably one of the most important skills a health practitioner can work on to improve their community development practice. Practitioners need to work in a way that ensures the cultural safety of all participants. They need to be able to communicate information and different viewpoints effectively and respectfully. Refer back to the cultural safety table (Chapter 2) for more detailed guidance on how to practise in a culturally safe manner.

Facilitating effective verbal and non-verbal communication requires highly developed interpersonal skills as well as knowledge about communication patterns in and between communities. Being aware of your own values and perspectives, including prejudices, expectations, ideologies, judgements and the need to control, is the first step. The personal skills required to communicate effectively include the ability to:

- ensure that the conversation is one of genuine dialogue and not a game of power and control
- create and maintain an atmosphere of mutual trust and acceptance
- be aware of cultural differences and sensitivities in communication
- listen carefully
- allow the other to speak before formulating your answer
- state one's message clearly using language that is readily understood
- use 'I' statements when speaking
- keep a conversation focused and directed where necessary

- understand the value of silence in communication
- be aware of the other person's time constraints and priorities
- be aware of the importance of the physical environment
- encourage the other to reflect on the implications of what is being discussed
- be prepared to share vulnerability and brokenness as well as courage.

Making use of story, such as lived experiences and everyday life stories, can be a powerful use of communication skills in community development practice. Stories can transmit culture and world views and express the status quo. Stories can also provide the basis for generating alternative options or solutions that start a course of change (Ledwith & Springett, 2010). The ability to draw the theoretical learning from a story and lead the transformation process is a high-level skill, which is discussed in more detail by Ledwith and Springett (2010).

3. Building consensus

In some cultures, consensus in decision making is the norm; in others, it is not. To reach a consensus, groups need to agree on a course of action that best meets the needs of the whole group. The decision may not be the preferred option of some, but diversity is respected and commitments are made to the action. The process of talking the issues through may take some time and skill; so health practitioners engaged in community development practice need skills in respecting, listening, empathising, reframing and communicating (Tesoriero, 2010, p. 263).

4. Using networking to promote collaboration

Health practitioners engaged in community development practice need to be able to develop cooperative strategies to assist communities to develop shared visions about the future. Some of the strategies include building trust, teams and community competence. There can be no community without some level of commitment to cooperation, which needs to be built over time (Farmer et al., 2012). Health practitioners may need to try to challenge the dominance of the competitive ethic which is so entrenched in many cultures (Verrinder, 2005). It is necessary to network with a wide variety of people and groups in and outside one's usual context (Kernot, 2010). Networks need to remain open and to involve people from the grassroots. This prevents the possibility of unofficial network elites forming.

5. Managing conflict

It is advisable to explore causes and forms of conflict to be able to work towards a negotiated resolution. At various times in community development practice there may be tension due to unclear expectations, broken agreements, irrational outbursts, conflicting agendas and so on. Conflict resolution techniques include controlled discussion, role reversal, hidden agenda counselling, and cooperative problem solving.

- Controlled discussion—designed to get combatants listening to each other. The health practitioner engaged in community development practice mediates an exchange of views. There are two rules: each person makes only one point at a time and each person restates the point to the other's satisfaction before replying.
- Role reversal—the health practitioner mediates an exchange of views with each person taking the other person's position.

- Hidden agenda counselling—each person is asked to state what he or she needs from the other by addressing an empty chair: this can uncover a hidden agenda that has nothing to do with the current situation.

- Cooperative problem solving—the health practitioner takes people through the diagnosis, treatment and follow-up problem-solving cycle. Each person must state clearly what the problem is, to what degree each is responsible, and if there are any other causes. Possible solutions are identified and an appropriate action plan, including an evaluation of the plan, is agreed on (Brown et al., 2005; Heron, 1999).

SOCIAL ENTERPRISE AND SOCIAL ENTREPRENEURSHIP

Throughout this chapter we have referred to the role of the health practitioner engaged in community development practice. In recent years the role of people that may not identify as health practitioners, and/or may not be employed in health- or community-related agencies, in community development practice has become more prominent. 'Social enterprise' and 'social entrepreneurship' refer to the development of sustainable social benefits in local settings through community-based social trade enterprise activities, where the resources are reinvested back into the community.

Social enterprise uses a community development approach with a business purpose to develop some form of trading activities, including community enterprises, voluntary organisations that trade products or skills, fair trade organisations and training programs (Farmer et al., 2012; Social Enterprise Alliance, 2010). One of the most widely known early social enterprise initiatives was the urban renewal project undertaken in Bromley by Bow, a disadvantaged and culturally diverse locality in inner London in the 1980s led by Andrew and Susan Mawson (Bromley by Bow Centre, n.d.). The Bromley by Bow Centre now offers a wide range of health and educational services and continues to function using the same social enterprise principles.

Social enterprise processes are the same as those outlined above for community development. Skill development and transfer are the same, but the tangible outcome is an exchange that may be goods or services with a commercial value that are developed and provided to others. The 'trade' may not involve money or the exchange may not be at usual commercial rates. Using social enterprise, community goals to overcome social inequalities and unmet needs are addressed using business growth or new venture principles, with a strong emphasis on building self-esteem and new skills. Income or resources are reinvested to secure enterprise sustainability (Sterling, 2012). Social enterprise can be a purpose and outcome of community development (Farmer et al., 2012; Kernot, 2010).

In recent times, some of the community development theory involving patient and careful work to build local networks and local knowledge has been bypassed by social entrepreneurs. Social entrepreneurs have taken more 'impatient' and innovative approaches to building community trust, community empowerment and social capital by making change on behalf of the community or setting up and putting a process or system in place that enables people to build their self-esteem and skills (Kernot, 2010). Examples include a range of programs to involve refugees or homeless people in food preparation and service, in a model showcased by Jamie Oliver and *The Big Issue* magazine run as a social enterprise (Sterling, 2012). Other examples of the growing number of social entrepreneurs include the 2016 winners of the Young Australians of the Year award, who started the Orange Sky Laundry offering a mobile, free laundry service to homeless people, and the siblings who were state finalists for commencing Fighting Chance, a program designed to build the self-esteem of young people living with disability through job skills training. Farmer and colleagues (2012) have documented the extensive social enterprise project across isolated rural communities in Scotland, Northern Ireland, Greenland, Sweden and Finland. In this project, a number of sustainable community social enterprises were developed.

Despite a different initial approach, in social entrepreneurship the principles of community development, of building community empowerment and trust over time, remain the same. Social entrepreneurs are people with passion and creativity who can bring about large-scale and durable social change from a basis of little resources. Social enterprise is a way that the volunteer sector can provide public services. Social entrepreneurs are usually successful at taking on seemingly insurmountable challenges and having the capacity to motivate and engage people who may have resources and/or imagination to be involved, to bring about a significant change in the social setting.

At first glance, social entrepreneurship seems like a top-down approach; it doesn't commence with immersion in a community of interest, taking time to develop community trust or undertaking a community assessment. A new social entrepreneurship initiative commences with a person or group with a social conscience wanting to make a difference. This top-down beginning frequently generates community-based bottom-up engagement and action that generates its own community empowerment, and thereby builds community capacity for the long term.

There are some notable international long-term community development initiatives commenced by social entrepreneurs that have changed the lives of the local community members who have taken part. The best known is the Grameen Bank in Bangladesh, where a rotating system of micro-credit loans allows the participants (usually poor, unskilled rural women) to receive interest-free funds to commence a small home-based business. These small micro-finance systems have proliferated around the world and have resulted in building the skills and empowering the poorest people to become self-sufficient.

Community social enterprises that arise from local community priority setting and action are attractive because they offer potential for enhanced services, often in the context of service loss. They 'feed on enthusiasms for community sustainability, ethical business and an interest in social capital as a means of building community capacity' (Farmer et al., 2012, p. 163). However, local community social enterprises can also be seen as 'mechanisms for offloading the expense of providing public services on to communities, particularly those in problematic situations such as rural settings where commercial provision may not be viable'. Community social enterprises need to be provided with a safety net that ensures service certainty and appropriate support and capacity building to enable them to meet the requirements of health and safety, quality and accountability. This is a key area where the professional networking and advocacy skills of a health practitioner engaged in community development practice will be useful in protecting community members' energy and goodwill from exploitation by being seen as a 'cheap' solution to an expensive 'problem'. Insights 6.3 and 6.4 highlight what can happen when a community is assisted to take risks.

There is no limit to who can be a social entrepreneur or start a social enterprise, or the issues that they may address. Initiatives can bring about change for women or men, disabled or able-bodied people in rural or urban areas in any country in the world; they can focus on diverse issues for disempowered community members, encompassing environmental action, homelessness, child trafficking, educational disadvantage and sanitation. Social entrepreneurs can be rich or poor, educated and unskilled, male or female, and from all cultural and religious groups. So while the social enterprise approach fits within

INSIGHT 6.3 Getting started with a community initiative

People and community groups often have 'great' ideas that will benefit people with a certain interest, or that will provide facilities or experiences for the wider community. Here are three examples of projects in Victoria that started with small community initiatives.

1. The Old Church on the Hill (https://www.theoldchurchonthehill.com/) is an old but attractive de-consecrated church in inner Bendigo, Victoria. It was purchased by a private benefactor and made available for community development purposes. The management committee works with the community to develop the spaces, including building a community kitchen and community gardens, and to build community networks and connections. There is a special focus on intercultural welcome and healthy eating and family-centred activities, including music.
2. Brim (https://www.wimmeramalleetourism.com.au/our-towns/brim-victoria) is a small town in the Wimmera region of Victoria, Australia, with a population in 2016 of 170. The Shire of Yarriambiack commissioned artist Guido van Helten to paint murals on some defunct wheat silos. The four characters depicted are 30 metres tall, and they have been a great attraction for visitors to the area. Nearby towns have also benefited significantly.
3. The Redesdale (https://www.redesdale.net) community in central Victoria attracted funding to complete a master plan for their recreation reserve. The community successfully attracted crowdfunding over a month to enable them to develop facilities for a pavilion to provide shelter for sports teams.

the health promotion principles of equity, social justice and empowerment, it is very difficult to define and describe practice guidelines, personality characteristics and training programs that advise or train people how to do it (Martin & Osberg, 2015).

As distinct from social change agents who, for instance, may go to a community to assist people to deal with challenges and expected changes, or to resolve conflict, there are no set methods for social entrepreneurs. Praszkier and Nowak (2012, p. 24) describe social entrepreneurs as people who can bring about small changes in a short time that reverberate through the social system to bring about significant changes in the long term. The characteristics of social entrepreneurs (Ashoka in Praszkier & Nowak, 2012, p. 24) include:

- having a new idea for solving a critical social problem
- being creative
- having an entrepreneurial personality
- envisioning the broad social impact of the idea
- possessing an unquestionable social fibre.

CHALLENGES FOR COMMUNITY DEVELOPMENT PRACTICE

There are a number of interrelated challenges, some operating at the global level, that have implications for community development practice. There is a tension between market economy processes and community development philosophy of empowerment, equity and fairness. In recent times, the rhetoric used by many governments around the world and large organisations, such as the World Bank, has been that 'community' and community

INSIGHT 6.4 Social enterprise in Girgarre

The small town of Girgarre in regional Victoria provides an inspirational example of small-town planning undertaken with a social enterprise philosophy. The dairy industry was struggling, local businesses were folding or leaving, the primary school was struggling. At a community visioning session, local people were encouraged to consider all options: 'there is no such thing as a bad idea'. The group decided to start a farmer's market, and to incorporate live music into the market format. Here is their story about perseverance. It is not a simple story.

Our town is alive and well thanks to a community's willingness to try something new. The one thing communities in a similar situation to ours need is an open mind—unless they have that, they're doomed! At the beginning, we had one group and one idea that seemed way-out at the time.

In a time when our whole lifestyle was under threat from drought, the global economic crisis and future uncertainty, we have a group of people from the city, willing to help us create this amazing weekend event. It is nothing short of spectacular. Girgarre is looking towards a spectacular and sustainable future. You have to take it in little chunks, and create a situation where people feel free to come forward and do as little or as much as they like.

During the running of the Farmer's Market, some 40 people aged from 10 to 70 volunteer to cook breakfast, squeeze juice, make tea and coffee, set up and pack up. People who had never volunteered before were driving over the district nailing up market signs in trees to advertise the day.

Having a place to gather has been important. Our hall was refurbished, and now there are over 160 events and hirings per year. What an impact the Moosic Muster has had on our town of just 200 people. Now we have nine subcommittees.

Some of the financial benefits for our community have included the funding of our community car (so necessary as there is limited public transport), upgrading of our CFA (fire brigade) facilities and the local school and the Recreation Reserve also receive vital financial support. The community becomes classless; people are judged by what they do, not by what they have. Their latest success is to attract significant funding through the Community Arts Victoria and Small Town Transformation grants for the community to establish 'Girgarre Revival: The Sound of Our Spirit Rising'.

Source: Written by Jan Smith. Read more details at http://girgarre.com.au/.

development processes are valued and have capacity to advance the wellbeing of the most marginalised groups. However, challenges to participation in civil society and to the strength of social capital have come from globally dominant neoliberal ideologies (discussed in Chapters 1 and 2). Values such as individualism, competitiveness and meritocracy, and governments have hijacked the language of community development while in reality offering simplistic and contradictory solutions to meeting the needs of the least powerful (Mooney, 2012; Talbot & Walker, 2007). The goals and processes that guide commercial activities and international markets are not based on equity (DeFilippis & Saegert, 2013).

The co-option of the language of community development by governments and powerful international organisations has meant that instead of working with communities to address the structural issues that determine their ill-health, communities have been encouraged to solve the problems without the resources or power to do so (Tesoriero, 2010). Community development may be used as a euphemism for 'oppression, domination, colonialism, racism, and the imposition of Western cultural values and traditions ...' (Campbell et al., 2007, p. 152). The language of governments masks not only the conflicts within communities, but also the inequalities in community development processes. The values and priorities of large non-government organisations (NGOs) and professional organisations may be at odds with small community-based organisations, social movements and self-help collectives that may have the greatest opportunity to build participation, but have no resources. Local community empowerment and control may not be possible because NGOs, government departments and bureaucrats are unwilling to relinquish control.

Community development may be seen as a way of getting something for nothing. Local involvement, priority setting, generating local action and providing social enterprise, services and resources clearly benefit organisations that may ordinarily pay to have these things done. The demands for local communities taking action without resources are enormous. The government discourse of empowerment through participation ignores the reality that communities are not homogeneous. Forming partnerships takes time and skill, and conflict arises within and between communities for the scant resources made available, and community members may see no benefit from the process or the outcomes (Lawson & Kearns, 2014). Can communities really take control, when they are financially and socially under-resourced and organisations that may benefit from the local action assume communities and individuals have resources of time, energy and money that are constantly renewable?

Community development should emphasise, not undermine, the importance of ensuring the cultural safety of the community. The rhetoric of mainstream services about empowerment through community development processes often masks values about expert knowledge, cultural imperialism and paternalism.

Community development can also be a way for governments to move responsibility for dealing with challenges to health or social dislocation back to individuals. This may occur when dealing with anti-social behaviours and chronic conditions in areas where community resources and funding are low including, for example, drought support and mental health assistance in rural and remote communities (Verrinder & Talbot, 2015).

Building trust in communities takes time, and will often take longer than the period of funding that has been allocated, or longer than the term of the government that made the policy decision. Building effective community participation is based on mutual trust (Labonté, 1997). Community members have to have reason to trust others; health practitioners engaged in community development practice need to work in ways that give community members reason to be trusted.

Community development is a process in which members of a community are enabled to work together to solve a problem they face and, through their participation, develop skills and achieve greater power over some of the issues that impact on their lives. However, as we have said, community development is not always used to empower communities and increase their access to a range of choices. In many instances, it may be used to increase the compliance of community members with a program being imposed on the community, as a means of increasing the success of that program.

Various authors (DeFilippis & Saegert, 2013; Tesoriero, 2010; Tones & Tilford, 1994) caution against seeing community development approaches with an uncritical eye. Community development approaches can be viewed as a continuum ranging from true community development as empowerment at one end through to the selective or limited use of community development strategies to impose the beliefs of practitioners, professional groups or politicians at the other end. When a more limited form of community development is used, it is worth asking whose interests are being served. To what extent is this type of community development likely to serve the needs of the disempowered in the community?

There may be times when the community may benefit from the imposition of good ideas, especially if the ideas are supported with financial and structural enterprises, as in social entrepreneurship. These ideas must also be accompanied by strategies that enable deep involvement with flexibility and choice for community members so they have capacity to make a lasting change in their lives. Without this, in the longer term the community may have become more, rather than less, dependent on the health practitioners and so the principles of health promotion in a comprehensive primary health care context may not be fulfilled. It is only when the principles of health promotion underpin community development and social entrepreneurship processes that community development can live up to its reputation for addressing the structural determinants of health and wellbeing.

Critical analysis of community development practice is therefore vital, including evaluation of the way in which the employing agency or funding body sees community development being applied. If unrealistic and/or manipulative uses of community development are suspected, clarification is needed. Some administrators and bureaucrats, like others in positions of power over decision making or funding, do not always understand the intention of the health promotion approach to community development.

Community development places emphasis on people working together as a group to achieve things for themselves and changing the structures that influence their lives at the local level. Governments might therefore support community development because it takes the focus of responsibility away from government, public policy and broad social change. Community development also provides a cheap option for government. In supporting community development for those reasons, governments may have little regard for its goals of empowerment and increased community competence. This may mean that they support community development in theory, but in practice support only limited forms (Cox, 1995). Further, governments may reject community development as an approach to health promotion because of its emphasis on drawing people together to address common issues. Governments may be nervous of an approach that encourages people to work for social change, as it is possible that people may start demanding increased accountability from government. The spread of neoliberalism made the need for community development even greater. Health practitioners implementing health promotion programs within a comprehensive primary health care context cannot afford to lose their focus on community development.

Community development approaches also have limitations. There has been a tendency to expect a great deal from community development. It is important to recognise that while community development processes can have some impact on power relationships and equity at a local level, these processes will not shift power relationships on a broad scale without a vision and a plan to create a social movement or structural change. Even with the best intentions in the world, these processes at the local level will not change widespread social, economic and political conditions that are creating health inequities, unless there is significant outward focus and concerted, collaborative effort to make policy change.

EVALUATING COMMUNITY DEVELOPMENT PRACTICE

In Chapter 4, the health promotion practice cycle from community assessment through to evaluation is presented. In this section we propose questions related to what to assess or measure in community development to indicate if community development goals and objectives have been achieved and whether the processes to achieve those have been empowering. Impact and outcome evaluation questions might include: Has the quality of life improved through the resolution of shared problems? Has social justice been achieved? Is there a stronger sense of community? These are difficult questions to answer. Process evaluation questions might include: Who is involved in the decision-making processes? Are community members being heard and valued? Who has identified the assets and needs of the community? Who has prioritised those assets and needs for action? Is the community actively engaged in all aspects of the health promotion program, from community assessment through to evaluation? Is there an active community advisory group? Who has received the benefits? Who is evaluating the successes? Evaluation might also consider the quality of partnerships that have developed, the forms of community learning, and other elements of empowerment processes, as well as whether there is a lasting benefit or difference for the community, or action in a broader sphere or setting.

Critical reflection is acknowledged as an important part of evaluation practice. The Marxist tradition uses 'praxis' to describe a cycle of doing, learning and critically reflecting. Through this process, a deeper understanding is achieved from which we can inform practice and build theory; this in turn creates further understanding of practice, community and social change. 'Reflective practice includes both reflection-on-action and reflection-in-action' (Lehmann, 2003, p. 83). It is a skill that can be learnt and can be an empowering experience for professional development and community development (Ledwith & Springett, 2010). Some practitioners put time aside to reflect on their practice, others keep a diary or talk things through with colleagues or friends, or read widely to contextualise practice. Tesoriero (2010) suggests that community values on particular issues will be reflected in policies, social commentaries and through the media and these can serve as points of reference that may be personally challenging. Critically reflecting on these challenges will enhance the quality of the community development practice undertaken by the health practitioner.

CONCLUSION

With the endorsement of community development as a health promotion strategy in the Ottawa Charter for Health Promotion, and recognition that it reflects the comprehensive primary health care approach due to its focus on working with people, and enabling their achievement of goals, health practitioners need to make it a central part of their practice. Health practitioners engaged in community development practice need a broad range of skills in order to support the communities they work with. Creating empowering conditions at the local level enables communities to work on the social and environmental determinants of their health. Empowered communities will also develop skills that may help bring about social change on a broader level. It is in this aspect of creating empowering conditions that social entrepreneurs have significant capacity to make a difference through diverse community development initiatives.

MORE TO EXPLORE

EXAMPLES OF COMMUNITY DEVELOPMENT

- The Go Goldfields (n.d.) project involves a collaboration between a number of agencies in Maryborough, Victoria, who are working together to overcome the effects of disadvantage experienced by many families in the area: 'Go Goldfields is about creating positive outcomes for children, youth and families in Central Goldfields Shire. We have come together around our shared vision of our community aspiring, achieving and living a full life'. While there were many individual efforts being undertaken to address different social determinants of ill-health in the past, with some successes, this is a unique place-based approach to community development that encompasses the entire shire. The 'collective impact approach' involves the groups sharing their knowledge, skills and resources, which is engaging community members and enabling a community-wide difference. Read more about this unique collaboration at http://gogoldfields.org

- A number of community development and community building examples are presented in *Community organizing and community building for health and welfare* (3rd ed.): Minkler (2012). This is a detailed text providing valuable discussion on key community development concepts and a range of examples from the field.

IUHPE Core Competencies for Health Promotion

The IUHPE Core Competencies for Health Promotion comprises nine domains of action. Each domain has a series of core competency statements and a detailed outline of the knowledge and skills that contribute to competency in that domain.

The content of this chapter relates especially to the achievement of competency in the health promotion domains outlined below.

1. Enable change	*1.2 Use health promotion approaches which support empowerment, participation, partnership and equity to create environments and settings which promote health*
	Determinants of health and health inequities
	Theory and practice of collaborative working including facilitation, negotiation, conflict resolution, mediation, teamwork
	Partnership building and collaborative working
	1.3 Use community development approaches to strengthen community participation and ownership and build capacity for health promotion action
	Theory and practice of community development including equity, empowerment, participation and capacity building
	Health promotion models
2. Advocate for health	*2.1 Use advocacy strategies and techniques which reflect health promotion principles*
	Advocacy strategies and techniques

	2.5 Facilitate communities and groups to articulate their needs and advocate for the resources and capacities required for health promotion action Methods of stakeholder engagement Health and wellbeing issues relating to a specified population or group Theory and practice of community development including empowerment, participation and capacity building
3. Mediate through partnership	*3.1 Engage partners from different sectors to actively contribute to health promotion action* Theory and practice of collaborative working including facilitation, negotiation, conflict resolution, mediation, teamwork, networking and stakeholder engagement
	3.2 Facilitate effective partnership working which reflects health promotion values and principles Principles of effective intersectoral partnership working
	3.3 Build successful partnership through collaborative working, mediating between different sectoral interests Collaborative working
	3.4 Facilitate the development and sustainability of coalitions and networks for health promotion action Facilitation and mediation
4. Communication	*4.1 Use effective communication skills including written, verbal, non-verbal, listening skills and information technology* Understanding of social and cultural diversity Applications of information technology for social networking media, and mass media
	4.4 Use interpersonal communication and groupwork skills to facilitate individuals, groups, communities and organisations to improve health and reduce health inequities Theory and practice of effective communication including interpersonal communication and group work Diffusion of innovations theory
5. Leadership	*5.1 Work with stakeholders to agree a shared vision and strategic direction for health promotion action* Principles of effective intersectoral partnership working
	5.5 Contribute to mobilising and managing resources for health promotion action Collaborative working skills Ability to motivate groups and individuals towards a common goal

6. Assessment	*6.5 Identify the health needs, existing assets and resources relevant to health promotion action*
	Social determinants of health
	Health inequalities
	6.7 Identify priorities for health promotion action in partnership with stakeholders based on best available evidence and ethical values
	Evidence base for health promotion action and priority setting
7. Planning	*7.1 Mobilise, support and engage the participation of stakeholders in planning health promotion action*
	Analysis and application of information about needs and assets
	Use of project/program planning and management tools
	7.3 Develop a feasible action plan within resource constraints and with reference to existing needs and assets
	Ability to work with: groups and communities targeted by the health promotion action; stakeholders and partners
8. Implementation	*8.1 Use ethical, empowering, culturally appropriate and participatory processes to implement health promotion action*
	Theory and practice of community development including: empowerment, participation and capacity building
	8.4 Facilitate program sustainability and stakeholder ownership through ongoing consultation and collaboration
	Use of participatory implementation processes
	Monitoring and process evaluation

In addition, IUHPE specifies knowledge, skills and performance criteria essential for health promotion practitioners to act professionally and ethically, including having knowledge of ethical and legal issues, behaving in an ethical and respectful manner and working in ways that review and improve practice. Full details are available at: http://www.iuhpe.org/index.php/en/the-accreditation-system.

Reflective Questions

1. Working in partnership with community groups is complex and can be time-consuming in practice. How would you go about developing a mutually respectful and supportive collaboration to work with a geographic community in your local area?

2. Reflect on the range of community practice roles, skills and attributes required to work effectively with communities. What skills and attributes are required for the different roles and of those which do you feel confident about and which do you feel you need development in? What strategies could you use to develop capabilities that you identified you need to develop to work effectively with communities?

3. Using Arnstein's Ladder of Citizen Participation as a framework for reflection, describe the aims and effectiveness of the community participation activities conducted by a number of organisations in your area.

REFERENCES

Alinsky, S. (1972). Rules for radicals. New York: Vintage Books.

Anderson, I., Baum, F., & Bentley, M. (Eds.). (2007). Beyond Bandaids: exploring the underlying social determinants of Aboriginal health. Papers from the Social Determinants of Aboriginal Health Workshop. Adelaide: Cooperative Research Centre for Aboriginal Health.

Archibald, M. M., & Clark, A. M. (2014). Twitter and nursing research: how diffusion of innovation theory can help uptake. Journal of Advanced Nursing, 70(3), e3. doi:10.1111/jan.12343.

Arnstein, S. R. (1971). Eight rungs on the ladder of citizen participation. In E. S. Cahn & B. A. Passett (Eds.), Citizen participation: effecting community changes. New York, NY: Praeger Publishers.

Asset-Based Community Development Institute. (2020). ABCD Institute. Retrieved from http://www.abcdinstitute.org/

AtKisson, A. (1999). Believing Cassandra: an optimist's look at a pessimist's world. Melbourne: Scribe Publications.

Aulich, C. (2009). From citizen participation to participatory governance in Australian Local Government. Commonwealth Journal of Local Governance, 2, 44–60.

Bromley by Bow Centre. (n.d.). Bromley by Bow Centre. Retrieved from https://www.bbbc.org.uk/

Brown, V. A., Grootjans, J., Ritchie, J., et al. (Eds.). (2005). Sustainability and health: working together to support global integrity. London: Earthscan.

Butler, P., & Cass, S. (Eds.). (1993). Case studies of community development in health. Melbourne: Centre for Development and Innovation in Health.

Campbell, D., Wunungmurra, P., & Nyomba, H. (2007). Starting where the people are: lessons on community development from a remote Aboriginal Australian setting. Community Development Journal, 42(2), 151–166. doi:10.1093/cdj/bsi072.

Cleland, C., Kearns, A., Tannahill, C., & Ellaway, A. (2016). Home truths: are housing-related events more important for residents' health compared with other life events? Housing Studies, 31(5), 495–518. doi:10.1080/02673037.2015.1094565.

Cox, E. (1995). A truly civil society. Sydney: ABC Books.

Craig, G., Mayo, M., & Popple, K. (2011). The community development reader history, themes and issues. Bristol: The Policy Press.

DeFilippis, J., & Saegert, S. (2013). The community development reader (2nd ed.). New York: Taylor and Francis.

Dwyer, J. (1989). The politics of participation. Community Health Studies, 13(1), 59–65.

Eckermann, A. K., Dowd, T., Chong, E., et al. (2010). Binan goonj: bridging cultures in Aboriginal health (3rd ed.). Sydney: Churchill Livingstone/Elsevier.

Farmer, J., Hill, C., & Munoz, S.-A. (2012). Community co-production: social enterprise in remote and rural communities. Cheltenham, UK: Edward Elgar.

Freire, P. (1974). Education for critical consciousness. London: Sheed & Ward.

Go Goldfields. (n.d.). About us. Retrieved from https://gogoldfields.org/about-us/.

Goetting, A., & Green, G. P. (2010). Mobilizing communities. Philadelphia, PA: Temple University Press.

Green, M., Moore, H., & O'Brien, J. (2009). When people care enough to act: asset based community development (2nd ed.). Toronto: Inclusion Press.

Heron, J. (1999). The complete facilitator's handbook. London: Kogan Page.

Jackson, T., Mitchell, S., & Wright, M. (1989). The community development continuum. Community Health Studies, 13(1), 66–73. doi:10.1111/j.1753-6405.1989.tb00178.x.

Kanekar, A. (2008). Diffusion of innovations theory for alcohol, tobacco, and drugs. Journal of Alcohol and Drug Education, 52(1), 3–7.

Kearns, A., & Mason, P. (2015). Regeneration, relocation and health behaviours in deprived communities. Health and Place, 32, 43–58. doi:10.1016/j.healthplace.2014.12.012.

Kernot, C. (2010). Social enterprises driving social innovation. Impact(Spring 2010), 18–21.

Kretzmann, J., & McKnight, J. L. (1993). Building communities from the inside out: a path toward finding and mobilizing a community's assets. Evanston, Ill: Center for Urban Affairs and Policy Research, Northwestern University.

Labonté, R. (1990). Empowerment: notes on professional and community dimensions. Canadian Review of Social Policy, 26, 64–75.

Labonté, R. (1997). Power, participation and partnerships for health promotion. Retrieved from https://www.vichealth.vic.gov.au/media-and-resources/publications/power-participation-and-partnerships-for-health-promotion.

Labonté, R., & Laverack, G. (2008). Health promotion in action: from local to global empowerment. Basingstoke, UK: Palgrave Macmillan.

Landcare. (2016). What is Landcare? Retrieved from http://www.landcarevic.net.au/help/how-to/what-is-landcare.

Lawson, L., & Kearns, A. (2014). Rethinking the purpose of community empowerment in neighbourhood regeneration: the need for policy clarity. Local Economy: The Journal of the Local Economy Policy Unit, 29(1–2), 65–81. doi:10.1177/0269094213519307.

Ledwith, M., & Springett, J. (2010). Participatory practice: community-based action for transformative change. Bristol, UK: Policy Press.

Lehmann, J. (2003). The Harveys and other stories: invitations to curiosity. Bendigo: St Luke's Innovative Resources.

Martin, R., & Osberg, S. (2015). Two keys to sustainable social enterprise. Harvard Business Review, 93(5), 86–94.

Mental Health First Aid Australia. (2019). Mental Health First Aid Australia. Retrieved from https://mhfa.com.au/.

Minkler, M. (1991). Improving health through community organization. In K. Glanz, F. M. Lewis, & B. K. Rimer (Eds.), Health behavior and health education: theory, research and practice. San Francisco, CA: Jossey-Bass.

Minkler, M. (2012). Community organizing and community building for health and welfare (3rd ed. Vol. 9780813553146). New York, NY: Rutgers University Press.

Mooney, G. (2012). Health of nations: towards a new political economy. London: Zed Books.

Munford, R., & Walsh-Tapiata, W. (2006). Community development: working in the bicultural context of Aotearoa New Zealand. Community Development Journal, 41(4), 426–442. doi:10.1093/cdj/bsl023.

Naidoo, J., & Wills, J. (2010). Developing practice for public health and health promotion (3rd ed.). Edinburgh: Bailliere Tindall/Elsevier.

O'Donahoo, F. J., & Ross, K. E. (2015). Principles relevant to health research among Indigenous communities. International Journal of Environmental Research and Public Health, 12(5), 5304–5309. doi:10.3390/ijerph120505304.

Paul Ramsay Foundation. (n.d.). Paul Ramsay Foundation: partnerships for potential. Retrieved from https://paulramsayfoundation.org.au/.

PepperGreen Farm Catering. (n.d.). PepperGreen Farm Catering. Retrieved from https://peppergreenfarmcatering.com.au/.

Praszkier, R., & Nowak, A. (2012). Social entrepreneurship theory and practice. Cambridge: Cambridge University Press.

Preston, R., Waugh, H., Taylor, J., & Larkins, S. (2009). The benefits of community participation in rural health service development: where is the evidence? Australian Literature Review. Paper presented at the 10th National Rural Health Conference, Rural Health, The Place To Be, Cairns, Australia.

Putnam, R. (1993). Making democracy work: civic traditions in modern Italy. Princeton, NJ: Princeton University Press.

Rifkin, S. (1986). Lessons from community participation in health programmes. Health Policy and Planning, 1(3), 240–249. doi: https://doi.org/10.1093/heapol/1.3.240.

Rogers, E. M. (2003). Diffusion of innovations (5th ed.). New York, NY: Free Press.

Rubin, H. J., & Rubin, I. S. (1992). Community organizing and development (2nd ed.). Boston, MA: Allyn and Bacon.

Rural & Remote Mental Health. (n.d.). Rural & Remote Mental Health. Retrieved from https://www.rrmh.com.au/.

Sanson-Fisher, R. W. (2004). Diffusion of innovation theory for clinical change. Medical Journal of Australia, 180(6), S55–S56.

Seabert, D. (2013). Diffusion of innovation theory. In D. Wiley & A. Cory (Eds.), Encyclopaedia of school health. Thousand Oaks, CA: Sage.

Skerratt, S., & Steiner, A. (2013). Working with communities-of-place: complexities of empowerment. Local Economy, 28(3), 320–338. doi:10.1177/0269094212474241.

Social Enterprise Alliance. (2010). Succeeding at social enterprise hard-won lessons for nonprofits and social entrepreneurs. San Francisco, CA: Jossey-Bass.

Steiner, A., & Atterton, J. (2014). The contribution of rural businesses to community resilience. Local Economy, 29(3), 228–244. doi:10.1177/0269094214528853.

Sterling, D. (2012). Social enterprise. Ethos, 20(2), 18–21.

Talbot, L., & Walker, R. (2007). Community perspectives on the impact of policy change on linking social capital in a rural community. Health and Place, 13(2), 482–492. doi:10.1016/j.healthplace.2006.05.007.

Tesoriero, F. (2010). Community development: community-based alternatives in an age of globalisation (4th ed.). Sydney: Pearson Australia.

Tones, K., & Tilford, S. (1994). Health education: Effectiveness, efficiency and equity (2nd ed.). London: Chapman and Hall.

Verrinder, G. (2005). Acting. In V. A. Brown, J. Grootjans, J. Ritchie, et al. (Eds.), Sustainability and health: working together to support global integrity. London: Earthscan.

Verrinder, G., & Talbot, L. (2015). Rural communities experiencing climate change: a systems approach to adaptation. In R. Walker & W. Mason (Eds.), Climate change adaptation for health and social services (pp. 179–199). Melbourne: CSIRO Publishing.

West Virginia Community Development Hub. (n.d.). What we do. Retrieved from http://wvhub.org/what-we-do/.

World Health Organization (WHO). (1986). The Ottawa charter for health promotion. Retrieved from https://www.who.int/healthpromotion/conferences/previous/ottawa/en/.

Introduction 326

Health education and health literacy 328

   Health education 328

   Health literacy 329

   Ensuring cultural safety 335

   Education for critical consciousness 336

   Criticisms of health education 337

Planning health education strategies 337

   Behaviour change theories and models 339

   Learning and teaching theory 344

Skills for educating groups and communities 351

   Developing learning goals and objectives 351

   Using adult learning principles 351

   Communicating effectively with adult learners 354

   Teaching–learning activities 355

Working with groups 359

   Group theory 360

   Types of groups 360

   Elements of successful group work 363

   Practical tips for working with groups 366

   Getting the group started 368

Conclusion 370

Reflective questions 372

References 373

COMPREHENSIVE PRIMARY HEALTH CARE

SOCIO-ECOLOGICAL APPROACH				
			SELECTIVE PRIMARY HEALTH CARE	
		BEHAVIOURAL APPROACH		BIOMEDICAL APPROACH
Healthy public policy to create environments and settings that support health and wellbeing	Community development action to support social and environmental change	**Health education and health literacy** to develop knowledge and skills for health and wellbeing action	Health information and social marketing to raise awareness about health and wellbeing priorities	Vaccination, screening, risk assessment and surveillance to monitor and reduce risk of disease conditions

Health promotion community assessment, program planning, implementation and evaluation

INTRODUCTION

Chapter 7 moves along the framework for health promotion practice to explore health education and health literacy, which aim to develop the knowledge and skills of people for health and wellbeing action. Health education and health literacy align with the developing personal skills action area of the Ottawa Charter for Health Promotion (WHO, 1986) and draw on a range of behaviour change approaches, including education strategies and capacity building.

Education plays a central role in the wellbeing of people, and learning in and of itself is health enhancing. Health education is a commonly used health promotion strategy. Building healthy public policy, community development, using the mass media, and working with individuals and groups also involve education in some form or another—whether it be education of policymakers, health practitioners or community members.

Health literacy is the outcome of effective health education and is empowering for people. Health education, when it builds personal health literacy, can enable people to gain better control over the factors that influence their own health and wellbeing, as well as the health and wellbeing of others in their lives. Health literacy extends beyond a focus on people being able to access, understand and use health-related information to make informed decisions about their health and wellbeing to the ability of health systems to foster health literacy and recognise it as a social determinant of health. In addition, the outcome of health and wellbeing knowledge is its use as a building block for health promotion action at a social and collective level, or in policy activism. Education is therefore inextricably linked with all other forms of health promotion. The skills outlined in this chapter build on the community development skills discussed in Chapter 6 and the community assessment activities presented in Chapter 4.

PUTTING THE OTTAWA CHARTER INTO PRACTICE

The following questions, arranged in the Ottawa Charter action areas, are presented to guide health promotion practitioners to reflect on and critically evaluate their professional role and practice, and the health promotion philosophy of their organisation. Content of this chapter will assist practitioners to develop the necessary professional knowledge and skills required to facilitate the development of knowledge and skills for health and wellbeing action with those with whom they work.

PUTTING THE OTTAWA CHARTER INTO PRACTICE FOR HEALTH EDUCATION AND HEALTH LITERACY

Build healthy public policy

- Are health education strategies supported by national and state health and wellbeing priorities?
- Are health education strategies directed at people who have the power to change the context of people's lives—where they live, work and play?
- Is health literacy recognised as a determinant of heath and included as a priority in organisational, strategic and other planning processes and documents?

Create supportive environments

- Will the use of a health education planning theory or model enable a socio-ecological health and wellbeing approach, rather than behavioural and biomedical approaches?
- What is being done by the organisation to develop the health literacy of its workforce?
- Do the health education strategies take account of the context of people's lives— are they enabling?
- Are you sure the health education strategies do not result in 'victim blaming'?

Strengthen community action

- Have the community members requested the health- and wellbeing-related information?
- Did community members decide what health information should be provided and what format it should take?
- Is health information accompanied by an 'action plan' that is achievable for the most disadvantaged and vulnerable recipients of the communication?
- Are there opportunities for peer education or 'train-the-trainer'?

Develop personal skills

- Do the health education strategies draw on and value the wisdom of the community?
- Does participation allow each person to enhance their self-esteem?

Continued

PUTTING THE OTTAWA CHARTER INTO PRACTICE Cont.

- Does the health education experience enable participants to build their health literacy?
- Is people's participation in decision making more than tokenism?
- Are participants able to develop personal and transferable skills by taking part in the activity(ies)?
- Could participants be the next round of educators?

Reorient health services

- Can you make the behaviour change strategy more health promoting; that is, can it address socio-ecological determinants of health and wellbeing?
- Are the health education strategies directed at capacity building for policymakers and agency management?

This chapter first presents an overview of health education and health literacy. Some of the behaviour change theories and models, and learning and teaching theory as a basis for planning health education strategies are then reviewed. Skills required for health practitioners to undertake effective education at group and community levels including using adult learning principles and a range of teaching–learning activities, and theory, tips and skills for working with groups are presented. Before starting the chapter, take some time to review *Putting the Ottawa Charter into Practice* on pp. 329–330.

HEALTH EDUCATION AND HEALTH LITERACY

Health education

As illustrated in the framework for health promotion practice, health education is one of a number of strategies used in health promotion within a comprehensive primary health care (CPHC) context. Health education has been defined as 'consciously constructed opportunities for learning involving some form of communication designed to improve health literacy, including improving knowledge, and developing life skills which are conducive to individual and community health' (WHO, 1998, in Koelen & van den Ban, 2004, p. 32). There are three important elements in this definition. The first is that health education entails much more than formal 'teaching' sessions, based on transmission of knowledge, which we may traditionally expect to undertake in a more conventional health education role. Health education can include educative sessions that are purposefully planned, but can also use and enhance opportunities for learning that arise in interactions, by watching, role modelling, reading or in other ways that may occur alone or with others. Opportunities for learning can be planned or they may arise unexpectedly; however, the decision for health practitioners to use them as a health education opportunity is a conscious one. Experiencing barriers to education is a social determinant of health, and basic literacy and numeracy skills a human right. Low literacy is associated with a number of risks to health and wellbeing, including poverty, risky use of alcohol, poor diet and lower use of preventive and screening health services (Australian Commission on Safety and Quality in Health Care, 2014; Berkman et al., 2011; Marmot, 2012).

The second important point in this definition is that the focus of health education must be on knowledge, skills enhancement, analysis and interaction to facilitate informed decision-making about health and wellbeing action. Health education is not a matter of 'telling' people what they 'need to know'. All health practitioners have an important role to play using a variety of different approaches to enhance health and wellbeing knowledge and understanding to assist people to make informed health and wellbeing decisions. Health practitioners require the skills to competently assess educational needs and enhance learning opportunities for individuals, groups and the communities they work with.

The final important point is that health education can occur at different levels. The description above focused on the individual or group as learner(s). For example, a person or group in a hospital ward, community health training room or standing around a BBQ are provided with an opportunity to learn more about a topic of interest and/or relevance to them. Health education also occurs at community-wide and political levels. Community-wide learning opportunities often use social marketing strategies to communicate health-related information which has considerable impact when the population needs the information such as in times of crisis. For example, in March of 2020 the Australian Department of Health launched the coronavirus (COVID-19) national social marketing campaign to inform Australians about the virus, including actions people can take to reduce risk to themselves and their families (Department of Health, 2020). Health education at a political level has the potential to influence policy; building the health literacy of policy advocates and politicians is a wise investment, because of the potential for improving health literacy across the wider population. Health education skills therefore form an essential component of the health practitioner's 'toolkit', which relates to the concept of health literacy.

Health literacy

Health literacy is a social determinant of health and wellbeing, a global priority (WHO, 2016, 2018) and an important component of health promotion action (Gugglberger, 2019). As the concept of health literacy has developed, so too have the ways in which it has been defined. Health literacy is an outcome of effective health education (Nutbeam, 2000, 2008) that has been defined from the perspective of the individual, as having

> ... the cognitive and social skills which determine the motivation and ability of individuals to gain access to, understand and use information in ways which promote and maintain good health. Health literacy means more than being able to read pamphlets and successfully make appointments. By improving people's access to health information and their capacity to use it effectively, health literacy is critical to empowerment.
>
> *(Nutbeam, 2000; WHO, 2012)*

Nutbeam (2000, pp. 263–264) described three levels of health literacy as outcomes of effective health education which highlight the importance of personal agency, that people or groups are active participants in decision making, and that the ultimate outcome is empowerment through health literacy:

1. *Basic/functional literacy.* This enables the individual to function effectively and make informed decisions about personal health and wellbeing.

2. *Communicative/interactive literacy.* This is a higher-level processing and analysis capacity that, together with social skills, enables the person to apply the knowledge to different situations.

3.   *Critical literacy*. This is a third level of cognitive capacity, where the person can critically analyse information and use it to influence change in wider community and social situations and events for collective action to address the underlying determinants of health and wellbeing.

Since the development of this broader definition of health literacy by Nutbeam there has been significant discussion of the concept (Kickbusch et al., 2013; Nutbeam, 2008; Sorensen et al., 2012). The WHO, in its Final Report on the Social Determinants of Health (WHO & Commission on Social Determinants of Health, 2008), advocated for a broader definition of health literacy that encompasses the ability to understand and communicate information about the social determinants of health (Guzys et al., 2015; Kickbusch et al., 2013). Begoray and Kwan (2012) described health literacy as including four core skills that reflect the degree to which people are able to access, understand, evaluate and communicate information in order to promote and maintain health across the life-course and a range of settings. This typology adds an additional layer to that in the Social Determinants of Health Report (WHO & Commission on the Social Determinants of Health, 2008) and the Nutbeam (2000) typology presented above, with the ability to pass on health information to others and to engage in dialogue for clarification and advocacy. This fourth level is somewhat similar to the concept of civic literacy proposed by Zarcadoolas and colleagues (2005) and Freire (1974) that encompasses the idea of citizens becoming aware of issues, participating in critical dialogue and becoming involved in decision-making processes for health and wellbeing. Health literacy therefore relates to people's ability to apply learning in health-enhancing ways, including using health literacy as a form of advocacy for change (Hill, 2011; Rowlands et al., 2012; Sorensen et al., 2012). By improving people's access to health information and their capacity to use it effectively, health literacy is critical to empowerment (Kickbusch et al., 2013).

More recent discourse on health literacy relates to the recognition that health literacy must also reflect the ability of health systems to foster health literacy; that is, the competency and ability of health professionals, educators and policymakers to enable people to be health literate (de Leeuw, 2011; Gugglberger, 2019; Rowlands et al., 2012).

> Health-literate professionals, service providers, and systems are able to provide relevant information to people in ways that improve their understanding and their capacity to be healthy and to effectively manage their health concerns.
>
> *(Gillis et al. in Rowlands et al., 2012, p. 4)*

A recent exploration of the relationship between health promotion and health literacy by Gugglberger (2019) identified the development of five relationship types—health literacy as a *foundation*, *outcome* and *partner* of health promotion, and as a *driver* and *informant* for health promotion. These relationships highlight the importance of health literacy in health promotion practice through the development of health promoting policy and programs inclusive of strategies that develop the health literacy of people, as well as the health literacy capability of health and health-related organisations and systems, including the workforce.

Importance of health literacy

It is well established that higher levels of health literacy result in better health outcomes for and health service utilisation of people, and considerable cost savings to the health system. People with low health literacy experience worse health outcomes because poorer health literacy affects disease risk reduction behaviour and personal health management (Hill,

2011; Kickbusch et al., 2013). Compared with people with higher levels of health literacy, those with poorer knowledge of health conditions have higher rates of hospitalisation and emergency care, their participation in health screening is lower, and the cost to the healthcare system is higher (Australian Commission on Safety and Quality in Health Care, 2014, pp. 13–17; Berkman et al., 2011; Kickbusch, 2001; Kickbusch et al., 2013). Around 60% of adult Australians have low health literacy (Australian Bureau of Statistics, 2006a). Research by the Australian Bureau of Statistics (2006b) found that people's ability to make health-related decisions and take appropriate actions is strongly associated with their general levels of education and literacy. The most vulnerable members of Australian society in terms of educational attainment, labour force participation and skill level, parental education, social or geographic isolation, and cultural minority status have the lowest health literacy. It is estimated the poor health literacy adds between 3 and 5% to the healthcare budget (Hill, 2011).

Health literacy is empowering for people whereby it develops capacity for decision making, enables people to enter into partnerships of care with healthcare providers, ensures better health of family members, and enables people to be advocates on behalf of others, of their community or for broader change to improve access to health services in the wider community. Health literacy is an asset for life; it builds personal and social capacity and it enables people to form partnerships with the healthcare system that improve the quality of care.

Health literacy is an important life skill transferable to different settings and life stages. It builds social capital in communities and can be the basis of social change (Kickbusch et al., 2013). Higher-level health literacy is empowering when it equips people for political or social lobbying to change things for society generally and to influence policymaking (Kickbusch et al., 2013; Nutbeam, 2008; Sorensen et al., 2012).

Measuring health literacy

There has been a growing body of work over the past two decades on how to measure health literacy. Baker (2006) reviewed various techniques to assess basic literacy, including education level and demographic factors, and specific tests to assess people's health literacy for reading print materials, including product labels. Other researchers have developed health literacy assessment tools—for a summary of these see Rowlands and colleagues (2012) and Guzys and colleagues (2015). A number of health literacy tests were found to be time-consuming to administer, only assessed functional literacy and had the potential to embarrass or alienate the person, making them impractical or unsuitable for most clinical settings and opportunistic health education events. Even when a simpler screening tool was developed and trialled, the learning outcomes were not necessarily better than when no prior assessment of health literacy was made. Baker (2006) and others recommend that health practitioners should assume all of their clinical patients or clients have poor health literacy, in both oral and print forms, and use good communication skills with varied and innovative resources to ensure health literacy is achieved.

Guzys and colleagues (2015) highlight that much of the discussion about health literacy, and guidance for improvements, focuses on individuals in clinical settings, whereas usual assessment techniques fail to capture the social and synergistic aspects of health learning and don't embrace the potential for health promotion approaches to health literacy in community settings.

Osborne and colleagues (2013) used a grounded theory approach to develop a health literacy measurement scale. After validation and field-testing, the Health Literacy

Questionnaire (HLQ) covers nine conceptually distinct domains of health literacy with a total of 44 items to assess the health learning needs and challenges of a wide range of people and organisations. This questionnaire has the advantage of being based in the lived experience of people as they navigate the healthcare system. It draws on Bloom's taxonomy of learning, presented later in this chapter, to ensure the concept statements are graded in complexity. It provides guidance for health professionals and health organisations about how they can make it easier for their clients to build health literacy. Domains of the HLQ encompass the three levels of health literacy described by Nutbeam (2000) presented earlier in this chapter, meaning that the health literacy capacity of the person or health organisation can be pinpointed accurately (Osborne et al., 2013). The HLQ is useful in better understanding the health literacy needs of population groups and as a means of evaluating the effectiveness of health education strategies (Osborne et al., 2013).

The Australian and New Zealand Governments took part in an international study of health literacy, using 91 items to assess people's knowledge of how to undertake health-related activities for health promotion, health protection, disease risk reduction (note, there is no dash between risk and reduction) and healthcare maintenance, and their ability to navigate health information sources. The results were comparable to those from Canada (Australian Bureau of Statistics, 2006a; Begoray & Kwan, 2012). Despite later acknowledge-ment that the ABS measurement of health literacy was outdated because it was based on a narrow medical-model definition of health literacy and the method was cumbersome, the research was important in highlighting Australia and New Zealand's poor levels of health literacy and the need for government investment in action to improve population health literacy.

Building health literacy

When health literacy is expressed as a competency to be achieved by members of the public as consumers of healthcare services, it implies characteristics of the healthcare system, including the people who work in it and those who make health policy (Baker, 2006; Rowlands et al., 2012). To achieve population-wide health literacy improvements, we must be able to rely on a health workforce that has the capacity for critical health literacy, and which includes system-wide knowledge of the entire health sector, as a means of reducing the fragmentation and inefficiencies in healthcare provision (Naccarella et al., 2015). A workforce that is health literate and has the knowledge and skills to ensure that health literacy as a social determinant of health is addressed in all health promoting policy and programs is essential.

Taking action to enhance the health literacy of community members is an important role for all health practitioners (Australian Commission on Safety and Quality in Health Care, 2014). In response to the evidence demonstrating low health literacy rates in Australia (Australian Bureau of Statistics, 2006a, 2006b), the Australian Commission on Safety and Quality in Health Care (ACSQHC) has developed the 'National Statement on Health Literacy: Taking action to improve safety and quality' which includes three key strategies:

1. *Embed health literacy into high-level systems and organisational policies and practices.*
2. *Ensure that health information is clear, focused and useable, and that interpersonal communication is effective.*
3. *Integrate health literacy into education for consumers and healthcare providers.*

(ACSQHC, 2014, p. 3; 2019)

The framework sets out the range of professional development and structural actions within the health system to build health literacy (Table 7.1). In 2015, the New Zealand Ministry of Health published *A framework for health literacy: A health system response* which specifies the expectations and actions for the health sector and workforce to embed health literacy as core business (Ministry of Health, 2015) and build health literacy for all New Zealanders.

At the 2016 Global Health Promotion Conference in Shanghai, health literacy was introduced as one of the three health promotion pillars and foci for health promotion action (WHO, 2016). Subsequent to this conference, the International Union for Health Promotion and Education (IUHPE) produced a Position Statement on Health Literacy in

TABLE 7.1 Actions that can be taken in the health system to address health literacy

Role	Possible actions
Consumers	• Discuss with healthcare providers any difficulties in understanding health information and services. • Ask family, friends or support services (such as translating services) for help with communication difficulties. • Ask for more information about any part of care that is unclear. • Be open and honest with healthcare providers about medical history and medications. • Improve knowledge and skills by participating in education. • Raise awareness among family, friends and the community about the importance of health literacy. • Become involved in the planning, design and delivery of health information and services for consumers.
Healthcare providers	• Recognise the needs and preferences of individual patients and consumers and tailor their communication style to the person's situation. • Assume that most people will have difficulty understanding and applying complex health information and concepts. • Use a range of interpersonal communication strategies to confirm information has been delivered and received effectively. • Encourage people to speak up if they have difficulty understanding the information provided. • Use ways of communicating risk information about treatment options to people that are known to be effective. • Participate in improvement projects aimed at reducing barriers to health literacy within the healthcare organisation's physical environment. • Participate in health literacy education and training, if available.
Organisations that provide healthcare services at a local level	• Develop and implement health literacy policies and processes that aim to reduce the health literacy demands of information materials, the physical environment and local care pathways. • Provide and support access to health literacy and interpersonal communication training for healthcare providers, including training methods in communicating risk. • Provide education programs for consumers aimed at developing health knowledge and skills.

Continued

TABLE 7.1 Actions that can be taken in the health system to address health literacy—cont'd

Role	Possible actions
Organisations that support healthcare providers	• Lead and coordinate action on health literacy within their profession. • Develop policies and position statements on health literacy. • Encourage and support professional development opportunities and influence education programs for healthcare providers in communication, health literacy and patient-centred practice in general. • Collaborate across the healthcare sector on health literacy activity, including sharing strategies and lessons learnt across and between professions and sectors.
Government organisations, regulators and bodies that advise on health policy	• Raise awareness about the issue of health literacy. • Embed health literacy principles into health policy development. • Support the design and delivery of policies, pathways and processes that reduce the complexity involved in navigating the health system including across sectors and settings. • Explore opportunities for including implementation of strategies to address health literacy as a core requirement of healthcare service design and delivery. • Work collaboratively across all levels of government to promote coordinated action on health literacy. • Advocate for funding and resource allocation for health literacy initiatives. • Implement, evaluate and share information about health literacy programs. • Develop partnerships to facilitate the exchange of information about health literacy research and programs between research and practice communities.

Source: ACSQHC, 2014.

2018 (IUHPE, 2018). This practical guide outlines seven action areas for health literacy development including:

1.   *Promoting a systems approach to health literacy*

2.   *Ensuring inclusion of health literacy in global, national, regional policies and strategies for health promotion and social determinants of health*

3.   *Recognising health literacy is content- and context-specific across the lifespan*

4.   *Emphasising health literacy action is a people/community-based process for empowerment*

5.   *Funding, producing and promoting research to contribute to a growing evidence base*

6.   *Workforce development strategies*

7.   *Identifying and engaging relevant stakeholders for collaborative health literacy action, research and policy.*

These action areas provide a useful framework for health practitioners to identify the scope of work required to enhance the health literacy of people and systems.

Health practitioners also have an advocacy role in ensuring their organisation provides opportunities for people to build their health literacy. As such, health practitioners from all disciplines have the responsibility to provide information and materials that meet the learning needs of their patients, clients and community groups. People have the right to accurate information about issues that affect their health, in a form that is accessible and appropriate to their learning needs. Without knowledge, people cannot make decisions about their own lives that enable them to reduce the risks to their health, they can't advocate on behalf of others and they can't make a plan that meets their specific needs (Kickbusch et al., 2013). The following are some ideas that can readily be included into health practitioners' everyday practice to build health literacy.

- Understand one's own level of health literacy and seek learning opportunities to build critical health literacy where needed.

- Use a structured, systematic approach to understand the health literacy level of those you work with, such as the Health Literacy Questionnaire outlined above.

- Use the teach-back technique to check a person's understanding by asking them to state in their own words what they need to know, or how they are going to manage their situation. It is a way for the health practitioner to confirm they have explained things in a manner that is understood.

- Ensure that printed materials are readily understood and then add to their impact by talking through the content, rather than just handing them to users.

- Promote informed decision making, such as with care planning and other aspects of self-management.

Ensuring cultural safety

Ensuring people from cultural and linguistic minority communities receive information about their health and wellbeing involves much more than just translating it into the language of the people. An essential aspect of overcoming the cultural imperialism that can easily permeate 'top-down' health education approaches is an awareness of the concept of 'worldview'. People's worldview, or their way of understanding and interpreting their world, is the product of the environmental and historical factors that have shaped their culture over time (Eckermann et al., 2010; Papps & Ramsden, 1996). Western medicine in nations such as Australia, New Zealand, the United States and Canada has been shaped by its origins in the British medical care system and the scientific research within this paradigm (Robson & Harris, 2005). It generated the medical model, and an organ system approach to diagnosing and treating illness. In contrast, Indigenous peoples in these nations have unique worldviews shaped by their strong spiritual links to the land, a sense of holism with each other and their land, and the absence of scientific research based on microbiological challenges to health (Hood, 2010, Chapter 10; Trudgen, 2000). In these nations, the Indigenous people's worldview is also shaped by the experience of colonialism and invasion, including incarceration and stolen generations; experiences that continue to underpin communication with authority figures, including with the healthcare system (Main et al., 1998). Consequently, there are many aspects of traditional didactic health education styles that alienate Indigenous peoples from the learning experience. Cultural learning preferences vary a great deal, but there are common elements, such as a strong oral tradition (Hood, 2010, Chapter 10). It is the responsibility of health practitioners, therefore, to ensure that they engage in practices that ensure the cultural safety of those they work with. Refer to Chapter 2 for a much more detailed discussion on cultural safety.

Education for critical consciousness

The concept of education for critical consciousness, critical consciousness-raising or conscientisation was developed in its original form by Freire (1974), although similar ways of working have also been developed by others. For example, the consciousness-raising techniques of the women's movement have much in common with Freire's education process. This approach to education offers a great deal to health promotion because of the focus on working with people, and because it provides a framework for action in dealing with the root causes of issues as recognised by people themselves. It provides an important link between the lives and experiences of individuals and change at a structural level.

Freire (1974, p. 13) criticised traditional notions of education for amounting to cultural invasion, as representatives of powerful groups impose their view of the 'facts' on less powerful members of society. He argued that education is never neutral because it in some way either confirms or challenges the status quo. On the basis of this premise, he argued for education that challenges the status quo and thus enables the empowerment of oppressed members of society and the development of a more just social system. Education for critical consciousness focuses on changing the environment rather than the individual alone, by working with people to examine the underlying issues behind their problems and to change the structures around them. An example might be that food and medication labels are made more readable in order to assist health literacy, rather than putting the onus completely on people to learn to understand complex language. This perspective has clear links to building higher levels of health literacy (ACSQHC, 2014; Nutbeam, 2000). Although this empowerment approach to teaching and learning may not be 'traditional', the outcomes are clear indicators of health literacy, and health educators can learn a lot from this perspective.

Freire (1974, in Minkler & Cox, 1980, p. 312) argued that social change can only be achieved by the active participation of the people collectively—strong leaders alone cannot achieve it. Therefore, action for change must be built on critical reflection and action by everyone concerned. Freire describes this process of critical reflection and action 'dialogue' as a two-way process occurring between 'teachers' and 'learners'. Education for critical consciousness is a process of problem-posing that leads people through analysis of their personal situation, then of the underlying social issues, to make a plan for action to address the issues they have discovered. The four steps involved in the process are:

1. *Reflecting upon aspects of their reality (e.g. What are the problems underlying poor health, housing, poor medication compliance, etc.?)*

2. *Looking behind these immediate problems to their root causes (What are the barriers?)*

3. *Examining the implications and consequences of these issues (What could be changed?), and finally*

4. *Developing a plan of action to deal with the problems collectively identified.*

(Minkler & Cox, 1980, p. 312)

As the four steps indicate, before a learning partnership can develop, health practitioners need to listen carefully to the learning needs articulated by community members, and also observe the dynamics of the groups and individuals concerned to determine what sense of belonging or community exists. Some sense of community or group belonging seems to be important for the conscientisation process to work effectively (Minkler & Cox,

1980, p. 320). It is for this reason that education for critical consciousness is regarded as an essential component of community development, as set out in Chapter 6.

Education for critical consciousness as described by Freire may not fit every learning situation. However, the principles of problem-posing, two-way communication and sensitivity to people can be used in any learning situation, so that it becomes an enabling process for the people involved. Freire's guidelines are congruent with adult learning principles presented later in this chapter.

Criticisms of health education

There has been some criticism of the use of health education strategies, particularly when they are conducted instead of, or at the expense of, social and structural changes through policy and community action. The first criticism is that health education with a narrow focus on behaviour change relates to the concept of 'victim blaming', addressed in Chapter 2. When individuals are expected to take responsibility for protecting their health and preventing factors and behaviours that make illnesses more likely, there is potential to 'blame' those who are unable to make these changes for their 'failure'. The inference here is that because a person knows that a behaviour, such as smoking, is not good for their health, they will be able to change this behaviour, and it is their own fault if they do not. The implication of these so-called 'lifestyle choices' is that people have the necessary knowledge, social support, money and motivation to make the changes and sustain them. It takes no account of the underlying reasons why people are engaging in the behaviour, the challenges of addiction, or the personal and social circumstances that affect the choices people are able to make (Nutbeam, 2000).

The second criticism is that expenditure on health education for behaviour change diverts attention and priority from the social and structural causes of health and wellbeing that are more amenable to long-term improvements through social policy change. There is an argument that health education strategies provide a short-term political outcome while avoiding decisions about implementation of broad long-term healthy public policies. Behaviour change approaches can be more expediently implemented during the course of one political term and they are more readily evaluated than the social policy change and community-building strategies outlined in Chapters 5 and 6. However, the evidence of the high rate of health illiteracy internationally, and the poorer health outcomes experienced by people with low health literacy, make a strong argument for retaining health education and social marketing as essential strategies in addressing the social determinants of health and wellbeing.

PLANNING HEALTH EDUCATION STRATEGIES

This section outlines health education planning frameworks and behaviour change theories to guide health practitioners to design health education strategies that support people to make informed and enhancing health and wellbeing decisions. In the past, the role of the health practitioner was to give (tell) people information so they would comply with the instructions from an expert. This can be represented by a simple linear diagram in Fig. 7.1.

It is clear that the assumptions inherent in Fig. 7.1 fail to encompass the complexity of what is required for people to adopt new health-enhancing behaviour(s). Some important questions to ask include:

- Is there accurate or inaccurate information about the risks to health?
- What factors influence the value a person places on the desired change—peer or social pressure, media?

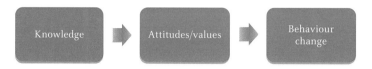

FIGURE 7.1 Historical assumptions about adoption of a behaviour change

- What factors enhance or inhibit the desire for change—costs, family social circumstance and previous education?
- What personal factors influence the person's readiness for change—motivation, self-efficacy, fear of alternatives?

However, this simple linear model does give insight into the empowering potential of health literacy. Knowledge is inherently empowering, but when a person is able to use that knowledge within the context of their lives and review their prior understanding and values about the relevant action, their communication or interactive health literacy is developed, and they have capacity for critical reflection to adapt their understanding and make the change to their behaviour.

When planning health education strategies for individuals and groups, it is useful to 'map' the activity to ensure it meets the educational needs of the group and that it enables them to make informed decisions about matters affecting their health and wellbeing. Familiarity with community-wide and individual health promotion practice frameworks and health education models and theories will assist practitioners' understanding of the characteristics of the learning audience and increase the range of health promoting strategies designed to meet learning needs (Bastable, 2014). Understanding the educational purpose is essential if it is to be effective in building health literacy. The purpose may be to design a program to increase knowledge or understanding of concepts, support personal growth and build capacity and resilience, or design an education session to enable a person or group to learn about a specific health and wellbeing topic or to develop a new skill.

Conceptual or theoretical models are commonly used to explain diagrammatically the links between a set of concepts (Brennan et al., 2014). Numerous conceptual models have been used in health education to understand the characteristics of the participants in a potential education activity or program, to involve them in planning it, and to enhance design of the approach and content, so their learning needs are met. In a diagrammatic model, bordered shapes, such as boxes, denote the concepts or factors of influence; the processes or relations between the concepts are delineated by lines or arrows. Lines indicate a link between factors of importance and arrows are used to indicate the direction and strength of the relations between concepts. In this way, a model presents a visual image of the reasoned explanation of a hypothesis about a series of abstract principles—a theory. Models are based on theories.

Four theoretical models widely used in planning and supporting individual health behaviour changes are described briefly here: the health belief model (Becker, 1974); the theory of reasoned action and planned behaviour (Ajzen & Fishbein, 1980); the transtheoretical (stages of change) model (Prochaska & Di Clementi, 1984); and social cognitive theory, developed from social learning theory by Albert Bandura (1986). They are illustrated because they have been extensively used and validated. Nutbeam and colleagues (2010) and Glanz and colleagues (2008) both provide very useful overviews of a range of commonly used planning models. The conceptual areas encompassed in health education planning models such as these can assist health educators to understand the needs and characteristics of their audience or learning community. When community members, and the wisdom of experience from the literature are used to guide the development of educational content, an empowering outcome will result; it will achieve basic health literacy and provide the basis for higher levels of health literacy (Nutbeam, 2000; Sorensen et al., 2012).

Behaviour change theories and models
Health belief model

The health belief model (Fig. 7.2) is based on social learning theory (Glanz et al., 2008; Nutbeam et al., 2010), and was developed to explain why some people take action to avoid a specific illness or condition and others do not. The model can be used to suggest health promotion actions that would make some individuals more likely to engage in health protective behaviours in relation to a specific condition. One of the strengths of the health belief model is that it guides the health educator to consider the social context of people's health behaviours (Becker, 1974). Nutbeam and colleagues (2010) caution that unless behavioural theories are put into the broader context of the lives of the individual or community, many factors that influence health will not be considered when planning the learning activity or they will remain unaddressed in the program content.

The health belief model illustrates that an individual is likely to take action based on the interaction between four conceptual areas. The model is still widely used in clinical and health promotion activities that have an individual behaviour change purpose (Bastable, 2014; Borowski & Tambling, 2015; Das & Evans, 2014; Donadiki et al., 2014; Sohler et al., 2015; Yue et al., 2015).

Refer to the diagrammatic arrangement of concepts set out in Fig. 7.2 as you read each description.

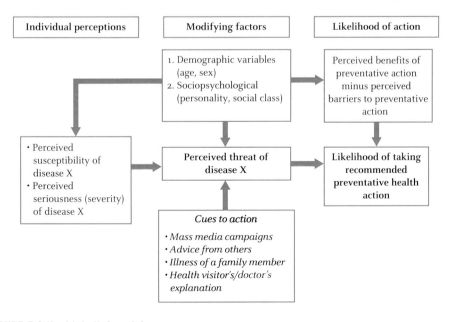

FIGURE 7.2 Health belief model

1. The individual's perceptions about the susceptibility of a given condition. Perceived susceptibility is a person's estimate of their probability or likelihood of encountering the health condition. This estimate is dependent on their knowledge, and thus an important function of health education is to provide accessible, reliable information as required.

2. The individual's perceptions about the seriousness or severity of the condition. Perceived seriousness relates to the difficulties that individuals believe a given health condition would create for them. These difficulties may include the implications for work, family and social life, so the emotional response of an individual to a condition is significant here. It is only when the perceived seriousness is manageable—neither too low to be insignificant, nor too challenging or frightening to contemplate—that a person can consider a change in behaviour. Thus, launching into a health education message when a person is overwhelmed by other issues and needs support is not only unethical but also likely to be ineffective.

3. The individual's perceptions about the benefits of taking action to reduce the risk of acquiring the condition or increase the likelihood of detecting the condition early in its development. The perceived benefits are important determinants of the recommended behaviour. For example, women who believe Pap smears can detect cancer early, and that this results in a good prognosis, are more likely to take part in screening.

4. The individual's perceptions about the barriers to taking action to reduce the risk of acquiring the condition or increase the likelihood of detecting the condition early in its development. Perceived barriers to the behaviour may be personal—such as the embarrassment or unpleasantness of having the procedure—or they may be social—such as cost, inconvenience or the frequency of the desired behaviours that are required, and the extent of life changes. Recent studies have highlighted that perceived barriers are especially important in influencing the likelihood that a person will undertake the recommended behaviours (Borowski & Tambling, 2015; Donadiki et al., 2014; Yue et al., 2015). These barriers give important guidelines for health educators on planning their sessions in order to acknowledge and address the needs and characteristics of their audience, especially with regard to providing strategies for overcoming the barriers. The types of strategies that can be useful are evolving along with the use of the internet as a source of health advice (Bastable, 2014).

People weigh up the benefits of taking the action against their perceptions about the risk and seriousness of having the condition and how difficult it would be for them to overcome the barriers to them taking the action to avoid the condition or situation. Perceived barriers may also provoke anxiety for the person, which prevents objective analysis of the choice of action. Hence, it is important to always provide an 'action plan', to provide a contact point, source of information or support, or a management program, when communicating a health education message.

The health belief model predicts that people's perceptions in these four areas are influenced by a range of modifying factors: internal factors, such as personality, education and resilience; and external factors, especially socio-demographic and cultural factors, which may include low health literacy. For example, women are more predisposed to risk reduction behaviours than men, peer groups can force conformity, and people with low health literacy are less likely to engage in health promoting action (Borowski & Tambling,

2015). Age, sex, income, education and health literacy have been correlated with health service use. To a lesser extent, perceptions about particular health conditions, and undertaking the recommended activity are also influenced by a number of internal and external cues (Das & Evans, 2014). It may be that an internal cue, such as a physical discomfort, or a feeling of discomfort when a person thinks about a threat to their health, triggers them to act. It may also be that an external cue, such as mass media, advice from others or the illness of another person, triggers the activity. The cues to action make the person aware of their own feelings about the health behaviour (Donadiki et al., 2014). It is not clear how strong the trigger needs to be or the specific timing. A good example of the use of cues has been the use of roadside billboards by the Transport Accident Commission (TAC, http://www.tac.vic.gov.au/road-safety) with information about the risks of speed or inattention used to prompt drivers to act safely.

When all these influences on health action are taken into account and understood about the participant group, it is then possible to make assumptions about their likelihood of engaging in health promoting behaviour. When these factors are identified in a discussion with the learner group, they can be used as a basis for planning the content and style of the learning experience. In-depth preparation for health education activities that considers the interaction between factors that will influence the success of a learning activity is important. Of course, health education alone may not be sufficient to overcome the barriers to change for some people. Issues such as addictions and social, educational, economic, environmental and psychological barriers may be understood by using the model, but they may not be able to be altered to a sufficient degree to enable the person to change their behaviour.

Theory of planned behaviour

The theory of reasoned action and theory of behaviour change have been refined over a number of years into this more integrated model, the theory of planned behaviour (Montaño & Kasprzyk, in Glanz et al., 2008; Nutbeam et al., 2010). This theory was developed to explain human behaviour that is under voluntary control; it is based on the premise that people make rational decisions about their behaviour, based on the information that is available to them at the time (Bastable, 2014). The major assumption in the model is that people's stated intention to act is the best determinant of behaviour. In recognition of the many things external to the person that can influence their ability, readiness and intention to make a behaviour change, the name of the theory is probably best described as the 'theory of planned behaviour' (Ajzen, 1991).

According to this model, behavioural intentions are influenced by:

1. people's attitudes to a behaviour—that the outcome will occur if the desired behaviour is followed and that the desired behaviour will be beneficial
2. subjective norms—what the person thinks other people think about the behaviour and their desire to comply with the wishes of others
3. people's perception of control they have over that behaviour.

The model predicts that a person is most likely to intend to adopt, maintain or change a behaviour if they believe the behaviour will benefit their health, is socially desirable, they feel social pressure to behave in that way, and they feel they have personal control over that behaviour (Nutbeam et al., 2010). Fig. 7.3 illustrates the relationship between concepts in this model. A number of recent studies have used the theory of planned behaviour as the basis for research on individual health-related behaviours, including texting while driving (Nemme & White, 2010), safe motorcycle riding (Chorlton et al., 2012), breakfast consumption (Kothe et al., 2011; Mullan et al., 2013), and fruit and vegetable

341

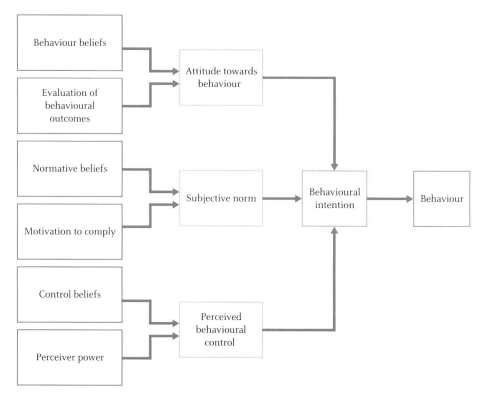

FIGURE 7.3 Theory of planned behaviour

consumption (Emanuel et al., 2012; Kothe et al., 2012). The theory has provided valuable guidance for the analysis of the behavioural intentions of the intended audience. The strength of prediction is greater if people feel they have more personal control over their behaviour. A person's stated intention with regard to changing a health behaviour is a strong predictor of the outcome (McDermott et al., 2015).

The theory highlights the need to take time to understand the beliefs and attitudes participants in a program or learning session have about the recommended behaviours, their barriers to making a commitment to change, and what has shaped those beliefs. It is also a useful model for analysing and addressing gender differences in response to certain health behaviour change strategies (Bastable, 2014; McDermott et al., 2015). This information is then used to identify and plan the components of a learning experience. It isn't as simple as assuming that lack of information is the only reason people don't adopt a health promoting behaviour. The theory is most successfully applied when all elements are researched and accounted for in the learning program that is offered. The third component of the theory related to self-efficacy, which was added later, highlights the importance of one-to-one coaching, counselling and support as components to assist behaviour change. This is especially important in situations where the behaviour may be life-threatening, or has an addictive or habitual element. Research by Côté and colleagues (2012), using the theory to explore nurses' intentions to incorporate research evidence into their clinical practice, highlighted the importance of subjective norms in the role of the nurse (codes of practice, professional values) that have influence on intentions to change practice. Similarly, Chorlton and colleagues' research (2012) about motorcycle riders' intentions to ride unsafely highlighted the importance of moral norms and beliefs about anticipated regrets in reducing their likelihood to ride dangerously. Given the power of beliefs to predict intentions, thorough assessment of the priority groups' beliefs about the behaviours, and incorporating these into strategies that clearly set out norms and expectations of group behaviour, can have a lasting influence (Bastable, 2014).

Transtheoretical or stages of change model

The transtheoretical or stages of change model was developed to bring together the concepts from a number of other behaviour change theories (Prochaska & Di Clementi, 1984) to describe and explain the different stages that occur during the process of changing a behaviour. The model recognises the personal challenge that sustaining a changed behaviour can pose for people, including having high enough motivation to consider a change and being physically ready and confident to make the change. The model has proved useful both as a basis for analysing health clients' readiness for learning (Brennan et al., 2014; Evers et al., 2012; Kelch & Demmitt, 2010; Lee-Lin et al., 2016) and as a framework for evaluating the outcomes of various programs to find out which health behaviour change approaches worked best (D'Sylva et al., 2012; Harrell et al., 2013; Karupaiah et al., 2015; Noordman et al., 2013).

The model expresses five distinct stages of change that are useful for the design and evaluation of behaviour change program activities. However, some researchers have found no clear delineation between the different stages of an individual's readiness for change (Bastable, 2014; D'Sylva et al., 2012).

Fig. 7.4 illustrates the different stages in a linear process, but it is also important to recognise that many people have 'false starts' to a change and the process may therefore be cyclical.

Five basic stages of change have been used in the model.

1. *Precontemplation*—this describes people who are not even considering changing behaviour, or are consciously intending not to change.

2. *Contemplation*—at this stage of readiness a person considers making a specific behaviour change.

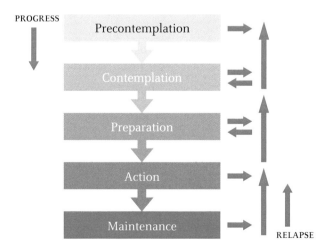

FIGURE 7.4 Stages of change model

3. *Preparation*—the person has a higher level of motivation and expresses an intention to change the behaviour in the next 30 days. They have taken some preparatory steps towards this decision.

4. *Action*—the stage at which the behaviour has commenced, but is not yet habitual (less than 6 months).

5. *Maintenance*—where the change is sustained and some of the anticipated health outcomes are occurring.

Relapse may also be the fifth stage.

Termination describes where there is no temptation to relapse, and this may be appropriate with some behaviours, such as those involving addiction. This is not a stage in the process of change, but describes a 'normal' state where a change to behaviour is not warranted.

The model is useful with individual and broader group or community program approaches (Evers et al., 2012; Kelch & Demmitt, 2010; Lee-Lin et al., 2016). The stages give useful guidance regarding sequencing the content and activities in a learning program and identifying barriers that can cause people to 'get stuck' and not be able to progress to the next stage (Nutbeam et al., 2010; Prochaska et al. in Glanz et al., 2008). Once again, the model emphasises the importance of working with, and understanding the intended audience before commencing and continuing to communicate effectively throughout the process. Many behaviour change therapeutic counselling approaches make use of this model (Kelch & Demmitt, 2010; Noordman et al., 2013).

Social cognitive theory

Social cognitive theory was originally called social learning theory (Bandura, 1986) and initially based on principles of learning through reinforcement, modified with a focus on learning from observing others and reinforcement with rewards. As social cognitive theory, cognitive factors such as beliefs, expectations and self-perceptions are included. Human behaviour is viewed as a dynamic interplay of three factors: a person's knowledge and understanding about the issue or behaviour (cognition); behavioural factors, including whether the person has the skills and self-efficacy to be able to perform the behaviour; and environmental factors, such as the setting, social norms about the behaviour, and the ability to change one's own environment. Each of the three factors has the potential to influence the others; a concept referred to in the theory as reciprocal determinism (see Fig. 7.5).

The model is used to guide health education planning and practice by building cognitive knowledge (emphasising goal setting, developing positive attitudes and setting realistic expectations), creating a suitable environment (fostering observational learning and choosing suitable positive community settings) and reinforcing behaviours (using the positive influence of others in role modelling and providing for practice of skills that build self-efficacy).

The social cognitive theory can be used to refine a health education program, such as diabetes education (Taylor et al., 2016). Understanding the audience perceptions about the components of the theory can give added insight into planning health literacy health promoting actions that assist behaviour change, such as increased exercise and improved nutrition (Basen-Engquist et al., 2013; Berlin et al., 2013; Heiss & Petosa, 2015; Taylor et al., 2016).

Learning and teaching theory

Once learning needs have been identified, preferably using a model to explore the content of the learning program, the health practitioner's role is to generate competence, help

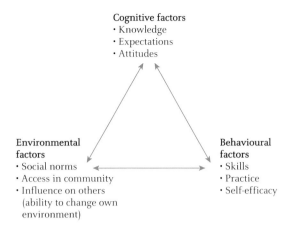

FIGURE 7.5 Social cognitive theory

build health literacy and assist people to access, analyse and apply their knowledge under changing conditions. There is now an added focus on what happens inside the 'learner', rather than what the 'teacher' does. Learners are not expected to be passive recipients of information delivered by experts. They have an active role in the teaching–learning process. Leddy and Pepper (in Hood, 2010, pp. 437–441) describe three key assumptions that should underpin effective teaching–learning.

1. Teaching–learning is a process, not a product; that is, new information and skills are not the only goals. How that learning occurs, how it is understood by the person and how it fits with their prior learning, are equally important and may contribute greatly to the learning process and the capacity for the learner to apply their knowledge and capacities in other dimensions of their life; that is, to become empowered by their health literacy.

2. The teaching–learning process occurs between people who all bring their own expertise to the situation, whether it be the expertise of personal and collective experiences or the more theoretical expertise of health educators.

3. The teaching–learning process needs to be built on effective communication and mutual respect.

These principles demonstrate the importance of a partnership approach to working with a learning community. Both the community member (or members) and the health educator contribute to the discovery of potential solutions in a supportive atmosphere in which learners assume responsibility for decisions they make. While it is clear that practitioners intuitively assess the person's stage of readiness for learning or change (Noordman et al., 2013), the aim is to make this assessment an activity that is more consciously prepared for. In such an approach, education is a guided problem-solving process in which both 'teacher' and 'learner' are open to learning from each other. It is worthwhile considering briefly the two major philosophical approaches to education that continue to underpin the way health education practitioners carry out their role—pedagogy and andragogy.

Pedagogy

Pedagogy is the art and science of teaching (Knowles et al., 2011). The premise behind this approach was based on the transmission of knowledge. Using this approach fits within traditional 'teaching' sessions where 'learners' are presented with information. Transmission of knowledge as the main form of education was only appropriate when the time-span of major cultural change was greater than the lifespan of individuals; that is, what people learned in their youth would remain valid and useful for the rest of their lives. This is no longer appropriate because of the rapid advances in knowledge and technologies, and in addition, a great deal more is now understood about the ways in which people construct their knowledge. See, for example, Vygotsky's constructivist theory of human learning (Gajdamaschko, 2015), in which social interaction plays a fundamental role in the development of cognition as learners 'construct' their understanding through interactions with the social environment, and teaching strategies are designed to provide variation in learning opportunities.

In some instances, using traditional pedagogical strategies—commonly a formal lecture—is appropriate, such as when learners are dependent on strong guidance, but they need to gain new knowledge or skills in order to progress. A key point in using this approach is that pedagogy should not be used by a 'teacher' who wants to keep the learners dependent (Knowles et al., 2011). The priority in health education is to assist learners to be self-directed in their enquiry, so the pedagogical lecture method is really only appropriate when the basic purpose is to disseminate information, the material is not readily available elsewhere, it is necessary to arouse interest in the subject or to provide an introduction or reinforcement about a topic.

Andragogy

Andragogy has been defined as the art and science of helping adults to learn. The term was used to describe the theory of adult learning by Malcolm Knowles where learning was more centred on the learner, rather than the teacher, and the relationships of power between teacher and learner are more equal. The core principles of adult learning have been refined by Knowles and colleagues (2011).

> *In adult learning, the learner:*
>
> - *is independent and self-directed; they take responsibility to meet their own learning needs*
> - *uses their prior knowledge and experience as a resource to add to their learning*
> - *has a strong focus on learning that will assist their social and professional roles*
> - *is motivated to learn straight away in order to solve a problem or to fill a knowledge gap. Learning is reinforced by immediate application of knowledge.*
>
> *(Bastable, 2014, Chapter 5)*

The andragogy–pedagogy approaches are not seen as dichotomous, but as two ends of a spectrum. Most realistic health education situations fall between the two ends, where the facilitator makes use of a variety of teaching and learning approaches to create the context most conducive for the audience to learn. However, because most audience members for a health education session or program will have reached educational maturity, a number of adult learning principles should guide education strategies.

Learning domains

Learning theories can help us to interpret the learners' behaviours, and to assist learners overcome learning barriers and meet their learning needs (Knowles et al., 2011). In this chapter so far, we have emphasised two important considerations when planning health education: first, to consider the social context of the learner and the factors that impinge upon them adopting health promoting behaviours; and second, that adopting that behaviour is much more complicated than merely being told to do it by an expert. The health education behaviour change planning models, presented earlier in the chapter, can be used to understand the learner's needs in their social context. Once the learner's current perceptions and factors influencing the likelihood to take action are understood, these can be used as a guide for what educational strategies can be used (Bastable, 2014). Accurate information, as a component of health literacy, is the basis on which a person develops their likelihood to take health-enhancing action, and to use this learning in other dimensions and times in their lives. Positive perceptions about taking a certain action are heavily influenced by interpersonal factors, such as motivation and self-efficacy and social cues, such as the advice or behaviour of others or the media. Educational approaches need to acknowledge the importance of these influences and assist the learners to negotiate their way through these challenges that get in the way of change (see Insight 7.1). Adopting different health behaviours frequently requires new personal or physical competencies and increased self-efficacy. Understanding how to influence these outcomes forms the basis of the health education models presented earlier (Knowles et al., 2011). Learning of facts does not necessarily alter behaviour. Personal attitudes and values about the health and wellbeing priority, and knowing you can do it, have the greatest influence on eventual health behaviour. In

INSIGHT 7.1 Educational approaches

- Holistic—complete, cooperative, integrated and all-encompassing.
  - Present an overview.
  - Demonstrate/model; ensure each component of session links.
  - Reinforce.
- Imaginal—relatively unstructured; consists of thoughts, images and experiences of learning. Learning is strongly linked with identity.
  - Provide for observation, imitation, shared experiences and incremental learning: incorporate stories.
  - Use concrete and visual images before concepts.
  - Allow for reflection and self-assessment.
- Kinaesthetic—tactile, through manipulation and movement.
  - Include hands-on experiences and movement.
  - Excursions and group activities, to allow alternative forms of presentation.
- Cooperative—emphasis on communal, shared and group learning.
  - Cooperation and collaboration rather than competition.
  - Allow for discussion; avoid singling out students, even for praise.
- Contextual—specificity and relevance are crucial.
  - Link content to specific context and application.
  - Aim for relevance to students' own lives.
- Person-oriented—family and personal relationships are fundamental to positive outcomes.
  - Learning is motivated by the person, rather than by authority or the nature of the task.
  - Relationship, personal connection and positive body language are crucial for successful assessments.

Source: Adapted from Main et al., 2000.

the following section, planning for the information, skills and emotional aspects of learning are separated into three domains. Although in practice we don't teach or learn in one domain in isolation, a separate analysis assists with understanding how learning can be built through a carefully planned process, and health knowledge can be built on to achieve health literacy (Bastable, 2014, Chapter 10; Honebein & Honebein, 2015).

Learning a new concept or skill may involve moving through progressive levels of understanding. Bloom (1964) developed a 'taxonomy of educational objectives' and argued that learning can be classified into three domains—cognitive, affective and psychomotor—according to the type of learning that is taking place. Each domain is further categorised according to the level or complexity of the concept that is being learned, progressing from the simple to the most complex. Classifying learning processes into these three domains serves to strengthen the understanding of the learning processes (Bastable, 2014). The domains can be used as a framework for writing learning objectives, based on the adult learning principles presented earlier. It is not usually appropriate to develop separate activities for learning knowledge (cognitive), attitudes (affective) and behaviour (psychomotor), because the concepts are interwoven. The domains are presented here in the sequence set out above as the simple linear relationship that knowledge builds emotional engagement with the topic and this builds interest and capacity for new skill development. However, learning can be just as effective when a new skill is gained first and this may then generate interest in learning more about it, perhaps with the desire to apply the knowledge in a different setting, and then developing the positive attitude or emotional commitment to it.

Each domain is related to a holistic process and can be applied to the specific learning needs and developmental tasks of the learner group. Each of the three domains is relevant to developing and facilitating the learning opportunities that may be identified when a health education planning model is used as the basis for preliminary assessment with the learning group.

Cognitive domain

The cognitive domain describes learning that relates to the recall and recognition of knowledge and the development of intellectual abilities. This is a hierarchical domain, in that each level of learning becomes more complex and builds on the learning processes of the prior level (Bastable, 2014; Bloom, 1964). The hierarchical arrangement with illustrative examples is set out in Table 7.2.

The levels of the cognitive domain are useful for setting or clarifying expectations, planning and writing learning objectives and assessment of cognitive abilities as the learning increases in complexity. The hierarchy demonstrates the way in which we put

TABLE 7.2 Taxonomy of cognitive learning domain

Level 1	Knowledge	Recall of facts, methods and procedures
Level 2	Comprehension	Combining recall and understanding
Level 3	Application	Using information in new specific and concrete situations
Level 4	Analysis	Distinguishing components and understanding relationships between components
Level 5	Synthesis	Putting the information into a unified whole
Level 6	Evaluation	Judging the value of ideas, procedures and methods

Source: Derived from Bloom, 1964.

into practice what we know and value. This domain underlies concept development. Conceptual knowledge allows the learner to adapt it readily to new learning situations and this is a quality of health literacy. Cognitive learning can be gained through a range of educational experiences and it forms the basis of most traditional teaching approaches. It is generally necessary to have cognitive understanding before the learner is able to effectively apply and analyse learning in the other domains (Bastable, 2014). Think of the concept of cross-infection; we learn basic information about modes of spread of micro-organisms, and then we apply that knowledge in diverse ways from food preparation and wound care to practising safe sex. Safe adaptation of the concept will only occur when it builds upon core knowledge.

Affective domain

The affective domain relates to changes in interest, attitudes, values and appreciation, and also to the ability to make adequate adjustments. The domain relates to the degree of a person's emotional response, their values and attitudes, to a topic or task. Attitudes and values are 'constructs'—terms that are used to explain things that cannot be observed directly. Attitudes are formed from people's knowledge and their feelings about an issue. Health education strategies based on the stages in affective learning outlined below have a powerful influence on moulding attitudinal change.

The stages in affective learning are:

1. *Receiving* (attending). Willingness to receive information; giving selected attention.

2. *Responding*. Displaying acquaintance with and comprehension of the message.

3. *Valuing*. Acceptance and internalisation of values and attitudes in question, by demonstrating the ability to apply the information personally.

4. *Organisation*. Conceptualisation of the value, and expressing a commitment and the ability to arrange the values in appropriate order.

5. *Characterisation*. The person gives a personal undertaking to adopt the behaviour that reinforces the attitude. The value becomes a philosophy of life. Practice reinforces the modified value system.

To enhance positive attitude formation, the educational experience must provide the person with:

- intellectual stimulation, in that they understand the message and it engages their emotions
- biological significance, in that they associate the message with themselves
- social significance in that the message is congruent with social values.

This domain is used by educators to help learners clarify, and perhaps adjust, their own attitudes and values (Bastable, 2014). Attitudes affect what people see and how they see it; using strategies that make people aware of their attitudes, and possibly how they contrast with social norms, is a valuable first step in people's acceptance of the need for change. Hyland (2010) draws parallels between the processes of mindfulness and those of building self-awareness through the affective domain, and argues that careful incorporation of strategies to build affective understanding is very important in the learning environment. Consider this point in relation to wider public acceptance of racial diversity or increasing intolerance of homophobia.

Creating learning experiences that resonate with the personal emotional or social experiences of the participants will assist in creating positive attitudes about a health and wellbeing priority. Learning activities that involve moral reasoning and those that debate ethical decision making assist learners to develop their personal value system. Using stories, pictures, cartoons and caricatures, YouTube clips and historical and recent videos and news items to illustrate and challenge double standards or provoke discussion are very useful teaching strategies for this. Group activities, including role-plays and case studies, can underpin group discussion around values clarification.

Psychomotor domain

The psychomotor domain is used in the observable performance of skills that require some degree of neuromuscular coordination. An individual uses the psychomotor domain when they apply accumulated knowledge and attitude to life situations. Three conditions are necessary:

1. The learner has the ability to learn a new skill.
2. The learner has a sensory image of how to carry out the skill (they can visualise or imagine the action).
3. The learner has the opportunity to practise.

The guided process of mentally preparing for a new skill, and the gradual development of competency through to creative adaptation of a behaviour is illustrated in Table 7.3.

The taxonomy clearly suggests the close link between the three domains: the affective component builds a positive value about the worth or usefulness of the skill and the cognitive domain means the learner understands the basic principles before they attempt the new skill. Key educational roles are to ensure cognitive and affective learning stages are met concurrently and as the psychomotor skill is developed, to provide appropriate encouragement and opportunities for learners/participants to take the risk and have a try. Consider the range of creative options for providing the learner with a visual image and demonstration, such as video, film, internet sources, diagrams and detailed description.

The different levels in each domain can be used as a framework for writing objectives for the learners, and as a guide for selecting the most appropriate strategies and sequencing

TABLE 7.3 Taxonomy of psychomotor learning domain

Level 1	Perception	The person understands the sensory cues that guide action; they can visualise what to do.
Level 2	Set	Readiness to act—position, equipment, physical capacity.
Level 3	Guided response	The new skill is performed along with demonstration—development may be incremental (one step at a time).
Level 4	Mechanism	With practice, the ability to perform the skills is habitual; smooth and uninterrupted. Movements are not complex; using the most effective method.
Level 5	Complex overt response	Skilled performance with economy of effort, smoothness of action, accuracy and efficiency, no wasted effort.
Level 6	Adaptation	Catering or adapting for special conditions.
Level 7	Origination	Origination of new movement patterns to suit particular circumstances—different setting, equipment, motor ability.

Source: Adapted from Quinn, 1995.

the learning activities. Domains of learning can also provide a framework for analysis of what works most effectively to assist learning (Honebein & Honebein, 2015).

SKILLS FOR EDUCATING GROUPS AND COMMUNITIES

This section provides guidance on a range of principles and approaches for planning and delivering health education strategies in a range of settings.

Developing learning goals and objectives

In Chapter 4 we presented guidelines for formulating SMART goals and objectives based on a health and wellbeing priority analysis, a component of health promotion planning. When there is a health education and health literacy goal, use a health education planning model to identify the learning needs of participants, then match the need with the level in each domain of learning to formulate program objectives and to sequence the content of the learning program. Formulating clearly expressed SMART objectives is very important for clarity to participants and funding agencies, and in providing a framework for evaluation (Bastable, 2014, Chapter 10). It may seem like a more complex process than is necessary, but it really is worthwhile to carefully document the links between learning needs and educational activities.

Using adult learning principles

The use of adult learning principles builds on the philosophical base of the teaching–learning process described earlier, and can be used to guide effective teaching and learning practice. Some general guidelines that can be applied to any teaching–learning situation are described below.

Allow people to direct the learning process

Active participation by learning community members in the education process is paramount to successful education leading to health literacy. A review of the extent to which healthcare providers involve patients in decision-making found that:

> Whatever the clinical context, few health-care providers consistently attempt to facilitate patient involvement, and even fewer adjust care to patient preferences. However, both shared decision-making interventions and longer consultations could improve this.
>
> *(Couët et al., 2013, p. 543)*

Health literacy will be enhanced when people come to the learning session or activity voluntarily, because they have recognised the need for new learning. Educators in any health setting need to involve the learners in planning, carrying out and evaluating their own learning (Couët et al., 2013; Knowles et al., 2011). Partnership in the education process is consistent with critical health promotion. People, including children, will learn most effectively when the learning opportunities address the questions raised by them and when they can decide on the learning processes they would prefer.

Individual or group-controlled learning is most likely to occur if people themselves set the goals of learning, and this is a key point in building to higher-level health literacy. Working with people, helping them to clarify just what it is they want to learn and barriers to their learning are very important parts of the teaching–learning process (Bastable, 2014; Knowles et al., 2011). Active participation in learning is fostered by maximising interactive teaching techniques and activities, rather than taking an 'empty vessel' approach and 'filling' passive recipients with information. People need to be able to have their say, use their initiative, experiment and find out what works for them to enhance their ability to analyse information and use it in different ways.

After identifying the learning needs, structuring the learning environment and activities to provide opportunities for learners to be active participants in the learning process is a priority. Which interactive techniques and activities are appropriate will vary depending on the learning priorities that have been identified (Bastable, 2014). Commonly used interactive styles include debating contentious issues, using structured group activities, planning action to address a problem and practising the action required (whether that be drafting a letter to a local government representative, role-playing the negotiation between work colleagues about smoking in the workplace, or preparing a nutritious and tasty meal).

Interactive techniques do not by themselves ensure higher-level learning, nor are they guaranteed to build health literacy. Inclusion of a short video, YouTube clip, picture or cartoon into a lecture as the basis for a short discussion or to prompt feedback can really enhance understanding of concepts and the learners' ability to transfer the understanding to a different situation or setting. How the teaching techniques are used that ultimately determines the extent and success of interactive learning and building health literacy. Emphasis should focus on how the health educator and learners make use of the techniques, rather than solely on which techniques are used.

Get to know the people's perspective

Teaching–learning is a communication process and as such is built on an understanding of the background and ideas of the audience/learners. New knowledge can be built on the basis of the learners' existing knowledge and prior experience in order to meet their need for additional information. Understanding the learner's perspective is often a long, slow process and not necessarily one that can be completed before the teaching–learning begins. Rather, facilitators need to be open to learning about the other person's perspective throughout the teaching–learning process, and to incorporate different approaches and content according to the learning needs they have identified. Learning can be unrewarding and unsatisfactory when this does not occur (Gravani, 2012). A person's attitudes towards relevant issues, their cultural background, their self-efficacy about the topic, their life experience and topics currently of priority for them may all influence their learning needs, their approach to learning and their ability to act on the information. To ensure that communication is effective, pay particular attention to the needs of people from culturally diverse backgrounds or who have impaired sight or hearing, low literacy skills or any other communication challenges. Ensuring cultural safety for the learner is highly important. Adult learning principles provide a useful framework for developing appropriate learning opportunities only within a context of respect for the values and worldviews of the learners (Hood, 2010, Chapter 11). Learners are frequently in a situation of powerlessness and low health literacy and thus it is not uncommon for culturally different worldviews to be ignored (Rosenberg et al., 2006; Schouten & Meeuwesen, 2006; Schouten et al., 2007). Refer back to the discussion on cultural safety in Chapter 2 for additional guidance.

Remember that the educator is often portrayed as the expert, and is in a position of power in the education setting. Educational activities will be underpinned by the facilitator's personal values and attitudes, which may be in conflict with those of the participants, so there is the potential to undermine the effectiveness of the learning.

Be aware of the context of people's lives

Encouraging people to be active in directing the learning process will help to ensure that education does not occur out of the context of their lives. Centre the learning experience on the real-life situations of the participants (Knowles et al., 2011). This will enable learning to be directed to the specific needs of the learners, taking account of such things as the particular barriers to learning or action that they need to address and any other issues that may be more important to them than those identified by health educators (Bastable, 2014; Schouten & Meeuwesen, 2006). Being aware of the whole situation people are dealing with will also help to identify other strategies that may be needed to address the issue at hand. For example, letters may be written to members of parliament regarding the re-routing of a main road, while road safety education may be conducted to deal with the problem in the short term. Making use of background information as part of the learning experience can assist the learner to achieve higher-level health literacy (Nutbeam, 2000).

Build on what people already know

Ensure that education starts from the point where it is easiest for people to begin to learn; their active participation in planning learning opportunities will assist. Build on what people already know, providing new material in a format and at a pace that is appropriate to the learner or learners. It may be necessary to provide information using a range of approaches and materials (ACSQHC, 2014). Finding out what people know in a way that does not leave them feeling vulnerable is an important skill here. Intersperse questions throughout teaching sessions to make the links to prior knowledge and to their individual experiences and to assess the level of understanding. For example, 'Can you tell me what you have heard about osteoporosis?' provides people with more scope to express ideas they are unsure of than asking people what they 'know' about the topic. Treat mistakes as occasions for learning.

Ensure planned achievements are realistic

Education is much more likely to be effective if realistic, achievable goals are set rather than expecting learners to achieve too much all at once. It will be useful, therefore, to spend some time with the people, finding out what they want to achieve and assisting them to adapt their plans if they seem unrealistically high or low. Helping people to plan what they want to achieve so that it is divided into a number of incremental, manageable pieces can also help them to keep track of their progress. Sometimes learners may not be embracing the topic with enthusiasm, there may be a range of barriers to learning and the information may feel overwhelming (Bastable, 2014). Think of the experience of being a newly diagnosed type 1 diabetic—so much to learn, internalise and adapt to, all while the learner may be feeling unwell and angry. No matter what topic is to be covered, it is essential that both client and educator share decisions about the learning process and sufficient time is allowed for thorough understanding to be achieved (Couët et al., 2013).

It is common for health educators, especially those new to the role, to 'over-plan' a health education session, and to include far too much information. The challenge is to be well prepared, but to leave the session details 'loose', so it can follow the learning needs and priorities of the group.

Take account of all levels of learning

Learning has traditionally been regarded as occurring on three levels: knowledge, attitudes and behaviour. While this schema has been criticised in recent years, as discussed above, it can be used to provide a useful guide for session content. It is easy to aim for high-level literacy without ensuring that the basic building block of individual learning is in place first. Consideration of whether knowledge development, attitudes and values clarification, or behaviour change and skill development, are needed will help determine on what level or levels learning needs to occur (Bastable, 2014). In reality, learning influences our understanding of knowledge, attitudes and behaviour concurrently, so attempting to separate them during the learning process is not always realistic. However, the three separate considerations can provide a useful guide when planning sessions and different learning styles. The earlier section on the domains of learning will assist in formulating broad educational objectives.

Use varied approaches and enable group learning

Put yourself in the learners' place and consider how easy it is to lose concentration when there is insufficient variation in the teaching and learning experience. Consider a change in teaching technique after around 10 minutes. Activities such as break-out discussions, posing a question and seeking responses, using images to illustrate a point, using hands-on techniques and showing a short video are all useful to meet different learning preferences and promote active learning. Participants will also learn a great deal from their colleagues when structured self-directed learning or discussion techniques are used for research around a topic and sharing results. There is a range of online tools to facilitate group learning that have the added benefit of providing flexible learning arrangements to meet the needs of many adults.

Present information in logical steps which draw on past experience

If people are to learn effectively, new ideas need to be provided in a logical sequence in which more complex ideas are built on simpler ones. Some planning is therefore needed to structure ideas so that they are presented in an ordered fashion (Knowles et al., 2011). Of course, these plans may be let go, to some extent, as learners direct the process through their questions and other activities, but the plan remains a useful framework. The notion of learning having to start with simple ideas before moving on to more complex ones has been questioned in recent years. As with the notion of starting with achievable issues in community development, there is growing recognition that people may be quite able to deal with complex ideas when they relate to their own experiences or the problem to be solved, without needing to discuss the simpler ideas first. In these instances, people are likely to be motivated to learn about the complex issues since they relate to the problem at hand.

Communicating effectively with adult learners

When working with any audience, including adult learners, it is important to value and respect the wisdom that participants bring to the learning environment (Schouten et al., 2007). Many learners are challenged and unnerved by being placed in a learning setting, especially if they are made to feel inferior. The following points provide guidance as to how the facilitator can manage the environment positively.

- Be a good listener. 'Hear' the participants, value their contributions and make links between their contributions and the key themes around the topic.
- Communicate effectively with warmth, respect and encouragement. A distant or superior attitude towards participants will make them less likely to contribute.
- Clarify points of difficulty or confusion. While a good knowledge of the topic is useful, the facilitator or educator should not expect to know 'everything'. Knowledge gaps can be treated as opportunities for exploration, without losing the respect of clients or participants. Learners will know very early when a facilitator is attempting to make the audience believe they have greater expertise than they really do.
- Be flexible to adjust to the needs of the learners. The pace of presentation and level of detail necessary to achieve understanding of a topic will vary according to the prior learning, including life experiences of the participants, and their need for the information at the time (Bastable, 2014; Couët et al., 2013).
- Don't 'own' the topic. One of the key skills health educators need to learn is to relinquish 'control' of the group and allow it to be led by the participants. A facilitator may need to 'steer' the discussion to ensure that topics the group decides are important are covered.

Teaching–learning activities

All the health promotion strategies described in this book so far can be useful for health education purposes. Community development, lobbying and advocacy, and group work can build health literacy for different groups of people. Likewise, the mass media, social media and social marketing campaigns can raise awareness and increase personal motivation for behaviour change. Teaching and learning strategies most appropriate for the learning need depend on the health and wellbeing priority at hand, needs of the learning community, the context in which the learning is taking place, and the particular skills of the teacher and learners. In addition, strategies can be adapted and new ones developed to better suit each situation. The following descriptions provide an introduction to some common education strategies that can be used to build capacity for empowerment through health literacy.

Talks and lectures

Talks and lectures are a relatively efficient way to pass on a lot of information to a group of people, and with the use of modern technology the learner groups may be located in a number of different, distant locations. Lectures can achieve great economies of scale, they allow an audience to participate passively and learn in a relatively unthreatening way (Bastable, 2014). However, their effectiveness can be limited (Knowles et al., 2011). First, people may attempt to provide too much information in a talk, swamping the audience in a way that tends to inhibit rather than foster learning. Second, unless combined with other strategies, talks tend to be one-way communication in which little interaction (and therefore little participative learning) occurs. However, it is also possible to combine talks and lectures with other interactive strategies, using a variety of approaches to get a message across.

Preparing and structuring a lecture

Formal lectures can easily become boring and fail to engage active learners. Some guidelines for making the content useful and accessible to learners follow.

1. Introduce the lecture.
   - Gain participant attention.
   - Establish rapport, perhaps with a warm-up exercise.
   - Provide motivational cues—explain why the ideas are important.
   - Set out the essential content.
   - Have only a few main points and summarise these with the use of objectives.
   - 'Pre-test' student knowledge to prompt awareness of relevant knowledge.

2. Deliver the body of the lecture.
   - Cover the content according to the objectives.
   - Provide a logical organisation—use the levels in domains of learning as a guide.
   - Maintain participant attention by showing enthusiasm for the topic, using humour if it is appropriate and comes naturally, inserting questions for the audience, being physically active (but not with irritating mannerisms) or providing handout material.

3. Conclude the lecture.
   - Recall the main ideas introduced earlier.
   - Specify what participants should now know.
   - Answer any questions.

Using a lecture is less appropriate when:
   - long-term retention is desired
   - the material is complex, detailed or abstract
   - learner participation is essential
   - higher cognitive objectives, such as analysis and synthesis, are being sought
   - learners have complex learning needs (Knowles et al., 2011).

Buzz groups (quick discussion in pairs to discuss an issue) may be used during long presentations to help energise the group, keep the presentation interesting, highlight key points and allow analysis of an issue. Increasing opportunities for people to combine their learning with social interaction builds health literacy (Nutbeam, 2000). Presenters may also use various social media techniques to test audience knowledge or provide a basis for discussion, within a lecture format. In these situations, it is also worth careful consideration of whether such a long formal presentation style is necessary.

Discussions and debates

Discussions and debates provide an opportunity for people to examine an issue by comparing a variety of views. They are useful to motivate intellectual and emotional exchange among learners, but must have a clear learning objective, and a process that allows analysis of the outcome of the discussion; otherwise the activity can be aimless or merely an opportunity for those with strongly held views to express them. Engaging in debate helps learners develop respect for the ideas and opinions of others as well as to acquire insight into a particular health- and wellbeing-related topic. Learners need to listen, communicate and analyse the topic of debate. Discussions and debates are a more participative approach to learning than talks and lectures, although care still needs to be taken to ensure that they are effective. First, discussion may need to be guided (perhaps through a series of questions) or provoked (such as through a challenging video or opinion). Second, if group discussion is to be a participative process for everyone, it may need to be facilitated so that everyone has a chance to participate. 'Speed-dating' is one way for learners to share their knowledge— pairs discuss a designated topic for a short while, then one changes partners and passes on their learning and continues the discussion in the next pairing (Murphy, 2005). Online discussion forums use similar strategies, but have the advantage of bringing together 'distant' participants.

Values clarification exercises

A number of activities can be designed to assist values clarification with participants. These processes are useful to assist learners to clarify their personal moral, ethical and social relationships, resulting in self-understanding and recognition of professional values and codes of practice. For example, the following strategies can be used for formulating one's value judgement:

- *rank order—the learner chooses among alternatives, or places alternatives in rank order*
- *voting on health issues, then comparing and discussing responses with other learners*
- *a values continuum where people identify and arrange values about issues on a continuum from one 'extreme' to the other*
- *a values whip, which forces participants to state how they arrived at their decisions; use interview techniques that elicit the opinions of others*
- *the use of devil's-advocate role-plays, where participants are required to take a stance in a role-play that is opposite to their preferred values*
- *autobiographical and biographical sketches—the use of 'stories' (participants' or others) can be powerful illustrators of the impacts of social values.*

(McAllister et al., 2015)

These methodologies are intended to help learners identify and clarify their thinking regarding health and wellbeing priorities, to understand their own values and those of others, and participate in wider debate and action (Knowles et al., 2011). Facilitators must not see these strategies as opportunities to indoctrinate participants or force their values on others, but providing opportunities for self-reflection will build learners' health literacy (Bastable, 2014).

Demonstration and practice of skills

Observing and then practising skills can be a valuable way to learn and may be vital when people are attempting to learn a new skill. If demonstration is to be effective, planning the demonstration as a series of logical steps and restricting explanation to key points will help simplify the process for learners. A range of multimedia resources are available to assist learning psychomotor skills, from preparing an insulin injection to using a condom.

Learners find such resources valuable for increasing their confidence when they are new to the clinical setting and for revision (Sole et al., 2013). These days, YouTube also provides almost instant access to a range of options on almost any 'How to … ?' topic. They are free, and the variations in technique can be an additional point of analysis and discussion in the development of higher-level health literacy skills. Refer back to the learning hierarchy set out in the psychomotor domain of learning as a guide for when to introduce demonstration into a learning occasion and, following this, ensure that adequate opportunities are available for participants to practise new skills.

Role-play

Role-playing often provides a useful opportunity for people to practise new or unfamiliar behaviour with others. It can also be used to provide an opportunity to explore values and feelings within a group and to allow learners to emotionally engage with a topic or perspective that may be new to them. Role-plays dealing with values, attitudes and emotions are a powerful strategy and can have unexpected outcomes. The role must be carefully structured; the facilitator needs to have knowledge and skill to lead the discussion in the desired direction, and to draw out the learning principles from the activity. Role-plays should only be used to explore emotional or challenging issues by health education practitioners with the knowledge and skills to assist in the development of a clearly defined and well-developed role, and who are able to assist participants to debrief and de-role at the end of the process. Otherwise, role-playing may do more harm than good (Heyward, 2010). Ruyters and colleagues (2011) outline a blended process where role-plays can be combined with a range of online group learning environments, such as wikis and blogs, to facilitate learning, discussion and de-briefing of law concepts.

Games

There is a variety of educational games available to trigger face-to-face learning. To be effective learning tools, games need to be relevant to the issue at hand and well facilitated. Like other teaching–learning strategies, games are not ends in themselves, and need to be integrated with other learning processes for full effect (Bastable, 2014). For example, a series of open-ended questions to guide discussion after a game may help draw out the key learning points, and link the message of the game to real-life experience. An additional use of games is to set students the task of developing the pilot of a new game for a specific purpose and audience. This process requires them to have a good understanding of the content material, and to think through and apply creative learning opportunities. They are demonstrating higher-level learning in the process. In reflection of rapidly evolving internet-accessible software and games technologies, there is a wide range of opportunities for using games to facilitate learning. These are outside the scope of this chapter, but valuable resources that outline a number of options are provided by Ingle and Duckworth (2013) and Felicia and Mallon (2014).

Self-contracting

Self-contracting provides a mechanism whereby people can contract with themselves to learn new information or to change their behaviour in some way. In learning environments such as schools and universities, knowledge of adult learning principles coupled with access to computers and the internet have made self-directed learning the norm. The priority is to build self-efficacy for lifelong learning. Self-contracting is a part of most group learning activities; individual learners each undertake to research a component of the topic and to share the information with their peers for mutual learning and other shared outcomes. In self-contracting for behaviour change, the achievement of a desired milestone, such as regular physical activity, may be supported by rewarding the behaviour in some way that has appeal to the person. It involves the person documenting the change, and the reward, and providing a duplicate for the supervisor. Building self-efficacy is the characteristic of both forms of self-contracting that is most valuable because it builds capacity to sustain the activity and is transferable to other learning and behaviour change challenges (Wilson & Narayan, 2016). The supervisor acts in a mentoring capacity to guide and assist the learner to achieve the designated goal.

Despite the discomfort some people feel with its behaviour modification origins, self-contracting has been found useful for people striving to change habitual personal behaviours. If using this process, it is very important that people determine what they should change and how they should support their new behaviour.

Action

Enabling people to act on an issue of concern can provide them with an opportunity to build health literacy and make a difference at the same time. Encouraging learners to take part in directing the learning activity is a key principle of adult learning, and it is particularly valuable for people with low reading capacity and for those who learn best by doing (Knowles et al., 2011). It forms the basis of many peer education strategies. Writing a letter about an issue of concern, planning and conducting a health and wellbeing survey or media campaign, or developing educational materials for use with peers, and assisting peers in safe medication administration are examples of action for change that can build lasting skills and enhance health literacy (Klein et al., 2014). Health educators may play an important role as resource people, but otherwise allow people to act independently.

Social media

While Facebook and other social media attract bad press and criticism, particularly with regard to their potential use for predatory behaviour and bullying, there is also great potential to use social media in health education activities and to build health literacy. Closed member groups can be created for a particular group, or around a specific topic. The process enables easy access, rapid debate and knowledge gain about a topic, and in most cases, participants censor inappropriate content, which in itself builds health literacy. Users/participants also report increased confidence in dealing with physically and emotionally challenging health issues (Ingle & Duckworth, 2013; Ruyters et al., 2011). For further discussion on social media see Chapter 8.

WORKING WITH GROUPS

Much health promotion, whether it is lobbying for political change, community development work or more formal health education, involves working with groups of people; community members, patient or client groups, work colleagues and sometimes managers and decision makers. Health educators work with groups that may be convened for other purposes, such as a parent-teacher group, and groups that meet specifically for an educational purpose, such as members of the public attending a training session, or a group of community members with diabetes. As in a one-to-one dialogue, group methods are used to assist people to identify their learning needs and collaboratively develop solutions to them

(Bastable, 2014; Koelen & van den Ban, 2004). Groups often have dynamics that are so much more than the sum of the individuals in them. It is possible, and advantageous, to develop an understanding of group dynamics and skills in working with a group, so that the group works effectively for what it is trying to achieve, rather than allowing its dynamics to work against it. The final section of this chapter provides a brief overview of the important components of group work process, along with some practical strategies for working with groups.

Group theory

Group theory has evolved since early in the 20th century, with several social psychologists researching the dynamics of group behaviour. Belief in the principles of democracy and collaboration underpins group theory and its application. Group methods have the advantage because they are learner-centred and focus on a specific topic; they enable direct feedback for the facilitator and participants about how information is received, whether it is relevant and useful, and if discussion of this topic should proceed (Bastable, 2014; Koelen & van den Ban, 2004). Group processes create awareness that participants are interdependent in enabling the discussion to be successful and the group to reach its mutual goal. Group work is compatible with comprehensive and selective primary health care approaches and has much to contribute to the practice of health promotion. Sometimes people may be brought together into a group somewhat unwillingly, at least at the start of a group process, but by recognising and working with the principles of group dynamics, health practitioners can help group members to enhance their health literacy through group participation.

Types of groups

Community groups will be created, sustained and facilitated in different ways, but the facilitator needs to find a balance between recognising the autonomy of the participants, building the benefits of cooperation and shared decision making, and maintaining control in 'steering' the group when needed. The two main types of groups used in health promotion practice are community action groups and self-help and support groups. Refer back to the principles of community empowerment presented in Chapter 6 for further guidance in working with groups of this nature.

Community action groups

These groups come together to engage in direct action for social change on priorities of concern to them. The groups are communities of interest who perhaps share the same occupation, beliefs or concerns and who meet regularly to take action. They include new society action groups, community development groups and organisational or occupational action groups.

New society action groups

New society action groups are consciousness-raising groups where cultural and ecological priorities for social action are identified. The priorities may be global or local, but thinking globally and acting locally are be the foundation of the group's action. There are many examples of issues-based new society action groups such as groups focusing on green consumerism, pollution, renewable energy, work cooperatives and so on.

Community development groups

Community development groups are local groups that work at the local level on local priorities with or without the support of local government and other organisations.

Organisational or occupational action groups

These groups work for organisational change. They may or may not have similar occupations but their aim is often for a better balance of hierarchy, cooperation and autonomy within an organisation. Workplaces provide an important setting for group health promotion activities, such as mentorship, advocacy and health enhancement.

Self-help and support groups

Self-help and support groups may be initiated by groups of peers or by health practitioners. Peer self-help groups work around a common issue for social change or for personal change in their members, or a combination of both. Their roles include mutual support, traditional education, advocacy, lobbying, research and information and service provision to both their members and other consumers of the health system. Mutual support is built within the group by members with similar issues of a personal nature that affect them directly and who share experiences and identify common needs and areas for social action for themselves or on behalf of others in similar situations (Klein et al., 2014). The issues may be anything from a particular condition affecting individuals, such as asthma, to psychosocial issues such as drug dependency, or life-stage issues such as retirement. As noted by Mechanic, 'interacting with others with comparable, or even greater problems than one's own can reduce the sense of isolation, increase feelings of receiving support, and provide a variety of useful coping approaches' (1999 cited in Koelen & van den Ban, 2004, p. 122).

With the increasing use of the internet, and especially social media, there has been growing popularity in people's use of 'virtual communities'—chat rooms, Facebook, Twitter and 'blogs'—to share information about a topic and provide peer-support. The group members can join and leave the discussion at any time, and there is not necessarily a designated facilitator to manage or lead the discussion, which may mean the group is not supportive or therapeutic, although there is often a high level of censorship if contributions are deemed inappropriate by other group members. An extension of this is the use of online support groups where membership is regulated to 'registered' participants. Online support groups are increasingly used in mainstream education and on a broad spectrum of physical and mental health topics (Felicia & Mallon, 2014; Ingle & Duckworth, 2013; Koelen & van den Ban, 2004; Ruyters et al., 2011).

Support groups within the health system form in response to inadequate services for their needs or other unmet needs. Whether they actively challenge the system or not, health practitioners may feel threatened by people addressing their own needs because they are unhappy with the way the system deals with them. Support groups may demand information from professionals when many are still unwilling to share it, and in so doing challenge the status and power differences between professional and client.

The main outcome of these groups is to gain shared insight into personal behaviour (their own or that of others) and to realise that they are not alone in dealing with the issues or challenges; peer learning can also be an important outcome. Consciousness-raising plays an important role in the development and function of many support and self-help groups and builds their health literacy (Klein et al., 2014). The insight or learning comes from the feedback of the group. Through talking together and sharing their experiences, members of these groups discover their shared ground and the common sources of health system oppression or indifference. Peer support and self-help groups may work to create their own alternative services or to change those already in operation (Durrant & Rieckmann in Bensley & Brookins-Fisher, 2009, Chapter 6; Egger et al., 2013). In either case, they often demand greater control over services so that they may better meet their needs.

Unless they are appropriately funded, peer support and self-help groups may be encouraged by government in a way that exploits the community members who join them, particularly those who put considerable energy into organising and running groups on a day-to-day basis. Governments may encourage support groups and peer self-help groups because they are a cheap option and because they assume the burden of responsibility for action in what are often difficult, time-consuming or previously ignored areas, especially emotional support needs. Health practitioners need to reflect critically on suggestions to encourage the development of self-help groups, to ensure these groups do not develop more for the benefit of the health system than the community itself.

Health practitioners have an important role to play with support groups and self-help groups in supporting them and acting as consultants, when groups request this. They should act as resources to further the groups' aim, but not take over the decision-making process. In deciding whether a peer self-help group should be established, health practitioners must consider whether the people concerned actually want such a group; that is, whether felt need is present. Attempts to impose formation of a self-help group from above are probably designed to meet the needs of the health system by removing a complex or costly management issue, but they are likely to be unsuccessful for the people concerned.

Another problem with some health practitioners' approaches to peer self-help groups is that they may be in favour of the idea of these groups being a peer-support group, but are less supportive of, and may even discourage, peer self-help groups that take on activities that try to have wider influence. However, supporting these groups for their peer-support work only, while discouraging social action, amounts to a form of social control in which group members are expected to put all their energy into achieving tasks that could perhaps be achieved legitimately by the health system, and are not supported in their work for the necessary policy or structural changes.

Sometimes the purpose of the group is achieved and the group runs its course, or it may disband for other reasons. This is a normal cycle for many groups. It is important that groups clearly establish their common purpose, celebrate the successes along the way, and recognise that the group may not last forever.

Several theorists have proposed that groups typically go through a series of stages as they establish themselves, develop and ultimately wind down. Probably the most commonly used model is Tuckman's 1965 model of group development (reviewed by Tuckman & Jensen, 1977). It has been further developed by others and is known now as a five-stage model, suggesting that a group typically goes through a series of stages in its life: forming, storming, norming, performing and adjourning. (For an overview of the history of its development and use see Bonebright (2010) and Tuckman and Jensen (1977).) The model continues to provide a useful basis for an initial understanding of the course of a group. Bonebright (2010) emphasises that it is now more common for groups to be facilitated for a specific purpose (such as working as a team, conflict management, mindfulness training) by people with specialist skills; group facilitation is a complex activity requiring high-level skills and careful management.

Elements of successful group work

Johnson and Johnson (2002) suggest that an effective group is one that accomplishes its goals, maintains good working relationships and develops in response to changing circumstances. Groups are more likely to be effective when:

- *goals are clear and relevant to all group members*
- *communication is accurate and clear, and two-way*
- *participation and leadership are shared among members*
- *decision-making procedures suit the issue being dealt with*
- *power and influence are shared, based on expertise not power*
- *controversy is encouraged, and creativity and problem solving promoted*
- *conflicts are resolved constructively.*

(Johnson & Johnson, 2002)

The criteria are appropriate when applied to a traditional face-to-face group that comes together or is brought together for a common goal or therapeutic purpose. When using these criteria to reflect on the characteristics of online virtual communities, it is clear the purposes and processes of the group may be markedly different. However, the number of online interactive group forums being created and moderated by recognised organisations is increasing and people are learning a great deal, contributing to the learning of others and finding great support and comfort from their participation in online groups. In observing a group, therefore, and deciding which aspects of its operations are effective and which may need improving, several issues are worth examining.

Tasks, maintenance and other functions of the group

The activities that a group performs can be roughly divided into three types: those that get the group's task done; those that maintain the life of the group and therefore may help it to get its tasks done; and those that individuals perform to look after their own needs. It is important that groups address these sets of activities. If members try to push through to accomplish their tasks while ignoring the needs of individuals, the group may soon become ineffective. If, on the other hand, a group concentrates on maintaining itself, people may communicate effectively and enjoy meetings for a while, but may leave the group without having addressed the issue that brought them to the group in the first place. They may leave feeling frustrated at the group's lack of achievement.

Of course, not all activities fit neatly into task functions or maintenance functions. Some activities may have components of both, and whether an activity is a task or maintenance function of a group may vary depending on the context and the particular group. For example, a support group's task activities may be the development of friendship and support networks, an activity that may be regarded in another type of group as having a maintenance function. To succeed, all groups need to address both their task functions and their maintenance functions, although there is no set proportion of activities that should be assigned to either category. What is important is for each group to strike a balance between the three types of activities. This balance will depend on the reason each group is meeting and, to some extent, on the individual needs of people in each group.

The following suggestions (adapted from Egger et al., 2013 and Roe et al., in Bensley & Brookins-Fisher, 2009, Chapter 11) provide useful preparation and process advice for ensuring a group meets its desired purposes.

- Plan the sessions/meetings in advance.
- Decide on the objectives for the group or the session.
- Prepare and circulate an agenda.
- Arrange for notes or minutes to be prepared.
- Attend to logistics—setting, seating, meeting rules.
- Use techniques for successful group processes:
  - a positive belief about the effectiveness of groups
  - an enquiring, interested attitude
  - use and expect respectful interaction
  - a sense of humour bolsters group effectiveness
  - maintain a commitment to capacity building for participants.
- Keep the group from getting too far away from its task.
- Refer to the objectives as the means of re-focusing when needed.
- Involve the group in seeking suggestions about how to deal with a problem.
- Make sure you or someone is available to summarise group discussion and reaffirm key points.
- Reflect on the processes and outcomes.
- Use specific strategies to involve people who do not seem to be participating.
- Plan to take time out to talk socially and find out how everyone is doing.
- Use simple (and informal) evaluation techniques to make sure the group is meeting participants' needs.

Leadership

The pattern of leadership within a group will reflect a great deal about how the group operates and how involved members are. Many people assume that the originator of the group is the only person who should exhibit leadership behaviours, but this is not so. Even in a group initiated by an external practitioner or facilitator, if the group is to be effective its leadership should be shared. Use the following questions to evaluate the leadership patterns in a group:

- What leadership behaviours are exhibited in the group?
- Is leadership shared by members of the group, or does one person maintain control?
- Who exhibits leadership behaviours and who does not?

Egger and colleagues (2013) and Bensley and Brookins-Fisher (2009) provide useful guidance for working with and facilitating peer support and other small groups.

Power and influence

Power and influence are very much linked to leadership in a group. Indeed, if the people with the power and influence in a group are not its leaders, conflict may result. The following questions provide useful indicators of power and influence in a group.

- Are there any people in the group whose opinions are listened to very carefully?
- Are there any people whose opinions are ignored?
- Are people with influence helping the group to achieve its goals?
- Are there conflicts between people with influence?

Decision making

There are several aspects of decision making that need to be considered when observing group processes:

- when decisions are made (timing)
- how decisions are reached (process)
- who is responsible (who monitors the decision-making process)
- what priorities are to be decided.

Timing of decision making reflects a number of important elements of group processes. How decisions are made may determine what degree of ownership is felt by group members over these decisions and help determine their level of satisfaction with the group's performance.

The following questions provide useful analysis of group decision making.

- How are decisions made in this group?
  - By one person?
  - By a small dominant group?
  - By simple majority?
  - By consensus?
- Who controls the decision-making procedures in a group?
- Are there issues that feature prominently in the group over which it has no decision-making power?

Group goals

A key issue in determining whether people feel involved in a group is the extent to which they share the group's goals. If the goals of an individual do not match the goals of the group, it is unlikely that he or she will be committed to it. It is important to establish a mutual goal before proceeding with group discussion.

The following questions provide a useful analysis of goal setting in a group.

- Does the group have clear goals?
- Who was involved in establishing them?
- Who 'owns' goals that are set?
- Are there members of the group who do not seem to share the group goals?

Communication

Patterns of communication in a group are extremely important. Distribution of leadership, participation, power and control, and conflicts of interest will all be reflected in observable patterns of communication. Communication is both verbal and non-verbal, and occurs between individuals and an individual and the group. It has a key role in facilitating the group's achievement of its tasks and group members' comfort and sense of belonging.

Use the following questions when observing communication in a group.

- Who talks and to whom?
- Who keeps the interaction going in the group?
- Are people silent, and if so, how does the group respond?
- Do people address the whole group when they talk or just some people?
- What non-verbal communication is happening?
- How powerful are the non-verbal messages?
- Is anyone giving mixed messages?
- Is more being not said than said?

Practical tips for working with groups

There are several practical tips that may make working with groups a more positive process for both facilitators and group members. The following tips for working with groups have been developed from Egger and colleagues (2013, Chapter 4), Bensley and Brookins-Fisher (2009, Chapters 6 & 11) and Scriven (2010, Chapter 13).

Numbers

In considering the optimal size of a group, the first consideration will be the purpose for which the group is meeting (Bastable, 2014). If it is a public meeting designed to canvass opinion on a priority, the actual size of the group may not influence effectiveness, and the same applies with online groups. If it is a structured face-to-face meeting, where members of several interested parties need representation, the size of the group may be determined by the number of such parties.

If, on the other hand, the group is a health education or peer-support group built on the principle of maximum participation by its members, it will be important to keep it to a manageable size. In such cases, the optimal size of a group is regarded as being between six (6) and 12 people. If there are fewer than eight (8) people in a group, people may feel exposed and be unwilling to participate. Moreover, an insufficient number of ideas may be generated in a problem-solving group. However, if there are more than 12 people in a group, it is difficult for everyone to get involved, and often the louder members will dominate (Bastable, 2014).

If there is a need to have more than 12 people in a face-to-face group, consider whether it can be split into smaller groups for discussion and activities. Alternatively, it may be worthwhile running two separate groups alongside each other. Which solution to choose will depend on the reason the group is meeting (can the topic 'cope' with a large group?) and the amount of resources you have (can you afford to run the same group twice?). If the group processes involve dealing with sensitive topics, it may be appropriate to have a group of fewer than eight (8) people to enable people to speak comfortably about the topic. In these cases, you may also consider whether it is more appropriate to discuss the topic on a one-to-one basis. With online forums, the number of participants actively engaged in discussion about a topic may be extremely variable, but generally this style of group works best when there are many potential participants, because this will result in rich and responsive discussion (Hernández-Ramos, 2004).

Timing

The length of time that a group meets for is very important in determining whether members feel it is valuable or not. Groups need to be together long enough to break the ice, settle down and achieve something, but not so long that people begin to get bored or feel they are wasting their time. Generally, between an hour and an hour and a half is a reasonable amount of time. Breaks or changes in the group's activity will enable it to stay fresh for that length of time, or even longer if necessary. However, meetings lasting more than one and a half hours would need to be well planned and demand a good reason to justify them. Planning the length of meetings with the participants will increase the likelihood that the duration planned is realistic and fits in with the other needs of group members.

The day and time that the group meets will have a considerable bearing on who will attend. There are some commonsense rules you can follow to ensure that the timing does not prevent people from attending. It makes good sense to check at the group's first meeting whether the day and time suit members and, if they do not, to negotiate a day and time that suit most of them. Not only does this increase the likelihood that people can attend the group, it also makes it quite clear that the group belongs to everyone, not just the group leader. Different meeting times could be trialled to maximise attendance and ensure that people who want to attend the groups are not consistently missing out because of poor timing.

Location

Location can also be negotiated. It is important that group members feel comfortable in the venue. Obviously, if people feel threatened, they are unlikely to continue going to the group. For example, many Aboriginal people have had negative experiences in hospitals and may not feel comfortable in a hospital or community health centre. If there is no local Aboriginal Medical Service, the local Aboriginal Land Council offices may be a comfortable place to meet.

Remember that hospitals and, to a lesser extent, community health centres may have a history of being authoritarian and of being places where people lose control over their own destiny. It may be difficult for these associations to be broken and thus a neutral meeting place should be used. Church halls, Country Women's Association halls, youth clubs, senior citizens' centres and people's homes are just some examples of possible meeting places. Which venue is most appropriate will depend very much on the members of the group.

Another important point about location is that it needs to be accessible to group members. Organising a group to meet in a venue that is not accessible to people using public transport, wheelchairs or walking aids, or with larger bodies, is likely to prevent some people from being able to attend. This is the great advantage for online groups and forums, because participants can choose the time that suits them best, and they don't need to travel to take part.

Seating

If a group is to work successfully, all members need to feel they have an equal right to participate. Ensure that you provide comfortable seating that caters to a wide variety of body sizes and physical abilities, including a variety of seating options such as sturdy chairs without arms and bench seating. Arrange the seating so that everyone can see and hear each other. Until group members get to know one another, barriers such as tables are sometimes useful because they stop people feeling exposed or threatened. Ensure that tables do not reduce accessibility or comfort for people with larger bodies or people with disabilities.

The position of the facilitator is important. They may sit opposite shy people in order to encourage them to speak, or next to someone who is talkative in order to minimise eye contact with that person, enabling others in the group to participate.

Getting the group started

How the group is established and the atmosphere that is created when it first meets will help determine whether or not people will go to future meetings. It is, therefore, important to start the group in a way that 'breaks the ice' and enables people to feel comfortable in their surroundings and with each other. This may be done fairly informally through introductions and discussion of the particular issues involved. However, for an educational or support group, it might be done more formally.

Icebreakers

Several things can be done at the beginning of a group's life, and at other times when necessary, to break the ice and help relax people into the group. These icebreakers may provide an opportunity for people to introduce themselves to one another in a fun way or discuss their reasons for being involved with the group and what they want to accomplish. There are several resources containing examples of icebreaker activities that can be useful in various groups. Some icebreaker activities can also serve as goal-setting activities, when they provide people with an opportunity to discuss why they have joined the group.

Introducing the group

Once the ice is broken and people are settled, the purpose is introduced and the group can discuss mutual goals. It is useful in the initial stages to ask participants to tell the group what they want to achieve from the group, and this information can be used in later discussion to plan together the group goals.

Experiential activity

Having met one another and determined which issues will be covered during the group's life, group members should leave the first meeting also having had a taste of what the group will be doing (Egger et al., 2013). Use an activity that demonstrates what the group will achieve. For example, a stress management group might discuss the particular stressors of its members and do a relaxation exercise. In this way members are able to leave the first meeting with some sense of whether the group is likely to be beneficial for them or not and whether or not they plan to return.

Facilitating group discussion

Very often people plan to have a discussion in a group, but they do not plan how it will actually happen. They assume that if they say, 'Let's discuss ...' a discussion will just begin. Unfortunately, the times when that will happen are more the exception than the rule. Most times, it is necessary to structure activities that will enable a discussion to develop (Bastable, 2014; Scriven, 2010). It will be necessary to have an idea of group members' attitudes to the topic before launching into a discussion to gain a sense of the best approach to take; whether it is appropriate to be provocative in order to encourage a vigorous debate, or wiser to begin gently and lead the group into the controversial areas. Consider this when planning discussion. Scriven (2010, pp. 185–188) suggests that the activities discussed below may be useful in encouraging discussion.

Using trigger materials

Show a film, read a personal account or play a game that touches on the key issues for the session. If it is slightly controversial, it will motivate people to discuss the issues. Ask specific questions to draw out the pertinent issues. Plan a set of questions before the event and ensure these are open-ended, so that participants are forced into giving comprehensive answers, not simply 'yes' or 'no' responses.

Debate

Break the group into two, provide both sides with information if necessary, give them time to prepare and then have them debate the issue. Often it is better to keep the debate informal to encourage spontaneous participation. Having group members argue the position they disagree with is one way of enabling them to clarify their views and hear the views of their 'opponents'.

Brainstorming

Brainstorming is a way of pooling everyone's ideas and coming up with innovative ones, especially if the aim of the session is to find solutions to a problem. It could be used, for example, to come up with ways to change the attitudes of local government councillors towards childcare facilities, convince businesses to become environmentally responsible, devise effective over-eating avoidance tactics or plan stress-release activities into a normal working day.

The typical strategy for brainstorming is as follows:

- put the problem or issue to the group
- ask participants to think up as many ideas as possible, without judging their own or other people's ideas
- accept all suggestions and write them down
- keep going until all ideas are exhausted and people cannot think of anything else.

The next step depends on the reason for the brainstorming. If the group is trying to find the most appropriate solution to a problem, the next step would be to prioritise the suggestions made. This may require group members simply to rate, prioritise or vote, or there may be lengthy discussion, depending on the issue and the philosophy of the group. If the brainstorming was designed to answer a question, you may simply want the group to arrange the answers into similar categories.

Rounds

Rounds ensure that everyone has an equal opportunity to participate. They can therefore be used both to encourage shy group members to speak and to prevent dominant group members from monopolising conversation. Scriven (2010, p. 187) suggests four rules that are necessary if rounds are to be successful.

1. No interruptions until each person has finished their statement.
2. No comments on anybody's contribution until the full round is complete (i.e. no discussion, praise, interpretation, criticism or I-think-that-too type of remark).
3. Anyone can choose not to participate. Give permission, clearly and emphatically, that anyone who does not want to make a statement can just say 'pass'. This is very important for reinforcing the principle of voluntary participation.

4. It doesn't matter if two or more people in the round say the same thing. People should stick to what they wanted to say even if someone has said it already; they do not have to think of something different.

Rounds can be valuable for beginning and ending sessions and getting feedback, or as a measurement of the entire group's opinion.

Buzz groups

Breaking the group into smaller groups to discuss a key issue may enable everyone to participate more fully in the group. As a rule, these small groups need only occur for relatively short periods of time, after which they can report back to the main group.

CONCLUSION

This chapter has briefly explored the role of health education and health literacy in health promotion practice within a comprehensive primary health care context. It is well established that higher levels of health literacy result in better health outcomes for and health service utilisation of people, and considerable cost savings to the health system. Health education enables learning about health and wellbeing, forming the foundation of health literacy. Two-way communication and respect, learning based around health and wellbeing priorities identified by people themselves and active learning build health literacy. There are different levels of health literacy but even assisting people to achieve a basic level has the potential to make a huge difference in their lives.

Health practitioners have much scope within their roles to incorporate health education into their work in a way that enables people to take greater control over their lives, and to use health literacy as a springboard to other health promotion strategies. International and national health literacy surveys at the population level provide good direction for where action is needed and there has been considerable progress on establishing health literacy measures. Health practitioners have a responsibility to be health literate about the healthcare system and to have appropriate skills to build health literacy. Making appropriate use of health education planning theories and models, and educational theory will enhance professional competency, especially for practitioners with health education as a key aspect of their role.

Awareness of group processes is an extremely useful component of working effectively with people with a learning need in common, and with teams, social action groups and participants in an education program. Working with groups in a supportive, enabling way is an important part promoting health and wellbeing withing a CPHC context, and the time spent developing group facilitation processes will be well rewarded.

MORE TO EXPLORE

BUILDING WORKFORCE HEALTH LITERACY

- Cuban literacy program comes to Indigenous Australians: Adult Learning Australia (2020)
- Indigenous Literacy: Indigenous Literacy Foundation (2020)
- Is health workforce planning recognising the dynamic interplay between health literacy at an individual, organisation and system level? (Naccarella et al., 2015)

- The *Investing in Health Literacy Report* from the European Observatory on Health Systems and Policies (2016) makes a clear argument that building health literacy in young children makes good economic sense and will make a sustained difference to the health of the population. In addition, there are co-benefits such as improved educational achievements, employment opportunities and lifetime economic benefits.

IUHPE Core Competencies for Health Promotion

The IUHPE Core Competencies for Health Promotion (International Union for Health Promotion and Education, 2016) comprises nine domains of action. Each domain has a series of core competency statements and a detailed outline of the knowledge and skills that contribute to competency in that domain.

The content of this chapter relates especially to the achievement of competency in the health promotion domains outlined below.

1. Enable change	*1.4 Facilitate the development of personal skills that will maintain and improve health* Health promotion models Behavioural change techniques for brief advice/interventions
2. Advocate for health	*2.1 Use advocacy strategies and techniques which reflect health promotion principles* Ability to work with: individuals and groups defined by gender, social and economic status, geography, culture, age, setting or interest; and those in own/other organisations/sectors
4. Communication	*4.1 Use effective communication skills including written, verbal, non-verbal, listening skills and information technology* Theory and practice of effective communication including interpersonal communication and group work Health literacy
	4.2 Use electronic and other media to receive and disseminate health promotion information Applications of information technology for social networking media, and mass media
	4.4 Use interpersonal communication and groupwork skills to facilitate individuals, groups, communities and organisations to improve health and reduce health inequities Diffusion of innovations theory
5. Leadership	*5.4 Incorporate new knowledge and ideas to improve practice and respond to emerging challenges in health promotion* Facilitation Ability to motivate groups and individuals towards a common goal

6. Assessment	*6.3 Collect, review and appraise relevant data, information and literature to inform health promotion action*
	Evidence base for health promotion action and priority setting
	Understanding social and cultural diversity
7. Planning	*7.2 Use current models and systematic approaches for planning health promotion action*
	Use and effectiveness of current health promotion planning models and theories
	7.3 Develop a feasible action plan within resource constraints and with reference to existing needs and assets
	Use of health promotion planning models
	Analysis and application of information about needs and assets
	7.4 Develop and communicate appropriate, realistic and measurable goals and objectives for health promotion action
	Use of project/program planning and management tools
	Ability to work with: groups and communities targeted by the health promotion action; stakeholders and partners
8. Implementation	*8.1 Use ethical, empowering, culturally appropriate and participatory processes to implement health promotion action*
	Use of participatory implementation processes
	Collaborative working

In addition, IUHPE (n.d.) specifies knowledge, skills and performance criteria essential for health promotion practitioners to act professionally and ethically, including having knowledge of ethical and legal issues, behaving in an ethical and respectful manner and working in ways that review and improve practice. Full details are available at: http://www.iuhpe.org/index.php/en/the-accreditation-system.

Reflective Questions

1. Review the website of a health-related organisation for evidence of actions focused on building health literacy. Refer to Table 7.1 for guidance on possible actions.

2. Select a specific health behaviour in a priority population. Use the social cognitive theory to identify the specific cognitive, environmental and behavioural factors that you would need to research as a foundation for planning a behaviour change strategy.

3. Identify a personal health-related behaviour that you would like to change. Reflect on the barriers and enablers to this change. Apply the stages of change model to determine which stage of change you are currently in, and propose strategies that would support you to move towards maintenance of the change in the behaviour.

REFERENCES

Adult Learning Australia. (2020). Cuban literacy program comes to Indigenous Australians. Retrieved from https://ala.asn.au/cuban-literacy-program-comes-to-indigenous-australians/.

Ajzen, I. (1991). The theory of planned behavior. Organizational Behavior and Human Decision Processes, 50(2), 179–211. doi:10.1016/0749-5978(91)90020-T.

Ajzen, I., & Fishbein, M. (1980). Understanding attitudes and predicting social behavior. Englewood Cliffs, NJ: Prentice-Hall.

Australian Bureau of Statistics. (2006a). Health literacy, Australia, 2006. Cat. no. 4233.0. Retrieved from http://www.abs.gov.au/AUSSTATS/abs@.nsf/mf/4233.0.

Australian Bureau of Statistics. (2006b). Re-issue 2008 Adult literacy and life skills (ALLS) survey, summary results. Cat no. 4228.0, Australia. Retrieved from https://www.abs.gov.au/ausstats/abs@.nsf/Previousproducts/4228.0Main%20Features22006%20(Reissue).

Australian Commission on Safety and Quality in Health Care (ACSQHC). (2014). Health literacy: taking action to improve safety and quality. Retrieved from https://www.safetyandquality.gov.au/sites/default/files/migrated/Health-Literacy-Taking-action-to-improve-safety-and-quality.pdf.

Australian Commission on Safety and Quality in Health Care (ACSQHC). (2019). National statement on health literacy—taking action to improve safety and quality. Retrieved from https://www.safetyandquality.gov.au/publications-and-resources/resource-library/national-statement-health-literacy-taking-action-improve-safety-and-quality

Baker, D. W. (2006). The meaning and the measure of health literacy. Journal of General Internal Medicine, 21(8), 878–883. doi:10.1111/j.1525-1497.2006.00540.x.

Bandura, A. (1986). Social foundations of thought and action: a social cognitive theory. Englewood Cliffs, NJ: Prentice Hall.

Basen-Engquist, K., Carmack, C. L., Li, Y., et al. (2013). Social-cognitive theory predictors of exercise behavior in endometrial cancer survivors. Health Psychology, 32(11), 1137–1148. doi:10.1037/a0031712.

Bastable, S. (2014). Nurse as educator: principles of teaching and learning for nursing practice (4th ed.). Burlington, MA: Jones & Bartlett Learning.

Becker, M. H. (Ed.) (1974). The health belief model and personal health behaviour. Thorofare, NJ: Charles, B. Slack.

Begoray, D. L., & Kwan, B. (2012). A Canadian exploratory study to define a measure of health literacy. Health Promotion International, 27(1), 23–32. doi:10.1093/heapro/dar015.

Bensley, R. J., & Brookins-Fisher, J. (2009). Community health education methods: a practical guide (3rd ed.). Sudbury, Mass: Jones and Bartlett Publishers.

Berkman, N. D., Sheridan, S. L., Donahue, K. E., et al. (2011). Health literacy interventions and outcomes: an updated systematic review. Evidence report/technology. Assessment No. 199. Publication Number 11-E006. Retrieved from https://www.ahrq.gov/downloads/pub/evidence/pdf/literacy/literacyup.pdf.

Berlin, L., Norris, K., Kolodinsky, J., & Nelson, A. (2013). The role of Social Cognitive Theory in farm-to-school-related activities: implications for child nutrition. Journal of School Health, 83(8), 589–595. doi:10.1111/josh.12069.

Bloom, B. S. (1964). Taxonomy of educational objectives: the classification of educational goals. London: Longman Group.

Bonebright, D. A. (2010). 40 years of storming: a historical review of Tuckman's model of small group development. Human Resource Development International, 13(1), 111–120. doi:10.1080/13678861003589099.

Borowski, S. C., & Tambling, R. B. (2015). Applying the Health Belief Model to young individuals' beliefs and preferences about premarital counseling. The Family Journal, 23(4), 417–426. doi:10.1177/1066480715602221.

Brennan, L. L., Binney, W., Parker, L., & Aleti, T. (2014). Social marketing and behaviour change: models, theory and applications. Cheltenham, UK: Edward Elgar.

Chorlton, K., Conner, M., & Jamson, S. (2012). Identifying the psychological determinants of risky riding: an application of an extended Theory of Planned Behaviour. Accident Analysis and Prevention, 49, 142–153. doi:10.1016/j.aap.2011.07.003.

Côté, F., Gagnon, J., Houme, P. K., et al. (2012). Using the Theory of Planned Behaviour to predict nurses' intention to integrate research evidence into clinical decision-making. Journal of Advanced Nursing, 68(10), 2289–2298. doi:10.1111/j.1365-2648.2011.05922.x.

Couët, N., Desroches, S., Robitaille, H., et al. (2013). Assessments of the extent to which health-care providers involve patients in decision making: a systematic review of studies using the OPTION instrument. Health Expectations, 18(4), 542–561. doi:10.1111/hex.12054.

D'Sylva, F., Graffam, J., Hardcastle, L., & Shinkfield, A. (2012). Analysis of the Stages of Change Model of drug and alcohol treatment readiness among prisoners. International Journal of Offender Therapy and Comparative Criminology, 56(2), 265–280. doi:10.1177/0306624X10392531.

Das, B. M., & Evans, E. M. (2014). Understanding weight management perceptions in first-year college students using the Health Belief Model. Journal of American College Health, 62(7), 488–497. doi:10.1080/07448481.2014.923429.

de Leeuw, E. (2011). The boulder in the stream. Health Promotion International, 26(suppl2), ii157–ii160. doi:10.1093/heapro/dar083.

Department of Health. (2020). Launch of the coronavirus (COVID-19) campaign. Retrieved from https://www.health.gov.au/news/launch-of-the-coronavirus-covid-19-campaign.

Donadiki, E. M., Jiménez-García, R., Hernández-Barrera, V., et al. (2014). Health Belief Model applied to non-compliance with HPV vaccine among female university students. Public Health, 128(3), 268–273. doi:10.1016/j.puhe.2013.12.004.

Eckermann, A. K., Dowd, T., Chong, E., et al. (2010). Binan goonj: bridging cultures in Aboriginal health (3rd ed.). Sydney: Churchill Livingstone/Elsevier.

Egger, G., Donovan, R., & Spark, R. (2013). Health promotion strategies and methods (3rd ed.). Sydney: McGraw-Hill.

Emanuel, A. S., McCully, S. N., Gallagher, K. M., & Updegraff, J. A. (2012). Theory of Planned Behavior explains gender difference in fruit and vegetable consumption. Appetite, 59(3), 693–697. doi:10.1016/j.appet.2012.08.007.

European Observatory on Health Systems and Policies. (2016). Investing in health literacy. Retrieved from http://www.euro.who.int/en/about-us/partners/observatory/publications/policy-briefs-and-summaries/investing-in-health-literacy

Evers, K. E., Paiva, A. L., Johnson, J. L. et al. (2012). Results of a transtheoretical model-based alcohol, tobacco and other drug intervention in middle schools. Addictive Behaviors, 37(9), 1009–1018. doi:10.1016/j.addbeh.2012.04.008.

Felicia, P., & Mallon, B. (Eds.). (2014). Game-based learning: challenges and opportunities. Newcastle upon Tyne, England: Cambridge Scholars Publishing.

Freire, P. (1974). Education for critical consciousness. London: Sheed & Ward.

Gajdamaschko, N. (2015). Vygotsky's sociocultural theory. In: J. Wright (Ed.). International encyclopedia of the social & behavioral sciences (2nd ed., pp. 329–334). Amsterdam, Netherlands: Elsevier.

Glanz, K., Rimer, B. K., & Viswanath, K. (Eds.). (2008). Health behavior and health education: theory, research, and practice (4th ed.). San Francisco: Jossey-Bass.

Gravani, M. N. (2012). Adult learning principles in designing learning activities for teacher development. International Journal of Lifelong Education, 31(4), 419. doi:10.1080/02601370.2012.663804.

Gugglberger, L. (2019). The multifaceted relationship between health promotion and health literacy [Editorial]. Health Promotion International, 34, 887–891.

Guzys, D., Kenny, A., Dickson-Swift, V., & Threlkeld, G. (2015). A critical review of population health literacy assessment. BMC Public Health, 15(1), 215. doi:10.1186/s12889-015-1551-6.

Harrell, P. T., Trenz, R. C., Scherer, M., et al. (2013). A latent class approach to treatment readiness corresponds to a transtheoretical ('Stages of Change') model. Journal of Substance Abuse Treatment, 45(3), 249. doi:10.1016/j.jsat.2013.04.004.

Heiss, V. J., & Petosa, V. J. (2015). Social cognitive theory correlates of moderate-intensity exercise among adults with type 2 diabetes. Psychology, Health and Medicine, 21(1). doi:10.1080/13548506.2015.1017510.

Hernández-Ramos, P. (2004). Web logs and online discussions as tools to promote reflective practice. Journal of Interactive Online Learning, 3(1).

Heyward, P. (2010). Emotional engagement through drama: strategies to assist learning through role-play. International Journal of Teaching and Learning in Higher Education, 22(2), 197.

Hill, S. (2011). The knowledgeable patient: communication and participation in health. Chichester, West Sussex: John Wiley & Sons.

Honebein, P. C., & Honebein, C. H. (2015). Effectiveness, efficiency, and appeal: pick any two? The influence of learning domains and learning outcomes on designer judgments of useful instructional methods. Educational Technology Research and Development, 63(6), 937. doi:10.1007/s11423-015-9396-3.

Hood, L. (2010). Leddy and Pepper's conceptual basis of professional nursing (7th ed.). Philadelphia, PA: Lippincott, Williams & Wilkins.

Hyland, T. (2010). Mindfulness, adult learning and therapeutic education: integrating the cognitive and affective domains of learning. International Journal of Lifelong Education, 29(5), 517–532. doi:10.1080/02601370.2010.512792.

Indigenous Literacy Foundation. (2020). Indigenous literacy. Retrieved from https://www.indigenousliteracyfoundation.org.au/what-is-indigenous-literacy.

Ingle, S., & Duckworth, V. (2013). Enhancing learning through technology in lifelong learning fresh ideas. Maidenhead: McGraw-Hill Education.

International Union for Health Promotion and Education. (2016). Core competencies and professional standards for health promotion 2016. Retrieved from https://www.iuhpe.org/images/JC-Accreditation/Core_Competencies_Standards_linkE.pdf

International Union for Health Promotion and Education (IUHPE). (2018). IUHPE position statement on health literacy: a practical vision for a health literate world. Retrieved from https://www.iuhpe.org/images/IUHPE/Advocacy/IUHPEHealth_Literacy_2018.pdf.

International Union for Health Promotion and Education. (n.d.). The IUHPE Health Promotion Accreditation System. Retrieved from http://www.iuhpe.org/index.php/en/the-accreditation-system.

Johnson, D., & Johnson, F. (2002). Joining together: group theory and group skills (8th ed.). Englewood Cliffs, NJ: Prentice Hall.

Karupaiah, T., Wong, K., Chinna, K., et al. (2015). Metering self-reported adherence to clinical outcomes in Malaysian patients with hypertension: applying the Stages of Change Model to healthful behaviors in the CORFIS study. Health Education & Behavior, 42(3), 339. doi:10.1177/1090198114558588.

Kelch, B. P., & Demmitt, A. (2010). Incorporating the Stages of Change Model in solution focused brief therapy with non-substance abusing families: a novel and integrative approach. The Family Journal, 18(2), 184–188. doi:10.1177/1066480710364325.

Kickbusch, I. (2001). Health literacy: addressing the health and education divide. Health Promotion International, 16(3), 289–297. doi:10.1093/heapro/16.3.289.

Kickbusch, I., Pelikan, J. M., Apfel, F., & Tsouros, A. D. (2013). Health literacy: the solid facts. Retrieved from https://apps.who.int/iris/bitstream/handle/10665/128703/e96854.pdf.

Klein, L. A., Ritchie, J. E., Nathan, S., & Wutzke, S. (2014). An explanatory model of peer education within a complex medicines information exchange setting. Social Science & Medicine, 111, 101–109. doi:10.1016/j.socscimed.2014.04.009.

Knowles, M., Holton, E., & Swanson, R. (2011). The adult learner: the definitive classic in adult education and human resource development (7th ed.). Oxford: Butterworth-Heinemann.

Koelen, M., & van den Ban, A. (2004). Health education and health promotion. The Netherlands: Wageningen Academic Publishers.

Kothe, E. J., Mullan, B. A., & Amaratunga, R. (2011). Randomised controlled trial of a brief theory-based intervention promoting breakfast consumption. Appetite, 56(1), 148–155. doi:10.1016/j.appet.2010.12.002.

Kothe, E. J., Mullan, B. A., & Butow, P. (2012). Promoting fruit and vegetable consumption: testing an intervention based on the theory of planned behaviour. Appetite, 58(3), 997–1004. doi:10.1016/j.appet.2012.02.012.

Lee-Lin, F., Nguyen, T., Pedhiwala, N., et al. (2016). A longitudinal examination of Stages of Change Model applied to mammography screening. Western Journal of Nursing Research, 38(4), 441–458. doi:10.1177/0193945915618398.

Main, D., Nichol, R., & Fennel, R. (2000). Reconciling pedagogy and health sciences to promote Indigenous health. Australian and New Zealand Journal of Public Health, 24(2), 211–213.

Main, D., Talbot, L., Eltchelebi, W., & Pattison, S. (1998). Using primary health-care philosophy to promote cross-cultural awareness for tertiary students studying Aboriginal health. Health Promotion Journal of Australia, 8(1), 34–39.

Marmot, M. (2012). Fair society, healthy lives: the Marmot Review—strategic review of health inequalities in England post-2010. Retrieved from http://www.instituteofhealthequity.org/resources-reports/fair-society-healthy-lives-the-marmot-review/fair-society-healthy-lives-full-report-pdf.pdf.

McAllister, M., Rogers, I., & Lee Brien, D. (2015). Illuminating and inspiring: using television historical drama to cultivate contemporary nursing values and critical thinking. Contemporary Nurse, 50(2–3), 127–138. doi:10.1080/10376178.2015.1025470.

McDermott, M. S., Oliver, M., Simnadis, T., et al. (2015). The Theory of Planned Behaviour and dietary patterns: a systematic review and meta-analysis. Preventive Medicine, 81, 150–156. doi:10.1016/j.ypmed.2015.08.020.

Ministry of Health. (2015). A framework for health literacy. Retrieved from https://www.health.govt.nz/publication/framework-health-literacy.

Minkler, M., & Cox, E. (1980). Creating critical consciousness in health: application of Freire's philosophy and methods to the health care setting. International Journal of Health Services, 10(2), 311–322.

Mullan, B., Wong, C., & Kothe, E. (2013). Predicting adolescent breakfast consumption in the UK and Australia using an extended theory of planned behaviour. Appetite, 62, 127–132. doi:10.1016/j.appet.2012.11.021.

Murphy, B. (2005). Need to get your students talking? Try speed dating! The Teaching Professor, 19(7), 3–4.

Naccarella, L., Wraight, B., & Gorman, D. (2015). Is health workforce planning recognising the dynamic interplay between health literacy at an individual, organisation and system level? Australian Health Review, 40(1), 33–35. doi:10.1071/AH14192.

Nemme, H. E., & White, K. M. (2010). Texting while driving: psychosocial influences on young people's texting intentions and behaviour. Accident Analysis and Prevention, 42(4), 1257–1265. doi:10.1016/j.aap.2010.01.019.

Noordman, J., de Vet, E., van Der Weijden, T., & van Dulmen, S. (2013). Motivational interviewing within the different stages of change: an analysis of practice nurse–patient consultations aimed at promoting a healthier lifestyle. Social Science & Medicine, 87, 60–67. doi:10.1016/j.socscimed.2013.03.019.

Nutbeam, D. (2000). Health literacy as a public health goal: a challenge for contemporary health education and communication strategies into the 21st century. Health Promotion International, 15(3), 259–267. doi:10.1093/heapro/15.3.259.

Nutbeam, D. (2008). The evolving concept of health literacy. Social Science & Medicine, 67(12), 2072–2078. doi:10.1016/j.socscimed.2008.09.050.

Nutbeam, D., Harris, E., & Wise, M. (2010). Theory in a nutshell: a practical guide to health promotion theories (3rd ed.). Sydney: McGraw-Hill Australia.

Osborne, R. H., Batterham, R. W., Elsworth, G., et al. (2013). The grounded psychometric development and initial validation of the Health Literacy Questionnaire (HLQ). BMC Public Health, 13(1). doi:10.1186/1471-2458-13-658.

Papps, E., & Ramsden, I. (1996). Cultural safety in nursing: the New Zealand experience. International Journal for Quality in Health Care, 8(5), 491–497. doi:10.1093/intqhc/8.5.491.

Prochaska, J. O., & Di Clementi, C. C. (1984). The transtheoretical approach: crossing traditional boundaries of therapy. Homeward, IL: Down Jones, Irwin.

Quinn, F. M. (1995). The principles and practice of nurse education (3rd ed.). London: Chapman & Hall.

Robson, B., & Harris, R. (Eds.). (2005). Hauora: Maori Standards of Health IV—a study of the years 2000–2005. Wellington: TeRopu Rangahau Hauora a Eru Pomare.

Rosenberg, E., Richard, C., Lussier, M.-T., & Abdool, S. N. (2006). Intercultural communication competence in family medicine: lessons from the field. Patient Education and Counseling, 61(2), 236–245. doi:10.1016/j.pec.2005.04.002.

Rowlands, G., Begoray, D., & Gillis, D. (2012). Health literacy in context: international perspectives. New York: Nova Science Publications Inc.

Ruyters, M., Douglas, K., & Law, S. F. (2011). Blended learning using role-plays, wikis and blogs. Journal of Learning Design, 4(4), 45. doi:10.5204/jld.v4i4.88.

Schouten, B. C., & Meeuwesen, L. (2006). Cultural differences in medical communication: a review of the literature. Patient Education and Counseling, 64(1–3), 21–34. doi:10.1016/j.pec.2005.11.014.

Schouten, B. C., Meeuwesen, L., Tromp, F., & Harmsen, H. A. M. (2007). Cultural diversity in patient participation: the influence of patients' characteristics and doctors' communicative behaviour. Patient Education and Counseling, 67(1–2), 214–223. doi:10.1016/j.pec.2007.03.018.

Scriven, A. (2010). Promoting health: a practical guide (6th ed.). UK: Balliere Tindall/Elsevier.

Sohler, N. L., Jerant, A., & Franks, P. (2015). Socio-psychological factors in the Expanded Health Belief Model and subsequent colorectal cancer screening. Patient Education and Counseling, 98(7), 901–907. doi:10.1016/j.pec.2015.03.023.

Sole, G., Schneiders, A., Hébert-Losier, K., & Perry, M. (2013). Perceptions by physiotherapy students and faculty staff of a multimedia learning resource for musculoskeletal practical skills teaching. New Zealand Journal of Physiotherapy, 41(2), 58–64.

Sorensen, K., Van Den Broucke, S., Fullam, J., et al. (2012). Health literacy and public health: a systematic review and integration of definitions and models. BMC Public Health, 12. doi:10.1186/1471-2458-12-80.

Taylor, L. M., Raine, K. D., Plotnikoff, R. C., et al. (2016). Understanding physical activity in individuals with prediabetes: an application of social cognitive theory. Psychology, Health & Medicine, 21(2), 254–260. doi:10.1080/13548506.2015.1058486.

Trudgen, R. (2000). Why warriors lie down and die. Towards an understanding of why the Aboriginal people of Arnham Land face the greatest crisis in health and education since European contact: Aboriginal Resource and Development Services.

Tuckman, B., & Jensen, M. (1977). Stages of small-group development revisited. Group & Organization Management.

Wilson, K., & Narayan, A. (2016). Relationships among individual task self-efficacy, self-regulated learning strategy use and academic performance in a computer-supported collaborative learning environment. Educational Psychology, 36(2), 236–253. doi:10.1080/01443410.2014.926312.

World Health Organization (WHO). (1986). The Ottawa Charter for Health Promotion. Retrieved from https://www.who.int/healthpromotion/conferences/previous/ottawa/en/

World Health Organization (WHO). (2012). Track 2: Health literacy and health behavior. 7th Global Conference on Health Promotion. Retrieved from http://www.who.int/healthpromotion/conferences/7gchp/track2/en/.

World Health Organization (WHO). (2016). Shanghai Declaration on promoting health in the 2030 agenda for sustainable development. Retrieved from https://www.who.int/healthpromotion/conferences/9gchp/shanghai-declaration.pdf?ua=1.

World Health Organization (WHO). (2018). Declaration of Astana, global conference on primary health care. Retrieved from https://www.who.int/docs/default-source/primary-health/declaration/gcphc-declaration.pdf.

World Health Organization (WHO) & Commission on Social Determinants of Health. (2008). Closing the gap in a generation: health equity through action on the social determinants of health. Final Report of the Commission on Social Determinants of Health. Retrieved from https://www.who.int/social_determinants/thecommission/finalreport/en/.

Yue, Z., Li, C., Weilin, Q., & Bin, W. (2015). Application of the health belief model to improve the understanding of antihypertensive medication adherence among Chinese patients. Patient Education and Counseling, 98(5), 669–673. doi:10.1016/j.pec.2015.02.007.

Zarcadoolas, C., Pleasant, A., & Greer, D. S. (2005). Understanding health literacy: an expanded model. Health Promotion International, 20(2), 195–203. doi:10.1093/heapro/dah609.

8

Health information and social marketing to raise awareness about health and wellbeing priorities

COMPREHENSIVE PRIMARY HEALTH CARE

SOCIO-ECOLOGICAL APPROACH

SELECTIVE PRIMARY HEALTH CARE

BEHAVIOURAL APPROACH

BIOMEDICAL APPROACH

Healthy public policy to create environments and settings that support health and wellbeing

Community development action to support social and environmental change

Health education and health literacy to develop knowledge and skills for health and wellbeing action

Health information and social marketing to raise awareness about health and wellbeing priorities

Vaccination, screening, risk assessment and surveillance to monitor and reduce risk of disease conditions

Health promotion community assessment, program planning, implementation and evaluation

INTRODUCTION

In Chapter 8, social marketing approaches for health promotion are examined. The aim of social marketing in health promotion is to 'sell' the benefits of taking action to protect or enhance the health of individuals and their environments. Social marketing is often criticised because it focuses on individual action and not necessarily the context of people's lives, which may be a barrier to change, or the broader environmental determinants of health and wellbeing. However, social marketing is widely used, particularly by governments, as is the health promotion strategy most visible to the general public and other stakeholders.

Social marketing involves the use of techniques developed in commercial or business fields, and applied to non-commercial or social causes. This connection with commerce sometimes has negative connotations for people because they don't approve of the tactics or priorities used by some industries. But unlike other forms of marketing, where the benefit of the activity goes to the marketer, in social marketing the desired benefit is improved health and wellbeing for people or communities (Egger et al., 2013). Social marketing has contributed to raising levels of knowledge in the community about certain diseases and ways to reduce the risk of those diseases, and in creating a perception of the need to reduce the socio-environmental impacts of personal behaviour. Social marketing can be used to support the implementation of a change to policy, or as a means of advocacy for a desired social change. Social marketing most often has a focus on specific illnesses or specific risks to health using selective approaches to health promotion. However, social marketing strategies designed to encourage individual voluntary behaviour change may only address the end result of the issue, and not the root causes of the issues themselves. Social marketing alone is therefore ineffective at addressing the socio-ecological determinants of health, and reducing health inequities. It is most useful when used as an adjunct to health promotion strategies focusing on changes to the social, economic, political, built or

PUTTING THE OTTAWA CHARTER INTO PRACTICE

The following questions, arranged in the Ottawa Charter action areas, are presented to guide health promotion practitioners to reflect on and critically evaluate their professional role and practice and the health promotion philosophy of their organisation. Content of this chapter will assist practitioners to develop the necessary professional knowledge and skills.

PUTTING THE OTTAWA CHARTER INTO PRACTICE FOR SOCIAL MARKETING APPROACHES TO HEALTH PROMOTION

Build healthy public policy

- Is the social marketing strategy supported by other health promotion strategies to develop or implement policies, rules, regulations, codes and standards of practice?

Create supportive environments

- What environmental supports are required to enable the behaviours promoted in the social marketing strategy to be achieved by everyone?
- Are recruitment resources accessible in terms of readership, language, circulation and media sources?

Strengthen community action

- Are there opportunities for community members to provide input to the social marketing strategy from their own lived experiences?

Develop personal skills

- Does the information ensure the cultural safety of people?
- Does the information provide a realistic 'action plan' for the audience?

Reorient health services

- Is the service health promoting?
- Is there a clear rationale for the benefit of the strategy based on epidemiological and economic outcomes?

natural environments. For example, when directed at organisations and agencies that have the power to make policy and legislative change, social marketing can be used in conjunction with building healthy public policy to bring about structural changes. Social and structural changes enable people to achieve enhanced wellbeing because they reduce the barriers that vulnerable people experience (Egger et al., 2013).

The critical health promotion values of social justice, equity, community control and working for social changes do not necessarily underpin social marketing, and this is another important reason why it is best used in combination with other actions. If used alone, the health promotion strategies in the behavioural approach constitute selective primary health care because they concentrate on reducing the risk of diseases and conditions based on epidemiological evidence, although more recently, some population-wide social marketing strategies have been designed to take account of the broader environment and to bring about a health-enhancing social change over time. Before starting the chapter, take some time to review *Putting the Ottawa Charter into Practice on p. 383.*

SOCIAL MARKETING

Social marketing involves the systematic application of commercial marketing processes to the analysis, planning, implementation and evaluation of strategies designed to influence the voluntary or involuntary behaviour of particular people in the population in order to improve health and wellbeing (Donovan & Henley, 2010; French, 2009). The use of social marketing as a health promotion strategy emerged in Australia in the 1970s with the character 'Norm' and the 'Life. Be in it' campaign. This followed recognition of the relationship between so-called 'lifestyle' behaviours and epidemiological health outcomes, and the realisation that face-to-face teaching by health promotion practitioners was not the most effective way of communicating health messages to wider audiences (French, et al., 2009; Nutbeam, 2008).

The aim of social marketing is to use marketing strategies to influence people's attitudes, values and beliefs that contribute to health- and wellbeing-related behaviours. Social marketing is therefore underpinned by behavioural psychology—understanding what motivates people, what are the barriers to behaviour change, and how they can be persuaded to make a change for the sake of possible long-term health and wellbeing gains (Donovan & Henley, 2010; Egger et al., 2013; French et al., 2009). Social marketing strategies have the following commonalities:

- They harness the capacities of diverse commercial marketing approaches.
- They are designed for a social good.
- Their aim is to induce a change in behaviour.
- They use specific and detailed planning to understand the characteristics of the intended audience.
- They usually focus on individual behaviour changes, but can also be directed at agencies with the power to change policy.

The application of social marketing is broadening in a number of ways. It is changing the nature and speed of communication, and numerous benefits and limitations have been identified (Moorhead et al., 2013). Social marketing is increasingly being used by governments as the strategy for population-wide behaviour change, including improving nutrition, smoking cessation, sun protection and increasing physical activity. French (2009) argues that, when carefully designed to reach the intended audience, social marketing strengthens individual agency, or control over decision making, whereas traditional health education approaches have the potential to undermine self-efficacy through their use of expert-driven or paternalistic behaviour compliance models. Social marketing can also be used by governments to gain support for an idea, and then based on that support, create new policy that changes the environment or context of people's lives, such as protective design in manufacturing, thereby contributing to greater health equity. Social marketing that involves the people in its development so their specific needs are understood provides people with choice (like marketing of other products), engages people more effectively, and can be a form of empowerment (French, 2009).

Social marketing, social media and social networking

The term 'social marketing' is now also being used to mean 'social media marketing'. This involves marketing yourself or your product more effectively using social media, including social networking apps. Using social media is part of the suite of social marketing methods, and has been defined as 'a group of internet-based applications that build on the ideological and technological foundation of web 2.0, and that allow the creation and exchange of generated content' (Kaplan & Haenlein, 2010). Furthermore, Moorhead and colleagues (2013) draw a distinction between social media and social networking; social networking is said to be a two-way and direct communication between parties whereas a number of platforms are used in social media to deliver a message which involves asking for something. The platforms can be collaborative projects, content communities, social networking sites, and virtual game and social worlds.

The rapid uptake of new information technologies has contributed to significant changes in the ways people access health information, including as a result of social marketing. Several primary uses of social media for health communication have been identified by Moorhead and colleagues (2013). These include increasing interaction between people, and facilitating, sharing and obtaining health messages. People are now more likely to use the internet as a source of information and advice and to exchange information with others than at any time in the past. This capacity to collate, compare and be engaged is the basis of many new social marketing strategies, and these are being prepared in creative partnerships between the private and health sectors (French, 2009).

One example of a social marketing campaign developed by a private advertising agency for a public health authority is the 'Dumb Ways to Die' social marketing campaign. The campaign was commissioned by Metro Trains Melbourne as part of a broader health promotion program that aimed to reduce train-related deaths due to 'dumb' behaviours such as walking or driving around boom gates at level crossings, or careless behaviour on train station platforms. The central social marketing activity was a three-minute animated music video posted on YouTube. The video amassed 2.3 million views on YouTube in the first 48 hours, with zero advertising costs (Metro Trains Melbourne, n.d.). Since the launch of the video in November 2012, it has had almost 200 million views. Within a day of its launch, the song was in the iTunes top 10 chart in Australia and was played for free on many radio stations around Australia. As momentum around the song built, social marketing activities expanded to include posters displayed at train stations and some other public venues, billboards, a children's book, plush toys and a clothing line. Another campaign activity was the Dumb Ways to Die website at which people could pledge 'I solemnly swear to not do dumb stuff around trains'. By 2015, around 90 million pledges had been made. The social marketing campaign was widely hailed for its creativity. At the international Cannes Lions advertising festival in 2013 it become the most awarded campaign in the history of the awards. In 2014, the social marketing campaign released 11 more videos, which collectively amassed 25 million views. A Dumb Ways to Die Christmas single was released and made it into the top 10 in a couple of countries, reaching number six on the Australian charts for Christmas singles. The social marketing campaign also included the development of video games. By 2015, the first game had 97 million downloads and was played 1.6 billion times. The second game went to number one in 83 countries and in two weeks had over two million downloads. The social marketing campaign was the most visible but not the only component of this health promotion program. The strategy portfolio also included strategies to create supportive environments, such as new reporting hotlines and incentives to encourage drivers and station staff to report near misses, and strategies to develop personal skills, such as a primary school education program that used Dumb

Ways to Die messages in class-based activities implemented by Metro Trains Melbourne staff.

Social marketing is built on recognition of the powerful influence of the mass media on the choices that people make. Thus, a good understanding of marketing can be a valuable asset to health practitioners, and the following section builds on the common characteristics of social marketing presented above. There will be further discussion about social media later in the chapter.

Social marketing activities

Social marketing activities are designed to educate, motivate or advocate. If the purpose of the social marketing strategy is to educate, the activities will focus on the provision of information and demonstration of skills. The line between social marketing and health education (Chapter 7) is blurred. However, social marketing is generally more focused on the emotional aspects of the issue, and seeks to change the values and attitudes of a specific population group about the issue.

Social marketing activities may be designed to motivate people to take some type of action. The techniques used to do so often include the use of strong visual or sound methods. Sun Sound is one example of a social marketing campaign designed to motivate people to take action to protect themselves from the sun (see Insight 8.1).

Finally, social marketing activities may be designed to advocate for change by influencing the socio-political sphere. If well designed, social marketing activities can have a strong influence on people and organisations with the power to change the settings or experiences in other people's lives. The capacity of social marketing to influence social values, policy development and political decision making is especially valuable, because advocacy has the capacity to move the responsibility for change away from individuals and towards creating a supportive environment for health and wellbeing (Donovan & Henley, 2010; Egger et al., 2013).

Social marketing campaigns typically involve an organised set of communication activities, including advertising, publicity materials, edutainment, advocacy and lobbying. Advertising uses memorable visuals and slogans, which are repeated frequently to promote recognition of the message and association with the desired change. Perhaps most notable are well-funded national campaigns about key social health issues, such as safe driving and smoking cessation. Campaigns conducted in Australia by the Transport Accident

INSIGHT 8.1 Sun Sound

The aim of the Sun Sound program was to improve youth behaviour related to sun protection. The Cancer Council NSW partnered with a university, research and communication agencies, and local governments to develop, implement and evaluate Sun Sound in outdoor recreational settings. Formative research revealed that although youth knowledge around sun protection was good, their sun protection behaviour remained poor. The campaign focus was a musical jingle broadcast between 11 am and 3 pm at beaches and pools to remind young people to take sun protection action at the time and point of sun exposure. Evaluation of the pilot program found that it was an effective cue to action. The campaign demonstrated that it is possible to influence behaviour by focusing on audiences at the actual point that behaviour occurs, using research-informed insights and a relevant marketing mix (Potente et al., 2013).

Commission (n.d.), the Cancer Council Australia's QUIT (n.d.-a) and Sun Safety (n.d.-c), and the Smoking: Not Our Future campaign from New Zealand (Research New Zealand, 2008) have achieved prominence. Recently, advertising relating to reducing greenhouse emissions has also been prominent.

Advertising campaigns are usually complemented by publicity materials. Publicity materials include media releases, op-ed articles, as well as other media and products. Images, logos and slogans are used consistently across web pages, social media platforms, and give-aways such as stickers, T-shirts, fridge magnets, water bottles, hats, and many other creative options to promote wider awareness, and as a final prompt to a behaviour. For example, publicity materials are produced for the Cancer Council Sun safety programs including the Slip, Slop, Slap, Seek and Slide campaign for sun protection in schools (Cancer Council Australia, n.d.-b).

Edutainment involves using radio, television, or movies to promote or change social awareness about various issues. A portmanteau of 'education entertainment', edutainment takes advantage of people tuning into a program for the entertainment value and being exposed to health promotion messages along the way. Topics such as respect for people suffering mental health problems, safe sex, domestic violence and sun safety have all been proactively incorporated into radio, television and movie productions. Health promotion professionals provide advice in script development drawing on research evidence. For an excellent example of the successful and diverse use of edutainment, see the comprehensive descriptions of programs offered and evaluated by the Soul City Institute for Social Justice across Southern Africa. The Soul City television program was developed to reduce the spread and incidence of HIV infection. A range of additional social wellbeing themes are now covered, using television, radio, print, peer support and community health organisation partnerships for community members of all ages, schools and specific subpopulations. In addition, there is now a strong health promotion workforce capacity-building program through a university link, to ensure wide dissemination of health promotion messages and professional support for those seeking assistance. The Institute's annual report outlines the effectiveness of linking social marketing edutainment with community-based primary health care activities to bring clear health improvements over time (Soul City Institute for Social Justice, n.d.). The program provides an integrated multimedia communication platform carefully crafted by formative research and is well evaluated.

Social marketing activities may focus on advocacy and lobbying. There have been many social marketing campaigns advocating for specific causes and lobbying for specific actions. For example, GetUp (https://www.getup.org.au/) is an online social action organisation in Australia. This is a powerful form of organised advocacy, and in some cases has had a marked effect on new policy, policy direction or funding for specific projects. Less organised but sometimes just as powerful are spontaneous Twitter exchanges that have spread rapidly (gone viral) and in the process have changed social values about a topic and influenced people in positions of power. Letters to the editor and media releases, discussed later in the chapter, are also examples of advocacy and lobbying.

A brief background of social marketing

While they are seen as selective primary health care approaches because they focus on change (usually by an individual) around a selected issue or risk, social marketing strategies are aimed at a large well-defined audience.

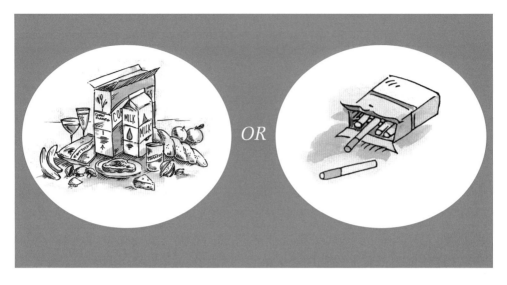

FIGURE 8.1 Three meals for two people OR one pack of cigarettes
Source: Drawn by Morris, P. Bendigo: La Trobe University.

At the national level, social marketing is an example of how national governments might become involved in health promotion. An integrated population health approach is demonstrated in health promotion strategies to improve fruit and vegetable consumption by school children, for example, or to reduce smoking. Social marketing has been used extensively in the anti-smoking campaigns of various state or national Cancer Councils, such as Quit in Victoria (http://www.quit.org.au/) and ASH New Zealand (Action on Smoking and Health, http://www.ash.org.nz/). Different messages have been used over the years, usually emphasising the personal, physical or wider social and financial costs of smoking and its complications (see Fig. 8.1). These social marketing approaches, which clearly emphasise individual behaviour change, have been supported by personal education and support services (like the Quitline telephone service), and progressive legislative changes, including increasing tax on cigarettes, restrictions on the sale of cigarettes to minors and restrictions on smoking in public places.

The term 'social marketing' suggests that in addition to providing health information, there is the 'selling' of a social idea, bringing about gradual change in personal and social values and attitudes to that issue. The Stayin' on Track project (Insight 8.2) is an example of a project that was piloted with young Indigenous men in their transition to fatherhood (Fletcher et al., 2015). A website was developed through a partnership between the University of Newcastle and the Young and Well Cooperative Research Centre (CRC), who engaged young Indigenous men as co-creators of the website to ensure that it met the needs of other young fathers-to-be. The statement 'I would never have thought that I would've been a dad. But now that I am a dad, it's the only thing that I want to do' suggests positive personal and social values can change with support.

Social marketing as part of the strategy portfolio

Social marketing can contribute positively to individual health and wellbeing (Freeman et al., 2015; Lauckner & Whitten, 2015; Moorhead et al., 2013; Wakefield et al., 2010), if

INSIGHT 8.2 Stayin' on Track project

Online resources for the Stayin' on Track project were created for, and delivered on mobile phones. Videos about emotions, the pride of being a father, tough times, and culture and fathers were made with the aim of building a peer-to-peer network to enable information sharing and support. Real-life stories about 'Before the Birth', 'After the Birth' and 'The Big Day' were made with young Aboriginal fathers from Newcastle, Tamworth and Moree in New South Wales. The videos were made by professional film-makers and the website was advertised through Indigenous websites and social media channels. SMS texts with information about father–infant care, supporting their partner, and taking care of themselves were sent to participants every day for six weeks. Mood Tracker and Dad Tracker texts were sent regularly to ask how they were going. If the Dad clicked 'I'm OK', he received an encouraging message. If not, the system alerted a mentor and the Dad received a call to link him to services if needed.

Source: Fletcher et al. (2015); Mengage (n.d.). Further information available from: http://www.mengage.org.au/Life-Stages/Becoming-A-Father/University-of-Newcastle-Stayin-On-Track

it is part of an integrated health promotion program (Egger et al., 2005; Wakefield et al., 2010). Sustained change for social and environmental protection can be achieved when activities are carefully planned and implemented, and if there are reasonable expectations of outcome given the context in which it is being used (McKenzie-Mohr, 2011). Social marketing activities may be aimed at individuals, networks, organisations, manufacturers and planners and at community or societal (policy) levels. Social marketing strategies may result in incidental effects (Wakefield et al., 2010) but alone, without complementary health promotion strategies aimed at building healthy public policy, creating supportive environments, and strengthening community action, they are likely to have little long-term impact on behaviour (Egger et al., 2013) or health and wellbeing outcomes.

It is important to bear in mind that the advertising industry conducts considerable market research and focuses its advertising very specifically to the groups it wishes to convince. There are problems inherent in trying to emulate the larger campaigns run by well-funded national advertisers. Health practitioners at a local level most often do not have the resources or the skills to match these activities. Local initiatives will have more impact when they are based on thorough knowledge of the prospective audience (Donovan & Henley, 2010; French et al., 2009; John-Leader et al., 2008; McKenzie-Mohr, 2011; Nelson et al., 2008). Added impact can be gained if local strategies can be planned to coincide with a national media campaign about the issue, or a national 'awareness week'. Calendars of national campaigns are available and can be a valuable resource to assist planning to make the greatest impact locally. However, at other times, especially where the budget is small, or it is a specific local issue, practitioners may need to get their message across by developing their own media resources. It may be more appropriate for a health practitioner to draw on the expertise of a graphic artist or advertising agency as well as potential participants than to prepare materials 'in-house'; the combined expertise will be more successful than acting alone.

Benefits of social marketing

Social marketing approaches can have a number of benefits for communities that may enable them to make sustained change in social conditions that enhance health.

- National awareness campaigns can be 'tagged' onto local community-driven activities, thus gaining greater awareness of the issue, enhancing the credibility of a local project and bringing efficiencies in program planning.

- Social marketing strategies can be used to reflect community values and create a sense of ownership towards significant issues in a community.

- Knowledge is itself enabling and empowering. Thus, social marketing messages should provide an 'action plan' informing the person what to do if they decide to take action on the issue, and thus social marketing can build health literacy (see Chapter 7).

- Social marketing fits very well with contemporary preferences for ways of accessing information and for adaptation to internet and social media uses. Six key overarching benefits have been identified with the use of social media: increased interaction with others; more available, shared and tailored information; increased accessibility and widening access to health information; peer/social/emotional support; public health surveillance; and the potential to influence policy (Moorhead et al., 2013).

- Social marketing makes use of strong visuals and simple language; these are critically important advantages for people with limited English language and reading capacities.

- Locally relevant social marketing approaches can bring forth a groundswell in networks seeking change in an issue affecting the community.

- At a national level, social marketing can enhance people's understanding of complex issues using short, accessible and memorable messages, especially groups who may not access more traditional health education resources. A national campaign can play a significant role by increasing social awareness about an emerging issue, or on changing social values about an emerging issue. Legislative or policy change may be more readily accepted as a result.

Ethical considerations in social marketing

A significant challenge for social marketing approaches is that most commercial products offer instant gratification (and potential long-term risk), whereas the benefits of health behaviour change are often delayed. One example of attempts to counterbalance the influence of advertising products that increase health risk in many high-income nations has been the banning of some advertising; most notably tobacco advertising. The introduction of plain packaging legislation for cigarettes in Australia is an extension of advertising restriction, which was vigorously opposed by the tobacco companies. As documented in Chapter 5, smoking rates in Australia are gradually falling. This decline reflects the strong legislative controls over advertising and sale of tobacco products. Tobacco companies have moved their advertising attention to low-income nations where the high smoking rate among very young children is an indication of the effectiveness of the tobacco industry's marketing strategies. To achieve comparable declines in the sales of other products that pose a health risk, similar legislative controls would be required. These would probably be vigorously opposed, because they would be regarded as seriously eroding people's expectations about freedom of speech and freedom of choice. Health behaviours are often at odds with social pressures. For example, harm minimisation approaches contrast with strong peer pressure to drink to excess (French et al., 2009).

Legislative control of advertising raises ethical questions about the right of the State to take over the life of the individual. It raises questions about who gets to decide what is right for the population, and whether the behaviour change is socially desirable? This is by no means a simple issue; after all, it is argued that mass media advertising manipulates people's free choice, often beyond recognition (Andreasen, 2002; French et al., 2009; Keleher & MacDougall, 2016). The ongoing debate about banning television advertising of energy-dense low-nutrient foods designed specifically to appeal to children during the after school programming time is an example of this dilemma for policymakers. In addition, health risk behaviours are often complex and involve several health and wellbeing determinants, as we have outlined in earlier chapters. Short messages are necessarily simplistic and cannot account for the complexities in individual situations.

Millions of dollars are spent annually on advertising products that are profitable but may compromise health and wellbeing. Health workers, even when they are supported by national media campaigns, are in no position to match the extent to which such products are marketed—they simply do not have the same financial resources at their disposal. However, social marketing strategies can be a form of advocacy directed at policymakers, manufacturing, commercial and government systems, and social structures and the media, just as readily as they can be directed at the individual (Buresh & Gordon, 2006; Egger et al., 2013; French et al., 2009). However, with individual and structural changes there can be unintended consequences, and social marketing, like other forms of health promotion, needs to be carefully evaluated and modifications made to strategies if they are warranted (Keleher & MacDougall, 2016).

Social marketing can be used effectively as part of health promotion practice in a comprehensive primary health care context, and can be empowering for those it is designed to assist (Buresh & Gordon, 2006; Lauckner & Whitten, 2015). Social marketing can be used as a reminder of health-enhancing behaviours and can therefore complement other health promotion strategies (Freeman et al., 2015; French et al., 2009; Lauckner & Whitten, 2015; McKenzie-Mohr, 2011; Moorhead et al., 2013; Potente et al., 2013). Social marketing can inform the public about the importance of new health policy or legislation at the same time that those changes are being implemented. It can be used to influence manufacturing, such as in safer vehicle design. However, social marketing is not inherently based on the principles of critical health promotion and comprehensive primary health care, and so it is up to governments, organisations and health practitioners to ensure that these principles are reflected in any social marketing strategies being planned, implemented and evaluated.

The whole notion of social marketing does not sit comfortably with everyone. The tactics advertising companies use are considered by some to be unethical because they are based on the idea of influencing people's choices, often without their awareness. Using the same tactics for social marketing raises some ethical concerns (Andreasen, 2006). Truss and White (2009, Chapter 9) sum up the ethical dilemmas in social marketing, stating 'if it can be used effectively for good, might not some agencies, authorities, or corporations seek to use it for less worthy purposes?' Keleher and MacDougall (2016, p. 250, citing Rothschild, 2001) provide a number of guidelines for ethical practice in social marketing, including: being sure that the underlying policy approach is ethical and equitable in the first place; using strategies that achieve the greatest good for the greatest number of people; allowing an option to choose or not to choose the change; making sure that social marketing is the best approach when compared with other behaviour-change methods such as health education or legislation; using methods that have been evaluated to be effective; and not consciously trying to manipulate the intended audience.

A great deal of mainstream media advertising is built on harmful stereotypes of people. Social marketing often accepts the stereotypes and builds on them unquestioningly, rather than challenging them. There is much work to be done in challenging these stereotypes, which themselves can contribute to narrow views of health and normality and reduced feelings of self-worth in individuals who don't fit the 'norm'. If social marketing builds on these stereotypes, rather than challenging them, the overall health benefit from any messages may be limited (Donovan & Henley, 2010; French et al., 2009).

Key criticisms and recommendations

The following are the key criticisms of social marketing.

- In order to generate wider appeal, the socially 'ideal' type of person is used in marketing images, namely young, white, able bodied, straight sized, cis gender, conventionally attractive, neurotypical, heterosexual people. The intended audience for the message may not associate themselves and their situation with the message. In the bigger picture, social marketing can perpetuate oppression through the cultural marginalisation and invisibility of people without these privileged identities.

- It may ignore the socio-ecological determinants of health. Messages are usually short and cannot accommodate wider social issues. This has potential to reinforce the disadvantage of vulnerable groups and raises the potential of 'victim blaming' (discussed in detail in Chapter 2).

- It has a single-issue focus, rather than emphasising holistic wellbeing.

- There is potential to manipulate vulnerable members of the intended audience.

- It has generally been used as an individual, behaviour change strategy.

- Limitations for social media specifically have been identified, which primarily centre on quality, lack of reliability, confidentiality and privacy (Moorhead et al., 2013).

Freeman and colleagues (2015) report that although social media is potentially effective in recruiting participants and motivating them to make 'small, concrete' behaviour changes and can be used for inexpensive small and large-scale projects, outcome evaluation models are needed. Wakefield and colleagues (2010) make several recommendations regarding media campaigns generally for governments, professional bodies and practitioners: comprehensive approaches to improving population health behaviours should include mass media campaigns; these campaigns should be based on sound research of the potential audience and pilot testing should occur; frequent and widespread messages over time require secure funding; complementary policies that support the change or disincentives for not changing should be considered; and outcomes should be rigorously evaluated.

STEPS OF SOCIAL MARKETING

In the context of the preceding discussion, it is clear that social media has the potential for both benefits and harms. Ensuring that the principles of critical health promotion and comprehensive primary health care, especially social justice, are integrated into social marketing strategies will enhance the potential for benefits and reduce the potential for harms. Thus, the principles of critical health promotion must be enacted throughout the planning, implementation and evaluation steps. There are a number of resources that can guide the process; for example, see Public Health Ontario's *Twelve Steps to Developing a Health Communication Campaign* (2012). Doug McKenzie-Mohr's (2011) five-stage community-based social marketing program, described in the following section, is an excellent guide to ensuring thorough planning of social marketing approaches that take into account the personal characteristics and social settings of the potential audience.

Step 1: Select behaviours

Many social marketing strategies are unsuccessful because insufficient background research is undertaken in the community assessment and planning phases of the health promotion practice cycle. Research, including direct observation, is needed to identify the specific actions that are contributing to the behaviour that has been identified as the health and wellbeing priority. Assumptions may be made by health practitioners that if more information is provided to people, their behaviour will change. Assumptions may be made by marketing companies that they understand the priority audience segment or that what worked elsewhere will be the same in each location. However, such assumptions may be incorrect. Each social marketing campaign will have unique characteristics (French et al., 2009). The first step in deciding on the specific focus of a social marketing strategy is to understand the priority audience.

Successful social marketing campaigns achieve their aim of creating awareness of an issue or bringing about change because they understand the characteristics of their audience; their knowledge, attitudes, values and beliefs. For example, age, gender and personality traits have been reported as influential in social media usage (Moorhead et al., 2013). Gathering information to clearly understand the priority audience enables the strategy to be specifically focused on a small, relatively homogeneous audience segment. The aim is to address and build on the existing knowledge and beliefs of the priority audience, and to correct misconceptions that are impeding the adoption of health-enhancing actions. Using a health behaviour change planning model (such as those set out in Chapter 7) at this stage of planning will enable a broad understanding of the priority audience. Understanding the characteristics of this specific audience segment who have relevant characteristics in common, and directing the message to them, will have more impact. Segmenting the audience in this way will mean the strategy is likely to reach the priority group, saving money and effort that could be wasted in a 'one-size-fits-all approach', and will help prevent the possibility of failing to engage with the group(s) that the strategy most wants to reach (Egger et al., 2005; Kotler et al., 2002).

Outlined below is the key information that needs to be identified about a priority audience in order to create the right message for them. McVey and Walsh (2009) and Donovan and Henley (2010) describe a similar process as generating 'insight'. For social marketing using advocacy for social or policy change, the themes would need to be modified accordingly.

- Demographic characteristics
    - Age range, gender distribution, work characteristics, income and education levels, where they live and work and specific cultural characteristics.
- Behavioural characteristics
    - What behaviour is currently putting them or their environment at risk?
    - What are the factors that reinforce the existing behaviours?
    - What are their perceptions about the risk or seriousness associated with their current behaviour?
    - What are their perceptions about the costs and benefits of the desired change?
    - What are their perceptions about the barriers to change?

- Psychological characteristics
    - What are their attitudes, values and beliefs about the issue or behaviour?
    - What are their main and preferred sources of health information—their media preferences?
    - What or who influences their readiness to change an existing behaviour?

McKenzie-Mohr (2011) identifies that the barriers to making a sustainable change in behaviour are often behaviour-specific; that is, one small step in the sequence of actions may be the barrier to change. He states the behavioural analysis must identify the 'end-state, non-divisible behaviours'; that is, understand each separate behaviour that contributes to the whole activity. Consider, for example, the many separate behaviours involved in 'reducing home energy consumption' or 'eating a nutritious breakfast'.

When this analysis is done, consider the potential impact and probability of changing each behaviour. What difference will each change make; what chance is there of it happening; and how will the program staff know if there has been a change?

Step 2: Identify barriers and benefits

This is the step that provides the evidence for chosen strategies. Doing this step thoroughly will enable development of appropriate strategies based on evidence, rather than on assumptions. The process of understanding the barriers to changing each of the non-divisible behaviours, and the benefits of it, is part of the community assessment stage presented in Chapter 4. In the same way, the sources of data can be:

- literature review/background papers
- direct observations (unobtrusive, active and non-active)
- focus groups to explore perceptions and current behaviours
- a survey to get generalisable community-wide advice.

In this step, different types of data are cross-referenced in order to gain an understanding of the complexity of an aspect of people's lives that results in certain behaviours (French et al., 2009). Detailed examination identifies the barriers to people making the changes and the potential, actual and perceived benefits of making that change (McKenzie-Mohr, 2011). Don't assume that the reason people will decide to change will be for the altruistic reasons that a program planner might espouse.

Step 3: Develop strategies

The activities involved in the first two steps constitute market or customer segmentation. Market segmentation involves dividing the potential audience for the behaviour change into segments according to their demographic and other characteristics (Step 1 above); selecting the segment of the audience who will be the specific focus of the messages (Step 2 above); and then developing a detailed marketing mix that will reach and engage the chosen audience (Donovan & Henley, 2010; French et al., 2009). The marketing mix is based on the 4Ps.

- *Product*: In social marketing, the product is the underlying benefit that change will bring to the person, rather than a tangible item. Product value will be augmented with additional offerings such as training, or monitoring equipment, and reinforced by a recognised symbol or logo, trusted endorsements, consistent messages.

- *Price:* In social marketing, price is about the cost of the behaviour change, including the financial, social, cultural or political cost. Social marketing must reduce the cost of making the change, such as offering inducements or making the change cheaper or easier to access or understand. The general principle is to reduce the costs of making the change and to increase the costs of not making the recommended change to behaviour.

- *Promotion:* It is important to find the mix of paid advertising, unpaid publicity, public relations and community events that will be most effective in reaching and engaging the chosen audience. A main point is to make the key message available just at the point of decision making between the desired behaviour and the alternative.

- *Place*: This refers to how, in what locations and when the message will be disseminated, and what other supports or activities may be necessary to enable people to understand and easily make the change (Donovan & Henley, 2010; French et al., 2009). Creating a setting where it is easier for people to make the change is essential. Understanding when people are more or less likely to perform the non-desired behaviour can assist with placement of cues.

Selecting and designing the mix of strategies is a complex process demanding thorough research, use of behaviour change theory, and careful, collaborative discussion. Some specific social marketing strategies relating to dealing with the media are presented in more detail later in this chapter, but the following is a summary of McKenzie-Mohr's advice (2011) about ways to enhance common approaches to make them most effective.

- Get a public and durable commitment. When people who have expressed an interest in making a change make a public commitment to that change in front of others, such as their family, the public or the media, they are more likely to make and sustain the change than if they make that commitment in private.

- Build community support, using social norms. When community members make public their decision to change behaviour this also creates a social norm about that action; people are more likely to adhere to a behaviour change when they observe others doing it.

- Foster social diffusion. Find ways to showcase the desirable behaviour and make it widely visible. One important strategy is to engage early adopters and use them through a range of media, as exemplars.

- Support the maintenance of a desirable change to a repetitive behaviour with the use of prompts, ideally at the site of the decision about the behaviour (on the fridge, on the rubbish bin, near the switch, next to the shower, etc.). This is where advertising prompts and 'give-aways' have their particular benefit.

- Communicate the message effectively using vividly presented simple information.

- Provide incentives which enhance motivation to act, especially where a once-only change is needed. Incentives should not be used to encourage compliance with a repetitive behaviour.

- Make it easy for the person to act, make it more convenient than before.

Step 4: Pilot testing the strategies

Pilot test the strategies once they have been designed using exactly the same methods as would be used in a wider roll-out. Only trial what can realistically be replicated on a population-wide basis in relation to cost and staffing. This is where process evaluation discussed in Chapter 4 is conducted and will be discussed further in this chapter in relation to social media.

Step 5: Implement the successful strategies

In a broad-scale implementation and evaluation:

- use local media for added impact
- use research on barriers and benefits as the basis for evaluation planning
- give feedback to the community.

Using the five-step process outlined above, the following are some additional guidelines in order to make social marketing approaches more effective.

- The barriers to behaviour change are unique for each desirable behaviour or particular action. Make the distinction between the behaviour and the component activities—barriers will reside in the level of the component actions.

- Do the barriers and benefits research for each behaviour; don't assume barriers are common across behaviours.

- The perceived benefits of a behaviour change do not have to have anything to do with the reason for taking action. For example, people are less convinced to take up cycling to work for the likely health benefits than they are by the evidence the cycling may be quicker.

- Barriers and benefits do not have to be real—just perceived. (For example, parents perceive that allowing their children to walk to school reduces their safety—when it might be that the threat of injury is just as great when being dropped off at a congested school gate.)

- Cost-effectiveness of a behaviour change strategy is an important consideration; graph and compare the potential of the various options before selecting strategies.

- Where possible make the behaviour change people are engaging in visible (invisible activities don't foster social norms).

- Consider strategies that make the desirable behaviour the default option— people have to opt out; policy change can support this approach.

- When suggesting behaviour change options, offer several choices and people are likely to do one of them. If the desired behaviour is not convenient this will undermine the effectiveness of the program.

- Provide positive feedback when behaviours are repetitive and people are engaged, in order to sustain their behaviour. Give social approval for adopting a desired behaviour. Overt disapproval alienates people.

- Don't offer rewards for habitual behaviour because removal of the incentives will result in compliance levels equal to or lower than before the incentive was offered. Incentives for habitual behaviours undermine the person's internal motivation for change. Prompts will increase impact.

- Gaining attention is essential. If the activity doesn't capture the people's attention it is not worth the effort of doing and making it public. Publicise local success stories—it will add to the momentum of adoption which can be very slow at the start, but speed up over time (Andreasen, 2006; Donovan & Henley, 2010; McKenzie-Mohr, 2011).

INTEGRATING SOCIAL MEDIA AND SOCIAL MARKETING

Social media applications are now an integral part of social marketing strategies. Platforms such as Wikipedia, YouTube, Facebook, Twitter, Snapchat, TikTok, Instagram and virtual game and social worlds all form part of the 'social media ecology' (Kietzmann et al., 2011, in Moorhead et al., 2013). Thackeray and colleagues (2012) suggest that these applications may help put the consumer at the centre of the social marketing process because they may enable people to be engaged in a communication process. If this engagement is truly participatory, then it is consistent with the values and principles of critical health promotion. However, if it is used as a one-way 'output channel', then this would perpetuate the 'top-down' approach of selective health promotion. Neiger and colleagues (2012, p. 160) report that social media have been used in health promotion programs for the purpose of:

- communication with consumers for market insights (CDC, 2010; Neiger et al., 2012)

- establishment of a brand with consumers (Neiger et al., 2012)

- dissemination of critical information (CDC, 2010 in Neiger et al., 2012)

- expansion of reach to include more diverse consumers (CDC, 2010 in Neiger et al., 2012)

- fostering of public engagement and partnerships (CDC, 2010 in Neiger et al., 2012).

The social media ecology needs to be understood to ensure the quality and reliability of the information and ensure the confidentiality and privacy of the users. Drawing on the work of Butterfield (2003, cited in Moorhead et al., 2013), Webb (2004), Smith (2007, cited in Moorhead et al., 2013) and Kietzmann and colleagues (2011), and Moorhead and colleagues (2013) developed a honeycomb framework of seven building blocks for understanding and using social media, comprising:

- *identity—the extent to which users reveal themselves;*

- *conversations—the extent to which users communicate with each other;*

- *sharing—the extent to which users exchange, distribute and receive content;*

- *presence—the extent to which users know if others are available;*

- *relationships—the extent to which users relate to one another;*

- *reputation—the extent to which users know the social standing of others and content; and*

- *groups—the extent to which users are ordered or form communities.*

(p. 2)

Including social media in a social marketing strategy has been described as a four-step process (Thackeray et al., 2012). First, describe the audience and find out what social media the consumers use. This assessment will form part of your community assets and needs assessment (see Chapter 4). Second, identify the purpose of using such a strategy. What is the purpose of engaging with the consumers? Is it to ask for feedback about the organisation, program or products? Or is it to gauge the attitudes, beliefs or information about a particular issue? In this step, the purpose is to engage the potential participant and encourage them to talk to their friends and acquaintances, invite them to be participants in the social marketing strategy, support each other, and then 'recruit them to design products and services' (p. 167). This forms part of the planning stage, which involves designing the program and developing an action plan (see Chapter 4). The third step is to cement the relationship. Using the honeycomb framework outlined above will help the organisation be transparent about the approach; that is, the process, and the risks and benefits to the consumers. Ethical guidelines and how the strategy will be evaluated need to be clearly articulated by the organisation and to the participants. The final step is to choose the technology. The choice will be a response to the community assessment and proposed plan developed with community participation. Successful implementation of the technology will be demonstrated by the extent of audience engagement and whether real dialogue has been fostered. Neiger and colleagues (2012) provide an excellent discussion on process evaluation of social media applications in health promotion and outline the various metrics that can be used (see More to Explore at the end of this chapter).

SOCIAL MARKETING SKILLS

In this section, brief guidance is provided to ensure the effectiveness of some of the most common social marketing activities that health practitioners will initiate or take part in when engaged in health promotion practice in a comprehensive primary health care context.

Setting social marketing objectives

In Chapters 4 and 7, the development of SMART objectives (Specific, Measurable, Achievable, Relevant, Time-bound) was emphasised; that is, the importance of clearly defining what the activity will achieve. Social marketing objectives are primarily concerned with increasing knowledge about an issue, producing favourable attitudes to a desirable change, influencing social norms within the priority audience, influencing public opinion to be in line with changing social values, and producing modest behaviour change in vulnerable people. It is very easy to set objectives that are too 'grand' for the style of message and/or the spread of the message. Health communication objectives will need to link to a wider social agenda (such as a national health priority area or national environmental strategy), a local govern-ment population health or environmental goal, or a community-based initiative. In this way, a strategy for a wider purpose will generate objectives for the social marketing component of the campaign.

Consider possible communication options

Selecting the mode of communication most likely to reach the priority audience is an important step. This decision needs to be balanced by budget considerations. These con-siderations reinforce the benefit of an analysis of all possible actions that would overcome the barriers to a specific behaviour change, and of analysing the costs and impacts of each potential strategy. Where possible, consider the multiplier benefits of 'tagging' a local campaign onto a national social marketing strategy; for example, have a local body liberation campaign on International No-diet Day. A very focused message will produce a good return if it can reach the desired audience (Buresh & Gordon, 2006; McKenzie-Mohr, 2011).

Make use of any 'free' opportunities for raising awareness about the issue, such as letters to the editor and editorials in newspapers, free social service announcements on radio and television, and news segments in agency newsletters in printed and online versions and other forms of online communication including YouTube, Facebook, Instagram, TikTok and Twitter. Some of these options may only be available in partnership with paid advertising. Consider whether the paid advertising will reach the priority audience and select the most cost-effective option based on market research (French et al., 2009; John-Leader et al., 2008; McKenzie-Mohr, 2011). For example, mass circulation newspapers have a very low readership in some audience segments but paid advertising on YouTube, Facebook or Instagram can boost the profile of a message to a younger audience who are less likely to be newspaper readers. Consider the following options.

- Newsletters. Identify how frequently a newsletter is published, what the publication requirements are and whether the readership fits with your strategy. Prepare the script and graphics to enable easy access for the reader.

- Media releases. Sometimes a media release is published 'as is', especially when photographs are provided at the time of submission, or a photo opportunity is identified. More details about writing a media release are provided in the next section.

- Internet media. A new, interactive website may be the mode of information-seeking preferred by some audiences. Internet sources are widely used as a means of individual research, and YouTube can demonstrate a desirable behaviour. Social media can provide very powerful commentary and endorsement. Information-exchange options such as group sessions, chat rooms and blogs are widely consulted. Consider using these means to engage an audience in the development phase also.

- Posters. In electronic and hard copy, these should contain the key messages in a form that attracts attention to the issue and the specific audience being sought. Posters should not be too complicated, but should contain contact information relevant to the theme. Many people now have the skills to create a web page and to load new material including poster-style pages and links onto them, and this provides an economical way of spreading a message that is more attractive than a simple email or text.

- Static displays. Displays that are designed to interest a passing audience are useful at venues where people congregate, such as shopping centres and farming field days. They can be very effective in showcasing early adopters and success stories. Interest is enhanced when there is an additional 'hook' to attract the audience, such as health screening or free items. These sites can also be very useful for market research about social issues and community values.

- Brochures, pamphlets and fact sheets. Distribution can be in hard copy or via email. They may be used to engage participants and/or to provide more detailed information that supports a social marketing campaign. They should always contain contact information. More detail about their preparation is provided in the next section.

- Promotional materials. Distributed free or for sale, these can be produced relevant to the characteristics of the market, and are especially useful as prompts to reinforce or remind habitual behaviours. They can be useful to showcase those who have adopted a change, or to enhance formation of a social norm about a particular behaviour. People are attracted to free items, such as stickers, writing pads, pens, fridge magnets, bookmarks, T-shirts, drink bottles and so on. The items are often costly to produce, but the advantage is that the message is retained. Consider engaging the audience in selection, design and production of the materials.

- Advertising. Print, television, radio, outdoor, or online options may be considered. Consider cost and audience preferences.

Using the mass media skilfully

Working effectively with the mass media requires skill. Communication skills are fundamental to the success of social marketing; these include having an outgoing personal style or presence; that is, being confident and verbally articulate and having good skills at written communication. Using the mass media strongly and articulately can raise the social value of health practitioners as knowledgeable and skilful in health promotion practice; this increases the credibility of their messages, as Buresh and Gordon (2006) have demonstrated with raising the professional profile of the nursing profession. Chapter 5 provided guidance for advocacy in policy change, and the media strategies described there will be applicable when working with a range of mass media in social marketing. As with any other specialty, it is wise to seek out the support and advice of experts when planning a major media campaign, especially in the area of graphic design and developing materials suited to online audiences. The following hints are suggested to help health practitioners develop an effective working relationship with local media outlets.

Preliminary work

An important first step in using the mass media is establishing contact with the people who make the decisions in local newspapers, radio stations and television stations, as well as the writers and production people (Buresh & Gordon, 2006; Egger et al., 2013; French et al., 2009). Getting to know these people may increase the chance of the articles or stories being accepted. Find out how to present the stories so that they are more likely to be accepted. Find out about the deadlines for copy. It can be very frustrating to miss the deadline and to have the story or campaign run too late for other elements of the program. Similarly, it is useful to explore the organisations that are willing to provide free social marketing advertising, to create a link to a social marketing campaign or website, or to canvass social marketing issues through their interactive web contacts such as Twitter. These media and organisational contacts may also be able to provide some valuable advice on how to improve media presentation skills.

Check the local paper and radio station to see if particular journalists or interviewers seem to have an interest in health issues, and then establish a working relationship with them. Working with those people will be much more useful, since they are the ones most likely to be interested in health promotion programs. They may also be more inclined to call for information about other issues should they need it. Establishing an ongoing relationship in this way can be useful for both health workers and media professionals (Buresh & Gordon, 2006; Egger et al., 2005).

A word of warning, however; check the workplace protocol for media releases or other media material linked to the organisation. Many health agencies require all contact with the mass media, and all media resources, including online media communications, to be approved by the chief executive officer or a designated representative. Similarly, web content and social media posts may be managed through a single office. If that is the case, use the correct channels and prepare the material sufficiently in advance to enable it to be reviewed and passed on. Most organisations using social media (rather than private users) have now developed a social media policy which sets out protocols for loading materials, using them in other forums and dealing with the need for censorship.

Elements of a newsworthy item

News is supposed to be an event or statement which is interesting, important, exciting or informative for anyone who might be affected by it. Regularly monitoring various forms of news reporting will highlight the different types of items being reported—some will report the dramatic or unique, some will report the health risks or benefits of technology, some will report on costs and so on (Buresh & Gordon, 2006, Chapter 6).

It is important to present items on health topics in a fashion that makes them just as interesting as items about other topics such as fashion or sport, or to prepare them in a way that fits with the style of the media where the item would ideally be placed. Elements that can help make an item newsworthy include the following.

- Information. The item will need to give information that is new to people or provide a new angle on what they know.

- Timeliness. The item will need to be presented at a time that fits in with other local or national events. Indeed, part of the skill in producing newsworthy items is in taking advantage of other events that have already proved newsworthy by 'dovetailing' into them. If the item is to be timely, it will also need to be presented far enough ahead of any action in which people are being encouraged to become involved, so that they have the opportunity to plan for participation if they wish to. Perhaps the greatest advantage of online interactive communications is their ability to provide almost instant commentary and feedback on a social issue. It takes little time to pose the question or raise the topic, and the range and strength of response can be a means of changing social perceptions about an issue (and censoring what are perceived as unacceptable views) and the responses can provide very valuable evidence to support ancillary social marketing, and other health promotion strategies designed to address the health and wellbeing priority.

- Significance and relevance. If the relevance may not be obvious to the whole of the audience, the item should outline the significance of the issues to that particular audience segment.

- Scope. The item will need to be relevant to many community members or a significant group in the community, or a number of different media are used in order to reach a wider cross-section. Having influential Twitter followers can disseminate ideas very widely and rapidly. See also the notes earlier in this chapter on market analysis and segmentation.

- Interest. The item will need to be interesting to the audience. Items can be made more newsworthy by linking the story to a national or historical issue. Create an opportunity for photojournalism—images can make a story come alive.

- Human interest. The item is more likely to be newsworthy if it is made directly relevant to the lives of ordinary people or the life of the community; where appropriate, use quotes from experts or local people who are affected by the news item, or pose a question that challenges people to understand more.

- Uniqueness. The item is more likely to be newsworthy if it presents an angle not found in other stories about the issue or it uses unique visuals or other media.

Addressing as many of the abovementioned elements as possible increases the likelihood of the item being accepted for use in any media. Remember, however, that these are a guide only, and an item that really stands out on one or two of these points may be more newsworthy than an item that just satisfies each point. Decisions about mainstream newsworthiness are made more on the perception of the editor than the application of any equation. The way in which the story is presented and how it appeals to the editor will be a key factor. Another key factor in mainstream media will be the time that a story is submitted and what other stories have come in that day. It is not uncommon for an item not deemed newsworthy by mainstream media to 'go viral' or generate very wide awareness and commentary on social media, and then emerge later on radio or television.

In print, radio and television, some days are easier for having stories accepted because they are less likely to be days when the media is dealing with many stories. Get to know the usual patterns of the media in the local geographic area, and get to know the journalists. One additional technique that has been used with success, particularly in regional areas, is to arrange sponsorship of health promotion activities by mass media outlets.

Writing to persuade: writing letters to the editor and others

Advocacy and lobbying techniques include writing letters and media releases. The key to success when writing a media release, a letter to the editor of a media outlet, or a letter to a member of parliament is to write persuasively. Writing persuasively takes some practice, but there are a few simple tips to increase the chance that the written material will present a persuasive argument (Egger et al., 1993).

- Use a simple, readable font (such as Arial), double spacing and a wide margin.
- Keep sentences short and sharp.
- Use plain language rather than complex language; write to express not impress.
- Keep the message simple, clear and as brief as possible; avoid unnecessary words (examine the length of letters previously published for guidance).
- Bring a new angle to a controversial topic.
- Discuss the wider impact of an issue, rather than just providing personal comment.
- Present constructive criticism, rather than simply being critical; avoid using excess emotional language.
- Tie in with your reader's experience where possible.
- Use terms your reader can picture; prefer the familiar word.
- Put verbs (action) into the language for added impact.
- Make full use of variety.
- Make your comments amusing, where appropriate.
- Check the media outlet to which you are writing for any guidelines on presentation of letters.
- If you wish to have your letter published anonymously, you can request this, but you will still need to supply your name and address, explaining why you want your name withheld.
- If your letter does not appear, you can contact the letters editor to find out why. It is not unusual for letters to take a number of weeks to be published.

Writing media releases

Rather than merely letting a journalist know that an important event is soon to occur, or that a particular issue warrants discussion, and hoping that they will write an article about it, you can write your own media release. This increases the chance that the story will run, because most of the work has already been done for the media outlet. A well-structured and persuasive media release may provide all the information that convinces the editor that the item is newsworthy. Editors will often reject potential news items simply because they do not have enough information at their fingertips to warrant pursuing the story.

As well as being clearly written, the media release must be well structured. There are four main steps in the development and structure of a persuasive writing style suitable for these purposes. These guidelines for structure break 'the rules' of a usual essay structure, which traditionally presents the background, develops a logical argument by presenting the evidence in a systematic manner and makes recommendations for action in the conclusion. The sequence is reversed in a media release:

1. Get the reader's attention.
2. Arouse the reader's interest.
3. Tell the reader what action to take.
4. Motivate the reader to take action.

Get the reader's attention

The first piece of information presented in a media release is the most newsworthy; what has been discovered, what new opportunity for participation is available, or what emerging issue needs to be addressed. This most interesting point will also provide the suggested title for the media story.

Two additional ways in which to get the reader's attention are to use an attractive layout, and make the content relevant to the reader. The layout of the document will give the reader an idea of whether they want to read it, and this is therefore very important. It includes a title that grabs the reader's attention, together with the use of headings and white space to help break up the document. These will be discussed in more detail below. Making the content relevant to the reader starts with being clear about whom the article is intended for, and writing with that audience in mind.

Arouse the reader's interest

The reader's interest will be aroused with the first sentence, which also outlines the audience group for the item. This is followed by a brief outline of why the item is relevant or important; which people would want to learn more or take part. Use direct quotations to achieve maximum impact. It is usual for the person writing the media release to write the entire text, with quotations, and then seek approval from the person being quoted. Direct quotes must be attributed to the speaker (Buresh & Gordon, 2006).

Tell the reader what action to take

If the aim is to encourage people to act on an issue, tell them what action they can take. If this isn't done, they may feel more informed when they have finished reading, but no more certain of what to do. It is important that they know what they can do to make a difference. Although raising the topic and highlighting the issue may have convinced the reader that the message is valid, the aim is often to do more than that, and it is important to provide an easy action plan straight after the initial message.

Motivate the reader to take action

Present a succinct summary of the issues in a way that helps the reader to work through the facts and come to an opinion. This can be done by arranging evidence or background information in a logical order, explaining where necessary and documenting any new or contentious information that is presented. This is available for people who have decided the issue is relevant for them and they need the full story. Presenting the background early in an article can be a turn-off to people reading the full article and deciding whether the behaviour change is achievable. In addition to the persuasive writing tips above, the following tips for writing media releases specifically will be beneficial (Loeffler & Winston, 2014).

- Write the media release on a computer, with a regular margin (2 cm), double spacing and a regular font such as Calibri or Times New Roman. Convert the document to a PDF and attach to a covering email.
- Use company letterhead so that the organisation presenting the release is clearly identifiable.
- Ensure that the release is clearly dated, or that the date for publication of the material is provided. Ideally, only send material for immediate release.
- Clearly mark the document with the heading 'Media Release'.
- Suggest an attractive title; one that grabs immediate attention, is short but has high impact.
- Keep the release short—no more than a page is recommended.
- Include quotations from relevant people—create links to local people and events.
- Include a contact name and phone number, and be prepared to be contacted.
- Provide details of events for photo opportunities.
- The first sentences are the most important—summarise the story, commencing with the more noteworthy outcome.
- Answer the 'who-what-where-when-why-how' of the story.
- Try to write the media release in the way you would like to see it reported.

Using photographs

Whether submitting a media release to a journalist, or media outlet or simply asking them to cover a particular issue, providing a photograph or advising of a photo opportunity, will help the story in two ways. First, it will increase the chance that the story will be published, because it will be a more interesting piece to publish. Second, because the story has visual appeal, more people are likely to read it when it appears. Photographs can attract a reader and persuade just as successfully as words, and sometimes even more so. If you are providing a photograph, it must be a high resolution. Be sure to refer directly to the topic of the photo in the media release and provide details for the caption (Loeffler & Winston, 2014).

Preparing for a radio or television interview

Radio and television interviews are useful means of getting across a message to a wide audience. However, the pace is usually fast, and complex issues are often not given the depth they may require. Thorough preparation is important to ensure the desired message is presented accurately and persuasively (Buresh & Gordon, 2006; Egger et al., 2005; Egger et al., 1993).

Wherever possible, present the interviewer with a list of the questions that need to be asked to cover the topic. Clarify the basic points with the interviewer beforehand. There is nothing worse than a two-minute interview disappearing without the message being put across because the interviewer did not understand a basic point and subsequently asked irrelevant questions.

In addition to presenting the interviewer with questions, prepare the answers, even on familiar topics. It is very easy to become nervous and forget the message. Also, because of the pace, the most important things must go first. There is no shame in not doing totally off-the-cuff interviews; indeed, only very experienced interviewees do this successfully.

If it is not possible to prepare questions beforehand, discuss what the interviewer plans on asking you. Use this discussion as an opportunity to suggest other appropriate questions. Interviewers usually appreciate any suggestions that will improve the quality of the interview.

Find out if the interview is going to be pre-taped or live. If it is pre-taped, there may be an opportunity for it to be edited if necessary. This is useful and it may be possible to request that the interview be pre-taped. Many interviewers will be happy to oblige if it is possible. A word of warning—never assume that something that is said is 'off the record'.

Always make eye contact with the interviewer. Maintaining eye contact with the interviewer, rather than continually reading notes, is enough to help keep your voice sounding conversational rather than monotone. Talking directly to the interviewer as much as possible will help keep your voice interesting. Buresh and Gordon (2006, p. 231) provide some simple guidelines in this area:

- Prepare, prepare, prepare.
- Prepare three short memorable phrases or messages.
- Be credible.
- Be enthusiastic.
- Speak with conviction.

Controversial issues and media interviews

Since health issues can so often involve differences of opinion, it is a good idea to go into every interview expecting the unexpected. The important thing to remember when being interviewed on a controversial topic is to stay focused on the issue and not get caught up in the controversy that is being created. Repeat the main point for emphasis, rather than being distracted. This takes some self-discipline but is well worth it in order to avoid clouding the issues.

Preparing health communication materials

Using the media to support or strengthen a personal health behaviour change message is increasingly part of health promotion work. It is vital, therefore, to be able to critically review the available materials to determine whether they are appropriate. If nothing suitable is available, the following general principles may guide the way in which local materials are produced for maximum effect. It is advantageous to involve members of the intended audience in the development of the draft materials and essential to pre-test the materials before publication.

Written materials

Written materials, such as brochures, posters and booklets, can provide useful reinforcement for other health information materials and enable people to take information home with them. With any written materials, a few key elements can make the difference between a readable, appealing document and one that does not invite the potential reader to go beyond a casual glance. These are:

- white space
- variety of font sizes
- readable language
- drawings and photographs.

White space

White space is simply the amount of empty space left in the document. It is very important because without adequate white space, a document can seem crowded and difficult to read. Space between words and paragraphs helps potential readers to see that the document is unlikely to swamp them, and will help them to work their way through it.

Variety of font sizes

Varying the font size and style judiciously, through the use of headings, in particular, helps to break up text. Headings that stand out also act as a summary of the document for people flipping through it, and so enable them to see if they would like to continue reading. Using rhetorical questions as headings also signals to the reader what is included in each section.

Readable language

No amount of variety in font size will counteract words that are difficult to understand or unreadable by the people the materials are supposedly designed for. So many written materials produced for health promotion contain language that makes the information in them inaccessible to many people. Research shows that texts with a high number of polysyllabic words require higher comprehension skills (Hawe et al. (1990). It is therefore essential to pre-test the materials to ensure that your materials are comprehensible for the audience with which you are planning to communicate. Several formulas for assessing the readability of education materials are readily available on the internet. Hawe and colleagues (1990, pp. 70–72) have provided a step-by-step formula called the SMOG formula, which yields an approximate reading grade. To calculate readability, take the entire passage of text being evaluated and select 10 sentences in a row near the beginning, 10 sentences in a row in the middle and 10 sentences in a row near the end of the text. Then, count every word with three or more syllables in each group of 10 sentences—even if the same word appears multiple times. Next, calculate the square root of the number derived in the previous step, and round it off to the nearest 10. That number is your SMOG Index score. Generally, written materials should be pitched at a level of complexity suitable for senior primary school students which is a SMOG Index score of about 7 or 8. Involving some of the people who will be the audience for the materials in the development process will ensure that the materials are readable and are culturally and socially appropriate, and also acknowledge the expertise of these people in issues related to their own lives.

Drawings and photographs

Drawings and photographs are key ingredients in written health communication materials. Indeed, there are times when they may appropriately represent all the writing in the document. The old saying 'A picture is worth a thousand words' is relevant here. Drawings and photographs may tell the reader a great deal more than words alone could do, and this is the case not only for people who have difficulty in reading, but for all readers.

Drawings and photographs help to make sense of any words, and may clarify things that are expressed with difficulty in words. They also give the document appeal and break up any writing in much the same way as white space.

A word of caution about drawings, however; ensure that they make sense to the people who will be the audience for the material. Drawings, like words, have readability levels. Health workers have a range of knowledge about matters of health and illness, and it is easy to forget how much of this is not shared by members of the community.

General guidelines for 'take-home' health information material

Most readers will be familiar with the display board of pamphlets and brochures in the foyer of many health agencies. Closer observation will demonstrate that some materials are much more attractive or enticing to select, and/or they convince the reader to read the full details. At times health practitioners may be called upon to design a brochure or material to advertise a forthcoming health promotion activity. Drawing on the principles of persuasive writing presented above, the following guidelines may be useful when preparing take-home material.

1. Work in partnership with members of the prospective audience to select and design the style of material and develop the wording.
2. Be as concise as possible to present the simplest possible message, using simple language. Get rid of any wasted words.
3. Short sentences help the development of an argument. They help the flow and are easier to fit into the layout of pamphlets.
4. Avoid jargon because it limits the audience and it dates the material.
5. Avoid too many definitions and too much background.
6. Use headings as 'signposts' and use a verb in the headings.
7. Pilot-test the material with other prospective clients of the resource.
8. Get feedback from minority groups who may not understand the language.
9. Allow plenty of time, prepare a draft, leave it, then return to edit it.
10. Check for completeness—ensure it provides an action plan: contact details, links to relevant agencies, and details of time and location where relevant.
11. Consider the requirements for agency or sponsor logo. Size and placement are important to agencies and sponsors. Unauthorised use or alteration of a logo may be subject to legal penalty. Agency logo placement and size may also need to reflect the size of their sponsorship of the social marketing strategy.

Audiovisual materials

Videos and audiotapes can provide useful health information in a form that is often more interesting than written materials and more accessible to people, particularly those who do not have good literacy skills, and certain age groups. They may also be preferred by those people who learn more readily through listening and watching than through reading (see Insight 8.2 Stayin' on Track and Insight 8.3 FaceSpace). Amateur productions may be quite successful if made by members of the group whose needs are being addressed, and can be very useful teaching tools—YouTube and TikTok provide a powerful illustration of this point. Materials produced by community members themselves are more likely to address a group's needs and be acceptable to it. However, presentation skills are required. Some people are better at communicating or performing in this medium than others.

> ## INSIGHT 8.3 FaceSpace: using social networking to promote safer sex to higher-risk groups
>
> The aim of the FaceSpace project was to use social networking sites (SNS) to deliver health promotion messages primarily through videos about safer sex to two key groups: people between 16 and 29 years of age (Youth Arm) and men who have sex with men. The process and impact evaluation focused on the extent to which SNS reached and engaged with these groups; the extent to which SNS increased sexual health knowledge and health-seeking behaviour; and provided recommendations for appropriate outcome evaluation. Over an 18-month period in 2009–10 fictional characters were used to interact and post content on various SNS, with sexual health promotion messages embedded within some of these postings.
>
> The results for the Youth Arm included:
>
> - Success in reaching a sample of the intended audience.
> - A total of 900 fans were reached across five Facebook pages.
> - Fans were more likely to become fans of a character of the same gender.
> - Fans reported positive feedback on the characters and narrative; interactions with the pages included posts, comments and 'likes', and the highest level of interaction occurred in the early stages of the project.
> - Interactions with fans primarily followed the uploading of videos, and peaked at 1161 unique page views in a week (approximately early January) coinciding with Facebook advertisements for the baseline survey.
> - A reduction in fan interactions with the project over time.
> - Challenges in finding the balance between educational and entertaining content (some fans reported that the health promotion messages were unclear).
> - Significant increases in sexual health knowledge between baseline and follow-up surveys (23% versus 42%, $p < 0.01$); however, no changes in sexual risk behaviours (i.e. condom use) over time.
> - A small proportion (11%) of fans reported learning something new and nearly a third (28%) reported being reminded of something they already knew.
>
> *Source: Burnet Institute (2020). For further information see Gold and colleagues (2011).*

Furthermore, producing a commercial-quality video can be expensive. It is possible to keep the costs down somewhat by engaging a producer to take on the role of consultant.

Adapting material from state or national campaigns to a local area

There are times when health promotion practitioners are asked to implement a social marketing campaign developed at a regional or national level. Materials may be provided as part of that program. These materials will need to be assessed for suitability to the local conditions. If they are not, they may be able to be adapted.

CONCLUSION

Social marketing has a powerful influence on people's lives and the manner in which they view the world. Using social marketing approaches in health promotion practice within the comprehensive primary health care context is therefore of considerable potential value. Mass and social media offer considerable scope in the promotion of health, whether it be attempting to reframe health issues in the public eye to raise awareness of public policy issues or to encourage a positive health change. As with other health promotion strategies, there is much to be gained by working in partnership with community members being mindful of the fact that media coverage of health issues, even successful media coverage, is not an end in itself, but a means to achieving health promoting change. This is also an area of health promotion where it is very useful to draw on the skills of media communication and graphic design specialists to ensure the right message reaches the desired audience.

MORE TO EXPLORE

SOCIAL MARKETING

- Comprehensive introduction to community-based social marketing: (McKenzie-Mohr, 2011).
- Systematic review on use of social media for health communication: (Moorhead et al., 2013).
- Evaluation of social media in health promotion: (Neiger et al., 2012).

IUHPE Core Competencies for Health Promotion

The IUHPE Core Competencies for Health Promotion comprises nine domains of action. Each domain has a series of core competency statements and a detailed outline of the knowledge and skills that contribute to competency in that domain.

The content of this chapter relates especially to the achievement of competency in the health promotion domains outlined below.

2. Advocate for health	*2.2 Engage with and influence key stakeholders to develop and sustain health promotion action*
	Health promotion settings approach
	Behavioural change techniques for brief advice/interventions
3. Mediate through partnership	*3.1 Engage partners from different sectors to actively contribute to health promotion action*
	Advocacy strategies and techniques
	Methods of stakeholder engagement
	Health and wellbeing issues relating to a specified population or group
4. Communication	*4.1 Use effective communication skills including written, verbal, non-verbal, listening skills and information technology*
	Stakeholder engagement
	4.2 Use electronic and other media to receive and disseminate health promotion information
	Communication skills
	Use of electronic media and information technology
	Use of print, radio, TV and social media

5. Leadership	*5.1 Work with stakeholders to agree a shared vision and strategic direction for health promotion action*
	Health literacy
	Emerging challenges in health and health promotion
	5.4 Incorporate new knowledge and ideas to improve practice and respond to emerging challenges in health promotion
	Applications of information technology for social networking media and for mass media
6. Assessment	*6.3 Collect, review and appraise relevant data, information and literature to inform health promotion action*
	Evidence base for health promotion action and priority setting
8. Implementation	*8.2 Develop, pilot and use appropriate resources and materials*
	Understanding social and cultural diversity
	Ability to work with groups and communities
	Process evaluation
9. Evaluation and research	*9.4 Use research and evidence-based strategies to inform practice*
	Knowledge of different models of evaluation and research

In addition, IUHPE specifies knowledge, skills and performance criteria essential for health promotion practitioners to act professionally and ethically, including having knowledge of ethical and legal issues, behaving in an ethical and respectful manner and working in ways that review and improve practice. Full details are available at: http://www.iuhpe.org/index.php/en/the-accreditation-system

Reflective Questions

1. Select a current national, government-led social marketing campaign. Using the 4Ps framework, identify the product, price, promotion, and place for the campaign. Describe the range of communication resources included in the promotion component of the campaign.

2. Critique the same social marketing campaign selected for reflective question 1 using Table 4.1 Health promotion values and principles. For each of the values and principles, assess the extent to which the campaign reflects a critical or selective health promotion approach.

3. Select a health and wellbeing priority issue that you feel passionate about. Write a persuasive letter to your local member of parliament advocating for the issue.

REFERENCES

Andreasen, A. (2002). Marketing social marketing in the social change marketplace. Journal of Public Policy & Marketing, 21(1), 3–13. doi:10.1509/jppm.21.1.3.17602.

Andreasen, A. (2006). Social marketing in the 21st century. Thousand Oaks, CA: Sage.

Buresh, B., & Gordon, S. (2006). From silence to voice: what nurses know and must communicate to the public (2nd ed.). Ithaca, NY: ILR Press/Cornell University Press.

Burnet Institute. (2020). FaceSpace: using social networking to promote safer sex to higher risk groups. Retrieved from https://www.burnet.edu.au/projects/69_facespace_using_social _networking_to_promote_safer_ssex_to_higher_risk_groups.

Cancer Council Australia. (n.d.-a). QUIT smoking. Retrieved from http://www.cancer.org.au/ preventing-cancer/reduce-your-risk/quit-smoking.html.

Cancer Council Australia. (n.d.-b). Slip Slop Slap Seek Slide. Retrieved from http://www.cancer .org.au/preventing-cancer/sun-protection/campaigns-and-events/slip-slop-slap-seek-slide.html.

Cancer Council Australia. (n.d.-c). Sun safety. Retrieved from http://www.cancer.org.au/ preventing-cancer/sun-protection/.

Centers for Disease Control and Prevention (CDC). (2010). The health communicator's social media toolkit. Retrieved from https://www.cdc.gov/healthcommunication/toolstemplates/ socialmediatoolkit_bm.pdf.

Donovan, R., & Henley, N. (2010). Principles and practice of social marketing: an international perspective. Cambridge: Cambridge University Press.

Egger, G., Donovan, R., & Spark, R. (2005). Health promotion, strategies and methods (2nd ed.). Sydney: McGraw-Hill.

Egger, G., Donovan, R., & Spark, R. (2013). Health promotion strategies and methods (3rd ed.). Sydney: McGraw-Hill.

Egger, G., Spark, R., & Donovan, R. (1993). Health and the media: principles and practices for health promotion. Sydney: McGraw-Hill.

Fletcher, R., Kelly, B., Gwynne, J., et al. (2015, May 27–30). The stayin' on track project— supporting young Aboriginal fathers through a user-developed website. Poster. Paper presented at the 13th National Rural Health Conference, Darwin.

Freeman, B., Potente, S., Rock, V., & McIver, J. (2015). Social media campaigns that make a difference: what can public health learn from the corporate sector and other social change marketers? Public Health Research & Practice, 25(2), e2521517. doi:10.17061/phrp2521517.

French, J. (2009). The case for social marketing. In J. French, C. Blair-Stevens, D. McVey, & R. Merritt (Eds.), Social marketing and public health: theory and practice. Oxford: Oxford University Press.

French, J., Blair-Stevens, C., McVey, D., & Merritt, R. (2009). Social marketing and public health: theory and practice. Oxford: Oxford University Press.

Gold, J., Pedrana, A. E., Sacks-Davis, R., et al. (2011). A systematic examination of the use of online social networking sites for sexual health promotion. BMC Public Health, 11 (583). https:// doi.org/10.1186/1471-2458-11-583.

Hawe, P., Degeling, D. E., & Hall, J. (1990). Evaluating health promotion: a health worker's guide. Sydney: MacLennan and Petty.

John-Leader, F., Van Beurden, E., Barnett, L., et al. (2008). Multimedia campaign on a shoestring: promoting 'Stay Active – Stay Independent' among seniors. Health Promotion Journal of Australia, 19(1), 22–28. doi:10.1071/HE08022.

Kaplan, A. M., & Haenlein, M. (2010). Users of the world, unite! The challenges and opportunities of social media. Business Horizons, 53(1), 59–68. doi:10.1016/j.bushor.2009.09.003.

Keleher, H., & MacDougall, C. (Eds.). (2016). Understanding health (4th ed.). South Melbourne: Oxford University Press.

Kietzmann, J. H., Hermkens, K., McCarthy, I. P., & Silvestre, B. S. (2011). Social media? Get serious! Understanding the functional building blocks of social media. Business Horizons, 54(3), 241–251. doi:10.1016/j.bushor.2011.01.005.

Kotler, P., Roberto, N., & Lee, N. (2002). Social marketing improving the quality of life (2nd ed.). Thousand Oaks, CA: Sage.

Lauckner, C., & Whitten, P. (2015). The differential effects of social media sites for promoting cancer risk reduction. Journal of Cancer Education, 31(3), 449–452. doi:10.1007/s13187-015-0881-5.

Loeffler, R. H., & Winston, W. (2014). Guide to preparing cost-effective press releases. London: Routledge: Taylor & Francis.

McKenzie-Mohr, D. (2011). Fostering sustainable behavior: an introduction to community-based social marketing (3rd ed.). British Columbia, Canada: New Society Publishers.

McVey, D., & Walsh, L. (2009). Generating 'insight' and building segmentations—moving beyond simple targeting. In J. French, C. Blair-Stevens, D. McVey, & R. Merritt (Eds.), Social marketing and public health: theory and practice (pp. 1–366). Oxford: Oxford University Press.

Mengage (n.d.). University of Newcastle: Stayin' on Track. Retrieved from http://www.mengage.org.au/Life-Stages/Becoming-A-Father/University-of-Newcastle-Stayin-On-Track

Metro Trains Melbourne. (n.d.). Dumb ways to die. Retrieved from http://www.dumbwaystodie.com/about/.

Moorhead, S. A., Hazlett, D., Harrison, L., et al. (2013). A new dimension of health care: systematic review of the uses, benefits, and limitations of social media for health communication. Journal of Medical Internet Research, 15(4). doi:10.2196/jmir.1933.

Neiger, B. L., Thackeray, R., Van Wagenen, S. A., et al. (2012). Use of social media in health promotion: purposes, key performance indicators, and evaluation metrics. Health Promotion Practice, 13(2), 159–164. doi:10.1177/1524839911433467.

Nelson, D. E., Gallogly, M., Pederson, L. L., et al. (2008). Use of consumer survey data to target cessation messages to smokers through mass media. American Journal of Public Health, 98(3), 536. doi:10.2105/AJPH.2006.090340.

Nutbeam, D. (2008). The evolving concept of health literacy. Social Science & Medicine, 67(12), 2072–2078. doi:10.1016/j.socscimed.2008.09.050.

Potente, S., Rock, V., McIver, J., et al. (2013). Fighting skin cancer with a musical sound: the innovative Australian sun sound campaign. Social Marketing Quarterly, 19(4), 279–289. doi:10.1177/1524500413506583.

Public Health Ontario. (2012). At a glance: the twelve steps to developing a health communication campaign. Retrieved from https://www.publichealthontario.ca/en/eRepository/Twelve_steps_developing_health_communication_campaign_2012.pdf.

Research New Zealand. (2008). Measuring the impact of the 'Smoking Not Our Future' campaign: final report. Retrieved from https://www.hpa.org.nz/sites/default/files/SNOF-evaluation-phone-survey-fnl-081218.pdf.

Soul City Institute for Social Justice (n.d.) Annual reports. Retrieved from https://www.soulcity.org.za/about-us/annual-reports.

Thackeray, R., Neiger, B. L., & Keller, H. (2012). Integrating social media and social marketing: a four-step process. Health Promotion Practice, 13(2), 165–168. doi:10.1177/1524839911432009.

Transport Accident Commission. (n.d.). Transport Accident Commission. Retrieved from https://www.tac.vic.gov.au/road-safety/tac-campaigns/tac-latest-campaigns

Truss, A., & White, P. (2009). Ethical issues in social marketing. In J. French, C. Blair-Stevens, D. McVey, & R. Merritt (Eds.), Social marketing and public health: theory and practice (pp. 1–366). Oxford: Oxford University Press.

Wakefield, M. A., Loken, B., & Hornik, R. C. (2010). Use of mass media campaigns to change health behaviour. The Lancet, 376(9748), 1261–1271. doi:10.1016/S0140-6736(10)60809-4.

Webb, M. (2004). Social software consultancy. Retrieved from http://interconnected.org/home/2004/04/28/on_social_software.

9 Vaccination, screening, risk assessment and surveillance

COMPREHENSIVE PRIMARY HEALTH CARE

SOCIO-ECOLOGICAL APPROACH

SELECTIVE PRIMARY HEALTH CARE

BEHAVIOURAL APPROACH

BIOMEDICAL APPROACH

| *Healthy public policy to create environments and settings that support health and wellbeing* | *Community development action to support social and environmental change* | *Health education and health literacy to develop knowledge and skills for health and wellbeing action* | *Health information and social marketing to raise awareness about health and wellbeing priorities* | ***Vaccination, screening, risk assessment and surveillance* to monitor and reduce risk of disease conditions** |

Health promotion community assessment, program planning, implementation and evaluation

INTRODUCTION

In this chapter, four health promotion strategies designed to reduce the risk of disease are examined, including vaccination against diseases, screening for specific diseases, individual disease risk factor assessment, and surveillance of diseases. These strategies can make a significant contribution to the health status of the population. However, if they are the *only* health promotion strategies implemented by a primary health care service, the overall approach would be regarded as biomedical. In the biomedical approach, health is defined as simply the absence of disease or injury, rather than the broader definition of the World Health Organization (WHO, n.d.-a) discussed throughout this book, which includes the absence of disease or injury, but extends this to include the ability to cope with disease and distress, and the presence of good health and wellbeing. When the biomedical approach to health promotion is used, control over health promotion strategies is maintained by health professionals who are generally funded to concentrate on disease or risk factors for disease, with limited attention to the principles of holistic health and wellbeing, socio-ecological determinants, social justice, equity, community control, and working for social change. Most of the health promotion strategies discussed in this chapter are carried out in primary care services, such as community health centres and local government, by primary care providers such as community health nurses, general medical practitioners and allied health professionals. Before starting the chapter, take some time to review *Putting the Ottawa Charter into Practice* on p. 417.

VACCINATION

Immunisation is the process whereby a person is made immune or resistant to an infectious disease, typically by the administration of a vaccine. Vaccines stimulate the body's own immune system to protect the person against subsequent infection or disease. Immunisation

PUTTING THE OTTAWA CHARTER INTO PRACTICE

The following questions, arranged in the Ottawa Charter action areas, are presented to guide health practitioners to reflect on and critically evaluate their professional role and practice and the health promotion philosophy of their organisation. Content of this chapter will assist health practitioners to develop the necessary professional knowledge and skills to see these health promotion strategies in the comprehensive primary health care context.

PUTTING THE OTTAWA CHARTER INTO PRACTICE

Build healthy public policy

- Are the national vaccination and screening programs supported by local community-based health promotion activities that facilitate participation for vulnerable groups?

Create supportive environments

- Are people provided with necessary supports to participate in vaccination, screening and risk-assessment activities?
- Are the barriers to participation in vaccination, screening and risk-assessment activities being addressed?

Strengthen community actions

- Are there opportunities for community members to fully participate in decision making about vaccination, screening, risk-assessment and surveillance activities?

Develop personal skills

- Are community members provided with capacity-building skills to enable participation in programs designed to enhance vaccination, screening and risk assessment?

Reorient health services

- Are the vaccination, screening, risk-assessment and surveillance activities being implemented in conjunction with other health promotion activities across the health promotion practice framework?

reduces the risk of illness, disability and death from diseases categorised as 'vaccine-preventable'. At the individual level, vaccination is not a 100% guarantee that the person will not acquire the disease, and so the disease is not technically 100% preventable. But vaccination reduces the risk of acquiring a disease so significantly that the term prevention is used to describe the effect of vaccination at a population level.

According to the WHO (2019), vaccination currently prevents an estimated two to three million deaths around the world every year. It is one of the most cost-effective health promotion strategies available, and can be implemented in even the most hard-to-reach and vulnerable populations. For every $1 spent on vaccines, the return on investment is

$16, and when considering broader economic and social benefits, the return on investment is $44 (Hervey, 2020). Vaccination is a vital tool to improve health equality, promote peaceful and inclusive societies, and contribute to the achievement of the Sustainable Development Goals (SDGs) (United Nations, n.d.). SDG3 is focused on good health and wellbeing, and vaccination contributes directly to two targets in this goal:

- SDG target 3.3: by 2030, end the epidemics of AIDS, tuberculosis, malaria and neglected tropical diseases and combat hepatitis, waterborne diseases and other communicable diseases;

- SDG target 3.8: achieve universal health coverage, including financial risk protection, access to quality essential healthcare services and access to safe, effective, quality and affordable essential medicines and vaccines for all.

Vaccination also contributes directly and indirectly to the achievement of 13 other SDGs, including SDG1 No poverty, SDG2 Zero hunger, SDG4 Quality education, SDG5 Gender equality, SDG6 Clean water and sanitation, SDG7 Affordable and clean energy, SDG8 Decent work and economic growth, SDG9 Industry, innovation and infrastructure, SDG10 Reduced inequality, SDG11 Sustainable cities and communities, SDG13 Climate action, SDG16 Peace, justice and strong institutions, and SDG17 Partnerships for the goals (Gavi, n.d.).

Despite the huge success of vaccination programs over the years, equitable access to vaccines is still a major problem. To try and bridge this gap, the *Global Vaccine Action Plan 2011–2020* (GVAP) was endorsed at the World Health Assembly in 2012 (WHO, 2013b) to deliver the Decade of Vaccines vision of universal access to vaccines. Supported by WHO, UNICEF, Gavi The Vaccine Alliance and the Bill and Melinda Gates Foundation, 194 member states of the World Health Assembly endorsed the plan to deliver access to vaccines that reduce the risk of cervical cancer, diphtheria, hepatitis B, measles, mumps, pertussis, pneumonia, rotavirus diarrhoea, rubella, tetanus, and polio by 2020. The Bill and Melinda Gates Foundation committed US$10 billion to the GVAP—the largest charitable pledge ever made to a single cause—with the aim that the full benefits of vaccination be extended to every child on the planet. The GVAP targets are to achieve vaccination coverage of ≥ 90% nationally and ≥ 80% in every district by 2020. Halfway through the decade-long plan, WHO warned that five of the six GVAP targets (diphtheria–tetanus–pertussis (DTP3), polio, measles, hepatitis B, pneumococcal, rotavirus) were not on track to be achieved, and only the introduction of underutilised vaccines was showing sufficient progress to achieve the GVAP target by 2020. As part of the plan to achieve the GVAP targets, in 2016, WHO implemented Close the Immunization Gap, which is now an annual campaign to raise awareness of the critical importance of complete vaccination throughout life (WHO, 2019).

The 2019 Global Vaccination Action Plan Review (Strategic Advisory Group of Experts on Immunization, 2019) reported that ongoing progress on vaccination had been made since 2010, including:

- more children are being vaccinated each year than ever before including in low- and middle-income countries

- rubella has been eliminated in 81 countries

- only 12 countries globally have not yet attained maternal and neonatal tetanus elimination

- most low- and middle-income countries have introduced at least one new vaccine

- global child mortality has declined by a quarter.

Despite these achievements, the report noted that many of the GVAP goals were unlikely to be achieved by 2020. For example, with respect to childhood vaccination, 86% of infants worldwide were vaccinated with three doses of DTP3 vaccine and one dose of measles vaccine in 2018, but this level had not increased since 2010. This level of coverage is not sufficient and needs to be at around 95% to protect against outbreaks of these diseases. The 14% of children not vaccinated—about 20 million children worldwide—are those most at risk of poor health, including the poorest, the most marginalised and those affected by conflict. Almost half of unvaccinated children live in just 16 countries. If these children contract an infectious disease, they are the least likely to access lifesaving treatment and care.

The GVAP review also included data on the coverage of human papillomavirus (HPV) vaccine, which protects against cervical cancer. As of 2018, 90 countries had introduced the HPV vaccine into their national vaccination programs. This means that one in three girls worldwide are now vaccinated against HPV. Australia is on track to become the first country in the world to eradicate cervical cancer (Hervey, 2020). However, only 13 of the 90 countries that have introduced HPV vaccination are lower-income countries (Strategic Advisory Group of Experts on Immunization, 2019). As with childhood vaccination, those most at risk are the girls least likely to have access to the vaccine or treatment for cervical cancer.

Disparities in vaccination rates

Disparities in vaccination rates within and between countries are the result of limited resources, competing health priorities, poor management of health systems and inadequate monitoring and supervision, particularly in poor countries and regions hurt by ongoing conflict (WHO, 2019). In countries such as Australia and New Zealand, although the majority of children are fully vaccinated, subgroups of the population are vulnerable to disease outbreaks due to low vaccination coverage (Flego et al., 2012). National vaccination rates in Australia have continued to increase over the past 10 years for one-year-olds and five-year-olds, and are now just below the aspirational target of 95%. The vaccination rate for Aboriginal and Torres Strait Islander one-year-olds in 2019 was 92.61%, lower than the Australian average, but for five-year-olds was 96.87%, which was higher than the Australian average. It is recommended that healthcare providers establish the Indigenous status of their clients so they can offer the additional vaccines that may be required (Commonwealth of Australia, 2013). In New Zealand, the vaccination rate for one-year-olds in 2019 was 92%, and 88% for five-year-olds (Ministry of Health, 2020a). In 2009, 73% of Māori children in New Zealand received all vaccinations by two years of age, compared with 84% of non-Māori children, a difference of 11%. By 2015, this difference had reduced to two percentage points, with 92% of Māori children receiving all vaccinations by two years of age compared with 94% of non-Māori children (Health Quality & Safety Commission, 2015). However, from 2015 to 2018, vaccination rates for two-year-olds in New Zealand decreased overall to 92%, and declined more sharply for Māori children to 88%, thereby widening the gap again between Māori and non-Māori vaccination rates (Immunisation Advisory Centre, 2018). It is therefore important to look closely at vaccination rates, even if they are relatively high overall, because they may conceal a large number of under-vaccinated children in equity-based priority population groups (Dawson & Apte, 2015).

Vaccination policy

All levels of government have a role to play in administering or delivering vaccination programs. In Chapter 5, building healthy public policy is described as the development of legislation, policy, strategic plans or rules of operation of a sector of government or an organisation, made on behalf of the relevant population or group designed to protect their health. National governments provide overarching legislation, policy and strategic direction for vaccination, as do state governments. Some state governments in Australia have introduced additional legislation about coverage, and municipal governments often plan and coordinate vaccination programs that specifically meet the needs of their catchment area. The Australian Immunisation Handbook (Australian Technical Advisory Group on Immunisation (ATAGI), 2018) and the New Zealand Immunisation Handbook (Ministry of Health, 2018) provide information about vaccines and vaccination practice.

In some instances, legislation can require compulsory vaccination. For example, *No Jab, No Pay* legislation at the national level in Australia ties family assistance payments to childhood vaccination (Department of Health, n.d.), with parents and carers being required to demonstrate that their child is either fully vaccinated for their age, on a vaccination catch-up program, or unable to be vaccinated for medical reasons, before they enter early childhood services. Examples of similar legislation at the state level include Victoria's *No Jab, No Play* law (Department of Health and Human Services, n.d.) and the Public Health Amendment (Vaccination of Children Attending Child Care Facilities) Bill 2013 in New South Wales (NSW). These legislative requirements have raised debates about the right to parent autonomy versus a paternalistic public health approach. The National Health and Medical Research Council (NHMRC) in Australia recommends that workplaces implement a comprehensive occupational vaccination program in healthcare settings, particularly where there are vulnerable populations such as older people in aged care facilities and transmission of vaccine-preventable diseases such as influenza is likely. It is recommended that all programs comprise a vaccination policy, maintenance of current staff vaccination records, provision of information about the relevant vaccine-preventable diseases, and the management of vaccine refusal. NHMRC also recommends a pre-employment screening and immunisation risk management assessment where all Category A healthcare workers who have contact with blood or body substances are required to provide evidence of immunity or a vaccination history (National Health and Medical Research Council, 2019).

Community (herd) immunity

To control a vaccine-preventable disease, a sufficient pool of people must be immune to the disease to prevent the spread of that disease in the wider population. This is called herd immunity or community immunity. Community immunity is required to protect people who are not immune to the disease, including children too young to be vaccinated, people unable to be vaccinated for a range of medical reasons, and people for whom vaccination has not been fully effective. Achieving herd immunity for infectious diseases requires high vaccination rates. For example, measles is highly infectious so a vaccination rate of about 92% to 94% is required to prevent it spreading to people who are not immune. Political will and substantial resources are required to obtain community immunity. When both are in place, spectacular results in vaccine-preventable diseases can be achieved, such as the global eradication of smallpox and the reduction of measles-related deaths (WHO, 2015a).

Barriers to community (herd) immunity

Despite the investment by governments at all levels, in workplaces and with primary care providers, vaccination programs have not been able to reach a sufficient pool of people and create community or herd immunity to prevent the spread of some diseases. Disease outbreaks have been linked to travellers from countries where some diseases are endemic, the communication style of staff in health agencies, a lack of awareness from parents about the timing of vaccination, a variety of social reasons such as the importance of support from family (Ministry of Health, 2013) and 'vaccine hesitancy' (Dawson & Apte, 2015). In 2011, there were 23 confirmed cases of measles acquired over a two-month period in NSW. Twenty of the confirmed cases lived in one of four postcodes (Flego et al., 2012). In the same year, 168 cases of measles were identified in NSW. Of those affected, 104 were children and adolescents. Forty people had received the one-dose MMR (measles, mumps, rubella) vaccine but 95 of the remaining 128 had no history or an uncertain history of vaccination. Thirty-two of these cases reported vaccine refusal (Dawson & Apte, 2015). Government data indicate that pertussis remains highly prevalent in Australia and is the least well controlled of all vaccine-preventable diseases. Data show that epidemics occur every three to four years and in populations that are unvaccinated the outbreaks can be widespread. However, in populations with high vaccination coverage, outbreaks are smaller, and, as such, morbidity and mortality rates are significantly lower (Australian Technical Advisory Group on Immunisation (ATAGI), 2018).

Low vaccination coverage rates have been attributed to structural and cultural factors and low levels of knowledge. Access to vaccination services and knowledge, particularly for newly arrived immigrant populations, are key factors (Flego et al., 2012). Poor public transport, lack of flexibility in appointment times, and ineligibility for free healthcare for newly arrived immigrants hamper access to programs. Lack of awareness of programs, or knowledge of what the vaccine is preventing or where services are located also contributes to low vaccination rates. Cultural barriers include a tendency to seek medical help when there is a crisis rather than acting proactively to reduce the risk, or preferring traditional medicine rather than Western medicine (Flego et al., 2012). Other factors such as overcrowding and frequent exposure to overseas travellers contribute to low vaccination completion in immigrant populations. Cost efficiency, physician recommendation, attitudes towards vaccination, knowledge, parental approval and geographical location influence acceptability of some vaccines (Dickson-Swift et al., 2008). These potential barriers and enablers to vaccination uptake, and obtaining a sufficient pool to prevent the spread of a disease to the unimmunised, need to be taken into consideration in developing vaccination programs. In Chapter 4, we outline the steps needed to increase the likelihood of successful programs and argue that a broad range of approaches can be used that are grounded in critical health promotion in a comprehensive primary health care (CPHC) context. Strengthening partnerships between communities, practitioners, governments and researchers is recommended.

Vaccine hesitancy

'Vaccine hesitancy' is a term that describes the attitudes of individuals who are concerned about the safety of vaccines (Dawson & Apte, 2015). The reasons for hesitancy are diverse. Weighing up perceived benefits, trust of information sources, concerns about the effect on the immune systems of children, and 'sub-optimal interactions with healthcare providers' have been described as key factors (Dawson & Apte, 2015, p. 104). Vaccine-hesitant parents often start their search for information on unfiltered internet sites and through social media, where a great deal of misinformation exists. Furthermore, misinformation may be coming from health practitioners themselves. Philips and colleagues (2014) report that less than half of the healthcare providers surveyed in their study correctly identified that there was no association between MMR vaccine and autism, despite a large volume of evidence reliably dispelling the myth. Smith and colleagues (2016) report that nurses' influenza vaccination rates are suboptimal and that this relates to their knowledge of influenza and their perception of risks. They argue this knowledge also affects the advice they give patients, with vaccinated nurses being more likely to recommend vaccination than those who are unvaccinated.

Enablers for community (herd) immunity

In addition to the legislation and policies described above, numerous other strategies have been used to improve vaccination rates. Reminding people about the vaccination schedule has proven to be the most successful (Fraser et al., 2016; Vann & Szilagyi, 2005). A Cochrane review of 47 studies in high-income countries found that vaccination rates improved in both children and adults when a reminder system was used. Reminding people by telephone, letters or speaking to people personally all improved vaccination rates. Telephone reminders were found to be the most effective, and the more people who were reminded, the greater the rates of vaccination. Reminders worked whether they were from private doctors, medical centres or public health departments (Vann & Szilagyi, 2005). In Australia, considerable effort has been made by many national, state and local governments to increase vaccination rates. These strategies include asking parents what needs to be done to facilitate attendance at vaccination sessions for children. As a result of community participation in program planning, family-friendly times and venues have emerged to meet the needs of communities. This has resulted in increased vaccination rates within these municipalities. 'Catch-up' clinics have also been trialled. In Flego and colleagues' study (2012), a stakeholder group identified barriers and enablers of vaccination uptake in a Pacific Island population in Sydney, and developed an action plan to increase vaccination rates. This group comprised Youth Health Services, local GPs of Pacific Island background, and members of the Western Sydney Public Health Unit. The group worked with principals and community liaison officers in two schools and churches in the locality. Information sessions were conducted in each of these organisations, and invitations were extended to community members to attend the 'catch-up' clinics (Flego et al., 2012). A review of the HPV (human papillomavirus) vaccination program in New Zealand revealed that vaccination uptake was higher when there was integration and information sharing between the district health board, HPV team, vaccination coordinator, school-based delivery, primary care delivery and whānau engagement. Conversely, when there was limited integration between these sectors, there were lower rates of vaccination uptake (Ministry of Health, 2012). Dawson and Apte (2015) suggest that education of healthcare providers and attention to good communication between healthcare providers and parents is fundamental to maximising vaccination rates. Respectfully acknowledging parental concerns and providing them with reliable sources of vaccine information, in combination with the structural changes discussed above, have been shown to be successful strategies to improve community vaccination coverage. This approach is in line with the guidelines for building health literacy presented in Chapter 7.

Delivering local vaccination programs

Many program planners are involved in trying to improve the rates of vaccination. While the Australian Immunisation Handbook (Australian Technical Advisory Group on Immunisation (ATAGI), 2018) provides clinical guidelines for healthcare professionals such as nurses and doctors, on the safest and most effective use of vaccines in their practice, it is local governments that often are coordinating the organisation of vaccination in community settings, schools, maternal and child health centres, and workplaces. Environmental health practitioners working in local government often have the coordinating role. Sound program planning is likely to lead to successful health outcomes (see Chapter 4) and the advantages of intersectoral collaboration and partnerships are discussed in

Chapter 5. Organisations that have a role in settings such as schools, workplaces, healthcare facilities, and cultural and recreational venues come together to work on a health issue of mutual concern or to promote health across the population. The approach aims to draw on what works best in each setting and use the skills and strengths of the collaborating agencies to achieve the goal—in this case, improving vaccination levels.

POPULATION SCREENING

Screening is used to detect early development of a disease (such as breast or colon cancer), or changes that occur before the disease has developed, or symptoms are evident (such as for cervical cancer). Screening is also conducted with newborn babies for conditions that are treatable, but not clinically evident in the newborn period. Specific conditions that are screened for vary from country to country, but may include hearing loss, metabolic, hormone and haemoglobin disorders, skeletal anomalies and congenital heart disease. In some countries, pregnant women are screened for HIV.

Population screening refers to a test that is offered to all individuals in a specific group, usually defined by age, as part of an organised program. Population screening is not appropriate for all conditions or diseases. Wilson and Jungner (1968) published their seminal list of 10 principles to guide decision making about whether a population-level screening program is appropriate for a particular condition. Since then, these principles have been used around the world to inform population-level screening frameworks. Fifty years later the principles were updated after a systematic review of evidence followed by a consensus-building process with international experts in population-level screening (Dobrow et al., 2018). The 12 principles of population-level screening proposed by Dobrow and colleagues (2018) fall under three domains:

Domain: Disease/condition principles

1. Epidemiology of the disease or condition

The epidemiology of the disease or condition should be adequately understood, and the disease or condition should be an important health problem (e.g. high or increasing incidence or prevalence, or causes substantial morbidity or mortality).

2. Natural history of disease or condition

The natural history of the disease or condition should be adequately understood, the disease or condition is well-defined, and there should be a detectable preclinical phase.

3. Focus population for screening

The focus population for screening should be clearly defined (e.g. with an appropriate age range), identifiable and able to be reached.

Domain: Test/intervention principles

4. Screening test performance characteristics

Screening test performance should be appropriate for the purpose, with all key components specific to the test (rather than the screening program) being accurate (e.g. in terms of sensitivity, specificity and positive predictive value) and reliable or reproducible. The test should be acceptable to the focus population and it should be possible to perform or administer it safely, affordably and efficiently.

5.   Interpretation of screening test results

Screening test results should be clearly interpretable and determinate (e.g. with known distribution of test values and well-defined and agreed cut-off points) to allow identification of the screening participants who should (and should not) be offered diagnostic testing and other postscreening care.

6.   Postscreening test options

There should be an agreed-on course of action for screening participants with positive screening test results that involves diagnostic testing, treatment or intervention, and follow-up care that will modify the natural history and clinical pathway for the disease or condition; that is available, accessible and acceptable to those affected; and that results in improved outcomes (e.g. increased functioning or quality of life, decreased cause-specific mortality). The burden of testing on all participants should be understood and acceptable, and the effect of false-positive and false-negative tests should be minimal.

Domain: Program/system principles

7.   Screening program infrastructure

There should be adequate existing infrastructure (e.g. financial resources, health human resources, information technology, facilities, equipment and test technology), or a clear plan to develop adequate infrastructure, that is appropriate to the setting to allow for timely access to all components of the screening program.

8.   Screening program coordination and integration

All components of the screening program should be coordinated and, where possible, integrated with the broader healthcare system (including a formal system to inform, counsel, refer and manage the treatment of screening participants) to optimise care continuity and ensure no screening participant is neglected.

9.   Screening program acceptability and ethics

All components of the screening program should be clinically, socially and ethically acceptable to screening participants, health professionals and society, and there should be effective methods for providing screening participants with informed choice, promoting their autonomy and protecting their rights.

10.   Screening program benefits and harms

The expected range and magnitude of benefits (e.g. increased functioning or quality of life, decreased cause-specific mortality) and harms (e.g. over-diagnosis and overtreatment) for screening participants and society should be clearly defined and acceptable, and supported by existing high-quality scientific evidence (or addressed by ongoing studies) that indicates that the overall benefit of the screening program outweighs its potential harms.

11.   Economic evaluation of screening program

An economic evaluation (e.g. cost-effectiveness analysis, cost–benefit analysis and cost–utility analysis) of the screening program, using a health system or societal perspective, should be conducted (or a clear plan to conduct an economic evaluation) to assess the full costs and effects of implementing, operating and sustaining the screening program while clearly considering the opportunity costs and effect of allocating resources to other potential nonscreening alternatives (e.g. primary prevention, improved treatments and other clinical services) for managing the disease or condition.

12. Screening program quality and performance management

The screening program should have clear goals or objectives that are explicitly linked to program planning, monitoring, evaluating and reporting activities, with dedicated information systems and funding, to ensure ongoing quality control and achievement of performance targets.

(Dobrow et al., 2018, p. E427)

Priorities for population screening differ from country to country but are similar in high-income countries such as Australia, New Zealand, Canada, the United Kingdom and the United States. In Australia, there are three national population screening programs for adults—BreastScreen, National Bowel Cancer Screening Program and National Cervical Screening Program—and the newborn screening program. In New Zealand, the National Screening Unit is responsible for breast and cervical screening for adult women, HIV screening for pregnant women, and newborn screening.

Population screening programs result in significant health gains at the population level. For example, the breast cancer mortality rate has decreased significantly since BreastScreen Australia was introduced, from 74 deaths per 100,000 women aged 50 to 74 years in 1991 to fewer than 50 deaths per 100,000, a rate which has been sustained since 2010 (Australian Institute of Health and Welfare, 2020).

Effectiveness of population screening

Despite the body of evidence supporting population screening for specific conditions, controversy continues over the effectiveness of some programs. Based on the principles of population screening described above, there is evidence in support of population screening for breast, cervical, colorectal and lung cancers, but not ovarian, prostate and skin cancers as screening programs have not been shown to reduce the population mortality rates from those cancers (Division of Cancer Prevention and Control Centers for Disease Control and Prevention, 2019). Outside the national population screening programs, people may be offered screening tests by health providers based on the assumption that early detection of a disease will be the result. However, translating the principles of population-level screening to individual-level screening is not straightforward. Some procedures and providers are not well regulated and for the uninformed, 'Dr Google' may present a bewildering amount of information. Barratt and colleagues (2004) suggest that:

... relevant information, such as information about the increased risk of diagnosis with screening, is often counterintuitive. Benefits are relatively rare and often delayed, and the screening process can involve a whole series of interventions. The harms of screening are poorly understood by the public, and screening tests are often viewed uncritically.

(p. 507)

Large numbers of healthy people have to be tested in order for population screening to have an impact on population health outcomes. However, a reduction of mortality and morbidity is not automatically assured just because there is a screening test available. There are many reasons for this. For example, in cancer screening: 1. the cancer may have been curable had it been allowed to progress and present normally anyway; 2. despite screening, death may still occur; and 3. had screening not been carried out, the cancer might never have presented clinically in the individual's lifetime. This is a situation that applies to a certain extent to all cancers for which there are screening programs. This is different from 'lead time', which is bringing forward the time of diagnosis for a cancer that was destined to present clinically, and has been identified during screening (Miller, 2008). Screening decisions are complex, and according to Barratt and colleagues (2004, pp. 507–510), health workers need to be aware of the potential risks in population screening which include:

- over-detection and over-treatment
- invasive follow-up investigations and treatments
- harm is immediate and benefits are delayed
- few people experience benefits from screening compared with the number who would be expected to benefit from most treatments
- individual values and preferences are critical to screening decision making
- evidence base for screening decision aids is often limited
- public attitude is that early detection and/or prevention must be automatically good
- little regulation is in place to protect consumers from aggressive marketing, and there may be strong financial incentives to get people to participate in screening.

Decision aids for policymakers, health professionals and consumers have been suggested by Barratt and colleagues (2004). Edwards and colleagues (2013) conducted a Cochrane Systematic Review and reported that people who received personalised risk information made more informed choices about screening compared with participants who received generic risk information. The personalised risk communication did not significantly affect participants' anxiety levels. However, the review could not draw conclusions about the best strategies for delivering personalised risk communication. How much information to provide and how it should be provided will depend on the individual, the screening test and the context (Entwistle et al., 2008).

Barratt and colleagues (2004) provide further guidance about communicating information about screening:

- Present the chances of having pseudo-disease as well as clinically important disease detected by screening.
- Give information about the whole of the early detection and treatment process.
- Present balanced information about the cumulative chance of benefits and harms over equivalent time frames.
- Present very small numbers by using large and consistent denominators; for example, outcomes per 1000 or per 10,000 people screened.
- Ensure that decision aids for screening accommodate the potential for the outcomes of screening to be labelled as benefits or harms.
- Explicitly declare where high-quality evidence is lacking.
- Use ranges or some other method to convey uncertainty in numerical estimates.
- Explain that there is a choice and the reasons why people might decide to decline screening.

- Include information about financial gains to the organisation offering the screening test in decision aids for screening.

Child health screening

The NHMRC undertook a topic-by-topic systematic review of the available evidence for child health surveillance and screening (Centre for Community Child Health Royal Children's Hospital Melbourne for the National Health and Medical Research Council, 2002). The review considered children from birth to 18 years of age but did not include prenatal screening activities. The review found that:

- there was little evidence for the effectiveness of screening programs in many domains
- there was scant data about cost-effectiveness
- there were major issues of program quality, monitoring of compliance with referrals for assessment, and whether facilities exist in many communities for assessment and follow-up
- in some cases, there was little evidence that therapy altered outcomes.

The NHMRC (Centre for Community Child Health Royal Children's Hospital Melbourne for the National Health and Medical Research Council, 2002) reported that these findings should not be seen as diminishing the importance of attempts at early detection. Rather, the report provided evidence that the process of child health screening should be reconsidered. The NHMRC recommended screening and surveillance be 'designed to detect specific definable problems' and that 'further research and critical thinking around prevention of problems and promotion of health be undertaken' (p. 17).

Research concerning screening for specific definable problems in children is available for many disorders. For example, screening newborns for inherited disorders such as phenylketonuria (PKU) is conducted in many countries. If PKU is not detected and treated early in life, permanent brain damage occurs, resulting in severe learning and behavioural difficulties and diseases such as epilepsy. Early detection and treatment lead to vastly improved outcomes for this and other disorders, including skeletal disorders (Pitt, 2010). Early identification and intervention for hearing loss has also been shown to prevent the problems of speech and language development, educational achievement and general development as well as longer-term impacts on the quality of life (Zhelev et al., 2015). Screening for hearing loss in children is conducted in newborns and at school entry in many countries, although what is tested and the age at which children are tested varies (and is debated), and many countries do not have robust screening programs in place (Zhelev et al., 2015). Research regarding screening for more complex social problems is also emerging.

Family violence screening

Screening for family violence is defined as 'a process by which an organisation or professional attempts to identify victims of violence or abuse in order to offer interventions that can lead to beneficial outcomes' (Australian Institute of Health and Welfare, 2015). This is a systematic process where all people attending a particular service are asked about family violence, whether it is suspected or not. Screening to identify risk factors associated with family violence was introduced in Victoria, Australia, in 2009. The Victorian Family Violence Multi-Agency Risk Assessment and Management Framework was developed for use by professionals including maternal and child health nurses, family violence service providers, the police, the courts and professionals in other mainstream services (Victorian

Government, 2018). Research shows that family violence screening does not cause harm in the short term but there is insufficient evidence for the implementation of routine family violence screening of all women in healthcare settings (O'Doherty et al., 2015). There is weak evidence for screening those considered high risk (e.g. antenatal women and those attending abortion services). However, a scoping review of the literature conducted by Hooker and colleagues (2012) reported that there were a number of barriers to implementing family violence prevention programs and that screening may not occur as recommended. They also reported that there was controversy surrounding screening for family violence in healthcare settings and that complex social problems such as family violence require a multilevel systems approach, beyond routine screening (Hooker et al., 2012). Due to the high prevalence of domestic violence, NSW Health (2019) requires screening to be undertaken as part of routine assessment for:

- all women attending antenatal services
- all women attending child and family health services
- women aged 16 years and over who attend mental health services
- women aged 16 and over who attend alcohol and other drugs services.

In other programs such as women's health and sexual assault, screening is undertaken on an ad hoc basis and so is not regarded as population screening. The Judith Lumley Centre at La Trobe University has undertaken a number of studies that focus on family violence screening and supportive care for women and children. Insight 9.1 is an example of that work.

INSIGHT 9.1 Family violence screening in maternal and child health nursing practice

THE PROBLEM

Family violence (FV) is a common and harmful public health issue. In Australia, up to one in four women have experienced partner violence in their lifetime (Cox, 2016). Women and children are the most at risk of FV and suffer significant harm, including physical and mental health consequences (WHO, 2013a). Additionally, women's parenting capacity is diminished in the context of abuse with subsequent detrimental impacts on the mother–child relationship (Hooker et al., 2016). The economic costs of FV to the nation are substantial.

Evidence suggests routine screening for FV does not improve health outcomes for women and children, with some exceptions, such as pregnant women (O'Doherty et al., 2015). Despite this, governments have implemented screening policies in an attempt to prevent and reduce FV and its harmful effects. However, policy often does not translate into practice. In reality, many healthcare professionals have not had FV training in their pre-registration education programs, feel unprepared to address FV with clients and face significant individual and structural barriers to engaging in FV work (Feder et al., 2009). Screening rates of FV are low and few screening programs are sustainable (O'Campo et al., 2011). To address this problem, researchers from La Trobe University trialled an enhanced model of FV screening to improve and sustain screening rates and supportive care for abused women and children.

INSIGHT 9.1 Family violence screening in maternal and child health nursing practice—cont'd

THE PROGRAM

The MOVE (improving maternal and child health nurse care for vulnerable mothers) randomised controlled trial assessed the efficacy of an enhanced model of nurse FV screening and supportive care within the Victorian maternal and child health (MCH) service. Study aims included increased asking and disclosure rates, safety planning by nurses and referral of clients to services. Additionally, researchers wanted to identify the prevalence of FV in the MCH population, to ensure nurse safety and to cause no harm (Taft et al., 2015).

SUSTAINABILITY

Any new clinical practice that aims to improve health outcomes needs to be sustainable. Evidence suggests there is a significant gap between what we know works and what is currently being delivered in clinical practice (Grimshaw et al., 2012). The use of theory in research that explores implementation processes can bridge the knowledge-to-action gap (McEvoy et al., 2014). Furthermore, engaging knowledge users in the process of implementing new clinical practices can facilitate implementation and knowledge translation and exchange. To ensure sustainable FV screening, the MOVE study included a six-month participatory action research phase with MCH nurse consultants to help develop practical FV resources and promote engagement in the FV work. MOVE researchers used an overarching implementation theory (normalisation process theory) in the design, intervention and evaluation phases of the trial to enhance sustained FV screening and care (Hooker & Taft, 2016).

OUTCOMES

The MOVE model enhanced screening rates and safety-planning discussions with women attending MCH services and caused no harm to clients. Up to 14% of women had experienced partner violence in the past 12 months. Two years on from the MOVE trial, screening rates have increased and intervention MCH nurse teams are four times more likely to complete safety plans with women than those in the control group (Taft et al., 2015).

PRACTICE IMPLICATIONS

MOVE success can be attributed to action research and partnerships with nurses, strong design and extensive use of implementation theory to encourage sustainable change. The use of implementation theory helps identify contextual barriers and facilitators essential for new practices to be normalised into everyday care and may assist future program replication and scale up. Recent recommendations by the WHO to routinely screen all pregnant women for FV (WHO, 2013c) means ongoing work is needed to support midwives and maternity services to provide evidence-based care.

Source: Written by Leesa Hooker, PhD.

INDIVIDUAL RISK FACTOR ASSESSMENT

Risk factor assessment is a process of determining biological, psychological or behavioural risks for diseases or injury. The assessment can be a comparison of national or international data to inform health policy or identifying health risks in an individual. The terms 'screening' and 'assessment' are often used interchangeably; however, they are different processes.

In the case of family violence discussed in Insight 9.1, risk assessment is said to be 'the process of identifying the presence of risk factors and determining the likelihood of an adverse event occurring, its consequence, and its timing' (Australian Institute of Health and Welfare, 2015; Braaf & Sneddon, 2007), whereas screening is a systematic process where all people attending a particular service are asked about family violence whether it is suspected or not. Comparing national or international data to inform health policy enables governments and organisations to assess overall risks to health and plan strategies to reduce the burden of disease from these risk factors. For example, in Australia funding has been provided for health promotion programs in workplaces. Individual risk factor assessment forms part of many workplace health promotion programs. The aim is to reduce chronic disease by increasing levels of physical activity, raising the intake of fruit and vegetables to recommended levels, reducing harmful levels of alcohol consumption and encouraging smoking cessation (Department of Health, 2014). The strategy of focusing on individual risk factor assessment is strongly contested (Baum, 2016) as risk factors normally associated with coronary heart disease explain only a portion of disease outcomes. For example, the early work of Rose and Marmot (1981) demonstrated that cholesterol, smoking, blood pressure and other factors combined explained considerably less than half of the difference in mortality between different ranks of the civil service in Britain. Since then, it has been demonstrated comprehensively that risk factors for ill-health correlate strongly with socio-economic inequalities within countries (for example, see Commission on Social Determinants of Health, 2008; Wilkinson & Pickett, 2009; WHO, 2007, 2015b, n.d.h). Baum (2016) argued that the approach emphasises individual responsibility and could thereby perpetuate victim blaming. These findings and arguments led many health workers to question the efficacy of risk factor assessment programs used in isolation to improve health when there was no complementary action to reduce income disparities.

Workplace health risk assessment

The effectiveness of workplace health risk assessment (HRA) programs for chronic disease suggests that the HRAs are efficacious when used in combination with other workplace health promotion programs (Bellow et al., 2012; Dickson-Swift et al., 2014; Hooper & Bull, 2009; Russell, 2009). The WHO (n.d.-f) recommends increasing the scope of workplace health promotion programs to take a socio-ecological approach and incorporate action to address physical, psychosocial, behavioural and environmental determinants of health. Over the past decades, workplace health promotion practice has been more consistent with selective health promotion approaches, from occupational health and safety procedures, through to behavioural approaches that include HRA focusing on lifestyle diseases. More recently, however, initiatives have broadened and are moving towards more critical approaches. For example, *Generating Equality and Respect: Tools and Resources* (VicHealth, 2016) provides resources that workplaces can use to create and support gender equity in the workplace with an overall aim of preventing violence against women.

St George and colleagues (2012) surveyed large, medium and small organisations and found that prevalence and support for workplace health promotion varied with the size of the organisation. Barriers to implementing programs were primarily related to time and cost and so practical, low-cost activities were preferred. Employers found workplace health promotion toolkits very useful, whereas telephone advice and telephone coaching services were the least preferred types of assistance. Influenza vaccinations were the most common activity in large and medium-sized workplaces and providing free or subsidised fruit was the most common activity in small organisations (St George et al., 2012). Other activities included health promotion posters, gym subsidies, yoga or pilates programs, health seminars and walking programs. A review by Russell (2009) for the New Zealand Government found that individual risk assessment programs, coupled with individual counselling, health education and organisational change have included:

> *stress management, smoking cessation, skin assessments, back care, nutrition education, workplace safety, prenatal and well-baby care, CPR and first aid classes, employee assistance programmes (EAP), work/life balance policies, flexi-time, exercise/fitness groups, discounts to local fitness facilities, healthful food choices at work meetings, events, training programs, family friendly policies, and facilities (such as bicycle racks, showers, gym equipment).*

Programs that focus on non-communicable disease risk factors in workplaces are reported to have been successful at increasing employees' fruit and vegetable consumption, reducing tobacco and alcohol use and dietary fat intake, improving blood pressure and cholesterol levels, increasing employee engagement (Russell, 2009), and reducing emergency department visits, outpatient visits and inpatient hospital days over the longer term (Bellow et al., 2012). One local government provided bowel cancer information and free bowel cancer screening kits to male staff members over 50 years in the works department. Four of the 25 staff members who followed through and undertook the screening returned a positive result. Following this, sessions on preparing simple nutritious meals were well attended by staff from the area. Risk factor assessments have also been used as a part of an integrated disease risk reduction strategy. For example, providing workplace Pap smear screening has been used as an opportunity to provide women with information about risk factors for diseases other than cervical cancer. At an organisational level, individual HRA programs provide organisations with the opportunity to improve the organisational environment for employees and contribute to individual health improvement.

There are benefits for the organisation through cost savings and increased productivity (WHO & World Economic Forum, 2008). However, as we have discussed throughout this book, focusing on health risk assessment without addressing the underlying conditions that contribute to disease and injury has been shown to be ineffective in reducing the burden of poor health at a population level. Dickson-Swift and colleagues (2014) report that the benefits of a program that is broader in scope include increased productivity, staff retention, staff morale and loyalty and reduced absenteeism. Further, organisations that implement more-comprehensive workplace health promotion programs gain a reputation for being good places to work. The authors argue that 'providing a supportive environment and improving organisational culture within a workplace are essential to ensuring success' (Dickson-Swift et al., 2014, p. 150). Their model for improving employee health and wellbeing includes taking action on:

- personal relationships (providing counselling)
- rewards (employees need to feel valued)
- flexible work (to enable dedicated health promoting activities)
- two-way communication (between management and staff)
- management support for a health promotion program
- paying attention to the physical environment.

RISK ASSESSMENT OF LOCAL ENVIRONMENTS

Environmental risk assessments are conducted at the local or regional level to protect the population from hazards and create supportive environments for health. These are assessments of risks to human health posed by physical, chemical, biological and social factors in the environment and the identification of amenities that promote health. This process is part of the community assessment stage discussed in Chapter 4. The environments in which people live and work strongly influence the way in which they can interact with each other. Urban and rural environments have a profound impact on health; for example, transport causes air pollution, noise and traffic injuries and assessment of health impacts of policies, plans and projects are needed using qualitative, quantitative and participatory techniques (WHO, n.d.-e). SDG 11 (see Chapter 3) is to 'make cities inclusive, safe, resilient and sustainable' (United Nations, n.d.) and planning liveable communities (Chapters 3 and 6) creates co-benefits across the urban planning, public health and environment sectors. Contact with nature and access to urban green spaces promote health (Townsend & Weerasuriya, 2010). Examples of environmental issues that can be included in the community assessment include:

- a safe and adequate water supply
- safe and nutritious food
- safe and adequate sanitation
- clean air
- safe and suitable shelter
- urban planning that promotes health
- environmental management systems that protect health
- safe workplaces and practices
- safe recreational environments.

Health impact assessments

Health impact assessments (HIAs) are community-based risk assessment tools that provide information about how a policy or program may affect the health of people in a community (WHO, n.d.-e). HIAs are also discussed in Chapter 3. Harris-Roxas and Harris (2011) argue that the historical disciplinary fields from which HIAs emerged (environmental health, a social view of health, and health equity) stem from different concerns. They argue that environmental health assessments are concerned with the impact of the physical environment on human health and, as discussed in Chapter 3, rely on predictive reductionist methods based on epidemiological and toxicological approaches. The assessments stemming from the social view of health, also outlined in Chapter 3, have tended to focus on policies and programs and to be constructionist in their approach to evidence and causality. HIAs are also considered important in addressing health inequities and because they introduce a discussion of values as part of the assessment process. This approach also tends to take a social constructionist or structuralist approach in collecting evidence (Harris-Roxas & Harris, 2011). Harris-Roxas and Harris (2011) suggest there are four different forms of HIA: mandated; decision support; advocacy; and community led. They suggest that the procedural steps of HIA (screening, scoping, assessment, decision making and recommendations, and follow-up) are common across the various forms.

The assessment of the environmental rights and responsibilities listed above are sometimes enshrined in legislation and conducted by health and environmental health professionals. These assessments are mandated under environmental protection or public health legislation. Responsibilities for conducting HIAs are allocated to national, state or local government agencies and they are usually used for major project proposals. The decision-support HIA is carried out on policies, plans or programs with an aim of avoiding negative health impacts and maximising positive impacts. Arguably, these might work well at local or sub-regional levels where it is possible to directly influence implementation. The aim of advocacy HIAs is to give voice to the views of those whose health is most likely to be directly affected and who are under-represented in the decision-making processes. Finally, the community-led HIA is said to be 'a democratic and political process, rather than a technocratic or rational process' (Harris-Roxas & Harris, 2011, p. 401) where a community's health-related concerns are recognised.

It is necessary to understand the purpose and form of HIAs, in particular, to come to a shared understanding during the screening and scoping process (Harris-Roxas & Harris, 2011). Government agencies such as the Office of Health Protection (Department of Health, 2017) provide guidance to professionals, and the WHO provides information and tools to member states for HIAs and also for risk factor surveillance. The STEPwise program, for example, is a standardised method for collecting, analysing and disseminating surveillance data in WHO member countries that enables countries to monitor trends within their country and compare data across countries.

SURVEILLANCE

In the context of this book, public health surveillance is the continuous and systematic collection, analysis and interpretation of health-related data needed for the planning, implementation and evaluation of health promotion programs. Practitioners in many health and environmental fields at local, state and national levels contribute to this endeavour. For health promotion in a CPHC context, public health surveillance can:

- *monitor and clarify the epidemiology of health issues, to allow priorities to be set and to inform health promotion strategies.*
- *serve as an early warning system for impending public health emergencies;*
- *document the impact of a health promotion program, or track progress towards specified goals.*

(WHO, n.d.-g)

The WHO assists member states to respond to epidemics and other public health emergencies through an integrated global alert and response system. Biosafety, biosecurity and preparedness for outbreaks of dangerous and emerging pathogens and monitoring of non-communicable diseases through risk factor surveillance, such as STEPwise, are strengthened through standardised approaches, training and improving laboratory capacities at the national level. The WHO's approach to surveillance of communicable and non-communicable diseases internationally is consistent with critical health promotion. The WHO prioritises resource-poor countries, and supports the strengthening of national capacity for alert and response through a multi-disease or integrated approach. The WHO STEPwise approach to non-communicable disease enables low- and middle-income countries to build and strengthen their capacity to initiate and maintain disease surveillance programs (WHO, n.d.-i).

The WHO argues that governments have a responsibility for the health of their people, which can be fulfilled only by the provision of adequate health and social measures. The WHO addresses issues such as the unequal development in different countries in the promotion of health and control of disease, especially communicable diseases.

Globalisation, climate change, the growth of mega-cities and the explosive increase in international travel increase the potential for the rapid spread of infections. Many epidemics, such as COVID-19 and influenza, pose enormous challenges to health systems in countries with limited resources. Others, such as mosquito-borne diseases, have an increasing potential to create new pandemics. The emergence and rapid spread of infectious diseases increases treatment costs (WHO, n.d.-b).

Every country should be able to detect, rapidly verify, and respond appropriately to emerging disease threats when they arise, and minimise their impact on the health of the population (WHO, 2012). Global health security needs the involvement of many collaborators and the WHO members recognise that no single entity can bring it about on its own (WHO, n.d.-c). The Australian Health Protection Principal Committee (AHPPC) is the key decision-making committee for public health emergencies. Comprising all state and territory Chief Health Officers and chaired by the Australian Chief Medical Officer, the AHPPC's ongoing roles are to advise the Australian Health Ministers' Advisory Council on health protection matters and national priorities, and mitigate emerging health threats related to infectious diseases, the environment and natural and human-made disasters. The AHPPC works with all state and territory governments to develop and adopt national health protection policies, guidelines, standards and alignment of plans (Department of Health, 2020a).

Communicable diseases

Surveillance of communicable diseases is historically the responsibility of governments and is usually enshrined in legislation. The *National Notifiable Diseases Surveillance System* coordinates national surveillance of more than 50 communicable diseases/disease groups in Australia. Guidelines for public health units in each state have been revised in response to outbreaks. Management plans for pandemics have been developed, and each local government must have an emergency management plan that incorporates planning for pandemic infections as well as fires, floods and other natural disasters.

The *Australian Health Management Plan for Pandemic Influenza* is an example of a direct response to global concern about epidemics and pandemics (Department of Health, 2019). Each state and territory in Australia has a management plan in line with the national plan. The emergence of COVID-19 in China in December 2019, and its subsequent spread throughout the world and declaration as a Public Health Emergency of International Concern in January 2020 resulted in the rapid publication of the *Australian Health Sector Emergency Response Plan to Novel Coronavirus* (COVID-19) (Department of Health, 2020b). The plan described the following actions to be taken by the health system in Australia to address the outbreak:

- Monitor and investigate outbreaks as they occur.
- Identify and characterise the nature of the virus and the clinical severity of the disease.
- Research respiratory disease-specific management strategies.
- Respond promptly and effectively to minimise the novel coronavirus outbreak impact.
- Undertake strategies to minimise the risk of further disease transmission.
- Contribute to the rapid and confident recovery of individuals, communities and services.

At the time of writing this book, the pandemic had passed its peak in many countries, but was still escalating in others, and new measures were being enacted almost daily to try to reduce transmission in first and second waves of infection. A key recommendation

---

INSIGHT 9.2 COVID-19

In December 2019, a novel strain of coronavirus was first identified in Wuhan, Hubei Province, China. The virus resulted in an illness named COVID-19, which ranged from mild to moderate symptoms in the majority of people with the infection. However, severe symptoms, complications and death occurred, predominantly in elderly people and people who suffered from chronic diseases and lowered immunity. The pandemic caused enormous health, social and economic disruption around the world. At the time of writing, the infection rates were still increasing, in some countries exponentially, and the full effect of the pandemic is not yet known. However, the pandemic raises many questions that we need to reflect on. Responses will vary from country to country.

- What was the role of the World Health Organization (WHO) in addressing the pandemic?
- Was the WHO effective in undertaking this role?
- How did the health outcomes vary according to the strategies taken by different countries?
- Did economic concerns cause undue delays in countries taking action to protect health and safeguard the health system?
- Was having federal, state and local jurisdictions all involved in pandemic preparedness and response an advantage or disadvantage?
- To what extent did the different approaches chosen by federal and state governments introduce confusion or distrust, or engender compliance with recommendations and rules?
- Were there mechanisms in place to enable countries and states to learn from this experience?
- How were the learnings acted upon?

---

after the SARS and Ebola disease outbreaks was for countries to 'go early and go hard'; in other words to put highly restrictive measures in place very early on in the outbreak. However not all countries adopted this strategy. In countries that put stringent public health measures in place early in the outbreak, such as South Korea and New Zealand, the spread of infection was much slower than those countries that did not adopt this strategy, such as Italy and the USA. A thorough analysis of the impact of such strategies is not possible at the time of writing, but will make for an interesting and potentially devastating critique of the different responses around the world. Some of the questions we can ask about the COVID-19 pandemic are raised in Insight 9.2.

The management of arboviruses is another example of population surveillance. Surveillance of viruses and carriers such as mosquitoes occurs at global, national, state and local levels. From these data, research to improve disease prediction occurs and health promotion programs are developed.

Health professionals at the local level are responsible for the systematic collection of data for notifiable communicable diseases. Analysis, interpretation and dissemination of health data occurs at the national and state levels. Lists of notifiable diseases and case definitions are provided to environmental health and medical practitioners and other health professionals and agencies (Department of Health, 2020c; Ministry of Health, 2020b). The notification rates are then the catalyst for action and may prompt further legislation and strategic plans. Quarantine, for example, has been used globally since the 14th century (Lin et al., 2007) as a strategy to reduce the spread of communicable disease. In Australia, the *Quarantine Act 1908* can be invoked to close borders, ban public meetings, commandeer buildings to provide specific health services and quarantine people against their will (Baum, 2008, p. 77). For example, the COVID-19 pandemic in 2020 sparked a range of measures from governments that limited people's movement and contact with others, in order to try and reduce the spread of infections. However, as noted above, at the time of writing the pandemic was still in its ascendancy and so the impact of these strategies cannot be fully evaluated yet. Prior to COVID-19, the *Quarantine Act* was enforced following outbreaks of Hendra virus in Australia, preventing movement of people and animals from horse farms and between states. In New Zealand, the *Health (Protection) Amendment Act 2016* was adopted to improve the tracing of people who may have an infectious disease, or may have been exposed to one; increase the range of infectious diseases that are notifiable; and provide incremental options for the management of individuals with significant infectious diseases (Parliamentary Counsel Office, 2016).

Notification rates of communicable diseases can also be the prompt for the ongoing development of national strategies. For example, rates of sexually transmissible infections (STI) in Australia contributed to the redevelopment of the five National Blood Borne Viruses (BBV) and STI Strategies 2018–2022, including the Fourth National STI Strategy, Eighth National HIV Strategy, Fifth National Aboriginal and Torres Strait Islander BBV and STI Strategy, Third National Hepatitis B Strategy, and Fifth National Hepatitis C Strategy (Department of Health, 2018).

Non-communicable diseases

The WHO also provides surveillance data to countries for non-communicable diseases. The global school-based student health survey (GSHS), for example, assesses the behavioural risk factors and protective factors in 10 key areas among young people aged 13 to 17 years (WHO, n.d.-d). The program is a collaboration between WHO, UNICEF, UNESCO and UNAIDS with technical assistance from the Centers for Disease Control, with the aim of helping countries to develop priorities and establish health promotion programs for young people. The GSHS is implemented by a nominee of either the ministry of health or ministry of education in participating countries. A self-administered questionnaire is used to obtain data on young people's health behaviours and factors related to mental, physical and social health (WHO, n.d.-d). Health practitioners planning health promotion programs need to make themselves aware of what information is already available and the data sources and collation services to assist this process (see Chapter 4). Community profiles, social and economic indicators, and epidemiological profiles are readily available for many communities.

CONCLUSION

Health promotion strategies described in this chapter have produced important population health gains. Vaccination programs have reduced the spread of vaccine-preventable diseases across populations around the world. Screening, risk assessment and surveillance are primary and secondary disease prevention programs that use systematic methods of collecting and disseminating information. These strategies make a significant contribution to the health status of the population. However, if they are the *only* health promotion strategies implemented by a primary health care service, the overall approach would be regarded as biomedical and consistent with selective primary health care. All of the strategies described in this chapter are most successful when implemented in conjunction with strategies described in Chapters 5 to 8, to form a socio-ecological approach to health promotion. Evidence suggests that health improves and health inequities decrease in populations when the principles of social justice, empowerment and sustainability underpin health promotion in a comprehensive primary health care context.

MORE TO EXPLORE

IMMUNISATION

Fine and colleagues (2011) provide a historical, epidemiologic and theoretical public health perspective on herd immunity.

IUHPE Core Competencies for Health Promotion

The IUHPE Core Competencies for Health Promotion comprises nine domains of action. Each domain has a series of core competency statements and a detailed outline of the knowledge and skills that contribute to competency in that domain.

The content of this chapter relates especially to the achievement of competency in the health promotion domains outlined below.

1. Enable change	*1.1 Work collaboratively across sectors to influence the development of public policies that impact positively on health and reduce health inequities*
	Determinants of health and health inequities
2. Advocate for health	*2.2 Engage with and influence key stakeholders to develop and sustain health promotion action*
	Advocacy strategies and techniques
	Methods of stakeholder engagement
	Health and wellbeing issues relating to a specified population or group
3. Mediate through partnership	*3.3 Build successful partnership through collaborative working, mediating between different sectoral interests*
	Systems, structures and functions of different sectors, organisations and agencies
4. Communication	*4.1 Use effective communication skills including written, verbal, non-verbal, listening skills and information technology*
	Communication skills including written, verbal, non-verbal, listening skills and information technology
	Working with individuals and groups
	Use of electronic media and information technology
	Use of print, radio, TV and social media
	Ability to work with individuals, groups, communities and organisations in diverse settings

5. Leadership	*5.3 Network with and motivate stakeholders in leading change to improve health and reduce inequities* Stakeholder engagement *5.4 Incorporate new knowledge and ideas to improve practice and respond to emerging challenges in health promotion* Collaborative working skills
8. Implementation	*8.1 Use ethical, empowering, culturally appropriate and participatory processes to implement health promotion action* Use of participatory implementation processes Resource management Collaborative working Ability to work with: groups and communities participating in the health promotion action; stakeholders and partners; and team members Monitoring and process evaluation
9. Evaluation and research	*9.4 Use research and evidence-based strategies to inform practice* Data interpretation and statistical analysis

In addition, IUHPE specifies knowledge, skills and performance criteria essential for health promotion practitioners to act professionally and ethically, including having knowledge of ethical and legal issues, behaving in an ethical and respectful manner and working in ways that review and improve practice. Full details are available at: http://www.iuhpe.org/index.php/en/the-accreditation-system

Reflective Questions

1. Sometimes parents request health practitioners to provide a rationale for having their children vaccinated. What are the public health benefits of national vaccination programs?

2. Despite the huge success of vaccination programs over the years, equitable access to vaccines is still a major problem around the world. Discuss why this is the case and current global initiatives to respond to this situation, particularly for vulnerable communities.

3. Population screening programs result in significant health gains at the population level. Identify a current population screening program in your country. Discuss the screening program, for whom it is intended and the population health gains of the program.

REFERENCES

Australian Institute of Health and Welfare. (2015). Screening for domestic violence during pregnancy: options for future reporting in the National Perinatal Data Collection. Retrieved

from https://www.aihw.gov.au/getmedia/62dfd6f0-a69a-4806-bf13-bf86a3c99583/
19298.pdf.aspx?inline=true.

Australian Institute of Health and Welfare. (2020). BreastScreen Australia monitoring report
2019. Retrieved from https://www.aihw.gov.au/getmedia/cff20c99-cb24-4f4a-97d6
-e0e02919fc67/aihw-can-128-Breast-cancer-screening-in-Australia.pdf.aspx.

Australian Technical Advisory Group on Immunisation (ATAGI). (2018). Australian Immunisation
Handbook. Retrieved from https://immunisationhandbook.health.gov.au/.

Barratt, A., Trevena, L., Davey, H. M., & McCaffery, K. (2004). Use of decision aids to support
informed choices about screening. BMJ (Clinical research ed.), 329(7464), 507.

Baum, F. (2008). The new public health (3rd ed.). South Melbourne: Oxford University Press.

Baum, F. (2016). The new public health (4th ed.). Melbourne: Oxford University Press.

Bellow, B., St George, A., & King, L. (2012). Workplace screening programs for chronic disease
prevention: a rapid review. Retrieved from https://www.saxinstitute.org.au/wp-content/
uploads/04_Workplace-screening-programs-for-chronic-disease-preventi.pdf.

Braaf, R., & Sneddon, C. (2007). Family Law Act reform: The potential for screening and risk
assessment for family violence. Sydney: Australian Domestic & Family Violence
Clearinghouse, UNSW.

Centre for Community Child Health Royal Children's Hospital Melbourne for the National Health
and Medical Research Council. (2002). Child health screening and surveillance: a critical
review of the evidence. Retrieved from https://catalogue.nla.gov.au/Record/2158072.

Commission on Social Determinants of Health. (2008). Closing the gap in a generation: health
equity through action on the social determinants of health. Final Report of the Commission
on Social Determinants of Health. Retrieved from https://www.who.int/social_determinants/
thecommission/finalreport/en/.

Commonwealth of Australia. (2013). Vaccine preventable diseases and vaccination coverage in
Aboriginal and Torres Strait Islander people, Australia 2006–2010. Communicable Diseases
Intelligence, 37(Supplement). Retrieved from https://www1.health.gov.au/internet/
publications/publishing.nsf/Content/cda-cdi37suppl.htm/$FILE/cdi37suppl.pdf.

Cox, P. (2016). Violence against women: additional analysis of the Australian Bureau of Statistics'
Personal Safety Survey, 2012 (ANROWS Horizons: 01.01/2016 Rev. ed.). Retrieved from
https://www.anrows.org.au/publication/violence-against-women-in-australia-additional
-analysis-of-the-australian-bureau-of-statistics-personal-safety-survey-2012/.

Dawson, B., & Apte, S. H. (2015). Measles outbreaks in Australia: obstacles to vaccination.
Australian and New Zealand Journal of Public Health, 39(2), 104–106. doi:10.1111/
1753-6405.12328.

Department of Health. (2014). Healthy workers initiative. Retrieved from http://www
.healthyworkers.gov.au/internet/hwi/publishing.nsf/Content/movemore.

Department of Health. (2017). What we do. Retrieved from https://www1.health.gov.au/internet/
main/publishing.nsf/Content/cda-about.htm

Department of Health. (2018). Fourth national sexually transmissible infections strategy
2018–2022. Retrieved from https://www1.health.gov.au/internet/main/publishing.nsf/Content/
ohp-bbvs-1/$File/STI-Fourth-Nat-Strategy-2018-22.pdf.

Department of Health. (2019). Australian health management plan for pandemic influenza
(AHMPPI). Retrieved from https://www1.health.gov.au/internet/main/publishing.nsf/Content/
ohp-ahmppi.htm.

Department of Health. (2020a). Australian Health Protection Principal Committee. Retrieved from
https://health.govcms.gov.au/committees-and-groups/australian-health-protection-princip
al-committee-ahppc.

Department of Health. (2020b). Australian health sector emergency response plan for novel
Coronavirus (COVID-19). Retrieved from https://www.health.gov.au/sites/default/files/
documents/2020/02/australian-health-sector-emergency-response-plan-for-novel-coronavirus
-covid-19_2.pdf.

Department of Health. (2020c). National notifiable diseases surveillance system. Retrieved from http://www9.health.gov.au/cda/source/cda-index.cfm.

Department of Health. (n.d.). No jab, no pay—new immunisation requirements for family assistance payments. Retrieved from https://www.health.gov.au/sites/default/files/no-jab-no-pay-fsheet.pdf.

Department of Health and Human Services. (n.d.). Frequently asked questions: No jab, no play. Retrieved from https://www2.health.vic.gov.au/public-health/immunisation/vaccination-children/no-jab-no-play/frequently-asked-questions

Dickson-Swift, V., Fox, C., Marshall, K., et al. (2014). What really improves employee health and wellbeing: findings from regional Australian workplaces. International Journal of Workplace Health Management, 7(3). doi:10.1108/IJWHM-10-2012-0026.

Dickson-Swift, V., Fox, C., Pitts, M., & Willis, J. (2008). What do young rural people know about Human Papillomavirus (HPV)? Young rural Victorians' knowledge and experience of Gardasil® vaccination and HPV. Paper presented at the Australian Sexual Health Conference, Sydney.

Division of Cancer Prevention and Control Centers for Disease Control and Prevention. (2019). Screening tests. Retrieved from https://www.cdc.gov/cancer/dcpc/prevention/screening.htm.

Dobrow, M. J., Hagens, V., Chafe, R., et al. (2018). Consolidated principles for screening based on a systematic review and consensus process. Canadian Medical Association Journal, 190(14), E422–E429. doi:10.1503/cmaj.171154.

Edwards, A., Naik, G., Ahmed, H., et al. (2013). Personalised risk communication for informed decision making about taking screening tests. Cochrane Database of Systematic Reviews, (2) CD001865. doi:10.1002/14651858.CD001865.pub3.

Entwistle, V. A., Carter, S. M., Trevena, L., et al. (2008). Communicating about screening. BMJ—British Medical Journal, 337(7673).

Feder, G., Ramsay, J., Dunne, D., et al. (2009). How far does screening women for domestic (partner) violence in different health-care settings meet criteria for a screening programme? Systematic reviews of nine UK National Screening Committee criteria. Health Technology Assessment, 13(16), iii–iv, xi–xiii, 1–113, 137–347. doi:10.3310/hta13160.

Fine, P., Eames, K., & Heymann, D. L. (2011). 'Herd immunity': a rough guide. Clinical Infectious Diseases, 52, 911–916.

Flego, K., Sheppeard, V., Scott, C., & Gabriel, S. (2012). Measles in Western Sydney: a symptom of excess burden of communicable diseases in Pacific Islanders? (poster). Paper presented at the Population Health Congress, Adelaide.

Fraser, A. C., Williams, S. E., Kong, S. X., et al. (2016). Public health amendment (Vaccination of Children Attending Child Care Facilities) Act 2013: its impact in the Northern Rivers, NSW. Public Health Research and Practice, 26(2). doi:10.17061/phrp2621620.

Gavi. (n.d.). Sustainable Development Goals. Retrieved from https://www.gavi.org/our-alliance/global-health-development/sustainable-development-goals.

Grimshaw, J. M., Eccles, M. P., Lavis, J. N., et al. (2012). Knowledge translation of research findings. Implementation Science, 7(1), 50. doi:10.1186/1748-5908-7-50.

Harris-Roxas, B., & Harris, E. (2011). Differing forms, differing purposes: a typology of health impact assessment. Environmental Impact Assessment Review, 31(4), 396–403. doi:10.1016/j.eiar.2010.03.003.

Health Quality & Safety Commission. (2015). A window on the quality of New Zealand's health care. Retrieved from http://www.hqsc.govt.nz/assets/Health-Quality-Evaluation/PR/window-on-quality-of-NZ-health-care-Nov-2015.pdf.

Hervey, A. (2020). A decade of vaccines. Retrieved from https://medium.com/future-crunch/a-decade-of-vaccines-7f86a432d771.

Hooker, L., Samaraweera, N., Agius, P., & Taft, A. J. (2016). Intimate partner violence and the experience of motherhood: a cross-sectional analysis of factors associated with a poor experience of motherhood. Midwifery, 34, 88–94. doi:10.1016/j.midw.2015.12.011.

Hooker, L., & Taft, A. J. (2016). Using theory to design, implement and evaluate sustained nurse domestic violence screening and supportive care. Journal of Research in Nursing, 21(5–6), 432–442. doi:10.1177/1744987116649633.

Hooker, L., Ward, B., & Verrinder, G. (2012). Domestic violence screening in maternal and child health nursing practice: a scoping review. Contemporary Nurse, 42(2), 198–215. doi:10.5172/conu.2012.42.2.198.

Hooper, P., & Bull, F. C. (2009). Healthy active workplaces: review of evidence and rationale for workplace health. Perth: Department of Sport and Recreation, Western Australia Government.

Immunisation Advisory Centre. (2018). National immunisation coverage for New Zealand. Retrieved from https://www.immune.org.nz/sites/default/files/publications/Immunisation%20coverage%20to%20June%202018.pdf.

Lin, V., Smith, J., & Fawkes, S. (2007). Public health practice in Australia: the organised effort. Sydney: Allen & Unwin.

McEvoy, R., Ballini, L., Maltoni, S., et al. (2014). A qualitative systematic review of studies using the normalization process theory to research implementation processes. Implementation Science, 9(1), 2. doi:10.1186/1748-5908-9-2.

Miller, A. (2008). Screening: evidence and practice. Bulletin of the World Health Organization. Retrieved from https://www.who.int/bulletin/volumes/86/4/07-048744/en/.

Ministry of Health. (2012). HPV Immunisation programme implementation evaluation. Retrieved from https://www.health.govt.nz/publication/hpv-immunisation-programme-implementation-evaluation.

Ministry of Health. (2013). Audience research: delayers of infant immunisation. Retrieved from https://www.health.govt.nz/publication/audience-research-delayers-infant-immunisation.

Ministry of Health. (2018). Immunisation handbook 2017. 2nd. Retrieved from https://www.health.govt.nz/publication/immunisation-handbook-2017.

Ministry of Health. (2020a). National and DHB immunisation data. Retrieved from https://www.health.govt.nz/our-work/preventative-health-wellness/immunisation/immunisation-coverage/national-and-dhb-immunisation-data.

Ministry of Health. (2020b). Notifiable disease surveillance: Public health surveillance information for New Zealand public health action. Retrieved from https://surv.esr.cri.nz/public_health_surveillance/notifiable_disease_surveillance.php.

National Health and Medical Research Council (NHMRC). (2019). Australian guidelines for the prevention and control of infection in healthcare. Retrieved from https://www.nhmrc.gov.au/about-us/publications/australian-guidelines-prevention-and-control-infection-healthcare-2019#block-views-block-file-attachments-content-block-1.

NSW Health. (2019). Domestic violence routine screening program. Retrieved from https://www.health.nsw.gov.au/parvan/DV/Pages/dvrs.aspx.

O'Campo, P., Kirst, M., Tsamis, C., et al. (2011). Implementing successful intimate partner violence screening programs in health care settings: evidence generated from a realist-informed systematic review. Social Science and Medicine, 72(6), 855–866. doi:10.1016/j.socscimed.2010.12.019.

O'Doherty, L., Hegarty, K., Ramsay, J., et al. (2015). Screening women for intimate partner violence in healthcare settings. Cochrane Database of Systematic Reviews (7) CD007007. doi:10.1002/14651858.CD007007.pub3

Parliamentary Counsel Office. (2016). Health (Protection) Amendment Act 2016. Retrieved from http://www.legislation.govt.nz/act/public/2016/0035/latest/DLM6223006.html.

Philips, L., Young, J., Williams, L. A., et al. (2014). Opportunistic immunisation in the emergency department: a survey of staff knowledge, opinion and practices. Australasian Emergency Nursing Journal, 17(2), 44–50. doi:10.1016/j.aenj.2013.12.003.

Pitt, J. J. (2010). Newborn screening. The Clinical Biochemist. Reviews, 31(2), 57.

Rose, G., & Marmot, M. G. (1981). Social class and coronary heart disease. British Heart Journal, 45(1), 13. doi:10.1136/hrt.45.1.13.

Russell, N. (2009). Workplace wellness: a literature review for NZWell@work. Retrieved from https://funding4sport.co.uk/downloads/well-at-work-workplace-wellness.pdf.

Smith, S., Sim, J., & Halcomb, E. (2016). Nurses' knowledge, attitudes and practices regarding influenza vaccination: an integrative review. Journal of Clinical Nursing, 25(19–20), 2730. doi:10.1111/jocn.13243.

St. George, A., King, L., Newson, R., et al. (2012). Implementing workplace health promotion initiatives: who should we target? Health Promotion Journal of Australia, 23(2), 134–140. doi:10.1071/HE12134.

Strategic Advisory Group of Experts on Immunization. (2019). The Global Vaccine Action Plan 2011–2020 review and lessons learned. Retrieved from: https://www.who.int/immunization/global_vaccine_action_plan/GVAP_review_lessons_learned/en/.

Taft, A. J., Hooker, L., Humphreys, C., et al. (2015). Maternal and child health nurse screening and care for mothers experiencing domestic violence (MOVE): a cluster randomised trial. BMC Medicine, 13(1), 150. doi:10.1186/s12916-015-0375-7.

Townsend, M., & Weerasuriya, R. (2010). Beyond blue to green: the benefits of contact with nature for mental health and well-being. Retrieved from https://das.bluestaronline.com.au/api/prism/document?token=BL/0817.

United Nations. (n.d.). About the Sustainable Development Goals. Retrieved from https://www.un.org/sustainabledevelopment/sustainable-development-goals/.

Vann, J., & Szilagyi, P. (2005). Patient reminder and patient recall systems to improve immunization rates. Cochrane Database of Systematic Reviews, (3) CD003941. doi:10.1002/14651858.CD003941.pub2.

VicHealth. (2016). Generating equality and respect—a world-first model for the primary prevention of violence against women: full evaluation report. Retrieved from https://www.vichealth.vic.gov.au/-/media/ResourceCentre/PublicationsandResources/PVAW/Generating-Equality-and-Respect-Full-evaluation-report.pdf?la=en&hash=79F91F773C804ED3A6CDF25EFCC0A270EFFE41E9.

Victorian Government. (2018). Family violence multi-agency risk assessment and management framework. Retrieved from https://www.vic.gov.au/sites/default/files/2019-02/MARAM-policy-framework-24-09-2018.pdf.

Wilkinson, R. G., & Pickett, K. (2009). The spirit level: why more equal societies almost always do better. London: Allen Lane.

Wilson, J. M. G., & Jungner, G. (1968). Principles and practice of screening for disease. Geneva: WHO.

World Health Organization (WHO). (2007). Civil society report on Commission on Social Determinants of Health. Retrieved from https://www.who.int/social_determinants/publications/civilsociety/en/.

World Health Organization (WHO). (2012). Rapid risk assessment of acute public health events. Retrieved from https://www.who.int/ihr/publications/WHO_HSE_GAR_ARO_2012_1/en/.

World Health Organization (WHO). (2013a). Global and regional estimates of violence against women: prevalence and health effects of intimate partner violence and non-partner sexual violence. Retrieved from http://apps.who.int/iris/bitstream/10665/85239/1/9789241564625_eng.pdf.

World Health Organization (WHO). (2013b). Global vaccine action plan 2011–2020. Retrieved from https://www.who.int/immunization/global_vaccine_action_plan/GVAP_doc_2011_2020/en/

World Health Organization (WHO). (2013c). Responding to intimate partner violence and sexual violence against women: WHO clinical and policy guidelines. Retrieved from http://www.who.int/reproductivehealth/publications/violence/9789241548595/en/.

World Health Organization (WHO). (2015a). Measles vaccination has saved an estimated 17.1 million lives since 2000. Retrieved from https://www.who.int/en/news-room/detail/12-11-2015-measles-vaccination-has-saved-an-estimated-17-1-million-lives-since-2000.

World Health Organization (WHO). (2015b). Social determinants of health—activities in 2015. Retrieved from https://www.who.int/social_determinants/social-determinants-health -activities-2015.pdf.

World Health Organization (WHO). (2019). Immunization coverage. Retrieved from https:// www.who.int/en/news-room/fact-sheets/detail/immunization-coverage.

World Health Organization (WHO). (n.d.-a). Constitution. Retrieved from https://www.who.int/ about/who-we-are/constitution.

World Health Organization. (n.d.-b). Emergencies preparedness, response. Retrieved from https:// www.who.int/csr/resources/publications/en/.

World Health Organization (WHO). (n.d.-c). Global Outbreak Alert and Response Network (GOARN). Retrieved from https://www.who.int/ihr/alert_and_response/outbreak-network/en/.

World Health Organization. (n.d.-d). Global school-based student health survey (GSHS). Retrieved from https://www.who.int/ncds/surveillance/gshs/en/.

World Health Organization (WHO). (n.d.-e). Health impact assessment. Retrieved from https:// www.who.int/topics/health_impact_assessment/en/.

World Health Organization (WHO). (n.d.-f). Healthy workplaces: a WHO global model for action. Retrieved from https://www.who.int/occupational_health/healthy_workplaces/en/.

World Health Organization (WHO). (n.d.-g). Public health surveillance. Retrieved from https:// www.who.int/topics/public_health_surveillance/en/.

World Health Organization (WHO). (n.d.-h). Social determinants of health: key concepts. Retrieved from https://www.who.int/social_determinants/thecommission/finalreport/ key_concepts/en/.

World Health Organization. (n.d.-i). STEPwise approach to noncommunicable disease risk factor surveillance (STEPS). Retrieved from https://www.who.int/ncds/surveillance/steps/riskfactor/ en/.

World Health Organization (WHO) & World Economic Forum. (2008). Preventing noncommunicable diseases in the workplace through diet and physical activity: WHO/World Economic Forum Report of a joint event. Retrieved from https://apps.who.int/iris/bitstream/ handle/10665/43825/9789241596329_eng.pdf;jsessionid=A1EC8D6DED8165E3FD71BE936B4F 8D0B?sequence=1.

Zhelev, Z., Hyde, C., Fitzgerald, J. E., et al. (2015). Tests for screening for hearing loss in children about to start school. Cochrane Database of Systematic Reviews, (11) CD011951. doi:10.1002/14651858.CD011951.

APPENDIX ONE
Declaration of Alma-Ata

On 12 September 1978, at Alma-Ata in Soviet Kazakhstan, representatives of 134 nations agreed to the terms of a solemn declaration pledging urgent action by all governments, all health and development workers, and the world community to protect and promote the health of all the people of the world. The climax of a major International Conference on Primary Health Care, jointly sponsored by WHO and UNICEF, this declaration stated:

1. *The Conference strongly reaffirms that health, which is a state of complete physical, mental and social wellbeing, and not merely the absence of disease or infirmity, is a fundamental human right and that the attainment of the highest possible level of health is a most important world-wide social goal whose realization requires the action of many other social and economic sectors in addition to the health sector.*

2. *The existing gross inequality in the health status of the people, particularly between developed and developing countries as well as within countries, is politically, socially and economically unacceptable and is, therefore, of common concern to all countries.*

3. *Economic and social development, based on a New International Economic Order, is of basic importance to the fullest attainment of health for all and to the reduction of the gap between the health status of the developing and developed countries. The promotion and protection of the health of the people is essential to sustained economic and social development and contributes to a better quality of life and to world peace.*

4. *The people have the right and duty to participate individually and collectively in the planning and implementation of their health care.*

5. *Governments have a responsibility for the health of their people which can be fulfilled only by the provision of adequate health and social measures. A main social target of governments, international*

organizations and the whole world community in the coming decades should be the attainment by all peoples of the world by the year 2000 of a level of health that will permit them to lead a socially and economically productive life. Primary health care is the key to attaining this target as part of development in the spirit of social justice.

6. *Primary health care is essential health care based on practical, scientifically sound and socially acceptable methods and technology made universally accessible to individuals and families in the community through their full participation and at a cost that the community and country can afford to maintain at every stage of their development in the spirit of self-reliance and self-determination. It forms an integral part both of the country's health system, of which it is the central function and main focus, and of the overall social and economic development of the community. It is the first level of contact of individuals, the family and community with the national health system, bringing health care as close as possible to where people live and work, and constitutes the first element of a continuing health care process.*

7. *Primary health care:*

   i. *reflects and evolves from the economic conditions and sociocultural and political characteristics of the country and its communities and is based on the application of the relevant results of social, biomedical and health services research and public health experience;*

   ii. *addresses the main health problems in the community, providing promotive, preventive, curative, and rehabilitative services accordingly;*

   iii. *includes at least: education concerning prevailing health problems and the methods of preventing and controlling them; promotion of food supply and proper nutrition; an adequate supply of safe water and basic sanitation; maternal and child health care, including family planning; immunization against the major infectious diseases; prevention and control of locally endemic diseases; appropriate treatment of common diseases and injuries; and provision of essential drugs;*

   iv. *involves, in addition to the health sector, all related sectors and aspects of national and community development, in particular agriculture, animal husbandry, food, industry, education, housing, public works, communication and other sectors; and demands the coordinated efforts of all those sectors;*

   v. *requires and promotes maximum community and individual self-reliance and participation in the planning, organization, operation and control of primary health care, making fullest use of local, national and other available resources, and to this end develops through appropriate education the ability of communities to participate;*

   vi. *should be sustained by integrated, functional and mutually supportive referral systems, leading to the progressive improvement of comprehensive health care for all, and giving priority to those most in need;*

vii. relies, at local and referral levels, on health workers, including physicians, nurses, midwives, auxiliaries and community workers as applicable, as well as traditional practitioners as needed, suitably trained socially and technically to work as a health team and to respond to the expressed health needs of the community.

8. *All governments should formulate national policies, strategies and plans of action to launch and sustain primary health care as part of a comprehensive national health system and in coordination with other sectors. To this end, it will be necessary to exercise political will, to mobilize the country's resources and to use available external resources rationally.*

9. *All countries should cooperate in a spirit of partnership and service to ensure primary health care for all people since the attainment of health by people in any one country directly concerns and benefits every other country. In this context the joint WHO/UNICEF report on primary health care constitutes a solid basis for the further development and operation of primary health care throughout the world.*

10. *An acceptable level of health for all the people of the world by the year 2000 can be attained through a fuller and better use of the world's resources, a considerable part of which is now spent on armaments and military conflicts. A genuine policy of independence, peace, détente and disarmament could and should release additional resources that could well be devoted to peaceful aims and in particular to the acceleration of social and economic development of which primary health care, as an essential part, should be allotted its proper share.*

The International Conference on Primary Health Care calls for urgent and effective national and international action to develop and implement primary health care throughout the world and particularly in developing countries in a spirit of technical cooperation and in keeping with a New International Economic Order. It urges governments, WHO and UNICEF, and other international organizations, as well as multilateral and bilateral agencies, nongovernmental organizations, funding agencies, all health workers and the whole world community to support national and international commitment to primary health care and to channel increased technical and financial support to it, particularly in developing countries. The Conference calls on all the aforementioned to collaborate in introducing, developing and maintaining primary health care in accordance with the spirit and content of this Declaration.

Source: *World Health Organization (WHO). (1978). The Declaration of Alma-Ata. World Health, August/September 1988, 16–17. http://www.who.int/publications/almaata_declaration_en.pdf.*

APPENDIX TWO
The Ottawa Charter for Health Promotion

The first International Conference on Health Promotion, meeting in Ottawa this 21st day of November 1986, hereby presents this CHARTER for action to achieve Health for All by the year 2000 and beyond.

This conference was primarily a response to growing expectations for a new public health movement around the world. Discussions focused on the needs in industrialized countries, but took into account similar concerns in all other regions. It built on the progress made through the Declaration on Primary Health Care at Alma-Ata, the World Health Organization's Targets for Health for All document, and the recent debate at the World Health Assembly on intersectoral action for health.

HEALTH PROMOTION

Health promotion is the process of enabling people to increase control over, and to improve, their health. To reach a state of complete physical, mental and social well-being, an individual or group must be able to identify and to realize aspirations, to satisfy needs, and to change or cope with the environment. Health is, therefore, seen as a resource for everyday life, not the objective of living. Health is a positive concept emphasizing social and personal resources, as well as physical capacities. Therefore, health promotion is not just the responsibility of the health sector, but goes beyond healthy life-styles to well-being.

Prerequisites for health

The fundamental conditions and resources for health are:

- *peace*
- *shelter,*
- *education,*

- *food,*
- *income,*
- *a stable eco-system,*
- *sustainable resources,*
- *social justice and equity.*

Improvement in health requires a secure foundation in these basic prerequisites.

Advocate

Good health is a major resource for social, economic and personal development and an important dimension of quality of life. Political, economic, social, cultural, environmental, behavioural and biological factors can all favour health or be harmful to it. Health promotion action aims at making these conditions favourable through advocacy for health.

Enable

Health promotion focuses on achieving equity in health. Health promotion action aims at reducing differences in current health status and ensuring equal opportunities and resources to enable all people to achieve their fullest health potential. This includes a secure foundation in a supportive environment, access to information, life skills and opportunities for making healthy choices. People cannot achieve their fullest health potential unless they are able to take control of those things which determine their health. This must apply equally to women and men.

Mediate

The prerequisites and prospects for health cannot be ensured by the health sector alone. More importantly, health promotion demands coordinated action by all concerned: by governments, by health and other social and economic sectors, by nongovernmental and voluntary organizations, by local authorities, by industry and by the media. People in all walks of life are involved as individuals, families and communities. Professional and social groups and health personnel have a major responsibility to mediate between differing interests in society for the pursuit of health.

Health promotion strategies and programmes should be adapted to the local needs and possibilities of individual countries and regions to take into account differing social, cultural and economic systems.

HEALTH PROMOTION ACTION MEANS:

Build healthy public policy

Health promotion goes beyond health care. It puts health on the agenda of policy makers in all sectors and at all levels, directing them to be aware of the health consequences of their decisions and to accept their responsibilities for health.

Health promotion policy combines diverse but complementary approaches including legislation, fiscal measures, taxation and organizational change. It is coordinated action that leads to health, income and social policies that foster greater equity. Joint action contributes to ensuring safer and healthier goods and services, healthier public services, and cleaner, more enjoyable environments.

Health promotion policy requires the identification of obstacles to the adoption of healthy public policies in non-health sectors, and ways of removing them. The aim must be to make the healthier choice the easier choice for policy makers as well.

Create supportive environments

Our societies are complex and interrelated. Health cannot be separated from other goals. The inextricable links between people and their environment constitutes the basis for a socioecological approach to health. The overall guiding principle for the world, nations, regions and communities alike, is the need to encourage reciprocal maintenance—to take care of each other, our communities and our natural environment. The conservation of natural resources throughout the world should be emphasized as a global responsibility.

Changing patterns of life, work and leisure have a significant impact on health. Work and leisure should be a source of health for people. The way society organizes work should help create a healthy society. Health promotion generates living and working conditions that are safe, stimulating, satisfying and enjoyable.

Systematic assessment of the health impact of a rapidly changing environment—particularly in areas of technology, work, energy production and urbanization—is essential and must be followed by action to ensure positive benefit to the health of the public. The protection of the natural and built environments and the conservation of natural resources must be addressed in any health promotion strategy.

Strengthen community action

Health promotion works through concrete and effective community action in setting priorities, making decisions, planning strategies and implementing them to achieve better health. At the heart of this process is the empowerment of communities—their ownership and control of their own endeavours and destinies.

Community development draws on existing human and material resources in the community to enhance self-help and social support, and to develop flexible systems for strengthening public participation and direction of health matters. This requires full and continuous access to information, learning opportunities for health, as well as funding support.

Develop personal skills

Health promotion supports personal and social development through providing information, education for health, and enhancing life skills. By so doing, it increases the options available to people to exercise more control over their own health and over their environments, and to make choices conducive to health.

Enabling people to learn, throughout life, to prepare themselves for all of its stages and to cope with chronic illness and injuries is essential. This has to be facilitated in school, home, work and community settings. Action is required through educational, professional, commercial and voluntary bodies, and within the institutions themselves.

Reorient health services

The responsibility for health promotion in health services is shared among individuals, community groups, health professionals, health service institutions and governments.

They must work together towards a health care system which contributes to the pursuit of health. The role of the health sector must move increasingly in a health promotion direction, beyond its responsibility for providing clinical and curative services. Health services need to embrace an expanded mandate which is sensitive and respects cultural needs. This mandate should support the needs of individuals and communities for a healthier life, and open channels between the health sector and broader social, political, economic and physical environmental components.

Reorienting health services also requires stronger attention to health research as well as changes in professional education and training. This must lead to a change of attitude and organization of health services, which refocuses on the total needs of the individual as a whole person.

Moving into the future

Health is created and lived by people within the settings of their everyday life; where they learn, work, play and love. Health is created by caring for oneself and others, by being able to take decisions and have control over one's life circumstances, and by ensuring that the society one lives in creates conditions that allow the attainment of health by all its members.

Caring, holism and ecology are essential issues in developing strategies for health promotion. Therefore, those involved should take as a guiding principle that, in each phase of planning, implementation and evaluation of health promotion activities, women and men should become equal partners.

COMMITMENT TO HEALTH PROMOTION

The participants in this conference pledge:

- *to move into the arena of healthy public policy, and to advocate a clear political commitment to health and equity in all sectors;*

- *to counteract the pressures towards harmful products, resource depletion, unhealthy living conditions and environments, and bad nutrition; and to focus attention on public health issues such as pollution, occupational hazards, housing and settlements;*

- *to respond to the health gap within and between societies, and to tackle the inequities in health produced by the rules and practices of these societies;*

- *to acknowledge people as the main health resource; to support and enable them to keep themselves, their families and friends healthy through financial and other means, and to accept the community as the essential voice in matters of its health, living conditions and well-being;*

- *to reorient health services and their resources towards the promotion of health; and to share power with other sectors, other disciplines and most importantly with people themselves;*

- *to recognize health and its maintenance as a major social investment and challenge; and to address the overall ecological issue of our ways of living.*

The Conference urges all concerned to join them in their commitment to a strong public health alliance.

CALL FOR INTERNATIONAL ACTION

The Conference calls on the World Health Organization and other international organizations to advocate the promotion of health in all appropriate forums and to support countries in setting up strategies and programmes for health promotion.

The Conference is firmly convinced that if people in all walks of life, non-governmental and voluntary organizations, governments, the World Health Organization and all other bodies concerned join forces in introducing strategies for health promotion, in line with the moral and social values that form the basis of this CHARTER, Health For All by the year 2000 will become a reality.

This CHARTER for action was developed and adopted by an international conference, jointly organised by the WHO, Health and Welfare Canada and the Canadian Public Health Association. Two hundred and twelve participants from 38 countries met from November 17 to 21, 1986, in Ottawa, Canada, to exchange experiences and share knowledge of health promotion.

The conference stimulated an open dialogue among lay, health and other professional workers, among representatives of governmental, voluntary and community organisations, and among politicians, administrators, academics and practitioners. Participants coordinated their efforts and came to a clearer definition of the major challenges ahead. They strengthened their individual and collective commitment to the common goal of Health for All by the year 2000.

This CHARTER for action reflects the spirit of earlier public charters through which the needs of people were recognised and acted upon. The CHARTER presents fundamental strategies and approaches for health promotion which the participants considered vital for major progress. The conference report develops the issues raised, gives concrete examples and practical suggestions regarding how real advances can be achieved, and outlines the action required of countries and relevant groups.

The move towards a new public health is now evident worldwide. This was reaffirmed not only by the experiences but by the pledges of conference participants who were invited as individuals on the basis of their expertise. The following countries were represented: Antigua, Australia, Austria, Belgium, Bulgaria, Canada, Czechoslovakia, Denmark, Eire, England, Finland, France, German Democratic Republic, Federal Republic of Germany, Ghana, Hungary, Iceland, Israel, Italy, Japan, Malta, Netherlands, New Zealand, Northern Ireland, Norway, Poland, Portugal, Romania, St. Kitts-Nevis, Scotland, Spain, Sudan, Sweden, Switzerland, Union of Soviet Socialist Republics, United States of America, Wales and Yugoslavia.

Source: *World Health Organization (WHO). (1986). The Ottawa Charter for Health Promotion, First International Conference on Health Promotion, Ottawa, 21 November, 1986. http://www.who.int/ healthpromotion/conferences/previous/ottawa/en/.*

APPENDIX THREE
Shanghai Declaration on Promoting Health in the 2030 Agenda for Sustainable Development

WE RECOGNIZE THAT HEALTH AND WELLBEING ARE ESSENTIAL TO ACHIEVING SUSTAINABLE DEVELOPMENT

On 21–24 of November 2016 in Shanghai, China, we formally recognize that health and wellbeing are essential to achieving the United Nations Development Agenda 2030 and its Sustainable Development Goals.

*We reaffirm health as a universal right, an essential resource for everyday living, a shared social goal and a political priority for all countries. The UN Sustainable Development Goals (SDGs) establish a duty to invest in health, ensure universal health coverage and reduce health inequities for people of all ages. **We are determined to leave no one behind.***

WE WILL PROMOTE HEALTH THROUGH ACTION ON ALL THE SDGS

*Healthy lives and increased wellbeing for people at all ages can be only achieved by **promoting health through all the SDGs** and by engaging the whole of society in the health development process. The transformative, practical, high impact and evidence-based strategies developed in the wake of the Ottawa Charter for Health Promotion provide us with a compass. We confirm their enduring relevance. This means acting decisively on all determinants of health, empowering people to increase control over their health and ensuring people centered health systems.*

WE WILL MAKE BOLD POLITICAL CHOICES FOR HEALTH

We face a new global context for health promotion. People's health can no longer be separated from the health of the planet and economic growth alone does not guarantee improvement in a population's health. Health security challenges are on the rise and powerful commercial forces work to counteract health. The wide spectrum of global health crises is a testimony of these rapid changes and requires an integrative response.

Unacceptable health inequities require political action across many different sectors and regions. They also require global collective action. If we are to leave no one behind this includes determined action on the rights of women, people on the move and of the increasing number of people affected by humanitarian and environmental crisis. We will prioritize good governance, local action through cities and communities, and people's empowerment by promoting health literacy. We will place a high priority on innovation and development to support people's enjoyment of a healthy life and give precedence to the health of the most vulnerable.

GOOD GOVERNANCE IS CRUCIAL FOR HEALTH

Policies for health and social justice benefit the whole of society. Failures in governance are too often detrimental to action to promote health, at national and at global level. The interdependence and universality of the SDGs offer great potential benefits from investing in all determinants of health.

We recognize that governments have a fundamental responsibility at national, local and global level to address the damaging effects of unsustainable production and consumption. This includes offsetting economic policies that create unemployment and unsafe working conditions, and enable marketing, investment and trade that compromise health. We also call on business leaders to demonstrate good corporate governance—profit must not stand above people's health. This is of particular concern in fighting the NCD epidemic.

We commit to

- apply fully the *mechanisms available to government* to protect health and promote wellbeing through public policies;
- *strengthen legislation, regulation, and taxation* of unhealthy commodities;
- *implement fiscal policies* as a powerful tool to enable new investments in health and wellbeing—including strong public health systems;
- introduce *universal health coverage* as an efficient way to achieve both health and financial protection;
- *ensure* transparency *and social accountability* and enable the broad engagement of civil society;
- *strengthen global governance to better address cross border health issues*;
- consider the growing importance and value of *traditional medicine*, which could contribute to improved health outcomes, including those in the SDGs.

CITIES AND COMMUNITIES ARE CRITICAL SETTINGS FOR HEALTH

Health is created in the settings of everyday life—in the neighbourhoods and communities where people live, love, work, shop and play. Health is one of the most effective markers of any city's successful sustainable development and contributes to make cities inclusive, safe and resilient for the whole population.

Together with city leaders we must address the toxic combination of rapid rural-to-urban migration, global population movements, economic stagnation, high unemployment and poverty as well as environmental deterioration and pollution. We will not accept that city residents in poor areas suffer ill-health disproportionately and have difficulty accessing health services.

We commit to

- prioritize **policies that create co-benefits** between health and wellbeing and other city policies, making full use of social innovation and interactive technologies;
- support cities to **promote equity and social inclusion**, harnessing the knowledge, skills and priorities of their diverse populations through strong community engagement;
- re-orient health and social services to **optimize fair access** and put people and communities at the centre.

HEALTH LITERACY EMPOWERS AND DRIVES EQUITY

Health literacy empowers individual citizens and enables their engagement in collective health promotion action. A high health literacy of decision-makers and investors supports their commitment to health impact, co-benefits and effective action on the determinants of health. Health literacy is founded on inclusive and equitable access to quality education and life-long learning. It must be an integral part of the skills and competencies developed over a lifetime, first and foremost through the school curriculum.

We commit to

- recognize health literacy as a **critical determinant of health** and invest in its development;
- develop, implement and monitor intersectoral **national and local strategies for strengthening health literacy in all populations and in all educational settings**;
- **increase citizens' control** of their own health and its determinants, through harnessing the potential of digital technology;
- ensure **that consumer environments support healthy choices** through pricing policies, transparent information and clear labelling.

CALL TO ACTION

*We recognize that health is a **political choice and we will counteract interests detrimental to health and remove barriers to empowerment**—especially for women and girls. We urge political leaders from different sectors and from different levels of governance, from the private sector and from civil society to join us in our determination to promote health and wellbeing in all the SDGs. Promoting health demands coordinated action by all concerned, it is a shared responsibility. With this Shanghai Declaration, we, the participants, pledge to accelerate the implementation of the SDGs through increased political commitment and financial investment in health promotion.*

Source: World Health Organization (WHO). (2016). Shanghai Declaration on Promoting Health in the 2030 Agenda for Sustainable Development. Retrieved from https://www.who.int/healthpromotion/ conferences/9gchp/shanghai-declaration.pdf?ua=1.

APPENDIX FOUR
Declaration of Astana on Primary Health Care

We, Heads of State and Government, ministers and representatives of States and Governments (as well as representatives of regional economic integration organizations), participating in the Global Conference on Primary Health Care: From Alma-Ata towards universal health coverage and the Sustainable Development Goals, meeting in Astana on 25 and 26 October 2018, reaffirming the commitments expressed in the ambitious and visionary Declaration of Alma-Ata of 1978 and the 2030 Agenda for Sustainable Development, in pursuit of Health for All, hereby make the following Declaration.

WE ENVISION

Governments and societies that prioritize, promote and protect people's health and well-being, at both population and individual levels, through strong health systems;

Primary health care and health services that are high quality, safe, comprehensive, integrated, accessible, available and affordable for everyone and everywhere, provided with compassion, respect and dignity by health professionals who are well-trained, skilled, motivated and committed;

Enabling and health-conducive environments in which individuals and communities are empowered and engaged in maintaining and enhancing their health and well-being;

Partners and stakeholders aligned in providing effective support to national health policies, strategies and plans.

    i.   *We strongly affirm our commitment to the fundamental right of every human being to the enjoyment of the highest attainable standard of health without distinction of any kind. Convening on the fortieth anniversary of the Declaration of Alma-Ata, we reaffirm our commitment to all its values and principles, in particular to justice and solidarity, and we underline the importance of health for peace, security and socioeconomic development, and their interdependence.*

ii. *We are convinced that strengthening primary health care (PHC) is the most inclusive, effective and efficient approach to enhance people's physical and mental health, as well as social well-being, and that PHC is a cornerstone of a sustainable health system for universal health coverage (UHC) and health-related Sustainable Development Goals. We welcome the convening in 2019 of the United Nations General Assembly high-level meeting on UHC, to which this Declaration will contribute. We will each pursue our paths to achieving UHC so that all people have equitable access to the quality and effective health care they need, ensuring that the use of these services does not expose them to financial hardship.*

iii. *We acknowledge that in spite of remarkable progress over the last 40 years, people in all parts of the world still have unaddressed health needs. Remaining healthy is challenging for many people, particularly the poor and people in vulnerable situations. We find it ethically, politically, socially and economically unacceptable that inequity in health and disparities in health outcomes persist.*

We will continue to address the growing burden of noncommunicable diseases, which lead to poor health and premature deaths due to tobacco use, the harmful use of alcohol, unhealthy lifestyles and behaviours, and insufficient physical activity and unhealthy diets. Unless we act immediately, we will continue to lose lives prematurely because of wars, violence, epidemics, natural disasters, the health impacts of climate change and extreme weather events and other environmental factors. We must not lose opportunities to halt disease outbreaks and global health threats such as antimicrobial resistance that spread beyond countries' boundaries. Promotive, preventive, curative, rehabilitative services and palliative care must be accessible to all. We must save millions of people from poverty, particularly extreme poverty, caused by disproportionate out-of-pocket spending on health. We can no longer underemphasize the crucial importance of health promotion and disease prevention, nor tolerate fragmented, unsafe or poor-quality care. We must address the shortage and uneven distribution of health workers. We must act on the growing costs of health care and medicines and vaccines. We cannot afford waste in health care spending due to inefficiency.

We commit to:

iv. **Make bold political choices for health across all sectors**

We reaffirm the primary role and responsibility of Governments at all levels in promoting and protecting the right of everyone to the enjoyment of the highest attainable standard of health. We will promote multisectoral action and UHC, engaging relevant stakeholders and empowering local communities to strengthen PHC. We will address economic, social and environmental determinants of health and aim to reduce risk factors by mainstreaming a Health in All Policies approach. We will involve more stakeholders in the achievement of Health for All, leaving no one behind, while addressing and managing conflicts of interest, promoting transparency and implementing participatory governance. We will strive to avoid or mitigate conflicts that undermine health systems and roll back health gains. We must use coherent and inclusive approaches to expand PHC as a pillar of UHC in emergencies, ensuring the continuum of care and the provision of essential health services in line with humanitarian principles. We will appropriately provide and allocate human and other resources to strengthen PHC. We applaud the leadership and example of Governments who have demonstrated strong support for PHC.

v. ***Build sustainable primary health care***

PHC will be implemented in accordance with national legislation, contexts and priorities. We will strengthen health systems by investing in PHC. We will enhance capacity and infrastructure for primary care—the first contact with health services—prioritizing essential public health functions. We will prioritize disease prevention and health promotion and will aim to meet all people's health needs across the life course through comprehensive preventive, promotive, curative, rehabilitative services and palliative care. PHC will provide a comprehensive range of services and care, including but not limited to vaccination; screenings; prevention, control and management of noncommunicable and communicable diseases; care and services that promote, maintain and improve maternal, newborn, child and adolescent health; and mental health and sexual and reproductive health. PHC will also be accessible, equitable, safe, of high quality, comprehensive, efficient, acceptable, available and affordable, and will deliver continuous, integrated services that are people-centred and gender-sensitive. We will strive to avoid fragmentation and ensure a functional referral system between primary and other levels of care. We will benefit from sustainable PHC that enhances health systems' resilience to prevent, detect and respond to infectious diseases and outbreaks.

THE SUCCESS OF PRIMARY HEALTH CARE WILL BE DRIVEN BY:

Knowledge and capacity-building

We will apply knowledge, including scientific as well as traditional knowledge, to strengthen PHC, improve health outcomes and ensure access for all people to the right care at the right time and at the most appropriate level of care, respecting their rights, needs, dignity and autonomy. We will continue to research and share knowledge and experience, build capacity and improve the delivery of health services and care.

Human resources for health

We will create decent work and appropriate compensation for health professionals and other health personnel working at the primary health care level to respond effectively to people's health needs in a multidisciplinary context. We will continue to invest in the education, training, recruitment, development, motivation and retention of the PHC workforce, with an appropriate skill mix. We will strive for the retention and availability of the PHC workforce in rural, remote and less developed areas. We assert that the international migration of health personnel should not undermine countries', particularly developing countries', ability to meet the health needs of their populations.

Technology

We support broadening and extending access to a range of health care services through the use of high-quality, safe, effective and affordable medicines, including, as appropriate, traditional medicines, vaccines, diagnostics and other technologies. We will promote their accessibility and their rational and safe use and the protection of personal data. Through advances in information systems, we will be better able to collect appropriately disaggregated, high-quality data and to improve information continuity, disease surveillance, transparency, accountability and monitoring of health system performance. We will use a variety of technologies to improve access to health care, enrich health service delivery, improve the quality of service and patient safety, and increase the efficiency and coordination of care. Through digital and other technologies, we will enable individuals and communities to identify their health needs, participate in the planning and delivery of services and play an active role in maintaining their own health and well-being.

Financing

We call on all countries to continue to invest in PHC to improve health outcomes. We will address the inefficiencies and inequities that expose people to financial hardship resulting from their use of health services by ensuring better allocation of resources for health, adequate financing of primary health care and appropriate reimbursement systems in order to improve access and achieve better health outcomes. We will work towards the financial sustainability, efficiency and resilience of national health systems, appropriately allocating resources to PHC based on national context. We will leave no one behind, including those in fragile situations and conflict-affected areas, by providing access to quality PHC services across the continuum of care.

vi. Empower individuals and communities.

We support the involvement of individuals, families, communities and civil society through their participation in the development and implementation of policies and plans that have an impact on health. We will promote health literacy and work to satisfy the expectations of individuals and communities for reliable information about health. We will support people in acquiring the knowledge, skills and resources needed to maintain their health or the health of those for whom they care, guided by health professionals. We will protect and promote solidarity, ethics and human rights. We will increase community ownership and contribute to the accountability of the public and private sectors for more people to live healthier lives in enabling and health-conducive environments.

vii. Align stakeholder support to national policies, strategies and plans.

We call on all stakeholders—health professionals, academia, patients, civil society, local and international partners, agencies and funds, the private sector, faith-based organizations and others—to align with national policies, strategies and plans across all sectors, including through people-centred, gender-sensitive approaches, and to take joint actions to build stronger and sustainable PHC towards achieving UHC. Stakeholder support can assist countries to direct sufficient human, technological, financial and information resources to PHC. In implementing this Declaration, countries and stakeholders will work together in a spirit of partnership and effective development cooperation, sharing knowledge and good practices while fully respecting national sovereignty and human rights.

- *We will act on this Declaration in solidarity and coordination between Governments, the World Health Organization, the United Nations Children's Fund and all other stakeholders.*
- *All people, countries and organizations are encouraged to support this movement.*
- *Countries will periodically review the implementation of this Declaration, in cooperation with stakeholders.*
- *Together we can and will achieve health and well-being for all, leaving no one behind.*

Source: World Health Organization (WHO). (2018). Declaration of Astana, Global Conference on Primary Health Care. Retrieved from https://www.who.int/docs/default-source/primary-health/declaration/ gcphc-declaration.pdf.

APPENDIX FIVE
Universal Declaration of Human Rights

On 10 December 1948 the General Assembly of the United Nations adopted and proclaimed the Universal Declaration of Human Rights, the full text of which appears in the following pages. Following this historic Act, the Assembly called upon all Member countries to publicise the text of the Declaration and 'to cause it to be disseminated, displayed, read and expounded principally in schools and other educational institutions, without distinction based on the political status of countries or territories'.

PREAMBLE

Whereas recognition of the inherent dignity and of the equal and inalienable rights of all members of the human family is the foundation of freedom, justice and peace in the world,

Whereas disregard and contempt for human rights have resulted in barbarous acts which have outraged the conscience of mankind, and the advent of a world in which human beings shall enjoy freedom of speech and belief and freedom from fear and want has been proclaimed as the highest aspiration of the common people,

Whereas it is essential, if man is not to be compelled to have recourse, as a last resort, to rebellion against tyranny and oppression, that human rights should be protected by the rule of law,

Whereas it is essential to promote the development of friendly relations between nations,

Whereas the peoples of the United Nations have in the Charter reaffirmed their faith in fundamental human rights, in the dignity and worth of the human person and in the equal rights of men and women and have determined to promote social progress and better standards of life in larger freedom,

Whereas Member States have pledged themselves to achieve, in co-operation with the United Nations, the promotion of universal respect for and observance of human rights and fundamental freedoms,

Whereas a common understanding of these rights and freedoms is of the greatest importance for the full realization of this pledge,

Now, Therefore THE GENERAL ASSEMBLY proclaims THIS UNIVERSAL DECLARATION OF HUMAN RIGHTS as a common standard of achievement for all peoples and all nations, to the end that every individual and every organ of society, keeping this Declaration constantly in mind, shall strive by teaching and education to promote respect for these rights and freedoms and by progressive measures, national and international, to secure their universal and effective recognition and observance, both among the peoples of Member States themselves and among the peoples of territories under their jurisdiction.

Article 1

All human beings are born free and equal in dignity and rights. They are endowed with reason and conscience and should act towards one another in a spirit of brotherhood.

Article 2

Everyone is entitled to all the rights and freedoms set forth in this Declaration, without distinction of any kind, such as race, colour, sex, language, religion, political or other opinion, national or social origin, property, birth or other status. Furthermore, no distinction shall be made on the basis of the political, jurisdictional or international status of the country or territory to which a person belongs, whether it be independent, trust, non-self-governing or under any other limitation of sovereignty.

Article 3

Everyone has the right to life, liberty and security of person.

Article 4

No one shall be held in slavery or servitude; slavery and the slave trade shall be prohibited in all their forms.

Article 5

No one shall be subjected to torture or to cruel, inhuman or degrading treatment or punishment.

Article 6

Everyone has the right to recognition everywhere as a person before the law.

Article 7

All are equal before the law and are entitled without any discrimination to equal protection of the law. All are entitled to equal protection against any discrimination in violation of this Declaration and against any incitement to such discrimination.

Article 8

Everyone has the right to an effective remedy by the competent national tribunals for acts violating the fundamental rights granted him by the constitution or by law.

Article 9

No one shall be subjected to arbitrary arrest, detention or exile.

Article 10

Everyone is entitled in full equality to a fair and public hearing by an independent and impartial tribunal, in the determination of his rights and obligations and of any criminal charge against him.

Article 11

1. *Everyone charged with a penal offence has the right to be presumed innocent until proved guilty according to law in a public trial at which he has had all the guarantees necessary for his defence.*

2. *No one shall be held guilty of any penal offence on account of any act or omission which did not constitute a penal offence, under national or international law, at the time when it was committed. Nor shall a heavier penalty be imposed than the one that was applicable at the time the penal offence was committed.*

Article 12

No one shall be subjected to arbitrary interference with his privacy, family, home or correspondence, nor to attacks upon his honour and reputation. Everyone has the right to the protection of the law against such interference or attacks.

Article 13

1. *Everyone has the right to freedom of movement and residence within the borders of each state.*

2. *Everyone has the right to leave any country, including his own, and to return to his country.*

Article 14

1. *Everyone has the right to seek and to enjoy in other countries asylum from persecution.*

2. *This right may not be invoked in the case of prosecutions genuinely arising from non-political crimes or from acts contrary to the purposes and principles of the United Nations.*

Article 15

1.   *Everyone has the right to a nationality.*

2.   *No one shall be arbitrarily deprived of his nationality nor denied the right to change his nationality.*

Article 16

1.   *Men and women of full age, without any limitation due to race, nationality or religion, have the right to marry and to found a family. They are entitled to equal rights as to marriage, during marriage and at its dissolution.*

2.   *Marriage shall be entered into only with the free and full consent of the intending spouses.*

3.   *The family is the natural and fundamental group unit of society and is entitled to protection by society and the State.*

Article 17

1.   *Everyone has the right to own property alone as well as in association with others.*

2.   *No one shall be arbitrarily deprived of his property.*

Article 18

Everyone has the right to freedom of thought, conscience and religion; this right includes freedom to change his religion or belief, and freedom, either alone or in community with others and in public or private, to manifest his religion or belief in teaching, practice, worship and observance.

Article 19

Everyone has the right to freedom of opinion and expression; this right includes freedom to hold opinions without interference and to seek, receive and impart information and ideas through any media and regardless of frontiers.

Article 20

1.   *Everyone has the right to freedom of peaceful assembly and association.*

2.   *No one may be compelled to belong to an association.*

Article 21

1.   *Everyone has the right to take part in the government of his country, directly or through freely chosen representatives.*

2.   *Everyone has the right of equal access to public service in his country.*

3.   *The will of the people shall be the basis of the authority of government; this will shall be expressed in periodic and genuine elections which shall be by universal and equal suffrage and shall be held by secret vote or by equivalent free voting procedures.*

Article 22

Everyone, as a member of society, has the right to social security and is entitled to realization, through national effort and international co-operation and in accordance with the organization and resources of each State, of the economic, social and cultural rights indispensable for his dignity and the free development of his personality.

Article 23

1. *Everyone has the right to work, to free choice of employment, to just and favourable conditions of work and to protection against unemployment.*

2. *Everyone, without any discrimination, has the right to equal pay for equal work.*

3. *Everyone who works has the right to just and favourable remuneration ensuring for himself and his family an existence worthy of human dignity, and supplemented, if necessary, by other means of social protection.*

4. *Everyone has the right to form and to join trade unions for the protection of his interests.*

Article 24

Everyone has the right to rest and leisure, including reasonable limitation of working hours and periodic holidays with pay.

Article 25

1. *Everyone has the right to a standard of living adequate for the health and well-being of himself and of his family, including food, clothing, housing and medical care and necessary social services, and the right to security in the event of unemployment, sickness, disability, widowhood, old age or other lack of livelihood in circumstances beyond his control.*

2. *Motherhood and childhood are entitled to special care and assistance. All children, whether born in or out of wedlock, shall enjoy the same social protection.*

Article 26

1. *Everyone has the right to education. Education shall be free, at least in the elementary and fundamental stages. Elementary education shall be compulsory. Technical and professional education shall be made generally available and higher education shall be equally accessible to all on the basis of merit.*

2. *Education shall be directed to the full development of the human personality and to the strengthening of respect for human rights and fundamental freedoms. It shall promote understanding, tolerance and friendship among all nations, racial or religious groups, and shall further the activities of the United Nations for the maintenance of peace.*

3. *Parents have a prior right to choose the kind of education that shall be given to their children.*

Article 27

1. *Everyone has the right freely to participate in the cultural life of the community, to enjoy the arts and to share in scientific advancement and its benefits.*

2. *Everyone has the right to the protection of the moral and material interests resulting from any scientific, literary or artistic production of which he is the author.*

Article 28

Everyone is entitled to a social and international order in which the rights and freedoms set forth in this Declaration can be fully realized.

Article 29

1. *Everyone has duties to the community in which alone the free and full development of his personality is possible.*

2. *In the exercise of his rights and freedoms, everyone shall be subject only to such limitations as are determined by law solely for the purpose of securing due recognition and respect for the rights and freedoms of others and of meeting the just requirements of morality, public order and the general welfare in a democratic society.*

3. *These rights and freedoms may in no case be exercised contrary to the purposes and principles of the United Nations.*

Article 30

Nothing in this Declaration may be interpreted as implying for any State, group or person any right to engage in any activity or to perform any act aimed at the destruction of any of the rights and freedoms set forth herein.

Source: United Nations. (1948). The Universal Declaration of Human Rights. Retrieved from http://www.un.org/en/universal-declaration-human-rights/index.html.

APPENDIX SIX
The Earth Charter Preamble

We stand at a critical moment in Earth's history, a time when humanity must choose its future. As the world becomes increasingly interdependent and fragile, the future at once holds great peril and great promise. To move forward we must recognize that in the midst of a magnificent diversity of cultures and life forms we are one human family and one Earth community with a common destiny. We must join together to bring forth a sustainable global society founded on respect for nature, universal human rights, economic justice, and a culture of peace. Towards this end, it is imperative that we, the peoples of Earth, declare our responsibility to one another, to the greater community of life, and to future generations.

EARTH, OUR HOME

Humanity is part of a vast evolving universe. Earth, our home, is alive with a unique community of life. The forces of nature make existence a demanding and uncertain adventure, but Earth has provided the conditions essential to life's evolution. The resilience of the community of life and the well-being of humanity depend upon preserving a healthy biosphere with all its ecological systems, a rich variety of plants and animals, fertile soils, pure waters, and clean air. The global environment with its finite resources is a common concern of all peoples. The protection of Earth's vitality, diversity, and beauty is a sacred trust.

THE GLOBAL SITUATION

The dominant patterns of production and consumption are causing environmental devastation, the depletion of resources, and a massive extinction of species. Communities are being undermined. The benefits of development are not shared equitably and the gap between rich and poor is widening.

Injustice, poverty, ignorance, and violent conflict are widespread and the cause of great suffering. An unprecedented rise in human population has overburdened ecological and social systems. The foundations of global security are threatened. These trends are perilous—but not inevitable.

THE CHALLENGES AHEAD

The choice is ours: form a global partnership to care for Earth and one another or risk the destruction of ourselves and the diversity of life. Fundamental changes are needed in our values, institutions and ways of living. We must realize that when basic needs have been met, human development is primarily about being more, not having more. We have the knowledge and technology to provide for all and to reduce our impacts on the environment. The emergence of a global civil society is creating new opportunities to build a democratic and humane world. Our environmental, economic, political, social, and spiritual challenges are interconnected, and together we can forge inclusive solutions.

UNIVERSAL RESPONSIBILITY

To realize these aspirations, we must decide to live with a sense of universal responsibility, identifying ourselves with the whole Earth community as well as our local communities. We are at once citizens of different nations and of one world in which the local and global are linked. Everyone shares responsibility for the present and future well-being of the human family and the larger living world. The spirit of human solidarity and kinship with all life is strengthened when we live with reverence for the mystery of being, gratitude for the gift of life, and humility regarding the human place in nature.

We urgently need a shared vision of basic values to provide an ethical foundation for the emerging world community. Therefore, together in hope we affirm the following interdependent principles for a sustainable way of life as a common standard by which the conduct of all individuals, organizations, businesses, governments, and transnational institutions is to be guided and assessed.

Principles

I. Respect and care for the community of life

1. Respect Earth and life in all its diversity.

   a. Recognize that all beings are interdependent and every form of life has value regardless of its worth to human beings.

   b. Affirm faith in the inherent dignity of all human beings and in the intellectual, artistic, ethical, and spiritual potential of humanity.

2. Care for the community of life with understanding, compassion, and love.

   a. Accept that with the right to own, manage, and use natural resources comes the duty to prevent environmental harm and to protect the rights of people.

    b.   Affirm that with increased freedom, knowledge, and power comes increased responsibility to promote the common good.

3.   Build democratic societies that are just, participatory, sustainable, and peaceful.

    a.   Ensure that communities at all levels guarantee human rights and fundamental freedoms and provide everyone an opportunity to realize his or her full potential.

    b.   Promote social and economic justice, enabling all to achieve a secure and meaningful livelihood that is ecologically responsible.

4.   Secure Earth's bounty and beauty for present and future generations.

    a.   Recognize that the freedom of action of each generation is qualified by the needs of future generations.

    b.   Transmit to future generations values, traditions, and institutions that support the long-term flourishing of Earth's human and ecological communities.

II. Ecological integrity

5.   Protect and restore the integrity of Earth's ecological systems, with special concern for biological diversity and the natural processes that sustain life.

    a.   Adopt at all levels sustainable development plans and regulations that make environmental conservation and rehabilitation integral to all development initiatives.

    b.   Establish and safeguard viable nature and biosphere reserves, including wild lands and marine areas, to protect Earth's life support systems, maintain biodiversity, and preserve our natural heritage.

    c.   Promote the recovery of endangered species and ecosystems.

    d.   Control and eradicate non-native or genetically modified organisms harmful to native species and the environment, and prevent introduction of such harmful organisms.

    e.   Manage the use of renewable resources such as water, soil, forest products, and marine life in ways that do not exceed rates of regeneration and that protect the health of ecosystems.

    f.   Manage the extraction and use of non-renewable resources such as minerals and fossil fuels in ways that minimize depletion and cause no serious environmental damage.

6.   Prevent harm as the best method of environmental protection and, when knowledge is limited, apply a precautionary approach.

    a.   Take action to avoid the possibility of serious or irreversible environmental harm even when scientific knowledge is incomplete or inconclusive.

    b.   Place the burden of proof on those who argue that a proposed activity will not cause significant harm, and make the responsible parties liable for environmental harm.

    c.   Ensure that decision making addresses the cumulative, long-term, indirect, long distance, and global consequences of human activities.

    d. Prevent pollution of any part of the environment and allow no build-up of radioactive, toxic, or other hazardous substances.

    e. Avoid military activities damaging to the environment.

7. Adopt patterns of production, consumption, and reproduction that safeguard Earth's regenerative capacities, human rights, and community wellbeing.

    a. Reduce, reuse, and recycle the materials used in production and consumption systems, and ensure that residual waste can be assimilated by ecological systems.

    b. Act with restraint and efficiency when using energy, and rely increasingly on renewable energy sources such as solar and wind.

    c. Promote the development, adoption, and equitable transfer of environmentally sound technologies.

    d. Internalise the full environmental and social costs of goods and services in the selling price, and enable consumers to identify products that meet the highest social and environmental standards.

    e. Ensure universal access to health care that fosters reproductive health and responsible reproduction.

    f. Adopt lifestyles that emphasize the quality of life and material sufficiency in a finite world.

8. Advance the study of ecological sustainability and promote the open exchange and wide application of the knowledge acquired.

    a. Support international scientific and technical cooperation on sustainability, with special attention to the needs of developing nations.

    b. Recognize and preserve the traditional knowledge and spiritual wisdom in all cultures that contribute to environmental protection and human wellbeing.

    c. Ensure that information of vital importance to human health and environmental protection, including genetic information, remains available in the public domain.

III. Social and economic justice

9. Eradicate poverty as an ethical, social, and environmental imperative.

    a. Guarantee the right to potable water, clean air, food security, uncontaminated soil, shelter, and safe sanitation, allocating the national and international resources required.

    b. Empower every human being with the education and resources to secure a sustainable livelihood, and provide social security and safety nets for those who are unable to support themselves.

    c. Recognize the ignored, protect the vulnerable, serve those who suffer, and enable them to develop their capacities and to pursue their aspirations.

10. Ensure that economic activities and institutions at all levels promote human development in an equitable and sustainable manner.

    a. Promote the equitable distribution of wealth within nations and among nations.

    b. Enhance the intellectual, financial, technical, and social resources of developing nations, and relieve them of onerous international debt.

    c.   Ensure that all trade supports sustainable resource use, environmental protection, and progressive labour standards.

    d.   Require multinational corporations and international financial organizations to act transparently in the public good, and hold them accountable for the consequences of their activities.

11.   Affirm gender equality and equity as prerequisites to sustainable development and ensure universal access to education, health care, and economic opportunity.

    a.   Secure the human rights of women and girls and end all violence against them.

    b.   Promote the active participation of women in all aspects of economic, political, civil, social, and cultural life as full and equal partners, decision makers, leaders, and beneficiaries.

    c.   Strengthen families and ensure the safety and loving nurture of all family members.

12.   Uphold the right of all, without discrimination, to a natural and social environment supportive of human dignity, bodily health, and spiritual wellbeing, with special attention to the rights of indigenous peoples and minorities.

    a.   Eliminate discrimination in all its forms, such as that based on race, color, sex, sexual orientation, religion, language, and national, ethnic or social origin.

    b.   Affirm the right of indigenous peoples to their spirituality, knowledge, lands and resources and to their related practice of sustainable livelihoods.

    c.   Honor and support the young people of our communities, enabling them to fulfil their essential role in creating sustainable societies.

    d.   Protect and restore outstanding places of cultural and spiritual significance.

IV. Democracy, non-violence, and peace

13.   Strengthen democratic institutions at all levels, and provide transparency and accountability in governance, inclusive participation in decision making, and access to justice.

    a.   Uphold the right of everyone to receive clear and timely information on environmental matters and all development plans and activities which are likely to affect them or in which they have an interest.

    b.   Support local, regional and global civil society, and promote the meaningful participation of all interested individuals and organizations in decision making.

    c.   Protect the rights to freedom of opinion, expression, peaceful assembly, association, and dissent.

    d.   Institute effective and efficient access to administrative and independent judicial procedures, including remedies and redress for environmental harm and the threat of such harm.

    e.   Eliminate corruption in all public and private institutions.

f. Strengthen local communities, enabling them to care for their environments, and assign environmental responsibilities to the levels of government where they can be carried out most effectively.

14. Integrate into formal education and life-long learning the knowledge, values, and skills needed for a sustainable way of life.

a. Provide all, especially children and youth, with educational opportunities that empower them to contribute actively to sustainable development.

b. Promote the contribution of the arts and humanities as well as the sciences in sustainability education.

c. Enhance the role of the mass media in raising awareness of ecological and social challenges.

d. Recognize the importance of moral and spiritual education for sustainable living.

15. Treat all living beings with respect and consideration.

a. Prevent cruelty to animals kept in human societies and protect them from suffering.

b. Protect wild animals from methods of hunting, trapping, and fishing that cause extreme, prolonged, or avoidable suffering.

c. Avoid or eliminate to the full extent possible the taking or destruction of non-targeted species.

16. Promote a culture of tolerance, nonviolence, and peace.

a. Encourage and support mutual understanding, solidarity, and cooperation among all peoples and within and among nations.

b. Implement comprehensive strategies to prevent violent conflict and use collaborative problem solving to manage and resolve environmental conflicts and other disputes.

c. Demilitarize national security systems to the level of a non-provocative defence posture, and convert military resources to peaceful purposes, including ecological restoration.

d. Eliminate nuclear, biological, and toxic weapons and other weapons of mass destruction.

e. Ensure that the use of orbital and outer space supports environmental protection and peace.

f. Recognize that peace is the wholeness created by right relationships with oneself, other persons, other cultures, other life, Earth, and the larger whole of which all are a part.

THE WAY FORWARD

As never before in history, common destiny beckons us to seek a new beginning. Such renewal is the promise of these Earth Charter principles. To fulfil this promise, we must commit ourselves to adopt and promote the values and objectives of the Charter.

This requires a change of mind and heart. It requires a new sense of global interdependence and universal responsibility. We must imaginatively develop and apply the vision of a sustainable way of life locally, nationally, regionally, and globally. Our cultural diversity is a precious heritage and different cultures will find their own distinctive ways to realize the vision. We must deepen and expand the global dialogue that generated the Earth Charter, for we have much to learn from the ongoing collaborative search for truth and wisdom.

Life often involves tensions between important values. This can mean difficult choices. However, we must find ways to harmonize diversity with unity, the exercise of freedom with the common good, short-term objectives with long-term goals. Every individual, family, organization, and community has a vital role to play. The arts, sciences, religions, educational institutions, media, businesses, nongovernmental organizations, and governments are all called to offer creative leadership. The partnership of government, civil society, and business is essential for effective governance.

In order to build a sustainable global community, the nations of the world must renew their commitment to the United Nations, fulfil their obligations under existing international agreements, and support the implementation of Earth Charter principles with an international legally binding instrument on environment and development.

Let ours be a time remembered for the awakening of a new reverence for life, the firm resolve to achieve sustainability, the quickening of the struggle for justice and peace, and the joyful celebration of life.

Source: Earth Charter International® www.earthcharter.org.

INDEX